AF764582

Focal Cortical Dysplasias

New advances for curing epilepsy

Copyright cover illustration: © Carlos Cepeda
Copyright page VII: All patients have given their authorization for the reproduction of their portrait.

ISBN : 978-2-7420-1705-8

Published by
Editions John Libbey Eurotext
30, rue Berthollet
Arcueil
www.jle.com

John Libbey Eurotext Limited
34 Anyard Road, Cobham
Surrey KT11 2LA
England

© 2022, John Libbey Eurotext. All rights reserved.

Unauthorized duplication contravenes applicable laws.
It is prohibited to reproduce this work or any part of it without the authorization of the publisher or of the *Centre Français d'Exploitation du Droit de Copie* (CFC), 20, rue des Grands-Augustins, 75006 Paris.

Focal Cortical Dysplasias

New advances for curing epilepsy

Edited by
Francine Chassoux
Andre Palmini

John Libbey Eurotext

Preface

Francine Chassoux, Andre Palmini

Why a book on Focal Cortical Dysplasias?

Although a lot have been done, and a large panel of experts have accumulated an impressive amount of data, we believe it is high time for a structured volume with the clear focus of combining data with the art and reflection of experts who have worked in the field for the last decades.

As we all know, papers are more and more succinct and objective, and often leave behind precious perspectives of experts who have faced different issues and reflected upon them over the years. When we thought about launching this initiative, the following came to our minds:

- 2021 marks the 50th anniversary of the famous description by Taylor and colleagues in 1971 of this bizarre lesion ("once seen, never forgotten!"). Thus, it is Taylor's type focal cortical dysplasia 50th birthday. Celebrating this event may help us check what has been done and where we are now. Let us look to the past with a look at improving the future.
- The field of FCD has witnessed an exponential advance in the last decades. Looking back 30 years, nobody could suspect that FCD would become perhaps the most relevant etiology of focal epilepsies in patients of all ages, particularly those with refractory seizures, nor that geneticists would unveil fascinating molecular mechanisms of production of dysplastic abnormalities that would be identified by ever improving skills of imaging specialists and their ingenious techniques. However, in the field of dysplasia – as in many others – there is a sort of disconnection between the fast production of knowledge and the pace of condensing and reporting such knowledge in a volume that is truly useful in the clinic.
- Despite major advances in all fields, FCD remain a mystery. More than ever, we must join efforts to better understand the mechanisms of epileptogenicity and the natural course of FCD, to recognize their many faces, and determine the best care. Curing epilepsy due to FCD should be our common challenge ("impossible n'est pas français!"). We are in the middle of the river, and the book may help us reach the other side.
- There are several unresolved issues and framing these aspects in a straightforward way may help clinicians to be attentive to further advances in the field. Why many patients with reasonably well controlled seizures suddenly become extremely refractory? Why surgical outcome is still not as good as we wish, despite better imaging and neurophysiology? Why may patients relapse many years after seizure freedom from apparently successful surgery? What is the effective functionality and plasticity of the dysplastic cortex and the "dysplastic brain"? How to determine the best trade-offs in FCD located around eloquent cortex, balancing resection of epileptogenic tissue with the need to preserve functionality? Should the surgical strategy be influenced by the histological FCD subtype? These and other questions need very focused approaches, from people producing knowledge that impacts patients around the world every day.
- Progress may include some disappointing outcomes. Elegant and audacious hypotheses have not been confirmed, while unlikely leads have opened the way to unsuspected findings. Some confusion may result from the divergent/contradictory advances, and we need clarifications about what is well established (no doubt), what remains to be further investigated and what should be abandoned.

Hence, we believe the time is ripe for a volume condensing the "practical knowledge" about FCD – knowledge that can be applied by clinicians taking care of the large number of patients with this epilepsy etiology worldwide.

We did our best for this book to be attractive, easy to read, well-illustrated and informative for clinicians searching a solution for their patients, as well as helpful for decision making. We hope readers will take this as a collaborative journey that, in the end, will help people at all levels to deal with patients with FCD.

Preface

Acknowledgements

Many thanks to our patiens who help us do better.
These smiles tell everything, pushing us to work, study, think, discuss, write
- the best reward for the efforts put forth by all authors of this book!

Milena

'She had no life' (with more than 30 seizures a day, since age 1). 'Now, without seizures, we discover each day how fantastic is the kid we have at home (sic 'Mom').

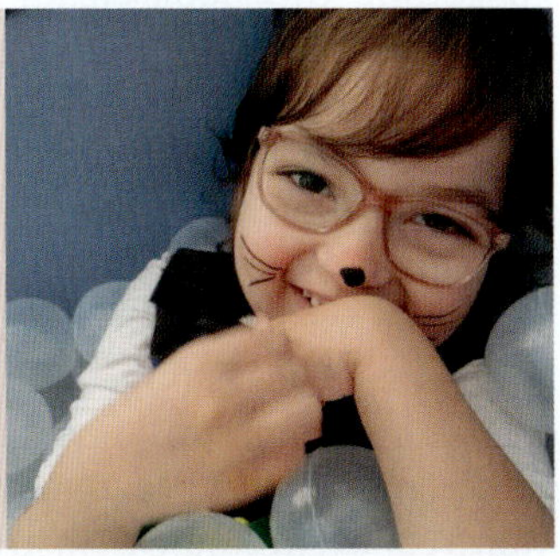

Reda

Reda had intractable epilepsy at the age of 15, limiting schooling and life projects. Operated at 20 for a small parietal FCD, he has been free to travel around the world to make up for lost time, held a position of responsibility in the industry and plans to found his own company.

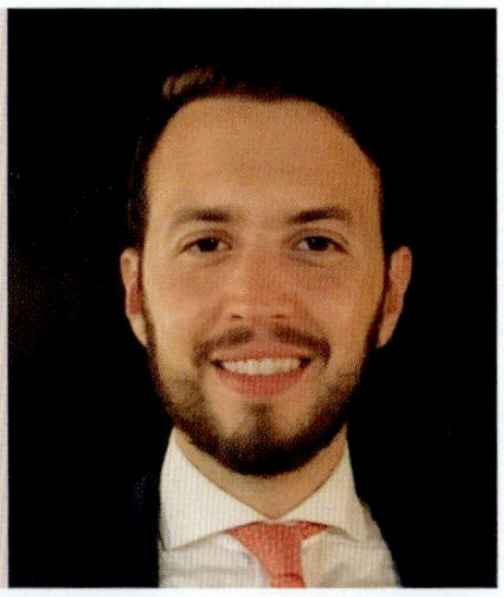

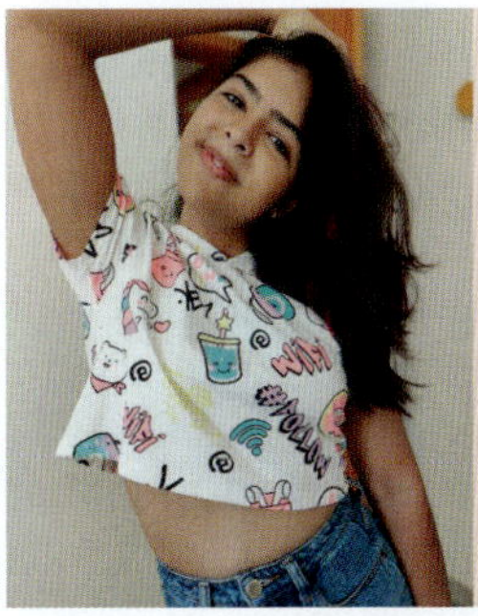

Beatriz

Seizures started at age 4. So many when operated at age 7 that she could not join social activities – and felt ashamed to make friends. Now, without her left frontal lobe dysplasia and seizure free, she gives us this trademark Brazilian smile as a gift.

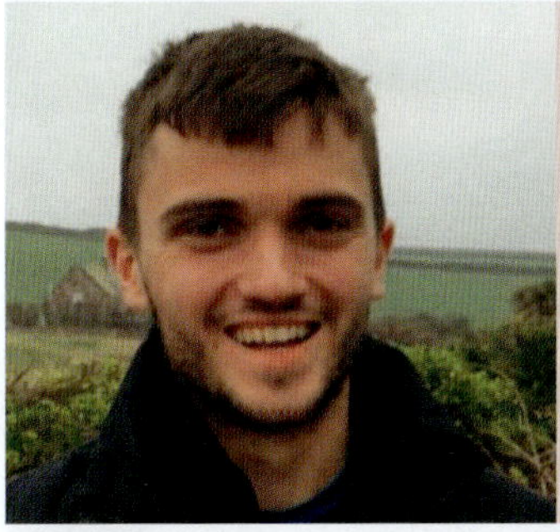

Max

Max was severely disabled by epilepsy from the age of 6 until surgery at 11. After the removal of a small central FCD, he feels incredibly healthy and is completing his legal training to be lawyer.

Geovana

Geovana was literally home-bound for more than a year, at age 17, because of many daily seizures due to a premotor FCD. No seizures in 4 years after surgery, now happy with a boyfriend.

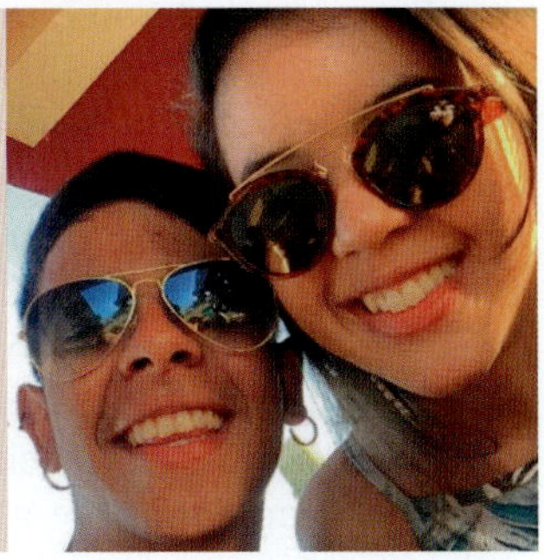

Camille

Camille was operated at age 7 for a frontal FCD. She had so many seizures that she couldn't walk. After surgery, she had a normal schooling and now enjoys the student life.

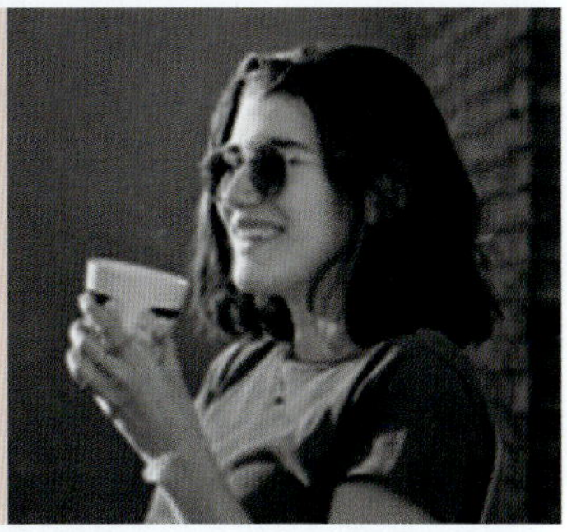

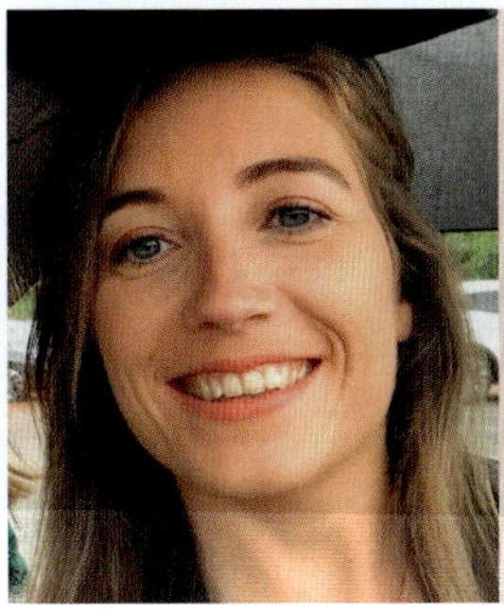

Charlène

Charlène had nocturnal seizures from the age of 4 and always felt as a sick child without future. Operated at 25 years for an opercular FCD, she is now seizure-free without drugs, and will be a mother when this book is published in July.

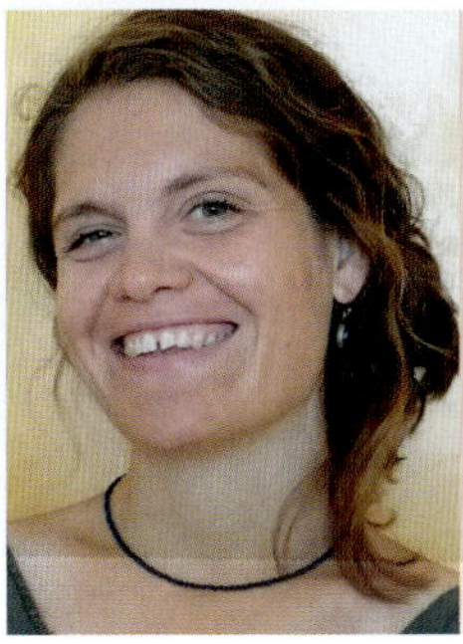

Margaux

Margaux had a severe epilepsy from the age of 2. Operated when she was 20 for a central FCD, she keeps her beautiful smile and is building her life without seizures.

Dedication

Frederick Andermann (1930-2019) and Pierre Gloor (1923-2003)

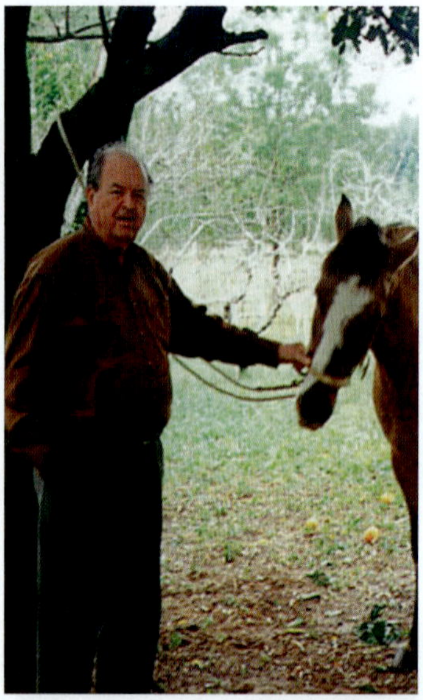

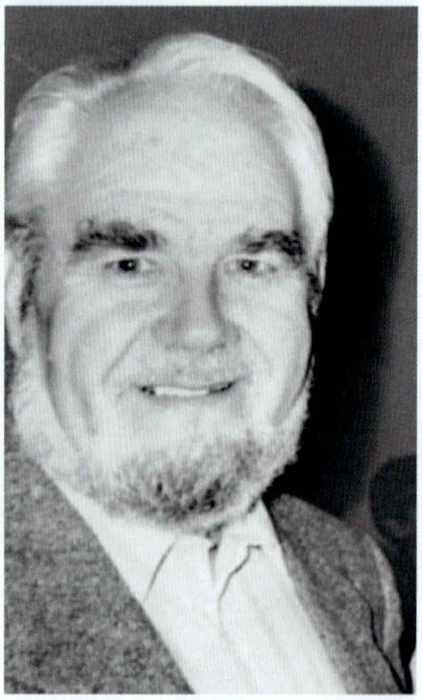

Co-editing this book closes a circle in my career, from describing series of patients with 'neuronal migration disorders' and their treatment in the beginning of the 90's through highlighting the intrinsic epileptogenicity of dysplastic tissue, then efforts at classification and finally focusing on surgical management following non-invasive investigation. All circles that close must have had a beginning, without which they would not exist. Therefore, this book is dedicated to those that guided me to start drawing this circle, my mentors at the Montreal Neurological Institute, Frederick Andermann and Pierre Gloor.

All authors of the chapters of this book knew Fred Andermann and I would wish all who will read it would have had the same privilege. Few people honour the honourable stance of a 'mentor', because it is hard to have the combination championed by Fred: always supporting your work, no matter what, always having ideas and insights beyond the obvious horizons – and always pushing you to 'just do it'. His mentorship was a marvellous gift that shaped my career.

Not all authors of this book knew Pierre Gloor. Yet, they and all people that will encounter this book would have marvelled at sitting with him to discuss epilepsy and seeing him interview a patient. A researcher of the highest caliber, he accepted me at the MNI at the time a neurology resident in Porto Alegre would use his poor English and a typewriter to address a letter to somcone he knew just from 'hard to get' xeroxed papers. His personal and scientific generosity took my understanding of epilepsy and EEG to a different level and the carefully performed electrocorticographies he always invited me to join has made, is making and will certainly make a difference to the lives of thousands of patients with bad epilepsies in a developing country.

Andre Palmini

Jean Talairach (1911-2007) and Jean Bancaud (1921-1993)

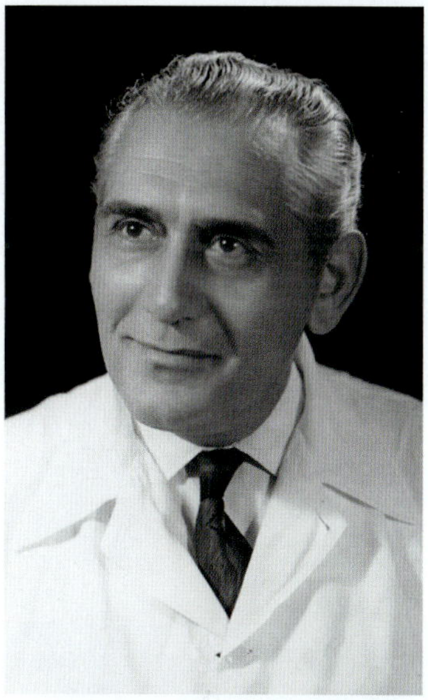

Psychiatrist by training, Jean Talairach was interested in the anatomy of the brain and became a neurosurgeon. Destined for philosophy, Jean Bancaud chose medicine and neurophysiology. The meeting of the two "Jean" was at the origin of a considerable evolution in the field of epilepsy.

The first one applied stereotaxy to the study of epilepsy, an original approach to reach any intracerebral target without opening the skull. The second elaborated the founding concepts based on the semiology of focal seizures and their spatio-temporal dynamics. Both passionate about rugby, they transformed their tries by developing an innovative method for the treatment of the most severe epilepsies based on stereoelectroencephalography (SEEG). The "Talairach system", a proper name that has become common, is today the essential reference for the study of the normal and pathological human brain. And SEEG courses organized by their followers, welcome specialists from all over the world who come to train in this methodology.

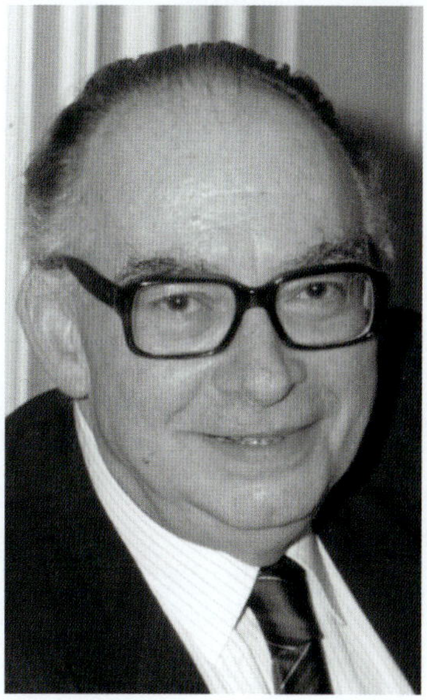

"I know that a patient is cured in the way he walks, he no longer hides, he raises his head, he is released" said the psychiatrist-neurosurgeon, confident in his art. "I always fear that a cured patient will have a seizure when entering my office" said the doctor-philosopher, praising doubt as a bulwark against error. Because the school of doubt was also that of high standards and rigor, its teaching remains our best guide for the patients' care.

This book is dedicated to them, in memory of what they taught us with patience and thoughtfulness, and which allowed us to continue their work.

Francine Chassoux

Editors

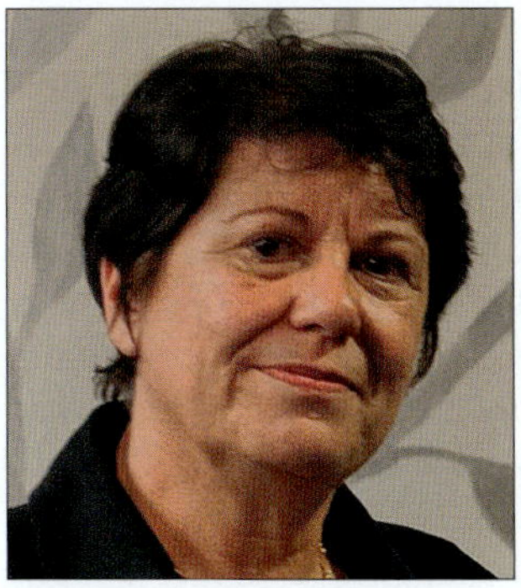

Francine Chassoux

Francine Chassoux is a neurologist, she had her epileptological training at Sainte-Anne Hospital in Paris with Jean Bancaud and Jean Talairach, focusing on pre-operative evaluation of patients with drug-resistant partial epilepsy, based on electro-clinical and anatomical correlations and intracranial recordings (SEEG). She headed the Epilepsy Unit in the Neurosurgery department in Sainte-Anne between 1993 and 2021 and collaborated with the Nuclear Medicine department (SHFJ-CEA, Orsay, France) from 1999.

Her main research topics are related to focal cortical dysplasias and other malformations of cortical development, hippocampal sclerosis and epilepsy surgery with a special interest for correlations between invasive techniques (SEEG, Wada test) and new imaging techniques (functional MRI, PET-scan, PET-MR). She was made Chevalier de la Légion d'honneur in 2013 for her medical and scientific work in epilepsy and especially in the field of focal cortical dysplasias. She authored or co-authored more than 110 peer-reviewed articles or book chapters (H index 35).

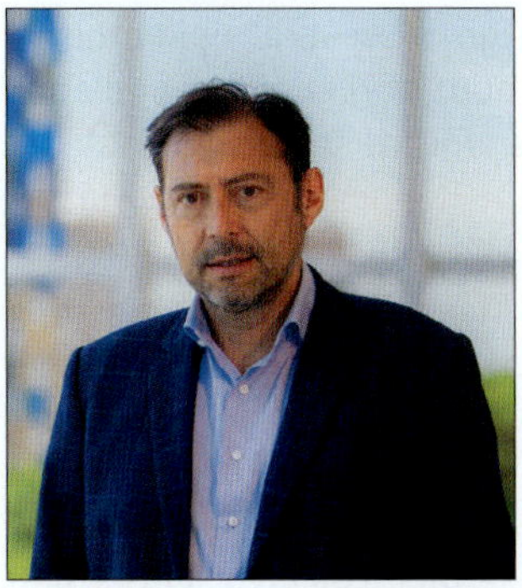

Andre Palmini

Andre Palmini is a neurologist in Porto Alegre, Brazil, trained in epileptology and clinical neurophysiology at the Montreal Neurological Institute from 1989 to 1991, under the guidance of Frederick Andermann and Pierre Gloor. That training was complemented over the years with post-docs in Neuroimaging of the Epilepsies at the Katholieke Universiteit Leuven in Belgium, from 2003-2004, and in Clinical Epileptology at the University College London, Queen Square in 2012. He has been visiting professor at the Chonbuk University in South Korea in 1993 and 1995 and is currently Professor of Neurology at the department of Clinical Neurosciences of the Pontificia Universidade Católica do Rio Grande do Sul (PUCRS), Head of the Service of Neurology and Clinical Director of the Epilepsy Surgery Program, at the Hospital São Lucas da PUCRS.

He has been mostly involved with practice and research on drug-resistant epilepsies, with a focus on focal cortical dysplasias, temporal lobe epilepsies, diffuse brain disorders leading to epileptic drop attacks and psychogenic non-epileptic seizures. He has written or co-written more than 120 peer-reviewed articles, 15 book charters, and two books.

Authors

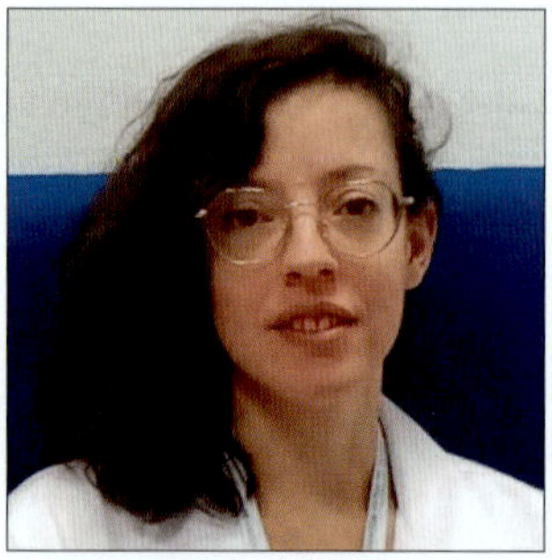

Belén Abarrategui

Belén Abarrategui has a medical degree in 2009 from the University of Alcalá de Henares and specialized in Neurology at Hospital Clinico San Carlos (Madrid, 2014), where she began her subspecialization in epilepsy. She has a PhD in Biomedical Sciences at Universidad Complutense (2017) on Epilepsy & Cognition, with short stints in Chicago (Rush University) and São Paulo (Hospital São Paulo). From 2019 to 2022, she worked as epilepsy fellow at Claudio Munari Center for Epilepsy Surgery, deepening the pre-surgical study for focal epilepsy surgery, focal cortical dysplasias, SEEG, multimodal functional mapping and interactions between epilepsy and language. Since 2022, she has been working as epileptologist at Hospital Puerta de Hierro (Madrid).

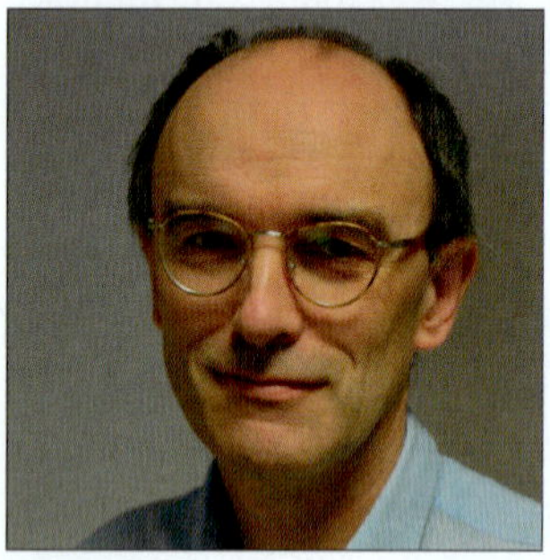

Jean-Michel Badier

Jean-Michel Badier is a research engineer. He obtained an engineering degree in biomedical engineering and a PhD from the University of Technology of Compiègne.

He has been involved in the design of several epileptology units. His research focuses on methods of recordings and analysis of epileptic networks. He has worked successively at the Sainte-Anne Hospital in Paris, at the Rennes University Hospital and at the Timone Hospital in Marseille.

He oversees the MEG platform in Marseille. He made possible the simultaneous recording of meg signal with SEEG recordings that today generate unique data set for the validation of MEG localization techniques.

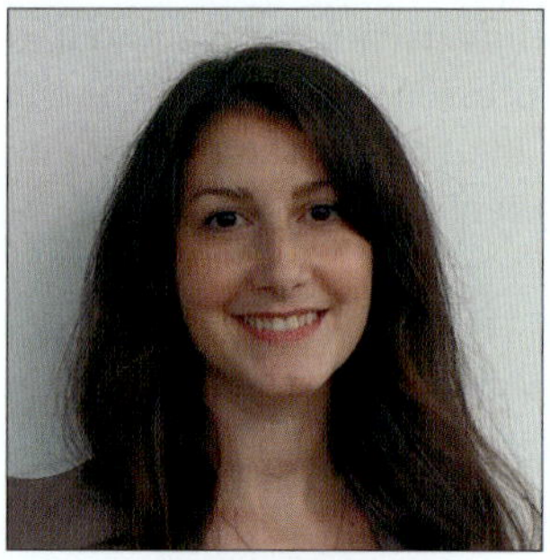

Sara Baldassari

Sara Baldassari obtained a PhD in Biomedical Sciences and Oncology from the University of Turin in 2017 and she was then trained as postdoctoral fellow at the Paris Brain Institute (ICM). She is now an Inserm tenured researcher in the laboratory of Dr Baulac at the ICM.

Her scientific research interests focus on the discovery of the genetic etiology of epilepsy with cortical malformations, and on the elucidation of the disease mechanisms through single-cell omics.

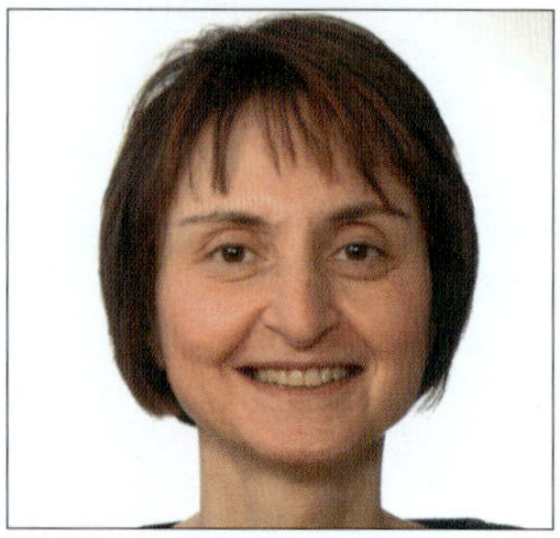

Carmen Barba

Carmen Barba is a child neurologist at the Neuroscience Department, Meyer Children's Hospital, Florence. She trained in neurophysiology and epilepsy surgery at the Neurological Hospital, Lyon, France with Jean Isnard and Francois Mauguiere and in invasive EEG recordings at the University Hospital, Grenoble, France with Philippe Kahane. She is Associate Professor in Child Neurology and Psychiatry, University of Florence and the Head of the Laboratory of Clinical Neurophysiology, Neuroscience

Department, Meyer Children's Hospital, Florence. She coordinated or participated in several projects on complex and rare epilepsies and epilepsy surgery. She is the author of more than 120 peer-reviewed articles and 10 book chapters (H index 26).

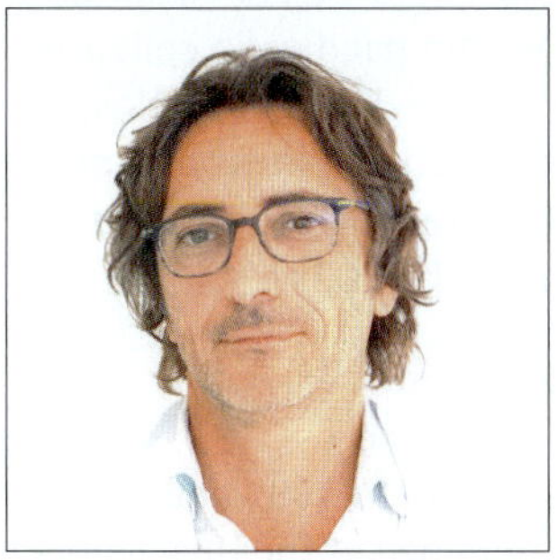

Fabrice Bartolomei

Fabrice Bartolomei is a neurologist specialized in epilepsy and professor at the University of Aix-Marseille (France) where he is head of the Epileptology and Cerebral Rhythmology Department (Timone Hospital, APHM). He is a member of the INSERM U1106 research unit (Institute of Systems Neuroscience, DYNAMAP team) and he is the coordinator of a university hospital research unit (RHU) «EPINOV» based on the study of individualized large-scale modeling in epilepsy surgery. He is particularly involved in the pre-surgical evaluation of patients with drug-resistant epilepsy and is a world leader in the analysis of Stereo-EEG recordings. He has published numerous studies in the field of epilepsy (>250), particularly developing the concept of «epileptogenic networks». He has long promoted the use of EEG/SEEG analysis and is co-inventor of the «Epileptogenicity Index», a method for assessing the epileptogenicity of brain regions.

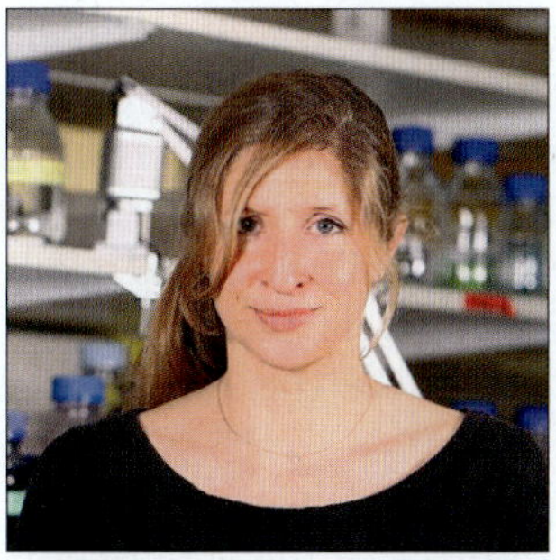

Stéphanie Baulac

Stéphanie Baulac is a research director at Inserm and Group leader at the Paris Brain Institute (ICM). Stéphanie Baulac's research focuses on genetics and somatic mosaicism of cortical malformations associated with focal epilepsies using a translational approach from genetic studies on resected epileptic brain tissues, to *in vitro* functional testing using patient-derived brain organoids, and *in utero*-based mouse models, with the ultimate goal to provide insights into targeted therapeutic opportunities.

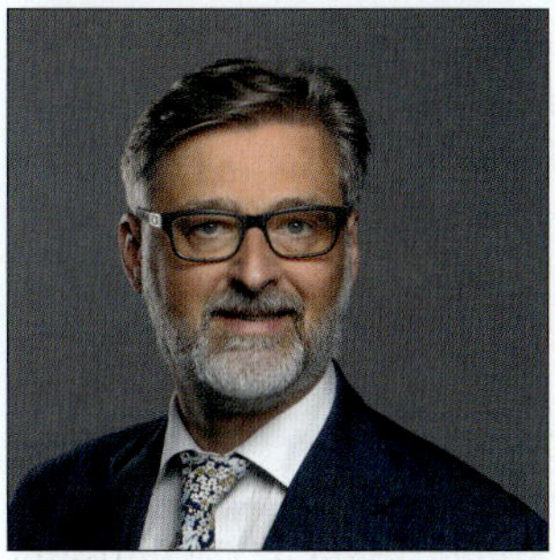

Ingmar Blümcke

Ingmar Blumcke is full professor and director of the department of Neuropathology at the University Hospital Erlangen in Germany. He graduated from medical school at Kiel University, Germany in 1991, and was a post-doctoral fellow in Marco Celio's lab at the University of Fribourg, Switzerland. Between 1994 and 2001, Dr Blumcke trained as resident in Neuropathology at the University Hospital in Bonn. Since then, his scientific interest addresses the clinical and molecular neuropathology of human epilepsies with particular emphasis on disease classification of Focal Cortical Dysplasia, hippocampal sclerosis and low-grade epilepsy-associated brain tumors.

He published more than 350 scientific papers in peer-reviewed journals, with a current H-factor of 74 (Clarivate Web of Science). Dr Blumcke received the Alfred Hauptman Award of the German Epilepsy Society in 2011, the International League against Epilepsy (ILAE) ambassador award in 2015 and the Dorothy Russell medal of the British Neuropathology society in 2018. He currently chairs the Education council of the ILAE and is an executive board member of the ILAE.

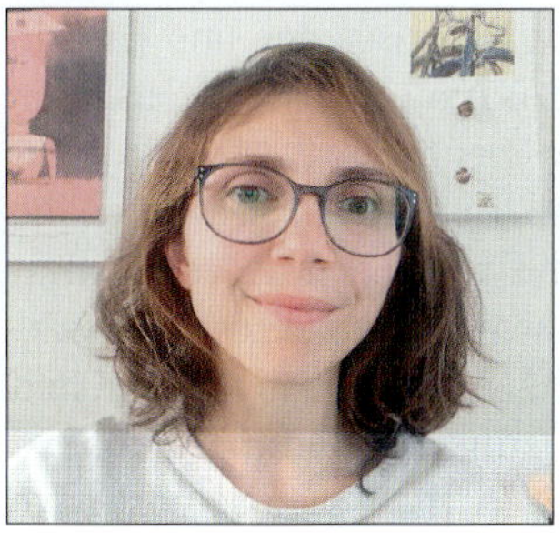

Francesca Bonini

Francesca Bonini is a neurologist trained in neurophysiology and epileptology at Timone Hospital, lecturer at Aix-Marseille Université and member of the Research Unit INSERM U1106. Her research interests include stereoelectroencephalography, magnetoencephalography as well as semiological and surgical aspects of epilepsy.

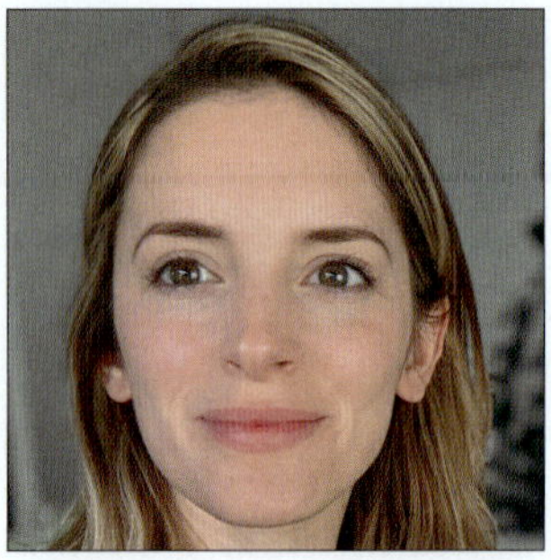

Sarah Buts

Sarah Buts is a paediatrician and paediatric neurologist from Belgium and is currently a clinical fellow in clinical trials and paediatric neurology at the Great Ormond Street Hospital in London, working on clinical trials within paediatric epilepsies. She had her paediatric training in the University Hospital Ghent in Belgium (2014-2019) and her paediatric neurology training in the Evelina London Children's Hospital and the University Hospital Ghent, Belgium (2019-2021).

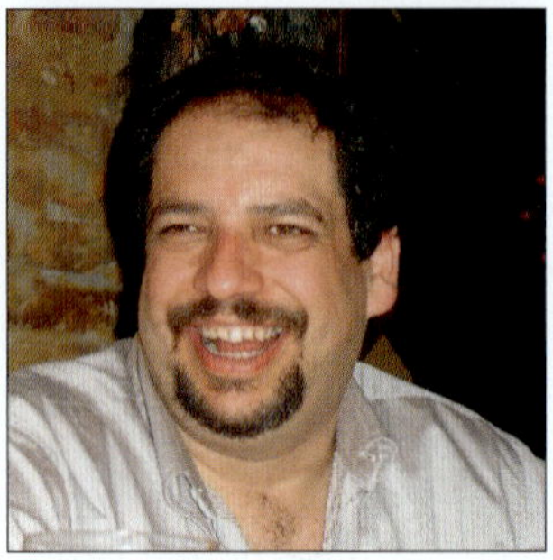

Francesco Cardinale

Francesco Cardinale had his medical degree in 1991 and his specialization in neurosurgery in 1996, obtained at the University of Bari, then obtained a fellowship for pediatric neurosurgery in Rome between 1995 and 1996 under the guidance of Prof. Anthony J Raimondi. He obtained a post-graduate master in biomedical statistics and epidemiology at the University of Pavia in 2005. Since 1998, he has been working as a neurosurgeon at the Claudio Munari Center for Epilepsy Surgery, Niguarda Hospital, Milan. His activity focuses on stereotactic methods for the implantation of intracerebral electrodes aimed at Stereo-EEG monitoring and on brain resective surgery. Dr Cardinale's research focuses mainly on advanced neuroimaging processing for lesion detection and surgical planning, and on robot-assisted neurosurgery. Dr Cardinale is also a PhD student in Neuroscience and works at the Dipartimento di Medicina e Chirurgia, Università degli Studi di Parma, and the Istituto di Neuroscienze, Consiglio Nazionale delle Ricerche, Parma, Italy.

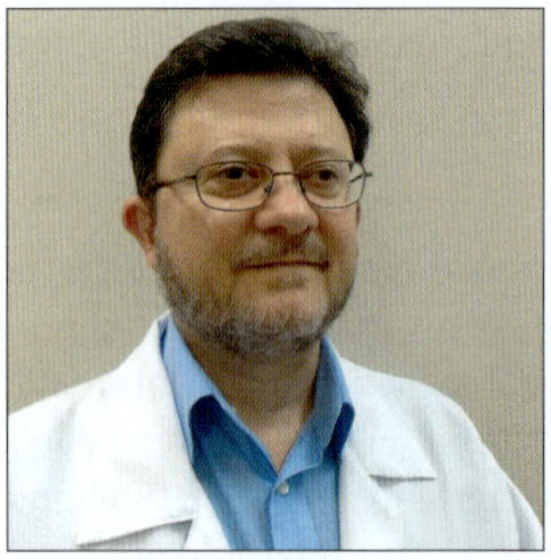

Fernando Cendes

Fernando Cendes is a full professor of the department of Neurology, State University of Campinas (UNICAMP), Brazil, and Coordinator of the Epilepsy Surgery Program at UNICAMP. He is board-certified in Neurology, in Clinical Neurophysiology, and in Diagnostic Neuroradiology. Dr Cendes is a former EEG (1989) and Epilepsy Fellow (1991-1997) at the Montreal Neurological Institute and received his Ph.D. degree in Neuroscience at McGill University, Canada, in 1996. He supervised 77 graduate students and 24 post-doctoral fellows in addition to his teaching activities with medical students and residents. He is the past Chair (2009-2013) and Treasurer (2013-2017), of the Diagnostic Methods Commission of the ILAE. He is an associate editor of the journals *Epilepsia* and *Frontiers in Neurology-Epilepsy*, and a member of the Editorial Board of several journals including *Neurology* and *Epilepsy Research*. His research is focused on Epilepsy, Neuroimaging, and Clinical Neuroscience, with more than 450 full papers published in peer-review journals, with 12,585 citations and an H index of 60 according to the Web of Science (http://www.researcherid.com/rid/C-1301-2012), and an H-index of 80 according to Google Scholar.

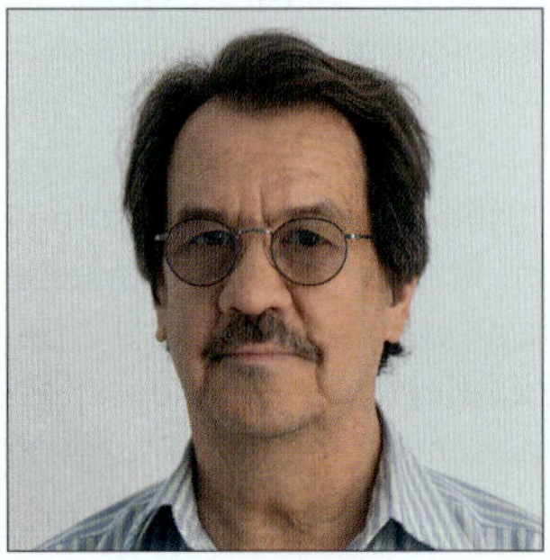

Carlos Cepeda

Carlos Cepeda is a professor of Psychiatry & Biobehavioral Sciences at the Semel Institute for Neuroscience and Human Behavior, University of California Los Angeles (UCLA). His main interest is to understand the basic mechanisms of neurological disorders such as epilepsy and Huntington's disease. He received his training in electrophysiology in Mexico, France, and the USA. He is proficient in a wide array of electrophysiological techniques including EEG, multi- and single-unit recordings. Since 1989, he has concentrated his research efforts on the examination of cellular and synaptic alterations in the cerebral cortex of children with pharmaco-resistant epilepsy. In particular, he used slices and whole-cell patch clamp recordings to unravel neuronal dysfunction in pediatric cortical dysplasia and tuberous sclerosis complex. His laboratory was the first to describe the membrane and synaptic properties of dysmorphic cytomegalic neurons and balloon cells. In parallel, he has been seeking new therapeutic avenues and tested a wide range of pharmacological compounds with potential antiepileptic properties. He has published over 200 peer-reviewed articles and 40 chapters. He has been funded by several NIH grants.

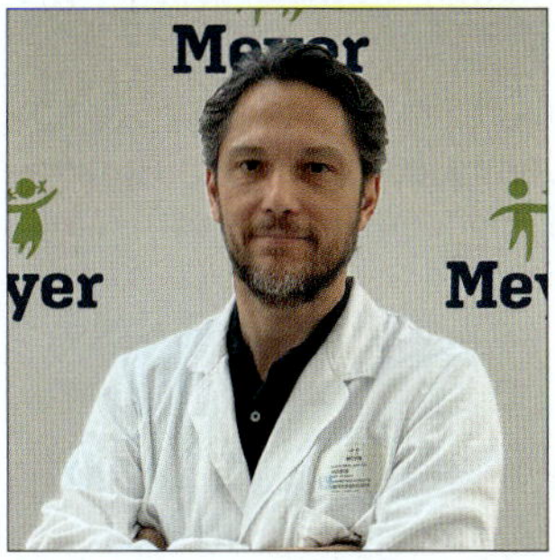

Valerio Conti

Valerio Conti is a geneticist and neurobiologist. He took his PhD at the University of Pisa characterizing ataxic mice models at genetic and morphofunctional level. As a visitor scientist, he trained in neurobiology at the Institut de Neurobiologie de la Méditerranée (INMED), Marseille, France with Carlos Cardoso and Alfonso Represa. He is the head of the Laboratory of Neurobiology at the Neuroscience Department, Meyer Children's Hospital, Florence.

His main research topics are related to functional characterization of pathogenic variants affecting known and novel genes associated with malformations of cortical development and developmental and epileptic encephalopathies in cellular and animal models. He co-authored more than 40 peer-reviewed articles and 4 book chapters (H index 19).

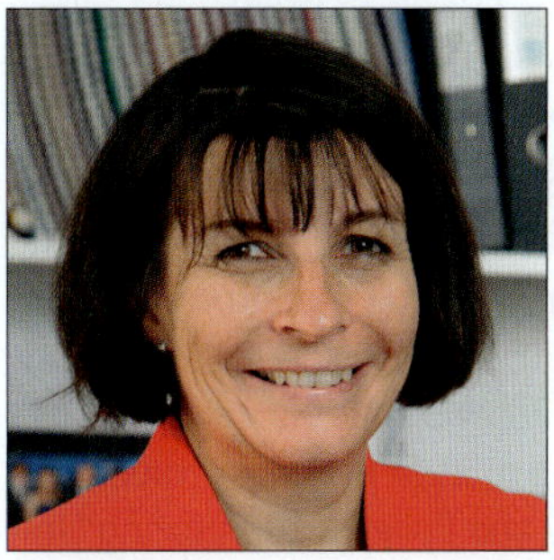

J. Helen Cross

Professor Helen Cross is The Prince of Wales's Chair of Childhood Epilepsy and Head of the Developmental Neuroscience Research and Teaching Department at UCL-Great Ormond Street Institute of Child Health, Honorary Consultant in Paediatric Neurology Great Ormond Street Hospital for Children NHS Foundation Trust, London and Young Epilepsy, Lingfield, UK. Her research has been targeted at improving outcomes in early onset epilepsy, specifically in assessing the role of surgery and ketogenic diet. She has held key leadership roles both nationally and internationally. She is currently President of the International League Against Epilepsy 2021-2025, Clinical Advisor to the National Children's Epilepsy Surgery Service, and was Clinical Advisor to the update of the NICE guidelines for Childhood Epilepsy 2018-2021. She developed, as Coordinator, the European Reference Network for Rare and Complex Epilepsies (EpiCARE) launched in 2017. She has published >400 peer reviewed publications, reviews and book chapters (H index 77). She received an ILAE Ambassador for Epilepsy award in 2007, and is a recipient of the American Academy of Neurology Sydney Carter Award, The International Child Neurology Association Frank Ford Award and the American Epilepsy Clinical Research Award. She received an OBE for contributions to childhood epilepsy in 2015.

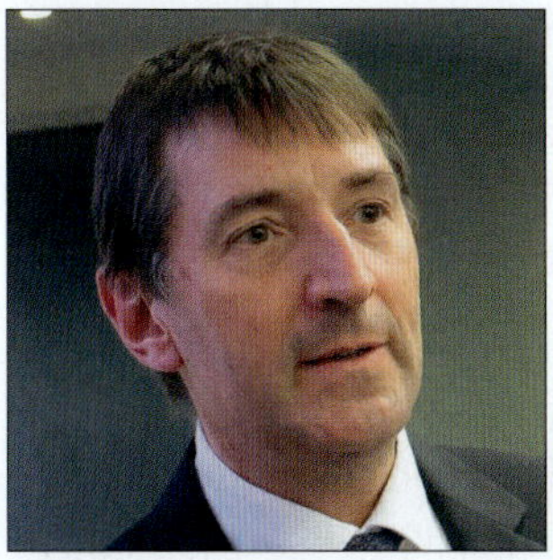

Bertrand C. Devaux

Bertrand Devaux is a neurosurgeon at Lariboisière Hospital in Paris, and professor of Neurosurgery at Université Paris-Cité. He trained in the department of neurosurgery at Sainte-Anne hospital in Paris, especially in stereotactic and functional neurosurgery, from 1986 and obtained his qualification in neurosurgery in 1989. He specialized in epilepsy surgery, developed the image-guided and robotic assistance for SEEG, and alternative techniques to resective procedures, such as multiple radiofrequency thermocoagulations. He was the head the department of neurosurgery at Sainte-Anne hospital from 2013 through 2021. At the Université Paris-Cité, he has been responsible for international students exchange (Erasmus program), and regional coordinator of neurosurgery residency program (2006-2015). His main research areas are epilepsy surgery in functional brain areas and the development of intraoperative optical imaging (full-field and dynamic OCT, multiphoton fluorescence) in cooperation with research laboratories. He received in 2014 the Chevalier de la Légion d'Honneur medal from the Ministery of Superior Education and research.

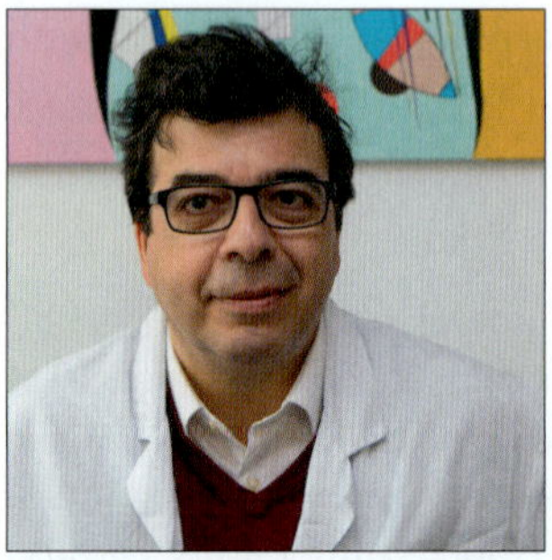

Georg Dorfmüller

Georg Dorfmüller is a pediatric neurosurgeon, specialized in epilepsy surgery. He is head of the department of pediatric neurosurgery at the Hôpital Fondation Rothschild in Paris, France.

Particular fields of expertise of this pediatric epilepsy surgery center are: SEEG explorations in young children, hemispherotomy procedures, and the surgical management of hypothalamic hamartomas.

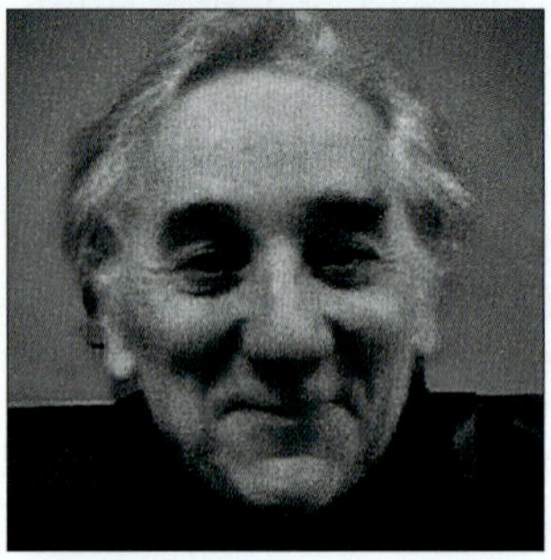

François Dubeau

François Dubeau is an associate professor of clinical neurology and member of the department of neurology and neurosurgery at McGill University. He obtained his degree in Medicine from the University of Montréal (1978), completed his neurology training also at UdeM (1985), and underwent a 3-year (1985-1988) post-doctoral fellowship in epilepsy, electroencephalography and neuropharmacology at the MNI. He is Fellow of the Royal College of Physicians of Canada since 1985. He joined the Montreal Neurological Hospital and Institute (MNH/MNI) and McGill University in 1990 and has worked there since. His clinical and research interests are centered on the analysis of the EEG and invasive EEG methods, mechanisms of epileptogenesis and seizure spread in humans, and functional imaging in the diagnosis and study of epilepsy. He worked in close collaboration with Jean Gotman, Birgit Frauscher, and Philippe Kahane from Grenoble-Alpes University, using the advantage of intracerebral EEG method to better define the epileptogenic zone (EZ) and the role of neurostimulation in the understanding of EZ. They have also created, together, an atlas of normal intracerebral physiology. From 2000 to 2016, he was Director of the EEG laboratory and Epilepsy Monitoring Unit at the MNH. He is author or co-author in over 300 peer-reviewed papers and book chapters.

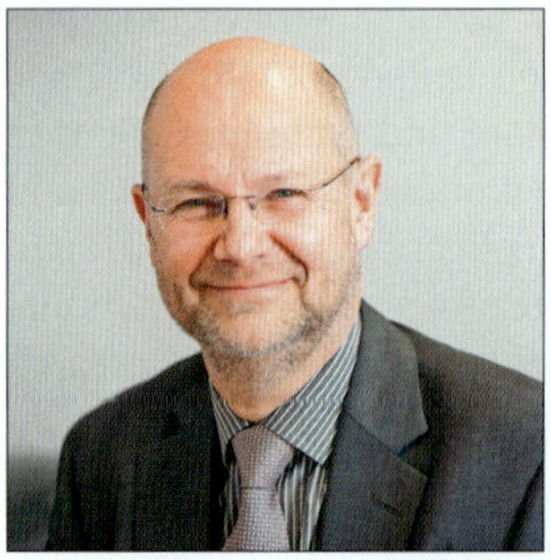

John S. Duncan

John Duncan is a consultant neurologist specializing in epilepsy, practicing at the National Hospital for Neurology and Neurosurgery, Queen Square, London and at Chalfont Centre for Epilepsy, His personal research focus is neuroimaging applied to epilepsy surgery.

He was appointed professor of Neurology at the UCL Institute of Neurology in 1998. From 2012 to 2018, he was clinical director of the National Hospital for Neurology and Neurosurgery. He is NIHR Senior Investigator and Governor of UCL Hospitals. In 2004, he received the annual Clinical Research recognition award of the American Epilepsy Society. He is past-President and past treasurer of the UK chapter of ILAE. In 2005, he was elected Ambassador for Epilepsy and to be a Fellow of the Academy of Medical Sciences.

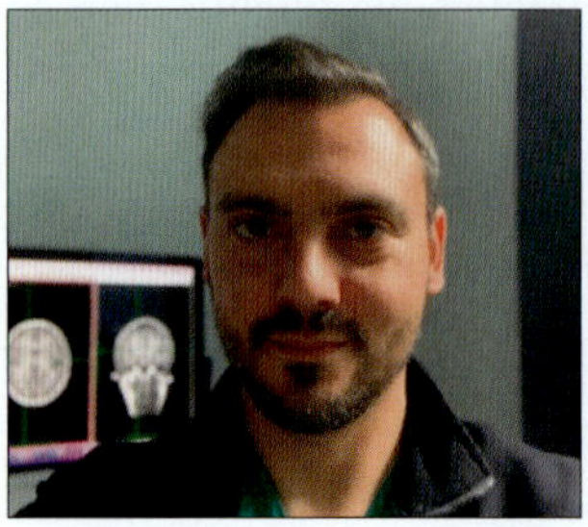

Piergiorgio d'Orio

Piergorgio d'Orio had his medical degree in 2011 from the University of Chieti, and his specialization in neurosurgery in 2017 obtained at the University of Milan. Since then, he has been working as a neurosurgeon at the Claudio Munari Center for Epilepsy Surgery, Niguarda Hospital, Milan, first as part of a fellowship at the Parma's National Research Council Institute of Neuroscience (2018-2021), then on staff at the hospital.

Dr d'Orio has particular interest in SEEG, biostatistics and neuro-imaging. He is also a PhD student in Neuroscience, working at the Dipartimento di Medicina e Chirurgia, Università degli Studi di Parma, and the Istituto di Neuroscienze, Consiglio Nazionale delle Ricerche, Parma, Italy.

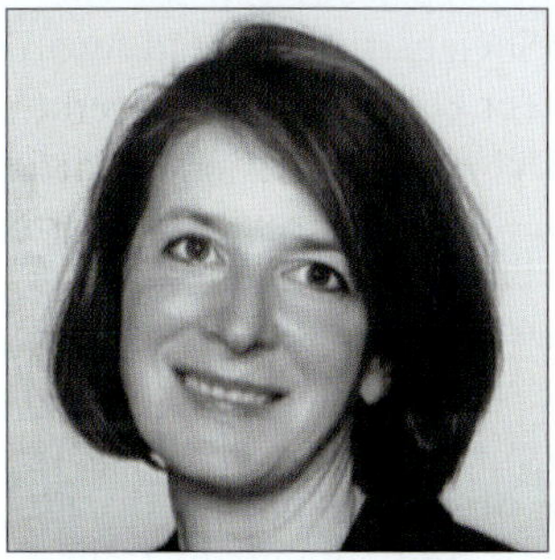

Susanne Fauser

Susanne Fauser is a neurologist and epileptologist. She had her epileptological training at the University Hospital Freiburg, Germany, focusing on the pre-operative evaluation of patients with drug resistant partial epilepsy. Moreover, she worked in the outpatient department for epilepsy patients (focusing on focal and generalized epilepsies) (2002 to 2012). Later on, she was senior physician at the department of Neurology, University Hospital Ulm, Germany, where she headed the Video-EEG-Monitoring Unit and the epilepsy ward between 2012-2015. From 2015 to 2021 she was senior physician at the Epilepsy Center Bethel, Bielefeld, Germany. In Bethel she headed the Video-EEG-Monitoring Unit for adult patients from 2018 to 2021 (mainly non-invasive and invasive presurgical work-ups, but also differential diagnosis). Since 2021 she is senior physician at the Clinic for Neurology, Ludwigsburg, Germany.

Her main research topics are related to Focal Cortical Dysplasias with special interest to postoperative outcome and predictive factors, histology and MRI findings. Moreover, she is interested in status epilepticus and in autoimmune encephalitis (i.e. Rasmussen encephalitis).

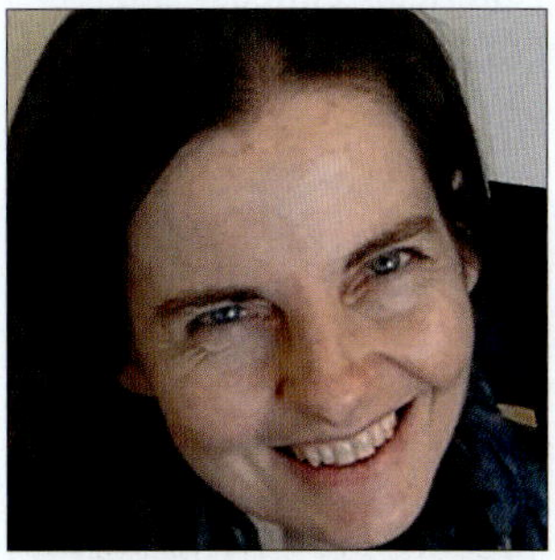

Martine Gavaret

Martine Gavaret is a neurologist, an epileptologist and a neurophysiologist in GHU Paris Psychiatrie et Neurosciences, Sainte Anne Hospital & Université Paris Cité & INSERM UMR 1266, IPNP, Paris. Her areas of expertise are epileptology, high resolution EEG and MEG source localization.

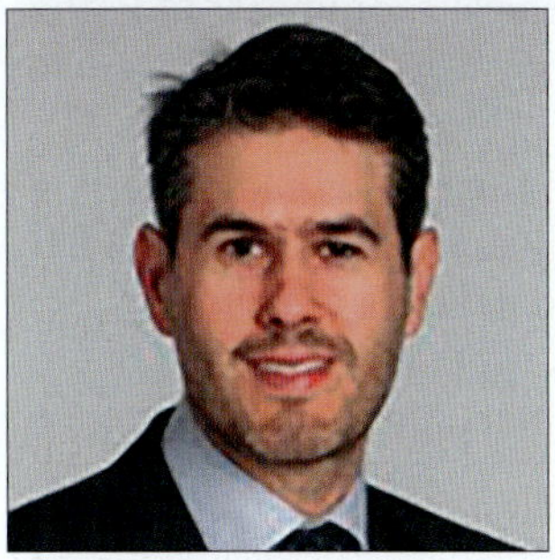

Jorge González Martínez

Jorge González Martínez is a neurosurgeon subspecialized in epilepsy and functional neurosurgery. He is the director of the Epilepsy and Movement Disorders Surgery at University of Pittsburgh Medical Center. Dr González Martínez is a medical pioneer in less invasive methods for treating medically refractory seizures such as stereo-electroencephalography, SEEG guided laser ablative procedures, neuromodulatory interventions and robotic guided surgeries, His particular field of interest and academic drive is related to neuro-electrophysiology, intracranial signal processing and behavioral neuroscience studies. Combined, the clinical and basic science efforts translate and pave the future for safer and more efficient methods for treating patients with severe seizures, promoting the improvement of symptoms, in combination with better functional and quality of life outcomes.

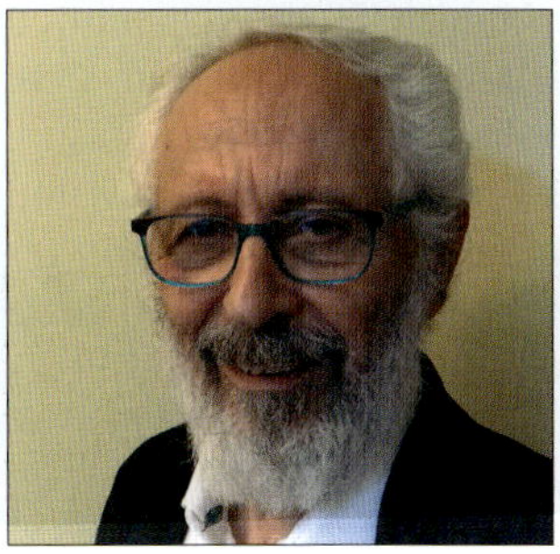

Jean Gotman

Jean Gotman is a professor at the Montreal Neurological Institute, McGill University. He received an engineering degree from the University of Paris and a PhD in Neuroscience from McGill. He pioneered the automatic detection of spikes and seizures during long-term EEG monitoring and made his methods widely available through Stellate, a company he created in 1986, which developed and sold all over the world equipment and software for EEG, epilepsy monitoring and polysomnography. He published over 340 peer-reviewed papers and 40 chapters. His research interests include analysis of the EEG, mechanisms of epileptogenesis, seizure generation and spread in humans, High Frequency Oscillations and functional imaging in the diagnosis and study of epilepsy.

He received the Research Recognition Award from the American Epilepsy Society, the Gloor and the Jasper Awards of the American Clinical Neurophysiology Society, the Penfield Award of the Canadian League against Epilepsy, was named Ambassador for Epilepsy by the International League against Epilepsy, and gave the Lennox-Lombroso lecture at the American Epilepsy Society.

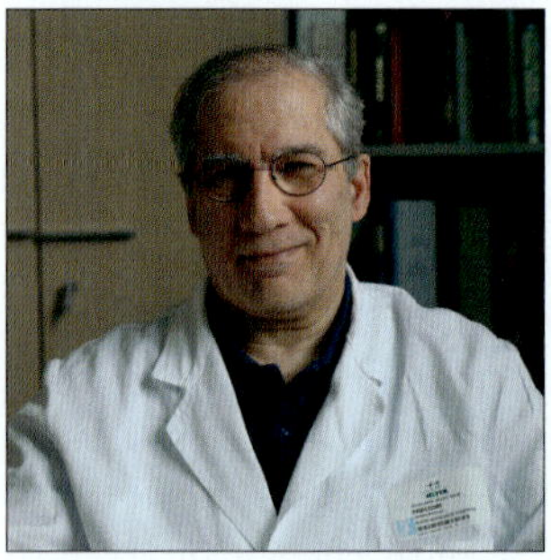

Renzo Guerrini

Renzo Guerrini is Director of the Neuroscience Department at the Children's Hospital A. Meyer, Florence, Italy. His previous academic positions include professorships at University of Pisa, King's College London and University College London. His research focuses on the neurophysiology, neurogenetics and the treatment of pediatric epilepsies. He has coordinated the Commission of Pediatrics of the ILAE and has been the principal investigator of DESIRE (Development and Epilepsy - Strategies for Innovative Research to improve diagnosis, prevention and treatment in children with difficult to treat Epilepsy), a major EU Research project.

He received the Ambassador for Epilepsy ILAE Award, 2003, the American Epilepsy Society's Clinical Research Recognition Award, 2012 and the Elisa Frauenfelder Prize on Research and Innovation, 2019. He has co-authored over 500 papers in peer-reviewed journals and 12 books (H index 108).

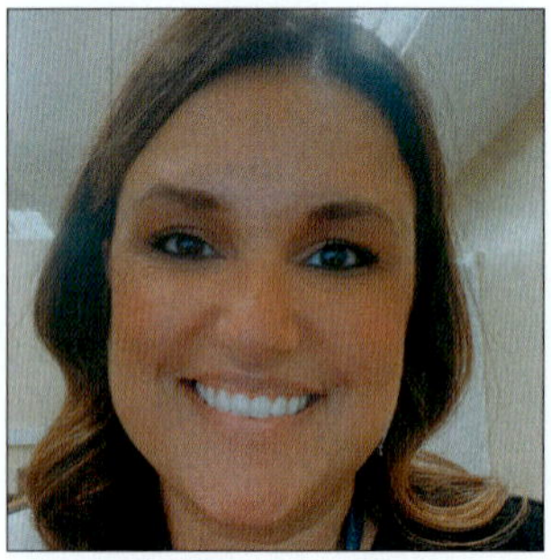

Francine Hehn

Francine Hehn de Oliveira is neuropathologist in Porto Alegre, Brazil, trained at University Hospital of Zurich, Switzerland. She is currently Professor of Pathology at the Pathology department of the Universidade Federal do Rio Grande do Sul (UFGRS) and Chief of Pathology department at Hospital de Clínicas de Porto Alegre. She is medical coordinator of Pathology, Genetics and Molecular Biology Lab of Hospital Moinhos de Vento, Porto Alegre, Brazil.

She is involved in diagnosing brain tumors, neurodegenerative autopsy cases and is responsible for around 500 diagnoses of epilepsy specimens since 2010. She has great interest in morphology, immunohistochemistry and genetics of epilepsy specimens. Author and co-author of more than 30 articles in the areas of neuroscience and neuropathology, she also authored a book on Pathology of Brain Tumors and three chapters of books in the field of pathology.

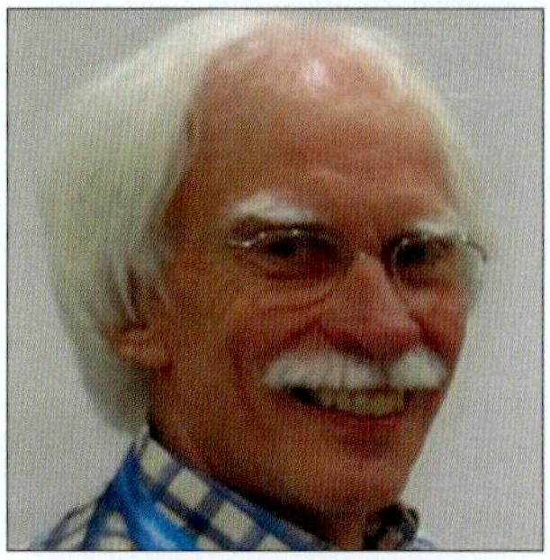

Hans Holthausen

Hans Holthausen is a pediatrician and neuropediatrician with more than 30 years of experience in pediatric epileptology. He got his education in Pediatrics and Neuropediatrics at the Ludwigs-Maximilian-University in Munich. He was appointed by the Epilepsy Center Bethel/Bielefeld (head at that time Peter Wolf) to become head of a pediatric section of a presurgical unit for Children and adults – after an EEG-fellowship and training in presurgical evaluation at the epilepsy center of the Cleveland Clinic, headed by Hans Lüders. After 10 years working in this position, he became head of the Center for Pediatric Neurology and Pediatric Neuro-Rehabilitation in Vogtareuth in the south of Germany. There, together with his coworkers and with generous support by the Bavarian government, managed to establish successfully another pediatric epilepsy center, which includes presurgical evaluation and epilepsy surgery. Hans Holthausen was the first chair of the Task Force of Pediatric Epilepsy Surgery of the ILAE. He is co-editor of 2 textbooks on Pediatric Epilepsy Surgery and author of numerous peer-reviewed publications and book chapters in textbooks, edited by renewed epileptologists. After his retirement from the position as head of the clinic, he is still affiliated with the center in Vogtareuth. He has kept until now his keen interest in pediatric epileptology, particularly in surgical and mental outcome of children with epilepsies in association with structural lesions.

Hans Holthausen is honorary member of the German chapter of the ILAE and honorary member of the Neuropediatric Society of the German speaking countries. He and is spending most of his time now on the analysis of the large body of data from the epilepsy center in Vogtareuth and in teaching and lecturing in many parts of world, in particular in Russia.

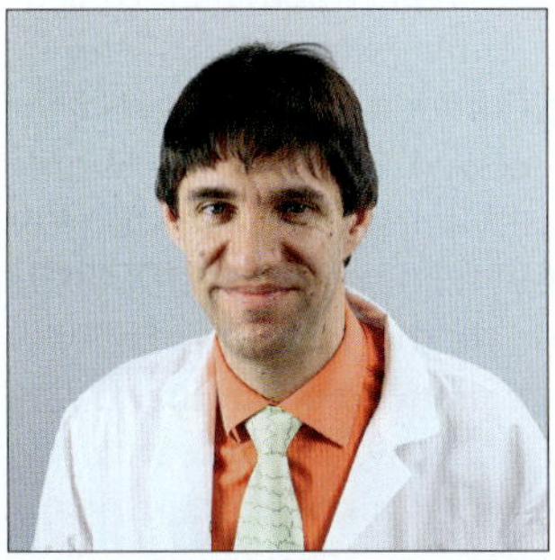

Pavel Kršek

Pavel Kršek is a paediatric neurologist and epileptologist, a professor of Neurology at Charles University in Prague, head of department of Paediatric Neurology, 2nd Faculty of Medicine and Motol University Hospital in Prague, and the current chair of Czech Society of Paediatric Neurology. His fields of clinical and research interest include drug-resistant epilepsy in children, epilepsy surgery (with special focus on focal cortical dysplasia and tuberous sclerosis), genetic causes of epileptic encephalopathies and malformations of cortical development, intraoperative monitoring, and quality of life of children with epilepsy. He has authored or co-authored over 110 papers in peer-reviewed scientific journals and participated in more than 30 grant projects including 3 international projects.

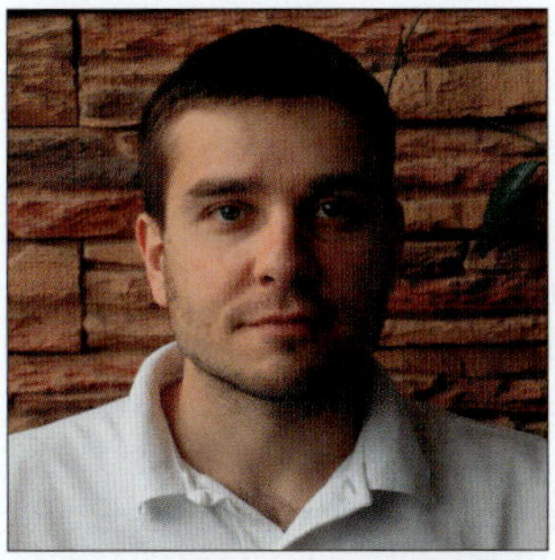

Martin Kudr

Martin Kudr is a paediatric neurologist focusing on epileptology and epilepsy surgery. Since graduating from Charles University in Prague, he has been working at the department of Pediatric Neurology, Motol University Hospital in Prague. The topic of his dissertation was SPECT in epilepsy surgery. He completed internships focused on epilepsy surgery at Miami Children's Hospital and University Hospital in Grenoble.

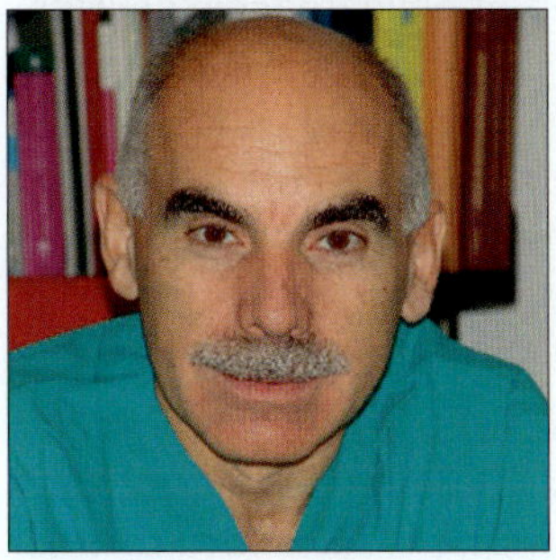

Giorgio Lo Russo

Giorgio Le Russo had his medical degree at the University of Turin in 1977 and specialized in Neurology and Neurosurgery (1987, 1982) at the University of Turin. He was a university researcher, at the Institute of Neurosurgery of Turin until 1993. He trained in Paris (Service de Neurochirurgie, Hôpital Sainte Anne, 1989-1990, with Prof. Talairach and Prof. Bancaud) and Grenoble (Service de Neurochirurgie, Centre Universitaire Grenoble 1991-1994, with Prof. Benabid) under the guidance of his Mentor Prof. Claudio Munari. He contributed to start the epilepsy surgery program in Grenoble and to found the Milan Center when Prof. Munari returned to Italy. He is currently in charge of the Claudio Munari Center for Epilepsy Surgery at Niguarda Hospital where he has been working since 1993.

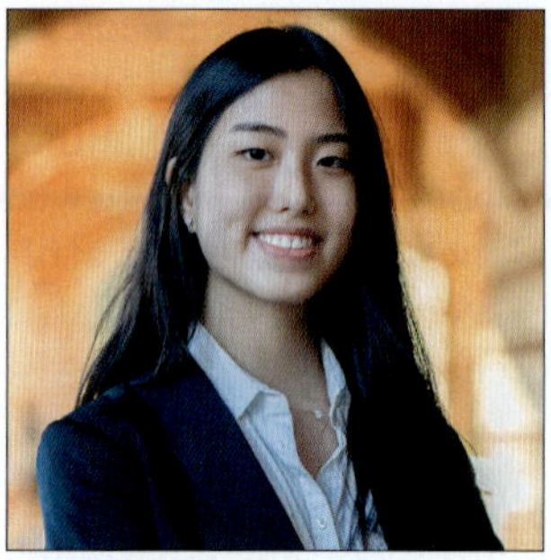

Daphne Marina

Daphne Marina graduated Magna Cum Laude with a Bachelor of Science degree in Physiological Science from the University of California, Los Angeles (UCLA). She is an aspiring M.D. candidate and has attended surgery and pediatric grand rounds at the UCLA Ronald Reagan Hospital. Currently, she is conducting quantitative analysis of non-neuronal cells present in Focal Cortical Dysplasia and tuberous sclerosis complex tissue samples to gain insights into their role in pediatric epilepsy. She was born and raised in Indonesia.

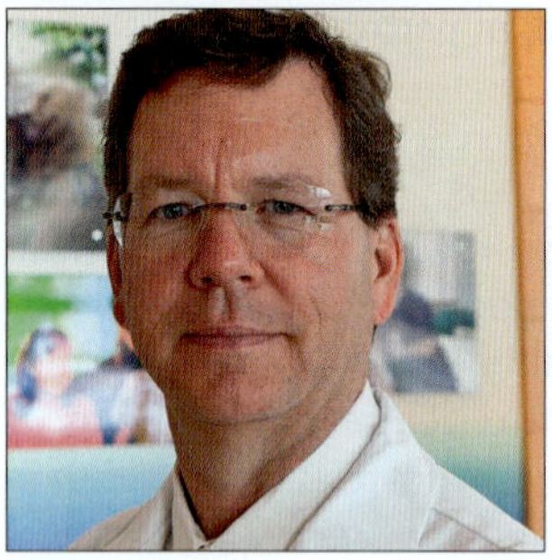

Gary W. Mathern

Gary Mathern is a professor in the departments of Neurosurgery and Psychiatry at the University of California, Los Angeles (UCLA) and the Davies/Crandall endowed chair for epilepsy research at UCLA. He received his medical degree from Case Western Reserve University and did a neurosurgery residency followed by an Epilepsy fellowship at UCLA. He became the neurosurgical director of the Pediatric Epilepsy Surgery Program in 1997, where he pioneered surgical treatment of children with refractory epilepsy. His research has involved histopathological and electrophysiological studies of resected human brain tissue, animal models of surgically treated epilepsy syndromes, and genetic studies of refractory epilepsy along with studies of neuroimaging in epilepsy. He has published more than 250 peer-reviewed papers and book chapters. He was awarded the Founder's award by the American Epilepsy Society and the Ambassadors award from the International League Against Epilepsy, and was Editor-in-Chief of Epilepsia.

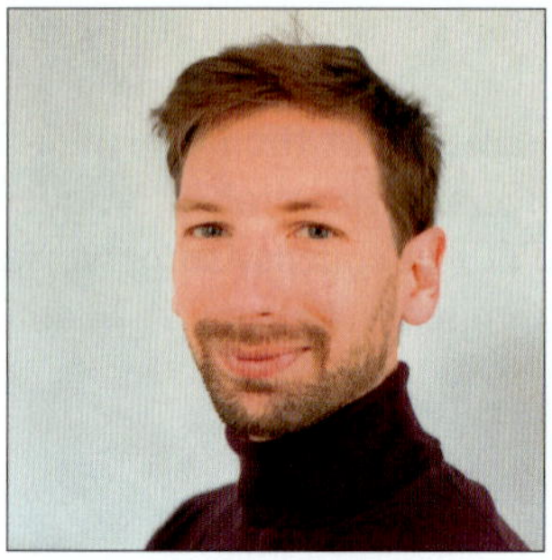

Charles Mellerio

Charles Mellerio is a neuroradiologist focused on two main areas: epilepsy and functional imaging. After completing his medical training and radiology residency, he specialized in cerebral imaging. His activities in Epilepsy imaging and clinical functional MRI began in 2008 at GHU Sainte-Anne (Paris) where he has post-processed over 2000 fMRI cases since then. He earned his PhD in neurosciences at Université de Paris and his thesis topic was "Optimization of advanced MRI tools in the detection and characterization of epileptogenic developmental lesions" with a special focus on focal cortical dysplasia imaging. He also developed these practices since 2016 at Centre d'Imagerie du Nord (CCN – Saint-Denis – France). He published around 50 peer-reviewed papers, several book chapters, and presented numerous scientific and educational presentations related to epilepsy and functional imaging.

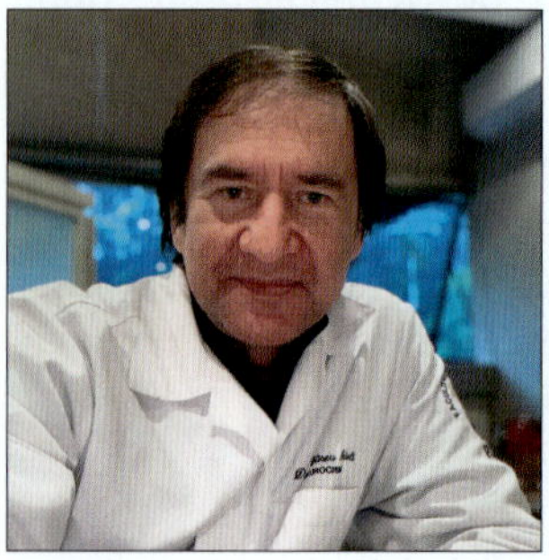

Eliseu Paglioli

Eliseu Paglioli is a neurosurgeon in Porto Alegre, Brazil, trained at the Instituto de Neurocirurgia, Hospital São José, Santa Casa de Misericórdia de Porto Alegre. He is currently Professor of Neurosurgery at the Department of Surgery of the Pontificia Universidade Católica do Rio Grande do Sul (PUCRS) and Surgical Director of the Epilepsy Surgery Program, at the Hospital São Lucas da PUCRS. He was head of the Neurosurgery Service of Hospital São Lucas from 2003 until 2021.

He has been strongly involved with surgical treatment of patients with drug-resistant focal and generalized epilepsies, having operated more than 2,500 patients with epilepsy over the last 30 years. His main focuses in surgical practice and research are the temporal lobe epilepsies and extratemporal focal cortical dysplasia operated under acute electrocorticography. Moreover, he has devised the technique and rationale for selective posterior callosotomy from epileptic drop attacks, which has also been an area of significant interest lately. He has written or co-written more than 75 peer-reviewed articles or book chapters.

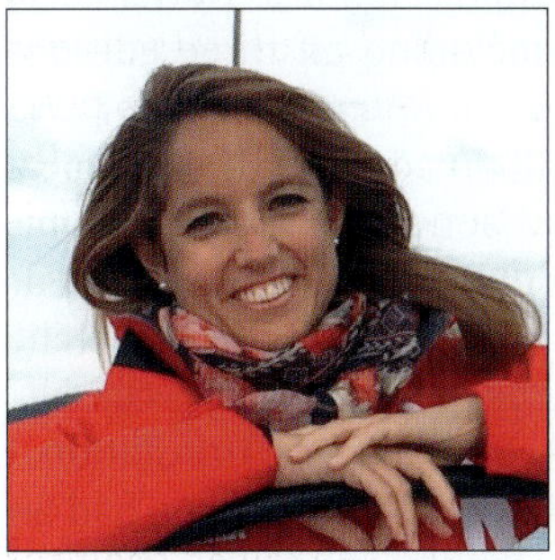

Martina Revay

Martina Revay had her medical degree in 2012 and her specialization in neurosurgery in 2020, obtained at the University of Milan. She obtained a fellowship for neurosurgery in Tolosa in 2017 under the guidance of Prof. Sol. She has been working as a neurosurgeon at the Claudio Munari center since 2018, first as part of a fellowship at the L. Sacco Biomedical and Clinical department of the Milan University (2018-2021), then on staff at the hospital. Dr Revay has a particular interest in SEEG, neurophysiological intraoperative mapping and monitoring, and neuro-imaging.

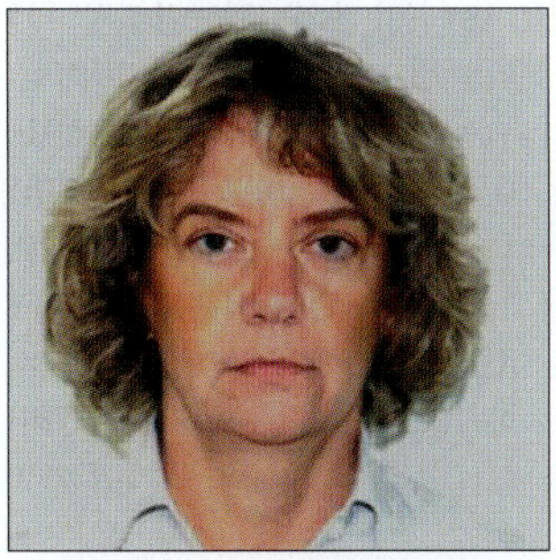

Ivana Sartori

After a medical degree in 1991, Ivana Sartori has her specializations in Neurophysiology (1995) and Neurology (2001) from the University of Pavia, and AISM examination for sleep medicine in 2000. She works as an epileptologist at the Claudio Munari Center for Epilepsy Surgery since 2001. Dr Sartori has a particular interest in SEEG and neurophysiological intraoperative mapping and monitoring. In addition, her research interests are concentrated in particular in neuroscience, thanks to a long collaboration with the Universities of Parma and Milan.

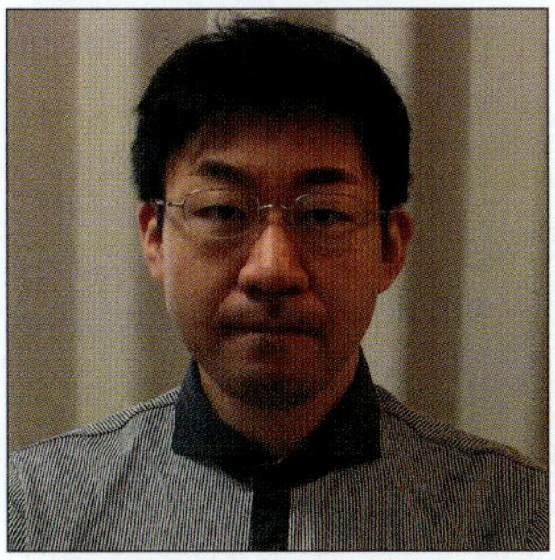

Masataka Tanaka

Masataka Tanaka is a chief doctor at the department of Neurosurgery, Yao Municipal Hospital, Japan. He received a medical degree from Akita University in 2008. He has been a board-certified neurosurgeon of Japan Neurosurgical Society since 2014. He specializes in functional and stereotactic neurosurgery. From 2020–2022, he joined Dr Jean Gotman's lab at the Montreal Neurological Institute, McGill University as a post-doctoral research fellow. As a neurosurgeon and researcher, his research interests include voxel-based morphometry, analysis of magnetoencephalography for Parkinson's disease, and EEG-fMRI for patients with epilepsy.

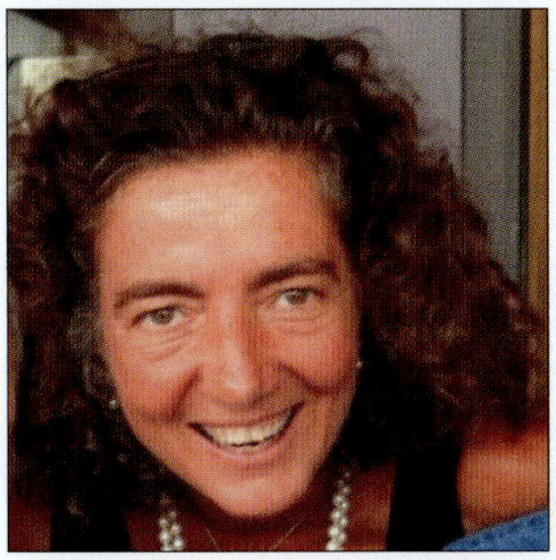

Laura Tassi

Laura Tassi graduated at the University of Milan, in 1988, becoming Neurologist in 1992. At present, she is a neurologist and neurophysiologist, as Hospital Practioner at the Claudio Munari Epilepsy Surgery Centre in Milano, in Italy. She is the responsible of the Long-Term monitoring Laboratory of the clinical epileptology program. She is acknowledged as an expert on pre-surgical assessment of drug-resistant epilepsies, including SEEG investigations, with about 30 years of experience in the field. Her area of research includes Malformation of cortical development, early indication for surgery, Thermocoagulation with intracerebral electrodes, characterization of ictal discharges during Stereo-EEG. She is the President of the Italian League Against Epilepsy.

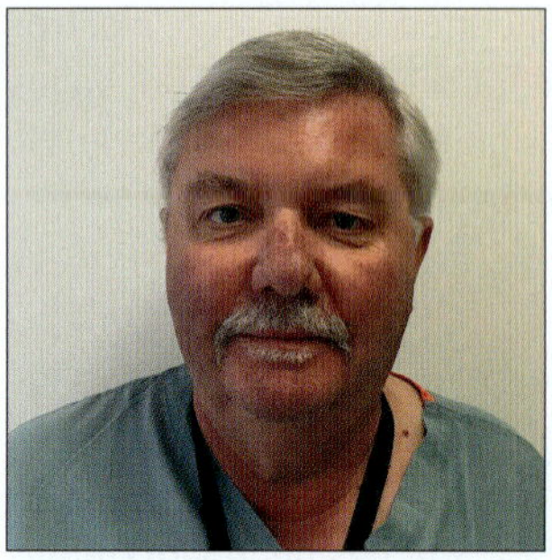

Harry V. Vinters

Harry V. Vinters has published more than 600 articles, reviews and book chapters on various aspects of neuropathology, ranging from its clinical aspects to issues of molecular pathogenesis, tissue culture and animal models. He has also co-authored or edited six books, including all three editions of the widely used *Neuropathology – a Reference Text of CNS Pathology* (Mosby, 3d edition, 2013). In addition to his clinical and teaching activities, he has had active research programs in several areas, including vascular dementias and the vascular component of Alzheimer disease (especially mediated through cerebral amyloid/congophilic angiopathy), neuropathologic substrates of intractable pediatric epilepsy, neurologic complications of AIDS, stroke and cerebrovascular disease—this work incorporates translational studies and investigation of animal models. In the early days of the AIDS epidemic, he had an active program in, and was among the first to characterize, the neurologic complications of HIV infection. In 1987, his laboratory contributed to discovery of one of the first 'neurotropic' strains of HIV. He was the recipient (in 2002) of the Research Award of the Alzheimer's Association of Los Angeles, Riverside and San Bernardino Counties. He served as Editor-in-Chief of 'Brain Pathology', from 2000-2006 and currently is lead investigator on a CIRM grant to study the neurologic complications of COVID 19. Dr Vinters' laboratory has hosted numerous international scholars and trainees—all of whom have gone on to distinguished careers in their home countries. He has served and currently serves on several editorial boards of major scientific journals, including *Neuropathology, Neuropathology & Applied Neurobiology*, and *Human Pathology*. In 2017, he received the Alfred Meyer Medal of the British Neuropathological Society and the Award for Meritorious Contributions to Neuropathology from the American Association of Neuropathologists.

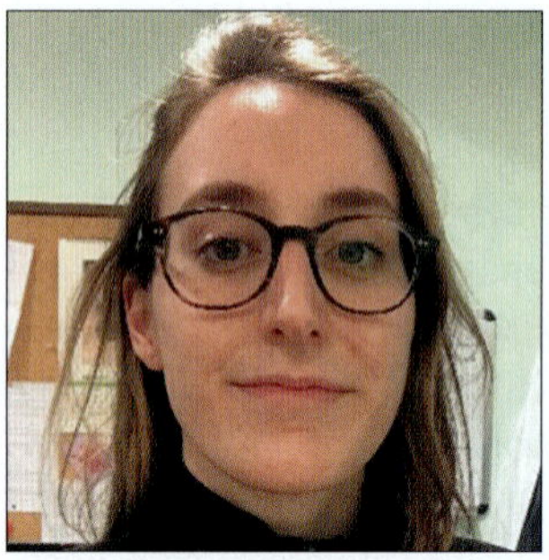

Flavia Maria Zauli

After a bachelor's degree in 2015 in Neurophysiopathology Techniques from Tor Vergata University of Rome, Flavia Maria Zauli had her Master's degree in Cognitive Science in 2018 from La Statale University of Milan. She is currently a PhD student in Mind, Brain and Reasoning at the L. Sacco Biomedical and Clinical department of the Milan University, practicing her clinical activity at the Claudio Munari Center. Dr Zauli has particular interest in high-density EEG with electrical source imaging and neurophysiological intraoperative mapping and monitoring.

She currently works at the Azienda Socio-Sanitaria Territoriale Grande Ospedale Metropolitano Niguarda, Claudio Munari Center for Epilepsy Surgery, as well as the Dipartimento di Scienze Biomediche e Cliniche L. Sacco and the Dipartimento di Filosofia P. Martinetti, Università degli Studi di Milano, in Milan, Italy.

SUMMARY

Preface
Francine Chassoux, Andre Palmini | V

Acknowledgements | VII

Dedication | VIII

Editors | XI

Authors | XII

Abbreviations | XXV

Part I. TOWARD A ROUTE IN THE LABYRINTH

Chapter 1 : A clinician's overview of the FCD
François Dubeau | 3

Chapter 2 : Classifications for FCD: evolution of concepts and current knowledge
Andre Palmini | 13

Chapter 3 : Neuropathology of FCD: a practical approach for clinical use
Ingmar Blümcke | 23

Part II. FROM GENES TO CLINICAL PICTURE

Chapter 4 : Genetics of FCD: an emerging scenario
Sara Baldassari, Stéphanie Baulac | 41

Chapter 5 : FCD and the mTORopathy spectrum
Valerio Conti, Carmen Barba, Renzo Guerrini | 51

Chapter 6 : Drug therapies in FCD: are they specific and why?
Sarah Buts, J. Helen Cross | 61

Chapter 7 : Electroclinical phenotypes in FCD
Francine Chassoux, Andre Palmini, Laura Tassi | 65

Chapter 8 : FCD in children: specific clinical findings and management
Pavel Kršek, Hans Holthausen | 75

Part III. NEUROPHYSIOLOGY OF FCD: THE PACEMAKER PATTERN

Chapter 9 : In search of the epileptogenic neuron in FCD
Carlos Cepeda, Daphne Marina, Harry V. Vinters, Gary W. Mathern | 91

Chapter 10 : Intrinsic epileptogenicity of FCD: insights from ECoG
Andre Palmini, Eliseu Paglioli | 103

Chapter 11 : Intrinsic epileptogenicity of FCD: insights from SEEG to scalp EEG
Francine Chassoux | 113

Chapter 12 : The epileptogenic zone in FCD: SEEG patterns in FCD subtypes
Fabrice Bartolomei | 125

Chapter 13 : MEG and HR-EEG in FCD: non-invasive localization of the epileptogenic zone
Francesca Bonini, Jean-Michel Badier, Martine Gavaret | 131

Chapter 14 : EEG-fMRI in FCD: mapping the epileptogenic networks
Masataka Tanaka, Jean Gotman | 143

Part IV. IMAGING OF FCD: THE DECISIVE STEP

Chapter 15 : The role of imaging in FCD: an overview
John S. Duncan | 151

Chapter 16 : Morphological and functional MRI for FCD in clinical practice
Charles Mellerio | 157

Chapter 17 : Critical perspective of automatic detection of FCD: what should the clinician use?
Fernando Cendes | 171

Chapter 18 : PET and SPECT: searching for FCD and identifying the epileptogenic zone
Francine Chassoux, Martin Kudr | 179

Part 1. PET in FCD | 179

Part 2. SPECT in FCD | 192

PART V. SURGICAL THERAPY FOR FCD: A CURATIVE PERSPECTIVE

Chapter 19 : Surgery for FCD: principles and outcome
Francesco Cardinale, Martina Revay, Piergiorgio d'Orio, Flavia Maria Zauli, Belén Abarrategui, Giorgio Lo Russo, Ivana Sartori | 203

Chapter 20 : Surgery for FCD without invasive monitoring: the role of ECoG
Eliseu Paglioli, Andre Palmini, Francine Hehn | 223

Chapter 21 : Surgery for FCD with invasive monitoring
Jorge Álvaro González Martínez | 231

Chapter 22 : Surgery for FCD in eloquent cortex
Bertrand C. Devaux | 243

Chapter 23 : Surgery for FCD in children
Georg Dorfmüller | 259

Chapter 24 : Long-term outcome after surgery for FCD
Susanne Fauser | 275

Conclusion
Francine Chassoux, Andre Palmini | 285

Abbreviations

AED	antiepileptic drug
ASD	anti-seizure drug
AI	artificial intelligence
ANN	artificial neural network
ASM	anti-seizure medication
BOLD	blood-oxygen-level-dependent
BOSD	bottom-of-the-sulcus dysplasia
DL	deep learning
CED	continuous epileptiform discharges
ECoG	electrocorticography
EEG	electroencephalography
EMSI	electromagnetic source imaging
ESI	electric source imaging
EZ	epileptogenic zone
fMRI	functional magnetic resonance imaging
FCD	focal cortical dysplasia
FDG-PET	fluorodeoxyglucose positron emission tomography
FBTCS	focal-to-bilateral tonic-clonic seizures
GABA	Gamma-aminobutyric acid
HFO	high-frequency oscillations
HME	hemimegalencephaly
HR-EEG	high resolution EEG
ICA	independent component analysis
IED	interictal epileptic discharge
LVFA	low voltage fast activity
mMCD	mild malformations of cortical development
mTOR	mammalian target of rapamycin
MAP	morphometric analysis program
MCD	malformations of cortical development
MEG	magnetoencephalography
ML	machine learning
MOGHE	mild malformation of cortical development with oligodendroglial hyperplasia in epilepsy
MRI	magnetic resonance imaging
MSI	magnetic source imaging
MUSEC	Multilobar Unilateral hypoplasia with emphasis in the posterior quadrant and severe epilepsy in children
MUSIC	multiple signal classification
NMD	neuronal migration disorders
NMDA	N-methyl-D-aspartate
PET	positron emission tomography subdural grid
SDG	subdural grids
SEEG	Stereo-electroencephalography
SOP	seizure-onset patterns
SOZ	seizure-onset zone
SRE	sleep related epilepsy
SPECT	single-photon emission computerized tomography
SPM	statistical parametric mapping
TSC	tuberous sclerosis complex

Part I. TOWARD A ROUTE IN THE LABYRINTH

CHAPTER

1. A clinician's overview of the FCD

François Dubeau

Keypoints

- Taylor and colleagues' description of FCD already contained all defining elements of the well characterized lesion that was later classified as FCD II.
- MRI identification of FCD transformed an apparent curiosity in one of the most frequent cause of drug-resistant epilepsy in children and adults.
- Crucially, identification of intrinsic highly epileptogenic patterns in FCD lesions helped to single out this pathology among the many causes of severe epilepsy.
- Molecular genetics, and particularly the discovery of the mTOR intracellular pathway as a regulator of neuronal development, are advancing the understanding of the biological bases of FCD II, or Taylor-type FCD.

Introduction

To open a book commemorating the 50th year of publication of the seminal paper by Taylor and colleagues describing focal cortical dysplasia (FCD) from a clinical perspective is both challenging and rewarding. The field has evolved in many directions, and very often neuroimagers, neurophysiologists, neurosurgeons, pathologists and basic scientists move to center stage, leaving the clinician apparently out of the main picture. However, clinicians are the ones that should suspect that the cause of severe epilepsy in their patients is indeed an FCD! There is no room for scientific advances if patients are not correctly diagnosed and managed. On the other hand, diagnosing FCD strengthens the doctor-patient-family relationship as a number of very important therapeutic and prognostic prospects are clearly laid out, not least the crucial role of the surgical treatment. Thus, it is very rewarding for clinicians to know that a correct diagnosis of FCD - and often a firm suspicion of a doubtful diagnosis - will streamline the diagnosis and treatment of their patients.

This chapter provides an overview of the journey of discovery in FCD, taken from the historical perspective of how each piece pf the puzzle came into place – and which pieces are still needed to complete picture. From the initial description of 50 years ago to the most modern refinements in diagnosis and biology, it gives a glimpse of what the reader will find in this book.

Historical landmarks

In 1971, David Taylor and his colleagues - MA Falconer, CJ Bruton and JAN Corsellis - from the Mausdley Hospital in London and the Runwell Hospital in Wickford, Essex, reported the first series of epileptic patients operated on because of refractory seizures with "*histological abnormalities as a particular form of localized cortical dysplasia*". The series comprised 10 subjects; 5 underwent a temporal resection, 2 an anterior frontal, 1 parietal, 1 occipital and 1 had first a temporal resection followed years later by frontal lobe surgery. Histologically, the authors described in 10/10 "... congregations of large, bizarre neurons, which were littered through all but the first cortical layer, and in most (7/10), grotesque cells, probably of glial origin, were also present in the depths of the affected cortex and in the subjacent white matter...". The authors emphasized that "the picture observed in these cases although reminiscent of tuberous sclerosis" (they recognized histopathological similarities with cortical tubers) was showing too many distinguishing clinical and pathological features and proposed that "the cases are looked on provisionally as comprising a distinct form of cortical dysplasia in which localized, exotic populations of nerve cells underlie the electrical and clinical manifestations of certain forms of epilepsy."

The 10 patients reported by Taylor and colleagues had drug-resistant focal epilepsies with an age at onset ranging from 2 to 31 years (mean age, 12.4 yrs). Scalp electroencephalogram (EEG) or per-operative electrocorticogram (ECoG) showed in all active, frequent, continuous or rhythmic interictal epileptiform anomalies. Radiological procedures (skull X-ray, pneumoencephalogram and carotid angiography) not surprisingly provided little information and were either normal or showing slight local enlargement or distortion of ventricles. Surgical outcomes were quite good: 7 patients became seizure-free or had only occasional attacks (Engel's class 1-2), 2 obtained marginal results (Engel's class 3-4) and 1 died in a status epilepticus. The cortical areas implicated and removed surgically in these 10 patients essentially comprised both at the macro and microscopic levels, the accepted characteristics now used to define and classify the focal cortical dysplasias. First, the part of the brain removed in each patient coincided with the area of the brain showing the maximal epileptiform abnormalities. Second, macroscopically, the specimens often showed no gross cortical anatomical abnormality but in certain cuts localized wide and "unusually thick" cortical ribbon and a poor gray-white matter differentiation were seen, with lesions limited to one lobe or a segment of the lobe. Third, at the microscopic level, the authors observed that the lesions could happen "at any point along or round a gyrus, but any one patch seldom stretched horizontally through the cortical ribbon for more than about 2.0 cm". They also described "... a clear junction between the normal and abnormal cortex ... and that the crown of the affected gyrus was often spared and the anomalies concentrated around the base of the sulcus" (e.g. cases 1, 2, 6, 7, 8, 9 and 10). The striking histological features were:
- a localized disruption and loss of the normal cortical lamination,
- congregations of large aberrant neurons distributed randomly in all cortical layers but the first and in the deeper layers
- adjacent white matter, large, distorted, ballooned cells with clear and opalescent cytoplasm.

All features consistent with what we now described as FCD type II (FCD II).

A gap in knowledge: 1971 to the 80s-90s?

This small series of patients, published at a time where brain imaging was unable to provide direct anatomical view of the gray and white matters, contained most of the clinical and electroencephalographic features, cortical lesion distribution, histological findings and post-surgical outcomes that will, two to three decades later, characterize series of pediatric and adult patients found to have focal cortical dysplasia. We now know that FCD is a frequent and highly epileptogenic developmental abnormality of the cerebral cortex, usually restricted to a lobe or segment of a lobe but that can be also multi-lobar, that may be associated with other histopathological abnormalities, and that presents with characteristic neuro-glial abnormal histological and organizational features (Mischel *et al.*, 1995; Tassi *et al.*, 2002; Palmini *et al.*, 2004; Barkovich *et al.*, 2005; Spreafico & Blümcke 2010; Blümcke *et al.*, 2011; *et al.*, 2018). Somewhat surprisingly, following the work of Taylor and colleagues it needed an additional 20 years before FCD came out as a distinct and frequent cause of intractable epilepsy. As discussed in the chapter by Palmini, that realization was somewhat slow, and it took some time before FCD were disentangled from neuronal migration disorders and individualized in the overall group of malformations of cortical development (MCD). As FCD became recognized as a specific developmental disorder, different classifications systems were proposed in attempts to achieve a unified nomenclature for this group of developmental malformations and obtain a better and more specific understanding of their clinical, neuroimaging, histopathology and biological characteristics (Mischel *et al.*, 1995; Tassi *et al.*, 2002; Palmini *et al.*, 2004; Barkovich *et al.*, 2005; Spreafico & Blümcke, 2010). The introduction of the consensus classification of the focal cortical dysplasia 40 years later by the International League Against Epilepsy (ILAE) diagnostic method commission in 2011 (Blümcke *et al.*, 2011) fostered further interest and efforts resulting in an increase knowledge both in the clinical and research domains. The following discussion is to briefly overview and summarizes the considerable progress made over the past five decades in understanding FCD mechanisms, diagnosis, epileptogenicity and treatment strategies.

Modern imaging made and continue to make the difference in detecting FCD

• FCD are not a rare cause of refractory seizures

In the series of Taylor, patients identified with an FCD represented over a period of 20 years, 3.3% of their cohort of patients operated for intractable epilepsy. By contrast, in 2017, the European Epilepsy Brain Bank consortium reported, 45 years later, the diagnoses made on the basis of resected brain specimens from over 9000 patients and obtained between 1990 and 2014 in 36 European centers (Blümcke *et al.*, 2017). Not surprisingly, adult's epilepsy patients requiring surgery (mean age at surgery, 28.1 yrs) had most commonly hippocampal sclerosis (44.5%). In children (mean age at surgery, 9.3 yrs), however, the most common histopathological diagnoses were the cortical malformations (39.3%) and FCD by far the most common, accounting for 70.6% of cases and FCD IIB (cortical dyslamination, dysmorphic neurons and balloon cells) representing almost half of them. The growing number of expert centers, advanced EEG recordings and new neuroimaging methods, and improved surgical approaches explain these findings. Neuroimaging plays an essential role in the diagnosis of MCD, and in the case of the FCD improved the *in vivo* recognition in an increasing number of patients (Bastos *et al.*, 1999; Bernasconi *et al.*, 2001; Besson *et al.*, 2008; Guerrini *et al.*, 2015; Severino *et al.*, 2020).

• Seeing the FCD

FCD are now more readily detected non-invasively with standard anatomical radiological approaches, and the additional use of quantitative MRI methods allows predicting the histological type with a greater accuracy (Adler *et al.*, 2017).

In the 1980s, MRI technology was still in its early development stages and routine clinical availability started in the mid 1980s – It is in 1985 that the Montreal Neurological Institute and Hospital (MNIH) acquired the first Canadian MRI scanner (a 0.5-Tesla scanner later replaced by a 1.5-Tesla machine). For our clinicians and researchers, it widely opened new fields of interest and particularly in the diagnosis and treatment of patients with intractable epilepsy. The opportunity was suddenly offered to literally "look" non-invasively the living brain and enabled to detect even subtle brain lesions known to be responsible for epileptic diseases (and as we will see with an increasing resolution). The very first original article from our institution using MR imaging showing structural changes suggestive of FCD was published in 1988 (Kuzniecky *et al.*, 1988). The series concerned only four subjects with motor seizures and rolandic epilepsy showing on MRI in 3 out of 4 "gross cortical architectonic abnormalities with localized macrogyria and high signal intensity lesion". Pathological material was eventually available in two of them with findings consistent with Taylor-type focal dysplasia of the cerebral cortex. This led to a great excitement and within few years resulted in the description and characterization of several types of MCD – including the FCD themselves and tuberous sclerosis, gray matter heterotopias and polymicrogyria. The MNIH contribution to the understanding of developmental malformations paralleled extraordinary efforts wide world, which during the following decade started to fill in the case of FCD, the gap left after Taylor and colleagues first description.

With the ongoing advances in neuroimaging, FCD is now relatively easier to identify, and improvements of MRI techniques such as high-field and ultra-high-field strength MRI (3 and 7 Tesla), the use of sophisticated post-processing methods and multimodal techniques facilitated not only their detection but also increased the ability of classifying subtypes of FCD, which help defining the epileptogenic zone (EZ) and ultimately guiding surgical decisions (Kim *et al.*, 2011; Duyn *et al.*, 2012; Opheim *et al.*, 2021). Other non-invasive methods, particularly functional imaging such as co-registered FDG-PET/MRI and EEG/fMRI proved to have high localizing value to detect the FCD and can be particularly helpful in the so-called MRI-negative patients (Chassoux *et al.*, 2010; Thornton *et al.*, 2011; Pittau *et al.*, 2017; Desarnaud *et al.*, 2018). EEG/fMRI also provides useful information on the complex relationship existing between the dysplastic tissue and the associated epileptogenic network, showing metabolic involvement of local and remote cortical and subcortical structures (Thornton *et al.*, 2011; Pittau *et al.*, 2017).

The diagnoses and classifications of the MCD, and FCD, are primarily based on neuropathological findings. However, the readily accessible data are based on MRI descriptions correlated with clinical features which include: patient's phenotypes, seizure and EEG characteristics in cases of associated epilepsy disorders, family history etc. To this classification scheme is now also attached genotypic and epigenetic or molecular characteristics, which on one hand should result in a better understanding of the mechanisms underlying the genesis and the impact of these lesions, but on the other hand, and at the same time, may add to the complex nature and heterogeneity of the MCD (Severino *et al.*, 2020) . Since neuroimaging represents the privilege avenue for FCD diagnosis and subtypes classification, high standardization and specificity of the imaging patterns are needed and should be readily accessible for clinical decision making; an issue particularly sensible in epilepsy patients with FCD, refractory seizures and poor associated developmental/cognitive outcomes (Jehi & Braun, 2021).

The neurophysiology of FCD refined the understanding of their epileptogenic mechanisms

• FCD are intrinsically and highly epileptogenic

FCD are more often associated with severe intractable epilepsy, seizures often start at a young age, and at a younger age compare to non-developmental lesions, and also even when compare to other MCD such as ganglioglioma and dysembryoplastic neuroepithelial tumor, polymicrogyria and gray matter heterotopia (Dubeau *et al.*, 1995; Leventer *et al.*, 2010; Blümcke *et al.*, 2017). Patients with FCD tend to have a large number of seizures, may be particularly prone to status epilepticus and show active epileptiform abnormalities (Desbiens *et al.*, 1993; Hirabayashi *et al.*, 1993; Kuzniecky *et al.* 1995; Tassi *et al.*, 2001). Palmini and colleagues (1995) and Gambardella and colleagues (1996) described an electrographic signature of FCD manifested by repetitive electrographic seizures or repetitive bursting discharges or continuous or quasi-continuous rhythmic spiking (Palmini *et al.*, 1995; Gambardella *et al.*, 1996). They reported the findings from per-operative electrocorticogram (ECoG) and scalp EEG recordings obtained from the same cohort of 34 patients investigated and operated at the MNIH for intractable epilepsy caused by FCD. This was the very first objective evidence that FCD seem to have a distinct electrophysiological behavior different compare to other epileptogenic brain lesions, and it was concluded that these changes reflected the highly epileptogenic nature of FCD. In addition, the rhythmic continuous discharges were found to be spatially restricted and co-localized with MRI-defined lesions, which led to the contention that dysplastic tissue could be intrinsically epileptogenic. In 2000, the group of Saint-Anne in Paris reviewed electrographic patterns in a series of 28 patients with FCD-proven histology studied by stereo-encephalography (SEEG) and, through these direct intralesional recordings, provided further evidence of the epileptogenicity of the dysplastic tissue (Chassoux *et al.*, 2000). As for the MNIH series, the majority of the patients had frontal and fronto-central FCD (16/28). The authors confirmed intra-lesional various patterns of rhythmic spiking activity: this activity was characterized by a continuous, rhythmic or pseudorhythmic spikes or polyspikes (20/26) or consisted of pseudoperiodic spikes or bursts of spikes briefly interrupted by depression or suppression of activity. They showed that the rhythmic activity co-localized in 86% of the cases with the FCD and the EZ (the site of subclinical ictal activity or onset clinical seizures) co-localized with the FCD in 82%. They also observed that FCD demonstrate a distinct and consistent low epileptogenic threshold, as suggested by low-frequency electrical stimulation of the dysplastic cortex. The group from Milan (Ospedale Niguarda and Istituto Carlo Besta), almost at the same time, published two articles reviewing a series of patients with FCD all operated on for drug-resistant focal epilepsy, and proposed a three-category classification of the FCD based on their neuropathological characteristics (Tassi *et al.*, 2002): The categories were identified as architectural dysplasia (AD, n = 31, dyslamination and ectopic neurons), cytoarchitectural dysplasia (CD, n = 6, dyslamination and giant neurons) and typical Taylor-type cortical dysplasia (TFCD, n = 15, dyslamination, dysmorphic neurons and balloon cells), precluding the future classification schemes of this group of MCD in FCD I (abnormal cortical layering or architectural abnormalities of the neocortex), and types II A-B (cytoarchitectural abnormalities of the neocortex) (Palmini *et al.*, 2004; Spreafico & Blümcke, 2010; Blümcke *et al.*, 2011; Najm *et al.*, 2018; Blümcke *et al.*, 2017). They described distinct clinical, EEG, imaging and surgical outcome: TFCD and CD were mostly extra-temporal, they were associated with a higher frequency of seizures but had a better surgical outcome compare to patients with AD. In addition, the lesion was found in the first group in the temporal lobe, and the distinctive rhythmic activity and signature previously described in FCD was seen only in the patients with TFCD. This Italian contribution was the basis of the Palmini classification of FCD, which was widely used in the first decade of this century (Palmini *et al.*, 2004).

• FCD are also network and signaling pathway disorders

FCD are localized regions of malformed cerebral cortex (Blümcke *et al.*, 2011). Although the epileptic activity appears co-localized with the visible MR lesion, the EZ often extends beyond this lesion involving other adjacent and even distant structures (Palmini *et al.* 1991; Palmini *et al.*, 1995; Chassoux *et al.*, 2000; Widdesh-Walsh *et al.*, 2007). This can be explained by the failure of neuroimaging, even when using sophisticated computational or post-processing methods, in showing the entire histological and epileptogenic abnormality (e.g. in FCD I). Another explanation could be related to the complex organizational nature of MCD (and FCD), and the finding of associated aberrant neuronal networks and signaling pathways described with them (Duchowny *et al.*, 2000; Jansky *et al.*, 2003; Crino 2015; Crino 2016; Lee *et al.*, 2022). These are important issues particularly in patients with drug-resistant epilepsies where a surgical approach is envisaged. Notwithstanding the fact that one should consider the region involved and whether or not eloquent cortex overlaps with the lesion and the EZ, the main question that always arises is how much tissue needs to be resected to achieve seizure-freedom; not only the lesion should be anatomically defined but the EZ organization and the functional involvement of the dysplastic tissue are essential components of an aberrant system that also need to be well characterized (Guerrini *et al.*, 2015). Several studies had demonstrated that complete resection of the lesion and EZ are essential, whenever feasible, to achieve a favorable seizure outcome (Palmini *et al.*, 1995; Chassoux *et al.*, 2000; Tassi *et al.*, 2002; Fauser *et al.*, 2004; Lerner *et al.*, 2009; *et al.*, 2009; Kim *et al.*, 2009).

We know that FCD may generate a characteristic electrophysiologic signature with combined features suggestive of an interictal-ictal continuum (Palmini *et al.*, 1995; Chassoux *et al.*, 2000; Tassi *et al.*, 2012). FCD are also associated with different intracerebral seizure-onset patterns (SOP). The group from Marseille identified six patterns in 53 patients explored by SEEG and distinguished two main patterns of activity: low voltage fast activity (LVFA preceded or not by paroxysmal potentials i.e. "pre-ictal" spiking or bursts of polyspikes or slow wave/DC shift) and slow rhythmic activity (rhythmic spikes or theta/alpha sharp activity). LVFA was recorded in 83% of the cases and seen in more than 90% of patients with FCD II vs ~65% of those with FCD I, while patterns with no LVFA (with slow rhythmic activity only) were essentially seen in FCD I (Lagarde *et al.*, 2016). More than one pattern can be generated by one type of FCD, and we had previously demonstrated that different types of developmental and non-developmental lesions can generate similar SOP suggesting that different pathological substrates can affect in the same way, and with a limited repertoire, mechanisms and networks underlying seizure expression (Perucca *et al.*, 2014). We also demonstrated however that specific high frequency oscillations (HFO) profiles suggest that seizures with different neurophysiological morphology likely have different mechanisms of generation: HFO (ripples and fast ripples, 80-500 Hz) are a specific biomarker of the seizure onset zone, and Ictal HFO density varied significantly across the different SOP. Interestingly, the highest HFO densities of both ripples and fast ripples were found in two SOP (bursts of polyspikes and delta brushes) known to be generated in FCD (Ferrari-Marinho *et al.*, 2016).

We have shown that FCD are intrinsically epileptogenic and able to generate distinctive epileptiform abnormalities. Several evidences also demonstrated that peri-lesional and distant cerebral structures are often engaged at seizure onset suggesting that FCD are part of a larger system or network organization. Aubert and colleagues (2009) using SEEG in a cohort of patients with FCD I and II (n = 30) and neurodevelopmental tumours (n = 6) analyzed the neurophysiological behavior of the lesion and several other adjacent (peri-lesional) and distant cortical areas at the time of seizure onset and early spread (Aubert *et al.*, 2009). They defined three different EZ organizations - focal, network or bilateral, based on the number of structures (lesional and non-lesional) able to demonstrate high epileptogenicity (they used the epileptogenicity index method as a relevant indicator of the epileptogenic nature of the recorded region or system (Bartolomei *et al.*, 2008)). The majority of the subjects had a network (61%) or bilateral (8%) EZ organization and only 31% had only one epileptogenic structure (with a strictly focal EZ). The great majority of those patients (87%) with a focal EZ organization became seizure-free after surgical resection (limits of resection where tailored for each patient based on SEEG findings) compared to 57% with a network organization and none with a bilateral organization. Although there were no significant statistical differences with regard to seizure outcome, there was a definite trend in favor of the focal organization group.

Understanding the molecular, synaptic and signaling pathways dysregulation of FCD: a significant step and further insights into their epileptogenesis

In the past decade, a better standardization of cortical development terminology and classification, important advances in molecular biology and genomics, and a better access to biological specimens have allowed a more precise exploration of the molecular and genetic disturbances of FCD. This included the effects of somatic and germline mutations, mutation load and mosaicism on the pathogenesis of FCD, resulting in a rapid identification of genes and signaling pathways and an unprecedented progress in our understanding of their perturbations.

FCD represents a neurodevelopmental disorder with specific histological features although its cause as well as the cellular mechanisms responsible for the profuse and aberrant intrinsic epileptogenicity observed in this cortical abnormality remain largely unclear. However, as detailed in chapter 4, although usually sporadic, FCD have been shown to be associated with diverse and specific molecular genetic abnormalities and sometimes there is a family pedigree (Sisodiya *et al.*, 2009). Furthermore, as nicely discussed in chapter 9, some of the mechanisms underlying the intrinsic epileptogenicity and exquisite drug resistance of FCD-related epilepsies are beginning to be unveiled.

These insights will help to understand the variable clinical presentation these patients may have, depending on histological type, brain location and size (Tassi *et al.*, 2002; 2001; 2012) – as well as why lesions can either be much localized and barely visible or restricted to one or two lobes or, alternatively, more diffuse and associated with structural and functional aberrations. Understanding such variation will be much helped by advances in imaging that now detects the dysplastic abnormality in most individuals (Severino *et al.*, 2020; Adler *et al.*, 2017). With a better definition of cortical development terminology and classification, important advances in molecular biology and genomics, and access to biological specimens the future is bright to the discovery of molecular and genetic disturbances that will result in an identification of genes and signaling pathways and to an unprecedented progress in our understanding of their perturbations (Sisodiya *et al.*, 2009; Barkovich *et al.*, 2012; Poduri *et al.*, 2013; Crino 2016; Adler *et al.*, 2017; Severino *et al.*, 2020; Lee *et al.*, 2022).

The causes of this highly epileptogenic lesion, most often leading to drug-resistant seizures (Palmini *et al.*, 1995; Gambardella *et al.*, 1996; Chassoux *et al.*, 2000) are probably numerous. They may be divided into genetic and acquired pathogenic mechanisms that play at different times in the pre- and post-natal brain, affecting cellular arrangement, plasticity and neuronal signaling. For instance, the association of a focal dysplastic cortex with epilepsy-prone lesions such as hippocampal sclerosis, neuro-glial tumors and vascular malformations or with acquired traumatic, hypoxic or infectious/inflammatory processes, suggests that a specific pathological entity, or an insult or a damage occurring at critical periods of the developing brain (ante-, peri- and postnatal) could result in histopathological changes and now classified as FCD III (Blümcke *et al.*, 2011; Crino 2015). On the other hand, FCD II can result from a genetic insult leading to dysregulation of the mTOR signaling pathway, sharing some similarities with the tuberous sclerosis complex (TSC) (Crino 2015; Crino 2016; Lee *et al.*, 2022). For instance, the relatively recent finding of pedigrees of familial focal epilepsy with FCD due to DEPDC5 mutations confirmed that this type of FCD is indeed associated with a dysregulation of the rapamycin (mTOR) signaling pathway thus including FCD II in the expanded group of disorders now referred as mTORopathies (Baulac *et al.*, 2015).

To date, several other genetic defects associated with dysregulations of the mTOR pathway have been described and apparently explain the majority of FCD cases (Lee *et al.*, 2022). Interestingly, for some time the dysmorphic neurons found in FCD II have been known to be the seizure generating cells (Cepeda *et al.*, 2005) and recent studies looking at dysplastic cells harboring mutations showed that the mutation load correlated with the electrophysiological phenotype: the density of dysplastic cells (dysmorphic neurons and balloon cells) is correlated with a high mutation and the highest load mutation is associated with the most active epileptiform abnormalities (Baldassari *et al.*, 2019; Lee, *et al.*, 2019). Hence, a localized high cell mutation load would explain the characteristic electrophysiological signature described in patients with intractable focal epilepsy due to FCD II. In contrast, regional differences with a low cell mutation load measured at the periphery or at distance from the main pathogenic area would possibly explain the inability for these regions to generate epileptic abnormalities. Similarly, one could hypothesize that an apparently identical FCD on neuroimaging found in an individual without seizures or epileptiform abnormalities, would have a relatively lower density of dysmorphic cells and a low mutation load in those cells.

In contrast to the advances in the understanding of FCD II, the current knowledge on FCD I, both in clinical and research domains, is far less robust. FCD I is a specific category with neocortical architectural disorganization without evidence of any other epileptogenic lesion – although often associated with drug-resistant epilepsy. Contrary to FCD II, it does not show the same distinctive and localizing neurophysiological and imaging markers. The lesion is often extensive or multilobar, and the cortical arrangement presenting mainly with abnormal cortical layering without major cellular and cytoarchitectural abnormalities explains the difficulties to recognize in vivo the dysplasia, even with sophisticated neuroimaging methods (Blümcke *et al.*, 2011). The paroxysmal EEG activity in FCD I is often widespread, and not focal, and does not have a signature, like in FCD II, allowing to differentiate this lesion from others. Finally, the pathogenic mechanisms responsible for this group of disorders are largely unknown although some evidence supports heterogeneity and a link with a variety of "acquired" insults occurring late during postmigrational development (Najm *et al.*, 2018; Coras *et al.*, 2021; Jesus-Ribeiro *et al.*, 2021). Also, no genetic mutation has been so far clearly associated with FCD I, and more investigations of the pathogenic mechanisms are clearly needed.

Questions that remain

The ability to stop seizures in patients with FCD and epilepsy resistant to drugs depends on the precision with which a given treatment, medical or surgical, can block or stop the dysregulated epileptogenic process generated by the dysplastic tissue i.e. "the seizure generating cells". In the past decades, in order to achieve this, the effort was to precisely target the region responsible for the seizures (with better and more precise neuroimaging methods and a better understanding of the neurophysiology of the lesion). We found that a well-designed surgical treatment strategy directly targeting the dysplastic tissue responsible for epileptogenesis and a precise determination and a complete removal of this epileptogenic lesion would lead to a satisfactory seizure outcome. Short and long term surgical outcomes for patients with focal epilepsy due to FCD are now relatively well established: in patients with FCD IIA and IIB the outcome is variable but can be satisfactory and even a fair number of those children and adult patients become seizure-free (Chassoux *et al.*, 2000, Tassi *et al.*, 2002; Fauser *et al.*, 2004; Lerner *et al.*, 2009; Krsek *et al.*, 2009; Kim *et al.*, 2009; Tassi *et al.*, 2012; Lamberick *et al.*, 2020). On the other hand, in patients with FCD I the outcome is typically more guarded in spite of the fact that the histological lesion would appear more «benign» (and does not contained high density of those dysmorphic cells and with higher mutation load that are believe to be the main contributors of epileptogenicity in FCD II) (Tassi *et al.*, 2002).

We know that conventional anti-seizure medications (ASM) that do not specifically target the pathogenic mechanisms associated with FCD, do not alter in a significant way the epilepsy process and, hence, clinical responses to ASM in patients with FCD are typically unsatisfactory (Fauser & Schulze-Bonhage 2006). More specific medical therapies targeting for instance the mTOR hyperactivation characteristic of the tuber and FCD II can reduce and maybe stop the epileptogenicity of these lesions (Crino 2016; Lee *et al.*, 2019; Lee *et al.*, 2022). Human data are so far only promising: partial results could be explained by the fact that these approaches at best can inhibit the pathological signalling system but do not remove, as surgery can do, the "seizure generating cells".

After Taylor and colleagues, a remarkable progress was made in our understanding and knowledge of FCD. We have improved the identification of the lesion, have better understanding of the mechanisms of epileptogenicity, and the diagnostic and therapeutic work up are more refined - resulting in a larger number of patients now readily candidates for more efficient treatments. Increasing accessibility to dysplastic tissue is providing new opportunities for research to directly study the cellular and synaptic mechanisms, and have already opened new windows to understand inhibition and activation of normal and pathologic neuronal systems. In spite of real progress, a large proportion of patients with FCD are treatment resistant. All these advanced methods and novel techniques aim to better define the epileptogenic tissue to be targeted, with the future hope that children and adults with FCD, and in a larger perspective with other MCD will benefit of innovative and improved therapies.

State of the art: what is this book about

In this book, all these issues are analysed in detail by most of the people who have produced the knowledge we have today. This introduction sets the stage for what the reader will get and describes the general aspects that have occupied the minds of clinicians and basic scientists dedicated to improve the lives of people with epilepsy due to FCD. If there is one aspect that links the issues raised in this introduction and that are tackled in the chapters that follow is that FCD is, by definition, an etiology of drug-resistant epilepsy. Thus, having FCD means having bad epilepsy and bad quality of life. The idea of curing these patients passes by the way these specialist-authors dwell deeply into the topics I have raised here, providing the state of the art of the knowledge about FCD. There could hardly be a better incentive for the new generations to get started on the field

This work is dedicated to Frederick Andermann, and to his pupils.

References

Adler S, Lorio S, Jacques TS, *et al.* Towards in vivo focal cortical dysplasia phenotyping using quantitative MRI. *Neuroimage* 2017; 15: 95-105.

Aubert S, Wendling F, Regis J, *et al.* Local and remote epileptogenicity in focal cortical dysplasias and neurodevelopmental tumors. *Brain* 2009; 132: 3072-86.

Baldassari S, Ribierre T, Marsan E, *et al.* Dissecting the genetic basis of focal cortical dysplasia: a large cohort study. *Acta Neuropathologica* 2019; 138: 885-900.

Barkovich AJ, Guerrini R, Kuzniecky RI, *et al.* A developmental and genetic classification for malformations of cortical development: update 2012. *Brain* 2012; 135: 1348-69.

Barkovich AJ, Kuzniecky RI, Jackson JD, *et al.* A developmental and genetic classification for malformations of cortical development. *Neurology* 2005; 65: 1873-87.

Bartolomei F, Chauvel P, Wendling F. Epileptogenicity of brain structures in human temporal lobe epilepsy: a quantified study from intracerebral EEG. *Brain* 2008; 158: 1818-30.

Bastos AC, Comeau RM, Andermann F, *et al.* Diagnosis of subtle focal focal dysplastic lesions: curvilineat reformatting from three-dimensional magnetic resonance imaging. *Ann Neurol* 1999; 46: 88-94.

Baulac I, Ishida S, Marsan E, *et al.* Familial focal epilepsy with focal cortical dysplasia due to DEPDC5 mutations. *Ann Neurol* 2015; 77: 675-83.

Bernasconi A, Antel SB, Collins DL, *et al.* Texture analysis and morphological processing of magnetic imaging assist detection of focal cortical dysplasia in extra-temporal partial epilepsy. *Ann Neurol* 2001; 49: 770-5.

Besson P, Andermann F, Dubeau F. *et al.* Small focal cortical dysplasia lesions are located at the bottom of a deep sulcus. *Brain* 2008; 131: 3246-55.

Blümcke I, Spreafico R, Haaker G, *et al.* Histopathological findings in brain tissue obtained during epilepsy surgery. *N Engl J Med* 2017; 377: 1648-56.

Blümcke I, Thom M, Aronica E, *et al.* The clinico-pathological spectrum of focal cortical dysplasias: a consensus classification proposed by an ad hoc task force of the ILAE diagnostic methods commission. *Epilepsia* 2011; 52: 158-74.

Cepeda C, Andre VM, Vinters HV, *et al.* Are cytomegalic neurons and balloon cells generators of epileptic activity in pediatric cortical dysplasia? *Epilepsia* 2005; 46(suppl. 5): 82-8.

Chassoux F, Devaux B, Landré E, *et al.* Stereoencephalography in focal cortical dysplasia. *Brain* 2000; 123: 1733-51.

Chassoux F, Rodrigo S, Semah F, *et al.* FDG-PET improves surgical outcome in negative MRI Taylor-type for cortical dysplasias. *Neurology* 2010; 75: 2168-75.

Coras R, Holthausen H, Sarnat HB. Focal cortical dysplasia type 1. *Brain Pathology* 2021; 31: el2964.

Crino PB. Focal cortical dysplasia. *Semin Neurol* 2015; 35: 201-8.

Crino PB. The mTOR signaling cascade: paving new roads to cure neurological disease. *Nature Review Neurology* 2016; 12: 379-93.

Desarnaud S, Mellerio C, Semah F, *et al.* 18F-FDG PET in drug-resistant epilepsy due to focal cortical dysplasia type 2: additional value of electroclinical data and coregistration with MRI. *Eur J Nucl Med Mol Imaging* 2018; 45: 1449-60.

Desbiens R, Berkovic SF, Dubeau F, *et al.* Life-threatening focal status epilepticus due to occult cortical dysplasia. *Arch Neurol* 1993; 50: 695-700.

Dubeau F, Tampieri D, Lee N, *et al.* Periventricular and subcortical nodular heterotopia. A study of 33 patients. *Brain* 1995; 118: 1273-87.

Duchowny M, Jayakar P, Levin B. Aberrant neural circuits in malformations of cortical development and focal epilepsy. *Neurology* 2000; 54: 423-8.

Duyn JH. The future of ultra-high field MRI and fMRI for study of human brain. *Neuroimage* 2012; 62: 1241-8.

Fauser S, Schulze-Bonhage A, Honegger J, *et al.* Focal cortical dysplasias: surgical outcome in 67 patients in relation to histological subtypes and dual pathology. *Brain* 2004; 127: 2406-18.

Fauser S, Schulze-Bonhage A. Epileptogenicity of cortical dysplasia in temporal lobe dual pathology: an elctrophysiological study with invasive recordings. *Brain* 2006; 129: 82-95.

Ferrari-Marinho T, Perucca P, Dubeau F, *et al.* Intracranial EEG seizure onset-patterns correlate with high-frequency oscillations in patients with drug-

Gambardella A, Palmini A, Andermann F, *et al.* Usefulness of focal rhythmic discharges on scalp EEG of patients with focal cortical dysplasia and intractable epilepsy. *Electroencephalogr Clin Neurophysiol* 1996; 98: 243-9.

Guerrini R, Duchowny M, Jayakar P, *et al.* Diagnostic method and treatment options for focal cortical dysplasia. *Epilepsia* 2015; 56: 1669-86.

Hirabayashi S, Binnie CD, Janota I, *et al.* Surgical treatment of epilepsy due to cortical dysplasia: clinical and EEG findings. *J Neurol Neurosurg Psychiatry* 1993; 56: 765-70.

Jansky J, Ebner A, Kruse b, *et al.* Functional organization of the brain with malformations of cortical development. *Ann Neurol* 2003; 53: 759-67.

Jehi L, Braun K. Does etiology really matter for epilepsy surgery outcome? *Brain Pathology* 2021; 31: el2965.

Jesus-Ribeiro J, Pires LM, Melo JD, *et al.* Genomics and epigenetic advances in focal cortical dysplasia types I and II: a scoping review. *Frontiers in Neuroscience* 2021; 14: 580357.

Kim DW, Lee SK, Chu K, *et al.* Predictors of surgical outcome and pathologic considerations in focal cortical dysplasia. *Neurology* 2009; 72: 211-6.

Kim YH, Kang HC, Kim DS, *et al.* Neuroimaging in identifying focal cortical dysplasia and prognostic factors in pediatric and adolescent epilepsy surgery. *Epilepsia* 2011; 52: 722-7.

Kobow K, Baulac S, von Deimling A, Lee JH. Molecular diagnostics in drug-resistant focal epilepsy define new disease entities. *Brain Pathology* 2021; 31: 1-9.

Krsek P, Maton B, Jayakar P, *et al.* Incomplete resection of focal cortical dysplasia is the main predictor of poor surgical outcome. *Neurology* 2009; 72: 217-23.

Kuzniecky R, Berkovic S, Andermann F, *et al.* Focal cortical myoclonus and rolandic cortical dysplasia: clarification by magnetic resonance imaging. *Ann Neurol* 1988; 23: 317-25.

Kuzniecky R, Morawetz R, Faught E, *et al.* Frontal and central lobe focal dysplasia: clinical, EEG and imaging features. *Dev Med Child Neurol* 1995; 37: 159-66.

Lagarde S, Bonini F, McGonigal A, *et al.* Seizure-onset patterns in focal cortical dysplasia and neurodevelopmental tumors: Relationship with surgical prognosis and neuropathologic subtypes. *Epilepsia* 2016; 57: 1426-35.

Lamberick HJ, Otte WM, Blümcke I, *et al.* Seizure outcome and use of antiepileptic drugs after epilepsy surgery according to histopathological diagnosis: a retrospective multicenter cohort study. *Lancet Neurol* 2020; 19: 748-57.

Lee WS, Baldassari S, Stephenson SEM, *et al.* Cortical dysplasia and the mTOR pathway: How the study of human brain tissue has led to insights into epileptogenesis. *Int J Mol Sci* 2022; 23: 1344.

Lee WS, Stephenson SEM, Howell KB, *et al.* Second-hit DEPDC5 mutation is limited to dysmorphic neurons in cortical dysplasia type IIA. *Ann Clin Transl Neurol* 2019; 6: 1338-44.

Lerner JT, Salamon N, Hauptman JS, *et al.* Assessment and surgical outcome for mild type 1 and severe type II cortical dysplasia. *Epilepsia* 2009; 50: 1310-35.

Leventer RJ, Jansen A, Pilz DT, *et al.* Clinical and imaging heterogeneity of polymicrogyria: a study of 328 patients. *Brain* 2010; 133: 1415–27.

Mischel PS, Nguyen LP, Vinters HV. Cerebral cortical dysplasia associated with pediatric epilepsy. Review of neuropathologic features and proposal of a grading system. *J Neuropathol Exp Neurol* 1995; 54: 137-53.

Najm I, Sarnat HB, Blümcke I. Review: the international consensus classification of focal cortical dysplasia – a critical update. *Neuropathology and Applied Neurobiology* 2018; 44: 18-31.

Opheim G, van der Kolk A, Bloch KM, *et al.* 7T epilepsy task force consensus recommendations on the use of 7T MRI in clinical practice. *Neurology* 2021; 96: 327-41.

Palmini A, Andermann F, Olivier A, *et al.* Focal neuronal migration disorders and intractable epilepsy: A study of 30 patients. *Ann Neurol* 1991; 30: 741-9.

Palmini A, Gambardella A, Andermann F, *et al.* Intrinsic epileptogenicity of human dysplastic cortex as suggested by corticography and surgical results. *Ann Neurol* 1995; 37: 476-87.

Palmini A, Najm I, Avanzini G, *et al.* Terminology and classification of the cortical dysplasias. *Neurology* 2004; 62(suppl. 3): S2-S8.

Perucca P, Dubeau F, Gotman J. Intracranial electroencephalographic seizure-onset patterns: effect of underlying pathology. *Brain* 2014; 137: 183-96.

Pittau F, Ferri L, Fahoum F, *et al.* Contributions of EEG/fMRI to assessing the epileptogenicity of focal cortical dysplasia. *Front Comput Neurosci* 2017; 11: 1-16.

Poduri A, Evrony GD, Cai X, Walsh CA. Somatic mutation, genomic variation and neurologic disease. *Science* 2013; 341: 43.

Severino M, Geraldo AF, Utz N, *et al.* Definitions and classification of malformations of cortical development: practical guidelines. *Brain* 2020; 143: 2874-94.

Sisodiya S, Fauser S, Cross JH, Thom M. Focal cortical dysplasia type II: biological features and clinical perspectives. *Lancet* 2009; 8: 830-43.

Spreafico R, Blümcke I. Focal cortical dysplasia: clinical implication of neuropathological classification system. *Acta Neuropathol* 2010; 120: 359-67.

Tassi L, Colombo N, Garbelli R, *et al.* Focal cortical dysplasia: neuropathological subtypes, EEG, neuroimaging and surgical outcome. *Brain* 2002; 125: 1719-32.

Tassi L, Garbelli R, Colombo N, *et al.* Electroclinical, MRI and surgical outcomes in 100 patients with type II FCD. *Epileptic Disord* 2012; 14: 257-266.

Tassi L, Garbelli R, Colombo N, *et al.* Type I focal cortical dysplasia: surgical outcome is related to histopathology. *Epileptic Disors* 2010; 12: 181-91.

Tassi L, Pasquier B, Minotti L. *et al.* Cortical dysplasia: electroclinical, imaging and neuropathologic study of 13 patients. *Epilepsia* 2001; 42: 112-1123.

Taylor DC, Falconer MA, Bruton CJ, Corsellis JAN. Focal dysplasia of the cerebral cortex in epilepsy. *J Neurol Neurosurg Psychiat* 1971; 34: 369-87.

Thornton R, Vulliemoz S, Rodionov R, *et al.* Epileptic networks in focal cortical dysplasia revealed using electroencephalography-functional magnetic resonance imaging. *Ann Neurol* 2011; 70: 822-37.

Widdesh-Walsh P, Jehi L, Nair D, *et al.* Subdural electrode analysis in focal cortical dysplasia. *Neurology* 2007; 69: 660-7.

CHAPTER

2. Classifications for FCD: evolution of concepts and current knowledge

Andre Palmini

Keypoints

- The clinical and experimental neuroscientific communities have been following in 'real time' the developments about the role of malformations of cortical development in severe epilepsies.
- From the broad scaffolding of neuronal migration disorders, the field moved toward a refined understanding of the MCD and singled out focal cortical dysplasia as the most frequently related to surgically remediable drug resistant epilepsy.
- The fact that histological abnormalities in FCD can variably involve cellular abnormalities, disruption of the laminar architecture or both has led to several attempts at classification in subtypes with meaningful clinical relevance.
- These classifications are an ongoing effort, progressively aided by advances in imaging, histopathology and molecular genetics, and may lead to better defined clinical entities

Introduction

MCD and, particularly, FCD, evolved from a poorly defined group of entities to a central role in epileptology. This exponential relevance has been catapulted by imaging, but backed by strikingly neurophysiological signatures and careful analyses of the underlying pathology.

Pari passu with the growing interest in FCD is the need to understand the nosological boundaries of these entities, ie, what is truly a dysplastic abnormality. Such considerations obviously do not apply to very well characterized Taylor-type FCD (FCD II), but do interest the field in what concerns the intricacies of dyslamination. In other words, what exactly it means to have a dyslaminated cortex in terms of epileptogenicity and pathogenesis continues to be a key issue, as much as this relates to the intimacy of the organization of cortical architecture, the disruption of which could have a variety of causes.

This chapter revisits the journey from the first reports to the current nosological understanding of FCD, focusing on the features that have been used to subclassify these lesions. By reviewing the main steps along the way, points that need clarification by further research are highlighted, with the hope to eventually reach a thorough understanding of the origin and the best ways to manage the epilepsy associated with these lesions.

Knowledge in the making

It is interesting to follow the evolution of knowledge. The exciting journey of charting unexplored territories and witness progress in the making is quite distinct from simply learning and accepting 'what is there'. Such has been the privilege of clinical and surgical epileptologists, imaging specialists and pathologists involved with the field of FCD over the last 3 decades. Developments followed an impressive accumulation of experience and technology and the pace of exchanges between specialists. Since the original description of Taylor and collaborators (Taylor *et al.*, 1971), the field went from an all-encompassing nomenclature (Palmini *et al.*, 1991) to very specific terminologies related to imaging-molecular diagnostic entities, which can inform timing and type of management (Palmini *et al.*, 2004; Blümcke *et al.*, 2011; Barkovich *et al.*, 2012; Harvey *et al.*, 2015; Holthausen *et al.*, 2022; Najm *et al.*,

2022, in press). Despite significant progress, the challenges ahead are significant, as would inevitably be with gaps in knowledge regarding what has become the most frequent etiology of drug resistant focal epilepsies. This chapter will point out the nosological journey so far and raise points that should be further studied as part of the rewarding process of eventually provide a cure for these epilepsies.

If one is to be faithful to the evolution of concepts regarding FCD, it is important to begin by analyzing a curious centripetal embryological-pathological perspective (**Figure 1**). In the beginning of the 'modern era', marked by the advent of magnetic resonance imaging (MRI), there was a concept that all malformations of the cerebral cortex could be subsumed under the 'umbrella mechanism' of abnormal neuroblast and glial migration to the cortex early in the embryonic period, leading to the terminology "neuronal migration disorders" (NMD) (Palmini *et al.*, 1991). That was the time of the seminal studies of Rakic on the formation of cerebral cortex, crystallized in the famous picture of neuroblasts migrating radially outward from the periventricular germinal matrix (Rakic 1988a, 1988b). Thus, at that time, malformations of the development of the cortex were virtually synonymous with disorders of neuronal migration.

Then the field moved ahead in a centripetal fashion – ie, from less to more precise conceptual terminology - through the realization that MRI and histopathology, once correlated, should be able to refine the pathophysiology of malformations and break down the umbrella term NMD into distinct mechanisms of interference with cortical development that went beyond neuronal migration. Through the careful work of a group of imaging specialists and epileptologists (Barkovich *et al.*, 1996), several anatomic subtypes of malformations were described, representing distinct mechanisms of interference with the formation of cerebral cortex. This led to the abandonment of the term NMD in favor of the more precise terminology MCD, highlighting the stages during the complex process of cortical development upon which pathological interferences could impact:

- neuronal–glial proliferation and differentiation,
- neuronal migration to the cortical plate (the 'true' NMD),
- the final stages of intracortical organization.

These distinct processes led to different types of MCD identifiable by MRI, which display variable degrees of epileptogenicity and, as later shown, have specific molecular etiologies.

To the crucial benefit of epileptology, the concept and recognition of different types of MCD helped reconcile the broad field of cortical malformations with the classical description of Taylor and colleagues of FCD as a surgical entity. After all, FCD were classically described based upon histopathological analysis of surgical tissue and, understandably, it was not very easy to conceive a small FCD as the same disorder, for instance, as diffuse pachygyria – although, both were initially 'grouped' as NMD (Palmini *et al.*, 1991b). Thus, breaking down the mechanisms of malformations allowed the conceptualization of FCD as one type of MCD, related mostly to abnormal proliferation and differentiation of neuroblasts and glia, with a component of impaired neuronal positioning within the cortical plate (Barkovich *et al.*, 2012).

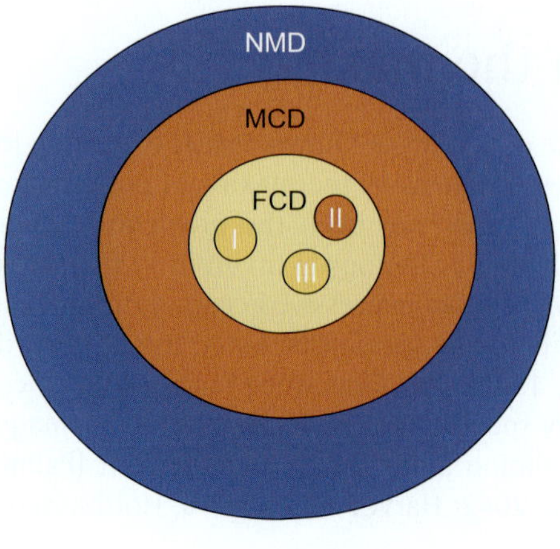

Figure 1

Evolution of concepts leasing to the understanding and current classification of FCD. NMD: neuronal migration disorders; MCD: malformation of cortical develeopment; FCD: focal cortical dysplasias.

This step has been of outstanding relevance for people with epilepsy because, even though *as a group* MCD are a major etiology of difficult-to-treat epilepsies, the specific type of MCD known as FCD is responsible for most surgically treatable epilepsies in patients with MCD.

FCD: Two intersecting axes to conceptualize, classify and make surgical decisions

From this point, two main axes have developed: one aimed at disentangling, understanding and classifying the main histologic features of FCD and the other concerning the relevance of distinct histopathological features to epileptiform abnormalities and seizure generation (**Figure 2**). The histological axis correlates the cellular intimacy of the FCD with clinical, imaging and fast developing genetic aspects, whereas the relation between histopathology and seizure generation should be key to inform surgical strategies.

• Axis 1. The histological axis: main histopathological features and the classification(s) of FCD

Histopathological features

Since the classical description of Taylor and colleagues, it has been a 'pathological imperative' to integrate three main histopathological features, variably seen in FCD lesions: *intracortical architectural changes* with loss of the usual laminated patter, *dysmorphic or dysplastic neurons and balloon cells*. Histopathological details, particularly the increasing role of immunohistochemistry and genetic markers will be covered in the chapter by I. Blümcke. Here, I will concentrate on the role played by each of these main features and related abnormalities in the classification of FCD.

The spectrum of dyslamination: from complete disorganization to milder forms of architectural changes in the pattern of cortical layering

The abnormal distribution of neurons in the six-layered cortex known as *dyslamination*, currently thought as a universal feature in FCD, is currently a key part of the debate on the best way to classify (and diagnose) these lesions (Najm *et al.*, 2018). The debate is particularly kindled by the fact that:

- the label 'dyslamination' accommodates several distinct abnormalities of cortical architecture;
- it is not clear whether dyslaminated cortex is itself epileptogenic (or always epileptogenic), particularly in connection with the distinct mechanisms that eventually lead to abnormal cortical lamination.

In the classical description of FCD, dyslamination referred to a 'haphazard', very disorganized distribution of neurons in such a way that a laminar pattern could not be discerned (Taylor *et al.*, 1971). Importantly, that pattern is seen in conjunction with dysplastic neurons and balloon cells, comprising the classical histopathology of 'Taylor-type' FCD – currently known as FCD II (see below). However, when these neuroglial cytological abnormalities are absent, several distinct dyslaminated patterns have been described, including the persistence of a striking columnar neuronal distribution, abnormal tangential laminations and reduced neuronal

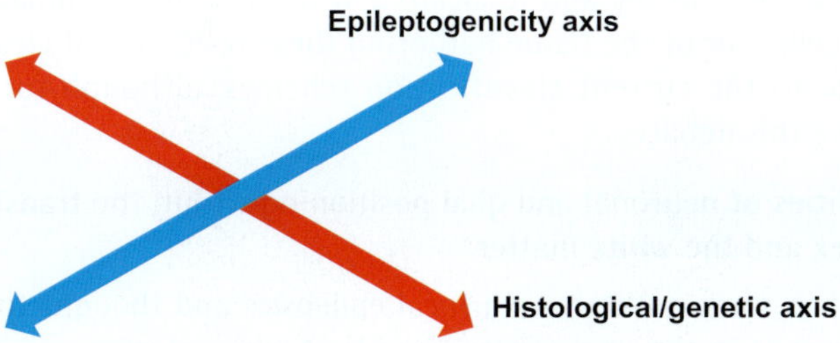

Figure 2
Intersecting axes to conceptualise and classify the FCD

population in specific cortical layers (Blümcke *et al.*, 2011). Some dyslaminated patterns are seen in isolation (Tassi *et al.*, 2010; Holthausen et al 2022) whereas others co-occur with non-dysplastic pathologies, such as hippocampal sclerosis, developmental tumors and gliosis (Blümcke *et al.*, 2011). However, several considerations should be made to contextualize the issue of dyslamination and its relevance in the classification of FCD. First, when formally studied, there has been only moderate interobserver agreement as to the presence of dyslamination in histological specimens (Chamberlain *et al.*, 2009). Then, experience with intracerebral recordings show that dyslamination can be found in portions of corticectomies that are included in resections but are not epileptogenic. Moreover, there is also the possibility that poorly oriented specimens sent to pathologists combined with neuronal loss may overestimate the occurrence of dyslamination. Because lesions such as hippocampal sclerosis or developmental tumours associated with dyslamination are in themselves epileptogenic and could secondarily lead to cortical architectural reorganization, the true dysplastic nature and intrinsic epileptogenicity of such associated dyslamination patterns is still debatable (Najm *et al.*, 2018; Najm *et al.*, submitted). Furthermore, in contrast to the amazing refinement of molecular genetics of FCD II, there are no unequivocal genetic markers for FCD solely characterized by dyslamination. Therefore, one should be cautious when discussing FCD only based on dyslamination and be opened to the possibility that classifications may have a whole different direction according to future research findings.

Cytological hallmarks of what Taylor and colleagues described as FCD

The FCD-defining abnormality from the classical perspective of Taylor and colleagues is the presence of 'dysplastic or dysmorphic neurons', described as large, dysmorphic cells, easily contrasted from normal neurons not only by their enlarged cell body and displacement of the nucleus, but also because they lack the usual orientation and are scattered throughout the abnormal cortex (Taylor *et al.*, 1971; Palmini *et al.*, 2004; Blümcke *et al.*, 2011). Their presence is associated with the haphazard intracortical distribution of neurons in a way that it is difficult to discern any layering when these dysmorphic cells are seen (see above). Additionally, some patients with FCD also have grossly abnormal ballooned cellular elements, closely related to the giant cells of tuberous sclerosis, known as 'balloon cells'. These are very immature cells, as suggested by the pattern of immunohistochemistry staining. Before the formal description of FCD, patients with these lesions were known as displaying a 'form fruste of tuberous sclerosis' (Perot *et al.*, 1966), exactly because of these ballooned cells. Impressively, almost 6 decades later, advanced molecular techniques are showing striking genetic similarities between FCD with balloon cells and tuberous sclerosis, through abnormalities in the mTOR complex pathway (Baldassari *et al.*, 2019). This is explained in detail elsewhere in this volume, in the very nice chapter by Baldassari and Baulac (chapter 4). As well described (Blümcke *et al.*, 2011), balloon cells can occur at any cortical location within the dysplastic lesion, are often found in the underlying white matter and can even be associated with MRI-negative brain tissue.

Importantly, there is still a borderzone regarding neurons that are not truly dysmorphic (dysplastic) neither on hematoxylin nor in immunohistochemical staining yet are larger than usual neurons and poorly oriented. Both in the 'Palmini classification scheme' and the ILAE consensus led by Blümcke (Palmini *et al.*, 2004; Blümcke *et al.*, 2011), these are described as immature neurons and associated with abnormal lamination. The epileptogenicity of these cells – or of the tissue harboring these cells - is not clear and they are not considered central to the current classification schemes, although further research may eventually rekindle this debate.

Related abnormalities of neuronal and glial positioning within the transition between the cortex and the white matter

A distinct element in some patients with focal epilepsies and thought to be related to FCD is an excess of neurons in the immediate subcortical white matter, accompanied or not by an excess of oligodendroglial cells, identified by immunohistochemistry. When these are the only histological abnormalities, they have been named mMCD (mild malformation of cortical development). The term 'dysplasia' has not been directly applied to these lesions as they lack both cortical dyslamination and cytological abnormalities. More recently, the recognition of the prominent epileptogenic role of these lesions when an excess of oligodendroglial cells is seen led to the description of a specific subtype of mMCD – mild malformation of cortical development with oligodendroglial hyperplasia in epilepsy (MOGHE) – which in a way revitalized the clinical relevance of the 'concept of mMCD' (Hartlieb et al 2019; Seetharam *et al.*, 2021, Mendes-Coelho *et al.*, 2021). Histologically, however, it is important to separate MOGHE from other situations in which there is an excess of neurons scattered in the subcortical white matter possibly related to a plethora of mechanisms, such as Zellweger and Dravet syndrome (Kaufmann *et al.*, 1986; Hayashi *et al.*, 2004). This note of caution is important to truly confine the term FCD or even 'dysplasia' to scenarios in which abnormalities of the formation of the cerebral cortex is the primary event – not an epiphenomenon of other molecular, metabolic or structural lesions that may secondarily affect the architecture of the cortex and the persistence of neurons in the white matter.

The classifications

During the 90's, examination of dysplastic lesions resected during epilepsy surgery showed several distinct combinations of histopathological abnormalities. Some lesions displayed only dyslamination, others had abnormal cortical layering associated with dysmorphic/cytomegalic neurons and still others had, in addition, balloon cells as a prominent feature. This realization was even more important because it had a clinical counterpart in that the distinct histopathological patterns had distinguishable epileptogenic features, from age of seizure onset and severity of the epilepsy to lesion location, pattern of electrophysiological abnormalities and imaging findings (Palmini *et al.*, 1995; Gambardella *et al.*, 1996, Krsek *et al.*, 2008; Lerner *et al.*, 2009). This made it clear that a classification *specific to FCD* (and certainly beyond the broader concept of MCD) was imperative.

Classifications, like concepts, are akin to geysers. Data, experience and insights from different people combine and progressively reach a boiling point, when they eventually surface. Not unlike the original description of FCD, in which the paper was led by a psychiatrist interested in the behavioral abnormalities of patients operated for intractable seizures, thus interacting with neuropathologists toward understanding what was happening in the brain (Taylor *et al.*, 1971), the first specific FCD classification (Tassi *et al.*, 2002; Palmini *et al.*, 2004) was also organized by clinicians who felt the pressing need to bridge the epileptological peculiarities of FCD with specific cellular and architectonic abnormalities. This effort surfaced mostly based on two sets of realizations that:

- there could be lesions with or without the dysmorphic neurons and balloon cells described originally by Taylor and colleagues, provided it could be accepted that architectural abnormalities in terms of cortical layering (ie, dyslamination) in itself did represent a form of FCD;
- dysplastic lesions with gross cellular abnormalities always had dysmorphic neurons, but could or could not have balloon cells.

This led to the "Palmini classification scheme" following a consensus reached in Cleveland and published in 2004: thus, type I FCD (FCD I) was characterized by cortical dyslamination without cytomegalic, dysplastic neurons, although absence or presence of hypertrophic yet not dysplastic neurons subclassified FCD I into FCD IA and FCD IB. On the other hand, type II FCD (FCD II) featured both abnormal architecture and dysplastic (dysmorphic, cytomegalic) neurons. The additional presence of balloon cells subclassified FCD II into FCD IIA (dysmorphic neurons without balloon cells) and FCD IIB (dysmorphic neurons combined with balloon cells). That scheme was widely used (Fauser *et al.*, 2004; Krsek *et al.*, 2008; Lerner *et al.*, 2009; Sisodiya *et al.*, 2009) and walked hand in hand with the explosion of publications on FCD during the subsequent years, fueled by better imaging and the progressive realization that it represented perhaps the most frequent pathology underlying refractory focal epilepsies. Such heightened interest in FCD also led to more detailed scrutiny of the histological abnormalities, including the application of immunohistochemistry to further understand the intimacy of these lesions and clarify, for instance, the distinction between large, immature, yet not dysplastic neurons (FCD IB) from truly cytomegalic, dysmorphic neurons defining FCD IIA. This coincided in time with the realization that distinct types of structural lesions – in themselves 'epileptogenic lesions' – could be further associated with cortical dyslamination (Tassi *et al.*, 2010).

Further detailing of histology and valuation of the cortical 'dyslamination' associated with distinct structural lesions – from hippocampal sclerosis to gliotic scars – led to another classification, this time with the input of a much larger group of clinicians, imaging specialists and, above all, pathologists (Blümcke *et al.*, 2011; Palmini, 2011). Details on this new, ILAE-endorsed, classification and a most recent 2022 update are given by Blümcke (chapter 3). Here, I just signal the main changes from the 'Palmini scheme':

- the subdivision of FCD I into three, instead of two subtypes (IA, IB, IC; according to the orientation of the dyslamination: radial, tangential or both;
- large, immature neurons were no longer the defining feature of FCD IB, which is now defined as tangential dyslamination;
- the addition of a third group, FCD III, combining dyslamination with other epileptogenic lesions, specifically hippocampal sclerosis (IIIA), tumors (IIIB), vascular malformations (IIIC), or gliotic scars (IIID).

At the time, the major reason behind creating a FCD III category was that FCD (or, at least, dyslamination) associated with these other lesions could prove pathogenically (and/or epileptogenically) distinct from the isolated types, and thus treatment approaches could be more specific. The other main goal of attempting to amend the initial classification was to open new avenues of research, including the putative addition of molecular genetics into the picture – always with a view to streamline diagnosis and aid therapeutic decisions. Importantly, this new classification somewhat downplayed the potential role of hypertrophic but not cytomegalic cells and immature pyramidal neurons in the epileptogenicity of these lesions. In other words, the hallmark histological characteristics defining FCD IB, based upon the presence of hypertrophic neurons in the 'Palmini classification scheme', were changed in the ILAE classification to a tangential dyslamination of the cortex, irrespective of the presence or not of those neurons. As suggested by recent evidence, reviewed by Cepeda and colleagues in this volume (chapter 9), immature pyramidal neurons may play a role in the epileptogenicity of dysplastic cortex, raising doubts of whether they should be left out of a more prominent role in the histological classification of these lesions. A decade onward from that revision, there is lively debate on the validity of some of the new 'FCD subtypes' proposed. On the other hand, genetics have clearly entered the picture, which has prompted an update and a critical reassessment of the subtypes added in the 2011 classification (Najm *et al.*, 2018; Najm *et al.*, in press).

• Axis 2. The epileptogenicity axis: relevance of distinct types of FCD to epileptiform abnormalities and seizure generation

Before FCD were thoroughly individualized from the larger group of MCD, several studies highlighted the fact that drug resistant epilepsy was much more common in relation to FCD than with other types of malformations, such as nodular heterotopia and polymicrogyria. Since the publication of 'Palmini classification scheme' a somewhat similar principle began to be applied to the distinct subtypes of FCD both prospectively and in retrospect (Palmini *et al.*, 1995; Chassoux *et al.*, 2000; Tassi *et al.*, 2002) – this time, however, in relation to mechanisms of epileptogenicity, neurophysiological features, imaging characteristics, lesion extent and surgical outcome. Many chapters in this book dwell on these specific scenarios and here I will just raise the issue, citing some seminal publications that paved the way to a plethora of others in the last decade.

Undoubtedly, a number of publications showed that different types of FCD have distinct clinical-epileptologic phenotypes, as well as lesion localization, extent, and distinction from surrounding cortex on MRI (Chassoux *et al.*, 2000; Tassi *et al.*, 2002; Sisodiya *et al.*, 2009). Some lesions have increased cortical thickness, blurring of gray-white transition, and abnormal signal (Barkovich *et al.*, 1997; Urbach *et al.*, 2002; Columbo *et al.*, 2012; Mellerio *et al.*,

2012). Others have less compelling features and may present only with shrinkage of the subcortical white matter or lie hidden within atrophic, partly destructive lesions, as detailed in the chapter by Mellerio in this volume (**chapter 16**). Similar differences are often detected on neurophysiologic evaluations, particularly the occurrence of exquisitely epileptiform patterns upon direct recording of some types of FCD, particularly FCD II (Palmini *et al.*, 1995; Chassoux *et al.*, 2000). Furthermore, clinical-histological-imaging intersections have been key to fuel the debate on the subtypes of FCD I (Tassi *et al.*, 2010; Holthausen *et al.*, 2022), to allow the characterization of a new dysplastic entity (MOGHE; Mendes-Coelho *et al.*, 2021) and to consistently bring molecular genetics into the picture (Baulac *et al.*, 2019; Blumcke *et al.*, 2021a).

Since the publication of the ILAE classification in 2011, which replaced the previous scheme and added several FCD subtypes, it has been a major endeavor to advance and refine the application of clinical-histological-imaging intersections to the many proposed subtypes (Blumcke *et al.*, 2021b, Najm *et al.*, 2018; Najm *et al.*, submitted). In particular, there is a significant issue with the objective identification of FCD I and III, even by experienced neuropathologists. As shown by studies probing inter-observer agreement, there is a wide disparity between the reliability of a diagnosis of FCD II – agreed by the vast majority of neuropathologists – and that of FCD I and III, agreed upon by a minority of specialists. This has been well shown by the most comprehensive and carefully conducted study to date with 'la crème de la crème'of epilepsy neuropathologists that further highlights the difficult issues of understanding the true dysplastic nature of many cases currently classified as FCD I/III (Blümcke *et al.*, 2021c).

This suggests that more work on the spectrum of dyslamination is needed – hopefully aided by molecular genetic studies - before firm conclusions can be drawn upon subtyping FCD I/III on the basis of cortical architectural abnormalities. As repeatedly discussed (Palmini, 2011; Najm *et al.*, 2018; Najm *et al.*, in press), this will be crucial to firmly establish FCD subtypes as relevant entities – or abandon those that prove irrelevant form a clinical, imaging, genetic and decision-making standpoints.

Challenges connected to current knowledge: from the solidly established Taylor-type (FCD II) to the struggle with the non-Taylor-type FCD

This long journey through the evolution of concepts, nomenclature and classifications have reached the point when it is clearer what the 'unclear issues' are. FCD II (Taylor-type) has beautifully stood the test of time and these 30 years have both witnessed and produced a host of confirmatory data on the uniqueness of this entity, which is easy to identify by histology ("once seen, never forgotten"), has well defined clinical, electrical, and imaging features, and excellent surgical outcome when the lesion can be fully resected. On the other hand, progress on imaging, immunohistochemistry, genetics and clinical observations raises inevitable challenges on the validity of FCD I and FCD III as truly representing dysplastic abnormalities, and hence considered epileptogenic lesions in themselves. The most relevant points are addressed in several chapters of this book by experienced authors, combining data with personal views. One important point discussed from distinct perspectives by Blümcke, Tassi and Holthausen (chapters 3, 7, 8) is which patterns of dyslamination truly represent dysplastic abnormalities and hence would be considered epileptogenic lesions in themselves. This applies, for instance, to FCD I, variably associated with very distinct scenarios such as reduced anterior temporal lobe volume in patients with focal seizures and normal cognition (Palmini *et al.*, 2004; Tassi *et al.*, 2010) and to children with very severe epilepsies and progressive deterioration associated with subtle but extensive MRI abnormalities (Holthausen *et al.*, 2022). Whether this large spectrum could be accounted for solely by the type of dyslamination or to something else entirely is the big issue here.

The other point is the sheer validity of type III FCD, i.e., whether abnormal dyslamination associated with diverse 'primarily' epileptogenic lesions (hippocampal sclerosis (HS), developmental tumors, vascular malformations and gliotic scars from early insults (Blümcke *et al.*, 2011) represent true malformations or could be due secondary tissue changes associated with the principal lesion and recurrent seizures. Indeed, it is interesting to observe how the FCD I/III puzzle relates to clinical observations. If one focus on temporal lobe epilepsy surgery, large consecutive series in which patients underwent anterior temporal lobectomy including the neocortex and the mesial structures described at least four scenarios, based upon the presence (or not) of HS and neocortical dyslamination (Tassi *et al.*, 2009; Tassi *et al.*, 2010; Mulhofer *et al.*, 2017):

- those with HS who:
  - had associated neocortical dyslamination (ie, FCD IIIA)
  - or did not have dyslamination ('pure HS');
- and those without HS who
  - had dyslamination (ie, FCD I) or
  - did not have neocortical dyslamination (no HS, no FCD).

Interestingly, surgical outcome in consecutive series of patients with HS undergoing selective amygdalo-hippocampectomy (ie, without removing, and thus without examining the histology of the temporal cortex) is the same or even better than anterior temporal lobectomy (Clussman *et al.*, 2002; Paglioli *et al.*, 2004; Schramm, 2008; Hemb *et al.*, 2013). This observation challenges the epileptological relevance of temporal neocortical dyslamination – alone or associated with other lesions, particularly HS. Perhaps this and other examples will keep kindling the debate on whether all that is currently considered as FCD – and thus included in a classification – should continue to be encompassed as a single pathology/denomination or could eventually come up as distinct entities.

References

Baldassari S, Ribierre T, Marsan E, *et al.* Dissecting the genetic basis of Focal Cortical Dysplasia: a large cohort study. *Acta Neuropathol.* 2019; 138: 885-900.

Barkovich AJ, Kuzniecky RI, Dobyns WB, Jackson GD, Becker LE, Evrard P. A classification scheme for malformations of cortical development. *Neuropediatrics.* 1996; 27: 59-63.

Barkovich AJ, Kuzniecky RI, Bollen AW, Grant PE. Focal transmantle dysplasia: a specific malformation of cortical development. *Neurology* 1997; 49: 1148–52.

Barkovich AJ, Guerrini R, Kuzniecky RI, Jackson GD, Dobyns WB. A developmental and genetic classification for malformations of cortical development: update 2012. *Brain.* 2012; 135: 1348-69.

Blümcke I, Pieper T, Pauli E, *et al.* A distinct variant of Focal Cortical Dysplasia type I characterised by magnetic resonance imaging and neuropathological examination in children with severe epilepsies. *Epileptic Disord.* 2010; 12: 172-80.

Blümcke I, Thom M, Aronica E, *et al.* The clinico-pathological spectrum of Focal Cortical Dysplasias: a consensus classification proposed by an ad hoc Task Force of the ILAE Diagnostic Methods Commission *Epilepsia.* 2011; 52: 158-74.

Blumcke I, Budday S, Poduri A, Lal D, Kobow K, Baulac S. Neocortical development and epilepsy: insights from Focal Cortical Dysplasia and brain tumours. *Lancet Neurol.* 2021a; 20: 943-55.

Blumcke I, Cendes F, Miyata H, Thom M, Aronica E, Najm I. Toward a refined genotype-phenotype classification scheme for the international consensus classification of Focal Cortical Dysplasia. *Brain Pathol.* 2021b; 31: e12956.

Blümcke I, Coras R, Busch RM, *et al.* Toward a better definition of Focal Cortical Dysplasia: An iterative histopathological and genetic agreement trial. *Epilepsia.* 2021c; 62: 1416-28.

Chamberlain WA, Cohen ML, Gyure KA, *et al.* Interobserver and intraobserver reproducibility in Focal Cortical Dysplasia (malformations of cortical development). *Epilepsia.* 2009.; 50: 2593-8.

Chassoux F, Devaux B, Landre E, Turak B, Nataf F, Varlet P, Chodkiewicz JP, Daumas-Duport C. Stereoelectroencephalog- raphy in Focal Cortical Dysplasia: a 3D approach to delineating the dysplastic cortex. *Brain.* 2000; 123: 1733–51.

Clusmann H, Schramm J, Kral T, Helmstaedter C, Ostertun B, Fimmers R, Haun D, Elger CE. Prognostic factors and outcome after different types of resection for temporal lobe epilepsy. *J Neurosurg.* 2002; 97: 1131-41.

Fauser S, Schulze-Bonhage A, Honegger J, *et al.* Focal Cortical Dysplasias: surgical outcome in 67 patients in relation to histological subtypes and dual pathology. *Brain.* 2004; 127: 2406-18.

Gambardella A, Palmini A, Andermann F, *et al.* Usefulness of focal rhythmic discharges on scalp EEG of patients with Focal Cortical Dysplasia and intractable epilepsy. *Electroencephalogr Clin Neurophysiol.* 1996; 98: 243-9.

Hartlieb T, Winkler P, Coras R, *et al.* Age-related MR characteristics in mild malformation of cortical development with oligodendroglial hyperplasia and epilepsy (MOGHE) *Epilepsy Behav.* 2019; 91: 68-74.

Harvey AS, Mandelstam SA, Maixner WJ, *et al.* The surgically remediable syndrome of epilepsy associated with bottom-of-sulcus dysplasia. *Neurology* 2015; 84: 2021-8.

Hayashi M, Sugai K, Kurihara E, Tamagawa K. An autopsy case of severe myoclonic epilepsy of infancy, who died of acute encephalopathy associated with influenza infection. *Epilepsia.* 2004; 45 (suppl 8): 65.

Hemb M, Palmini A, Paglioli E, *et al.* An 18-year follow-up of seizure outcome after surgery for temporal lobe epilepsy and hippocampal sclerosis. *J Neurol Neurosurg Psychiatry.* 2013; 84: 800-5.

Holthausen H, Coras R, Tang Y, *et al.* Multilobar unilateral hypoplasia with emphasis in the posterior quadrant and severe epilepsy in children with FCD ILAE Type 1A. *Epilepsia.* 2022; 63: 42-60.

Kaufmann WE, Theda C, Naidu S, Watkins PA, Moser AB, Moser HW. Neuronal migration abnormality in peroxisomal bifunctional enzyme defect. *Ann Neurol.* 1996; 39: 268-71.

Krsek P, Maton B, Korman B, Pacheco-Jacome E, *et al.* Different features of histopathological subtypes of pediatric Focal Cortical Dysplasia. *Ann Neurol.* 2008; 63: 758-69.

Lerner JT, Salamon N, Hauptman JS, *et al.* Assessment and surgical outcomes for mild type I and severe type II cortical dysplasia: a critical review and the UCLA experience. *Epilepsia.* 2009; 50: 1310–35.

Mendes Coelho VC, Morita-Sherman M, Yasuda CL, *et al.* Magnetic resonance imaging findings and clinical characteristics in mild malformation of cortical development with oligodendroglial hyperplasia and epilepsy in a predominantly adult cohort. *Epilepsia.* 2021; 62: 1429-41.

Muhlhofer W, Tan YL, Mueller SG, Knowlton R. MRI-negative temporal lobe epilepsy-What do we know? *Epilepsia.* 2017; 58: 727-42.

Najm IM, Sarnat HB, Blümcke I. Review: The international consensus classification of Focal Cortical Dysplasia - a critical update 2018. *Neuropathol Appl Neurobiol.* 2018; 44: 18-31.

Najm I, Lal D, Vanegas MA *et al.* The ILAE consensus classification of Focal Cortical Dysplasia (FCD): an update proposed by an ad hoc Task Force of the ILAE Diagnostic Methods commission. *Epilepsia* 2022, in press.

Paglioli E, Palmini A, Paglioli E, *et al.* Survival analysis of the surgical outcome of temporal lobe epilepsy due to hippocampal sclerosis. *Epilepsia.* 2004; 45: 1383-91.

Palmini A, Andermann F, Olivier A, *et al.* Focal neuronal migration disorders and intractable partial epilepsy: a study of 30 patients. *Ann Neurol.* 1991a; 30: 741-9.

Palmini A, Andermann F, Olivier A, *et al.* Neuronal migration disorders: a contribution of modern neuroimaging to the etiologic diagnosis of epilepsy. *Can J Neurol Sci.* 1991b; 18 (4 Suppl): 580-7.

Palmini A, Gambardella A, Andermann F, *et al.* Intrinsic epileptogenicity of human dysplastic cortex as suggested by corticography and surgical results. *Ann Neurol.* 1995; 37: 476-87.

Palmini A, Najm I, Avanzini G, *et al.* Terminology and classification of the cortical dysplasias. *Neurology.* 2004; 62: S2-8.

Palmini A. Revising the classification of Focal Cortical Dysplasias. *Epilepsia.* 2011; 52: 188-90.

Perot P, Weir B, Rasmussen. Tuberous sclerosis: surgical therapy for seizures. *Arch Neurol* 1966; 15: 498-506.

Rakic P. Defects of neuronal migration and the pathogenesis of cortical malformations. *Prog Brain Res.* 1988a; 73: 15-37.

Rakic P. Specification of cerebral cortical areas. *Science.* 1988b; 241 (4862): 170-6.

Schramm J. Temporal lobe epilepsy surgery and the quest for optimal extent of resection: a review. *Epilepsia.* 2008; 49: 1296-307.

Seetharam R, Nooraine J, Mhatre R, Ramachandran J, Iyer RB, Mahadevan A. Mild. malformation of cortical development with oligodendroglial hyperplasia and epilepsy (MOGHE): a widespread disease with an apparently focal epilepsy. *Epileptic Disord.* 2021; 23: 407-11.

Sisodiya SM, Fauser S, Cross JH, Thom M. Focal Cortical Dysplasia type II: biological features and clinical perspectives. *Lancet Neurol.* 2009; 8: 830–3.

Tassi L, Colombo N, Garbelli R, *et al.* Focal Cortical Dysplasia: neuropathological subtypes, EEG, neuroimaging and surgical outcome. *Brain.* 2002; 125: 1719-32.

Tassi L, Meroni A, Deleo F, *et al.* Temporal lobe epilepsy: neuropathological and clinical correlations in 243 surgically treated patients. *Epileptic Disord.* 2009; 11: 281-92.

Tassi L, Garbelli R, Colombo N, *et al.* Type I Focal Cortical Dysplasia: surgical outcome is related to histopathology. *Epileptic Disord.* 2010; 12: 181-91.

Taylor DC, Falconer MA, Bruton CJ, Corsellis JA. Focal dysplasia of the cerebral cortex in epilepsy. *J Neurol Neurosurg Psychiatry.*1971; 34: 369-87.

CHAPTER

3. Neuropathology of FCD: a practical approach for clinical use

Ingmar Blümcke

Key points

- It is good medical practice to subject every surgically removed tissue sample to a systematic neuropathological examination, to clarify the underlying disease diagnosis and confirm the likely pathomechanism.
- MCD are the most common causes of drug-resistant focal epilepsy in children and the third most common causes in adults submitted to epilepsy surgery.
- FCD represents 80% of all MCD lesions in epilepsy series.
- FCD II represents the single most common structural brain lesion in children with drug-resistant focal epilepsies submitted to surgical treatment.
- FCD I subtypes are less well defined at the clinical, pathological and genetic level.
- The first guiding principle in neuropathology is to acknowledge the rule of commonality for major disease entities, including specific clinical parameters.
- The second guiding principle is that of neuropathological pattern recognition defining each diagnosis by its specific structural correlate.
- The emerging third guiding principle is to integrate histopathology with available molecular-genetic findings from the same tissue sample, i.e. molecular neuropathology, in order to validate and confirm difficult-to-classify diagnoses, particularly in the realm of epilepsy surgery.

Introduction

Neuropathology is the medical specialty confirming a disease diagnosis in the central nervous system, the peripheral nervous system and the skeletal muscle. The most important examination method in neuropathology is the microscope, i.e., histopathology which is increasingly supported by integrated molecular pathology testing. It is good medical practice, however, to subject every surgically removed tissue sample to a systematic neuropathology examination to clarify the underlying disease diagnosis and confirm the likely pathomechanism, either being malformative, neoplastic, inflammatory or neurodegenerative in its nature. This knowledge is mandatory for any successful therapy and applies in particular to focal epilepsies.

MCD are the most common causes of drug-resistant focal epilepsy in children and the third most common causes in adults submitted to epilepsy surgery. Amongst all MCD disease entities, FCD represents 80% of all lesions. The chapter will follow through three guiding principles in neuropathology: the first is to acknowledge the rule of commonality for major disease entities, including specific clinical parameters such as common age at disease onset and common brain localization. A second guiding principle to be discussed herein is that of neuropathological pattern recognition defining each diagnosis by its specific structural correlate. Finally, the emerging third guiding principle is to integrate histopathology with available molecular-genetic findings from the same tissue sample, i.e. molecular neuropathology, in order to validate and confirm difficult-to-classify diagnoses in the realm of epilepsy surgery.

First guiding principle in histopathology

• Frequent is frequent and rare is rare...

... whom ever frequently diagnose a rare disease will frequently be wrong!

FCD II represents the single most common structural brain lesion in children with drug-resistant focal epilepsies submitted to surgical treatment (Blümcke *et al.*, 2017). In a large European cohort of almost 10.000 patients, FCD II was identified in 9% of all patients (top #3 ranking) and 17% of all children submitted to epilepsy surgery (top #1 ranking; **Table 1**). This example will be taken, therefore, to demonstrate the impact of the 1st guiding principle in neuropathology to scientifically define disease entities, as they commonly present with the same pattern of clinico-pathological and genetic signatures.

The first description of FCD II was by David Taylor and colleagues already 50 years ago (Taylor *et al.*, 1971) and characteristic histopathology patterns, electroclinical and neuroimaging findings evolved since then to a comprehensive disease definition (Palmini *et al.*, 1995, Chassoux *et al.*, 2000, Tassi *et al.*, 2002, Palmini *et al.*, 2004, Blümcke *et al.*, 2011, Najm *et al.*, 2018). The genetic foundation of FCD II has also been clarified with brain somatic mutations affecting mTOR pathway signaling genes as major causes, i.e. *AKT3*, *DEPDC5*, *MTOR*, *NPRL2*, *RHEB*, *TSC1* or *TSC2* (Baldassari *et al.*, 2019). These genetic abnormalities in mTOR signaling are most compatible with the common histopathology phenotype demonstrating enlarged dysmorphic neurons (DN) and enlarged balloon cells (BC). The ILAE classification specifies two subtypes of FCD II (Blümcke *et al.*, 2011), i.e. FCD IIA defined by DN and FCD IIB defined by DN and BC, and which will be further discussed below. The median age at disease onset of FCD II is two years (**Tables 1 and 2**), and the frontal lobe is affected in more than 51% of all patients. MRI abnormalities include a transmantle sign in many cases of FCD IIB, whereas FCD IIA may escape visual MRI detection. However, abnormalities in the cortical folding as well as cortical thickening can often be identified by post-processing or higher magnetic field strength (Wang *et al.*, 2020a, 2020b). Increasing knowledge about this clinico-pathological and genetic patterns will eventually guide clinical work-up and diagnosis during the pre-surgical evaluation.

FCD I subtypes are less well defined at the clinical, pathological and genetic level. However, a comprehensive clinico-pathological description was recently published for FCD IA (Holthausen *et al.*, 2022). It will herein be referred to as Holthausen disease, best described by early onset of severe epilepsy (**Table 2**) with unilateral multilobar hypoplasia on MRI, and emphasis of abnormal electroencephalography (EEG) patterns in the posterior quadrant, i.e. the occipito-parieto-temporal region (Holthausen *et al.*, 2022). This FCD subtype is rare, representing 3.8% of children submitted to epilepsy surgery in a specialized single center in Germany. It is envisaged that such microcolumnar organization resembles neuronal radial migration streams during corticogenesis (Mountcastle, 1997, Rakic, 1988) and may result, therefore, from delayed or arrested maturation at mid-gestation. However, experimental evidence has not yet been provided scientifically. Taking neurodevelopmental principles of the neocortical organization into consideration, the ILAE Task Force also acknowledged the possibility of abnormal horizontal layer organization, which has been assigned as FCD IB (Blümcke *et al.*, 2011). To date, however, no study conclusively described a clinical phenotype or syndrome for patients with FCD IB. Another FCD I subcategory was also established in the 2011 classification scheme, assuming a mixed phenotype of radial and horizontal cortical disorganization, i.e., FCD IC. Such a mixed phenotype has been indeed recognized by routine pathology in the neocortex affected by early perinatal lesions, such as large vascular malformations. Nonetheless, although the categories of FCD IB and IC are often used nowadays, we have not yet learned about specific clinical presentations. MRI is usually negative (Wang *et al.*, 2013b) and patients have not been reported before the 2011 ILAE classification of FCD was released. The true existence of these FCD subtypes, potential pathogenic cause and clinical features will require, therefore, further research efforts.

An important differential diagnosis of FCD I is that of MOGHE, defined as "mild malformation of cortical development with oligodendroglial hyperplasia in epilepsy" (**Table 2**, **Figure 2**). It was first described in 2017 (Schurr *et al.*, 2017) and recognized since then in additional case series (Gaballa *et al.*, 2021). As a principle guideline, the pattern of MOGHE is most consistent with early onset frontal lobe epilepsy (**Table 2**), and age-related MRI findings reveal blurred grey-white matter junction with difficult-to-delineate lesion borders (Hartlieb *et al.*, 2019). MOGHE is amenable to epilepsy surgery and currently more

Table 1

The spectrum of cortical malformations amenable for epilepsy surgery

MCD entities	All patients		Age at onset	Disease duration	12 m sz-free
FCD II	625	46.2%	2 (0.1-37)	11	65.2%
mMCD	207	15.3%	8 (0.3-37)	11	50%
FCD (NOS)	195	14.4%	4 (0.1-37)	10	52.3%
FCD I	142	10.5%	2 (0.1-45)	7	46.7%
PMG	70	5.2%	1 (0.1-15)	4	57.7%
MOGHE	54	4%	2 (0.1-18)	5	49.3%
cMCD	29	2.1%	0.1 (0.1-19)	3.5	58.8%
HME	21	1.6%	0.1 (0.1-0.7)	1	56%
HET	6	0.4%	0.1 (0.1-2)	12	88.9%
HH	4	0.3%	0.1 (0.1-0.9)	9	16.7%
Total	**1353 (19%) ***		**2 (0.1-37)**	**8**	**60.7% ****

Catalogue of 10 histopathology disease entities assigned to the MCD category in 7078 patients collected at the German Reference Center for Epilepsy Surgery, grouped according to their frequency.

FCD II: Focal Cortical Dysplasia ILAE Type II (syn. Taylor's dysplasia and Palmini FCD II); FCD I: Focal Cortical Dysplasia ILAE Type I (also including Palmini's FCD I, (Palmini *et al.*, 2004)); mMCD: mild malformation of cortical development; MOGHE: mMCD with oligodendroglial hyperplasia; HME: hemimegalencephaly; HET: nodular heterotopia; HH: hypothalamic hamartoma; cMCD: complex MCD incl. HME and HET or PMG; median age at epilepsy onset in years (including range); 12 m sz-free: complete seizure freedom 1 year after surgery. 48% of all patients were female (not shown)

* the MCD category represented 19% of the entire cohort;

** percentages calculated for subgroups with available outcome data.

Table 2

A revised FCD classification scheme (Blumcke *et al.*, 2021c) with common clinico-pathological and genetic findings in individual FCD subtypes

	FCD subtype	Age at disease onset#	Principal localization	Histopathology pattern	Molecular Pathology
FCD ILAE I	FCD IA	0.6 0.3-10) §	Posterior quadrant	Microcolumns & het. Neurons in wm	DNA methylation
	FCD IB	7.5 (0.1-32)	Temporal lobe	Horizontal dyslamination	Na
	FCD IC	na	Tbd	Vertical and horizontal dysorganization	Na
FCD ILAE Type 2	FCD IIA	2 (0.1-37)	Frontal lobe	Dysmorphic neurons	GATORopathy*
	FCD IIB	2 (0.1-32)	Frontal lobe	Dysmorphic neurons/ Balloon cells	MTORopathy**
FCD ILAE Type 3	FCD IIIA	6 (0.5-49)	Temporal lobe	With hippocampal sclerosis	DNA methylation
	FCD IIIB	1 (0.3-20)	Temporal lobe	With developmental brain tumour	DNA methylation
	FCD IIIC	12 (0.5-38)	Temporal lobe	With vascular malformation	DNA methylation
	FCD IIID	3 (0.3-31)	Temporal lobe	With lesion acquired during early life	DNA methylation
White Matter	mMCD	8 (0.3-37)	Temporal lobe	Het. Neurons in wm	DNA methylation
	MOGHE	2 (0.1-18)	Frontal lobe	Oligodendroglial hyperplasia/ het. Neurons in wm	SLC35A2

WM: white matter; het.: heterotopic; na: not available; tbd: to be determined, with not enough entries in the registry to calculate this figure;

median (with range) of age at disease onset in years, data obtained from the German Reference Center for epilepsy surgery of 7078 cases;

§ data taken from Holthausen *et al.* 2021;

* (Iffland *et al.*, 2019) ;

** (Blumcke and Sarnat, 2016).

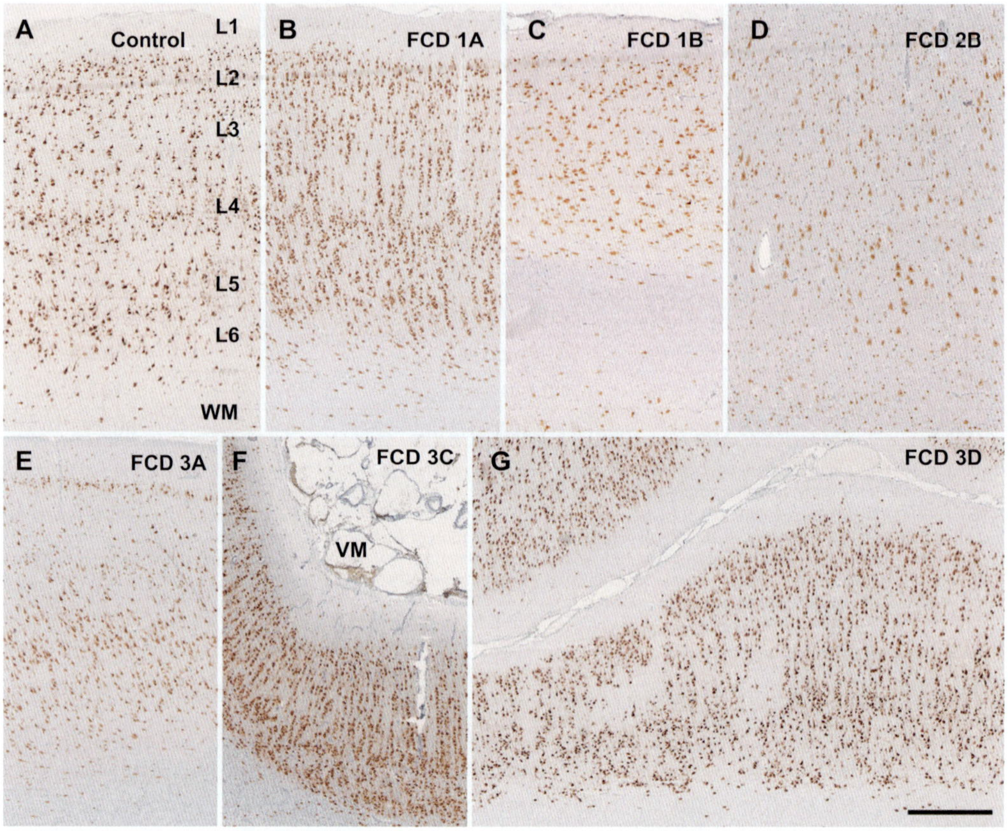

Figure 1

Patterns of architectural abnormalities defining FCD subtypes

A panel of classic examples all taken at the same objective magnification and with same immunohistochemical labelling (NeuN). A. Control neocortex obtained from the temporal lobe with its characteristic six neuronal cell layers (L2-L6) and the neuron sparse L1 on top and white matter at the bottom (WM). B. FCD IA of the occipital lobe is defined by abundant neuronal microcolumns with often small neurons vertically arrayed like parallel strings of pearls. C. FCD IB of the temporal lobe without any layered neocortical organization. Also note the dramatically thinned cortical diameter as compared to most other examples (but see F). D. FCD IIB of the frontal lobe is characterized by lack of any cortical layering. Instead, large dysmorphic neurons appear randomly placed from WM to L6. Balloon cells are not visible in this NeuN immunohistochemistry. E. FCD IIIA in the temporal neocortex of a patient with Hippocampal Sclerosis. Note the neuronal cell loss in supragranular layers L2 and L3. F. FCD IIIC in a patient with Sturge-Weber syndrome and a vascular malformation (VM), i.e., meningeal angiomatosis. The adjacent neocortex is thin and shows abundant microcolumns (as in FCD I A and FCD IIID). G. FCD IIID of the parieto-frontal region in a patient with perinatal stroke. Note the patchy disruption of cortical layers at many areas on the left and abundance of microcolumns of the right.
Scale bar = 500 µm, applies to all images.

than 60% of patients are seizure free one year after operation (Gaballa *et al.*, 2021), which is a significant progress from the first series from 2017, in which only 33% of patients had postsurgical seizure control. Most interestingly, 50% of patients with MOGHE reveal a brain somatic mutation in the SLC35A2 gene (Bonduelle *et al.*, 2021). SLC35A2 is a UDP-galactose transporter and the underlying pathomechanisms of MOGHE is thus likely different from FCD II and mTOR signaling. Accordingly, dietetic galactose supplementation can represent a successful therapy in genetically confirmed patients with SLC35A2 germline mutations (Witters *et al.*, 2020) and that is currently explored also for MOGHE with brain somatic mutations of the SLC35A2 gene.

mMCD is a topic less well studied and scientifically described (**Table 2, Figure 1**). Thus, it has not been recognized in the ILAE classification scheme of 2011 but will likely be re-introduced in the upcoming update (Blumcke *et al.*, 2021c, Blumcke *et al.*, 2021b). mMCD was defined

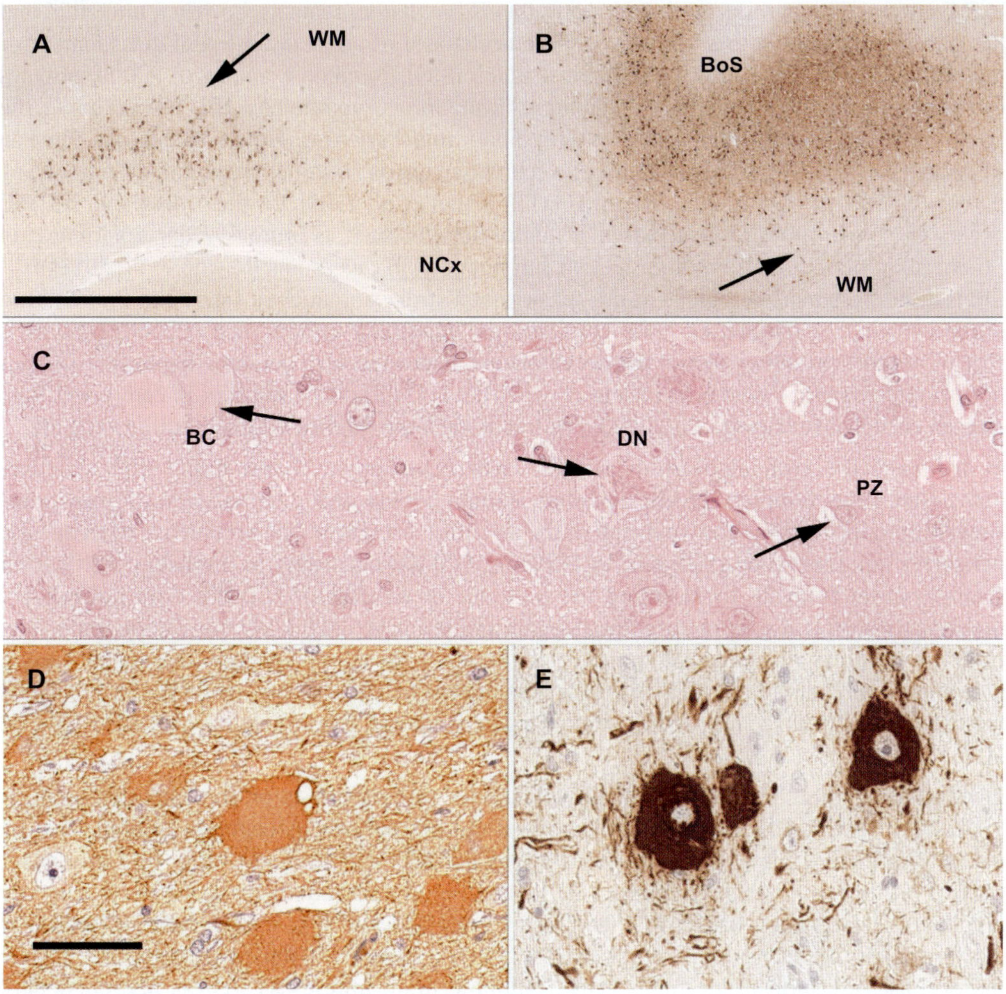

Figure 2

Cytoarchitectural abnormalities defining FCD II

A. 42-year-old female patient with frontal lobe epilepsy since age 5 years and histopathologically confirmed FCD IIA. The arrow points to the sharp border between the cortical FCD and the normal appearing white matter (WM). Normal 6-layered neocortex (NCx). Neurofilament-immunohistochemistry, scale bar = 2,5mm (applies also to B). B. 19-year-old female patient with frontal lobe epilepsy since age 9 years, and histopathologically confirmed FCD IIB at a bottom-of-sulcus (BoS). The boundary towards the white matter is less well pronounced (arrow). C. HE staining at higher magnification of FCD IIB with opalesque balloon cells (BC), enlarged dysmorphic neurons (DN), and normal appearing pyramidal cells (PZ). D. balloon cells frequently stain with antibodies directed against vimentin, but also pS6 or alpha-ß-crystallin. Scale bar = 50µm, applies also to C and E. E Neurofilament accumulating dysmorphic neurons in FCD II.

by the Palmini classification of FCD as an excess of heterotopic neurons in the white matter including an increase of ramifying neuronal processes best visible when using immunohistochemistry for the MAP2 epitope (Palmini *et al.*, 2004). This pattern has also been described as hallmarks in FCD IA and MOGHE and may play a general role in many other epilepsy surgery tissue samples (Emery *et al.*, 1997). However, the 1st guiding principal cannot yet been adequately applied for any mMCD cohort and will need further scientific clarification to define its clinical and structural presentation as well as its potentially epileptogenic features.

FCD ILAE Type 3 (FCD III) summarize a spectrum of architectural cortical abnormalities associated with principal lesions acquired during early life, i.e. disruption of the 6-layered horizontal organization and/or abundance of vertically oriented microcolumns (**Figure 1**). These histopathology patterns can be well differentiated from each other but mostly resemble architectural

FCD I patterns. The pathogenesis underlying this FCD category remains, however, uncertain and has been linked instead to a secondary pathomechanism of arrested postnatal development or maturational delay (Spreafico, 2010, Marin-Padilla, 1999). Common examples of FCD III subtypes exemplify the usefulness of the 1st guiding principle in neuropathology. FCD IIIA occurs in the temporal neocortex of 10% of patients with hippocampal sclerosis (**Figure 1**). Seventy-three % of patients with FCD IIIA had a history of a febrile seizure as an initial precipitating injury compared with 36% of HS patients without FCD IIIA (Thom *et al.*, 2009). On the other hand, FCD IIIC occurs in almost 100% of large vascular malformations, such as Sturge-Weber syndrome and other arterio-venous malformations (AVM), but not at all in cavernoma (Miyata *et al.*, 2022). FCD IIID is most prominent in regions of pre- or perinatal stroke and in close vicinity to the resulting porencephalic cyst (**Figure 1**). Another clinico-pathologically well-defined FCD IIID subtype is that of neocortical layer 4 loss in the occipital lobe associated with perinatal hypoxemic injuries occurring predominately in boys (Wang *et al.*, 2017). FCD IIID may also occur in early onset Rasmussen encephalitis (Wang *et al.*, 2013a) or traumatic brain injuries acquired during early life.

In contrast, the true association of FCD with developmental low-grade and epilepsy-associated brain tumours (LEAT), including ganglioglioma and dysembryoplastic neuroepithelial tumours, remains controversial in the scientific literature. The prevalence of dysplastic neocortex adjacent to or infiltrated by LEAT, i.e., FCD IIIB according to the ILAE classification scheme, varies from 25 to 75% and the presence or absence of FCD IIIB does not reliably predict post-surgical seizure outcome (Slegers and Blumcke, 2020). We must hope, therefore, that the progress in molecular-genetic technologies targeting epilepsy-associated human brain tissue will help to clarify if these cases represent true FCD or pro-epileptogenic molecular interactions of the tumor with surrounding peritumoral brain tissue (Slegers and Blumcke, 2020, Blumcke *et al.*, 2016a).

In conclusion, the 1st guiding principle challenges rare diagnosis of clinically, histopathologically or genetically less well characterized patient cohorts. A common example will be that of a patient with 1st seizure onset beyond the 2nd or 3rd decade of life. Any new onset MCD is rather rare in this patient as FCD shares a high epiletogenicity score and commonly manifests at early ages. In contrast, common causes of "late" first seizure onset is a vascular malformation, i.e., cavernoma, paraneoplastic limbic encephalitis or other acquired inflammatory diseases, high grade neoplasms, traumatic brain injuries as well as neurodegeneration in the elderly. It is common ground in medicine, however, that ultra-rare diagnosis will always occur. When such rare diagnoses become frequent in epilepsy centers, however, multidisciplinary teams should review all their diagnostic findings. An ILAE Task Force for FCD has discussed this situation and suggested to introduce a multilayered integrative classification scheme for FCD (Blumcke *et al.*, 2021b). This would allow the treating physician to collect all available diagnostic findings obtained from the multidisciplinary expert panel, including the clinical presentation, neuroimaging findings, histopathology and eventually also genetic studies, in order to achieve an integrated comprehensive final diagnosis during the (post-surgical) patient management conference.

Second guiding principle in histopathology

• The structural correlate of each specific diagnosis is obtained from recognition of microscopic patterns, which also define the underlying pathomechanism!

The concept of cellular pathology has been introduced in the early 19th century and marked the transition from Hippocratic medicine of medieval times to the evolution of modern medicine. It aroused from the systematic introduction of microscopy-based studies of human tissue showing an unambiguous association of cellular reaction patterns with root causes of the disease. A prominent example from these early times was the endemic infection with tuberculosis in Berlin during the 19th century, which caused necrotizing granuloma with giant cells of Langhans in the lung and many other organs including the brain. This pattern recognition strategy evolved further with the use of panels of newly available stainings and eventually led to the routine application of antibody-based immunohistochemistry in the beginning of the 1980's. This allowed lineage-specific identification of cellular profiles in pathologically severely compromised tissues, e.g., malformations or neoplasia. The current FCD classification scheme of the International League against Epilepsy (ILAE) is also based on this strategy to define patterns of abnormal cellular and/or architectural organization of the affected neocortex into specific FCD subtypes (**Figure 1**). Advanced genetic studies have nowadays confirmed that abnormal patterns of cortical malformations arise when neuro-glial precursor cells acquire specific post-zygotic gene alterations, i.e., mosaicism, at specific time points of their neurodevelopment (Blumcke *et al.*, 2021a).

FCD I is defined by the ILAE classification scheme as a purely architectural abnormality of the 6-layered neocortical organization. There is now ample evidence for an abundant micro-columnar organization in the epileptogenic neocortex of young children with early onset focal epilepsy, in particular of the posterior quadrant, as in Holthausen's disease, and which has been histopathologically confirmed as FCD IA (Holthausen *et al.*, 2022). This subtype represents, therefore, the best example for an abnormal and predominately vertically disorganized neocortex (**Figure 1B**). Cytopathological patterns as described further below were missing in this disease entity, however. There is also no genetic abnormality defined yet for FCD IA, although a recent research paper provided a specific DNA methylation pattern of FCD IA (**Figure 3**) which may help to objectively differentiate this subtype from other differential diagnoses, such as MOGHE and mMCD (Jabari *et al.*, 2021). Furthermore, the microcolumnar organization of the neocortex in FCD IA suggested that the cortical maturation is delayed or compromised in these patients, perhaps related to subtle prenatal hypoxemic injuries

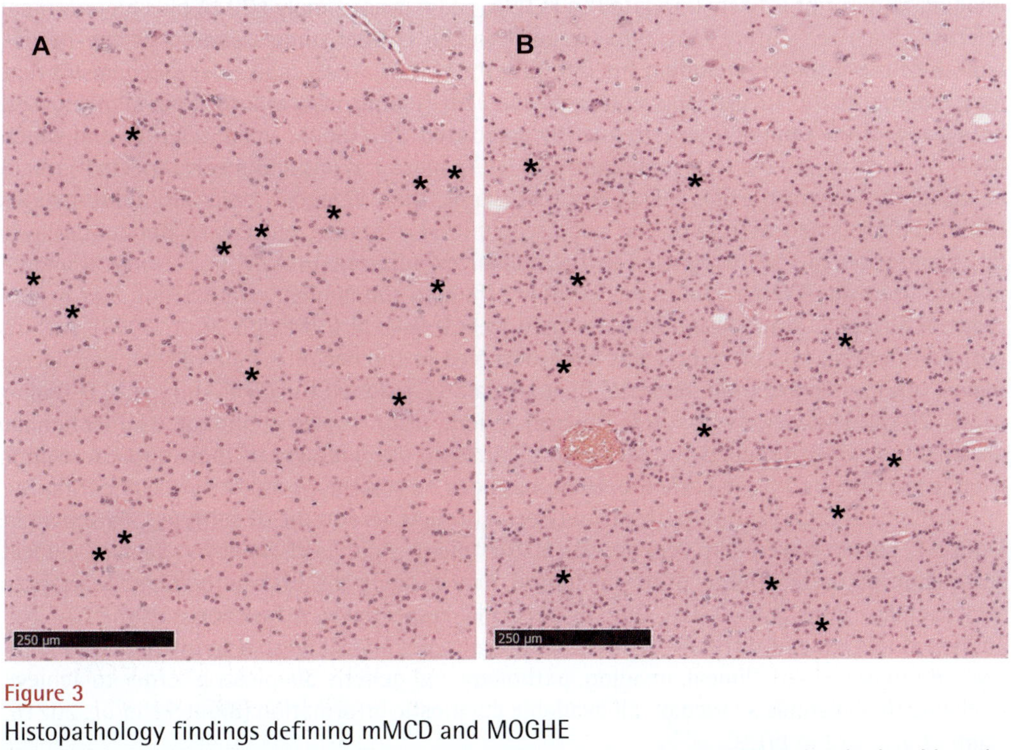

Figure 3

Histopathology findings defining mMCD and MOGHE

A. 27-year-old female patient with temporal lobe epilepsy and no hippocampal sclerosis. Asterisks point to abundant heterotopic neurons in the white matter, i.e., mMCD (>25 neurons/mm², normal values are 2-4 neurons/mm²; see (Emery *et al.*, 1997)). B. 5-year-old male patient with frontal lobe epilepsy, and a pathogenic brain mosaicism in the SLC35A2 gene. Note the increased oligodendroglial cell density, i.e., MOGHE, compared to the same magnification shown in A. Asterisks point to abundant heterotopic neurons in the white matter (>20 neurons/mm²). Upper borders of both images A and B represent grey-white matter boundaries. H&E staining of a 4µm thin FFPE section.
Scale bars = 250µm.

(Holthausen *et al.*, 2022). As a matter of fact, the human neocortex develops in a microcolumnar organized fashion, anatomically as well as functionally, until adolescence. These patterns cannot be microscopically recognized anymore in the adult brain but remain evident in children with severe epilepsy and cognitive impairment due to FCD IA.

In contrast to the microcolumnar dyslamination pattern of FCD IA, FCD IB could be recognized if the 6-layered (horizontal) neocortex does not show a clearly discernible layered organization (**Figure 1C**). Individually missing layers were most often observed for Layers 2 and 4. These layers are also most variable in the normal homotypic and heterotypic human cortical architecture as defined by the Brodmann map (Brodmann, 1908). The third FCD I subtype defined by the ILAE classification (Blümcke *et al.*, 2011) would then combine the findings in IA and IB, i.e., present both vertical and horizontal abnormal cortical architecture. This FCD IC histological feature, however, had not been described before the 2011 FCD classification scheme and patient cohorts have not yet been reliably identified since (see also 1st guiding principle in histopathology above).

Architectural abnormalities described for FCD IB and FCD IC can be most often recognized in the FCD ILAE Type III subtypes (**Figure 1E-G**). These occur, however, always in the vicinity of another principal lesion. A typical example is that of FCD IIIA in association with hippocampal sclerosis. Herein, the supragranular cell layers 2 and 3 are severely compromised as previously described as temporal lobe sclerosis (Thom *et al.*, 2009). This cortical pattern is always associated with hippocampal sclerosis, affecting approximately 5-10% of patients with that principal pathology. Intriguingly, it has not been observed in any other disease condition, lacks a specific MRI signature and, most importantly, does not have the same microcolumnar vertical dyslamination pattern described in FCD IA (Holthausen *et al.*, 2022). Thus, FCD IIIA, a debatable and frequent entity due to its association with hippocampal sclerosis and lack of an imaging fingerprint is likely unrelated to FCD IA, i.e., it is not simply FCD IA plus hippocampal sclerosis. Such realization may prove crucial to the correct understanding of the pathogenesis of this disorder, including the interpretation of whatever molecular mechanisms that may emerge in the future. This contrasts the MRI finding of temporo-polar blurring and hypoplasia of the temporal pole frequently associated with hippocampal sclerosis and which likely result from secondary degeneration of white matter axons and myelin sheets (Garbelli *et al.*, 2012, Demerath *et al.*, 2021). In other words, these temporal pole MRI abnormalities cannot be explained by FCD at the microscopic level. A similar pattern of horizontal layer disorganization can be recognized in the neocortex adjacent to AVM or meningeal angiomatosis in Sturge-Weber syndrome, variably affecting the laminar composition and occurrence of Layers 2, 3 and 4 and also assigned to FCD ILAE III C (Miyata *et al.*, 2022). A third pattern affecting loss of layer 4 has been observed in the occipital lobe of young children, mainly boys, suffering from perinatal hypoxemia and assigned to FCD ILAE Type III D (Wang *et al.*, 2017). The vicinity of these cortical lesions often shows abundant microcolumnar organization which supports the notion of an arrested development of these cortical regions when compromised during early life. There has been no systematic studies yet comparing the microcolumnar organization patterns between FCD ILAE IA and IIIC-D subtypes. As shown in **Figure 1**, patterns are likely very similar at the microscopic level, however. Lack of clinical knowledge of these remote principal lesions may prompt the histopathologist to classify such samples rather as FCD ILAE Type IB or FCD IC, respectively. A Task Force of the ILAE has addressed this issue of difficult-to-classify FCD subtypes and suggested to introduce a multilayered integration of clinical, imaging, pathology and genetic diagnosis in order to achieve a reliable final diagnosis based on all available diagnostic information (Blumcke *et al.*, 2021b; Najm *et al.*, 2022 in press).

FCD ILAE Type II lesions are defined by cytoarchitectural abnormalities, i.e., alterations in the 6-layered composition of the neocortex as well as at the cellular level of pyramidal neurons (**Figure 2**). The architectural abnormalities in FCD II subtypes rarely reflect those described above for FCD I or III. Instead, the neocortex may have no discernable layering with the exception of a cell-sparse Layer 1. The cytological abnormality in all FCD II lesions, i.e., FCD IIA and FCD IIB, is defined by the term of "dysmorphic neuron" (**Figure 2E**). These are large glutamatergic pyramidal cells anatomically not well oriented, i.e. their apical dendrite may not point to the cortical surface, and which also occur in cell clusters or were heterotopically displaced in the adjacent white matter (Muhlebner *et al.*, 2012). The latter would suggest a compromised migration during neurodevelopment, and which has been experimentally confirmed when introducing *MTOR* or *PIK3CA* gene alterations typically observed in FCD IIB specimens into the developing murine neocortex (D'Gama *et al.*, 2017). Another cyotarchitectural abnormality is that of BC, a cytomegalic cell type pathognomic for FCD IIB (**Figure 2D**). BC have been shown to express both neuronal and immature glial markers, indicating a failure to differentiate prior to migration into the cortex (Cotter *et al.*, 1999, Urbach *et al.*, 2002, Lamparello *et al.*, 2007). Several studies using *in vitro* electrophysiological recordings in surgical specimens from patients with FCD IIB have shown that BC are electrically silent, whereas dysmorphic neurons display hyperexcitable intrinsic membrane properties (Cepeda *et al.*, 2005, Rampp *et al.*, 2021). There is also a substantial amount of data demonstrating persistence of immature features (Avansini *et al.*, 2018), suggesting dysregulation of inhibitory synaptic transmission involving altered γ-aminobutyric acid (GABA)-A mediated currents (Blauwblomme *et al.*, 2019). The pathological features of FCD II also involves glial cells, including both oligodendrocytes and astrocytes. White matter pathology with depleted myelin and oligodendroglia represents a major feature of FCD IIB (Muhlebner *et al.*, 2012), indicating impaired oligodendroglial turnover and maturation. Reactive astrocytes and activated microglial cells were frequently represented in the FCD II lesion, contribute to the induction of major pro-inflammatory signaling pathways and alterations in the blood-brain barrier and extracellular matrix organization (Arena *et al.*, 2019, Zurolo *et al.*, 2011, Iyer *et al.*, 2010). Moreover, FCD II is also characterized by a prominent activation of adaptive immunity mechanisms involving T-lymphocytes (Iyer *et al.*, 2010, Xu *et al.*, 2018, Owens *et al.*, 2019).

MOGHE is a newly recognized disease entity histopathologically defined by patchy areas of oligodendroglial hyperplasia overlapping with areas of hypomyelination at the grey-white-matter boundary (Schurr *et al.*, 2017). As systematically measured by these authors, the oligodendroglial cell number is double compared to age- and location matched control cell densities and the myelin content is hypodense (**Figure 3**). Another histopathology hallmark is increased proliferation activity of oligodendroglial cells in the white matter as indicated by Ki67 immunohistochemistry (Schurr *et al.*, 2017). There are also many heterotopic neurons in the same white matter regions and microdissection studies revealed that aberrant SLC35A2 variants were present in both oligodendroglial cells and heterotopic neurons, suggesting a disease foundation by glio-neuronal precursor cells during neurodevelopment (Bonduelle *et al.*, 2021).

Finally, mMCD is histopathologically defined by abundant heterotopic neurons in the white matter of surgical tissue specimen when not associated with any other principal lesion (**Figure 3**). As mentioned above, this mMCD definition is the same introduced by the Palmini classification scheme of 2004 as mMCD Type 2 (Palmini *et al.*, 2004), and was continued as such by the ILAE FCD classification of 2011 without any further scientific amendments (Blümcke *et al.*, 2011). The diagnosis of mMCD is used, however, in many laboratories around the world and was also recognized in a recent FCD agreement trial launched by an ILAE Task Force (Blumcke *et al.*, 2021c). Heterotopic neurons occur at low density also in the normal, non-epileptic subcortical white matter (Rojiani *et al.*, 1996) but are frequently increased above a histopathologically defined threshold of 4 +/- 2 neurons/mm^2 as described by Emery and coworker for their patients with temporal lobe epilepsy using MAP2 immunohistochemistry (Emery *et al.*, 1997). The FCD classification of 2011 has specified an even higher density of >30 neurons/mm^2 in order to prevent an overuse of this diagnosis. Since this is such a common finding in many epilepsy surgery specimens with many different disease conditions, and yet without convincing research evidence towards an epileptogenic potential of these heterotopic neurons *per se*, the term "mMCD" should not be used as secondary or tertiary diagnosis if the epileptogenic condition can be microscopically explained otherwise by FCD, neoplasia or hippocampal sclerosis. In addition, there are yet no imaging findings consistent with the histopathology diagnosis of mMCD nor does genetic data further validate this entity. Those reports assigning the SLC35A2 mutation to mMCD have been partially reviewed and revised to MOGHE in all instances (Bonduelle *et al.*, 2021).

Third guiding principle in histopathology

• Integration of molecular pathology to obtain a reliable scientific diagnosis

In general, the histopathological work-up of epilepsy surgery specimens is based on routine Hematoxylin and Eosin (HE) staining with its many difficulties and pitfalls to reliably identify anatomical landmarks and cortical layering. This applies in particular to samples not resected anatomically *en bloc*, or when the sample is compromised by perioperative artifacts or diagnostic procedures such as intracranial EEG recordings, laser ablation or thermo-coagulation. Therefore, it has been a long-standing effort in histopathology to support microscopic diagnoses with objectively-measurable tools. The latter have evolved with the advancement of molecular pathology and are based on the recognition of gene driving mutations in specific diseases, i.e. IDH1 R132H mutation in glioma of astroglial or oligodendroglial cell lineage. Further progress has been made with the development of mutation-specific antibodies which can be used for routine histopathology stainings (see manual below). The next level of molecular pathology diagnostics was established by introducing DNA methylation-based disease classifiers in neuro-oncology (Capper *et al.*, 2018), but which can now also be applied for MCD (Jabari *et al.*, 2022). These human brain tissue-based diagnostic tools will have considerable impact on the reliability of histopathological diagnoses, fostering agreement amongst laboratories and colleagues and refining prediction of the results of treatment targets individualized for each patient, as an evolving 3rd guiding principle in neuropathology.

Interestingly, although FCD are the most common MCD recognized in epilepsy surgery series (Blümcke *et al.*, 2017, Lamberink *et al.*, 2020), the agreement of microscopic diagnoses remains ever challenging, as documented in a number of studies (Chamberlain *et al.*, 2009, Coras *et al.*, 2012, Blumcke *et al.*, 2016a, Blumcke *et al.*, 2021c, Blumcke *et al.*, 2019). Recently, the ILAE Task Force of FCD has launched a new approach combining histopathology and molecular genetics: neuropathologists iteratively reviewed a consecutive series of specimen resected from patients whose presurgical evaluation suggested some type of FCD (Blumcke *et al.*, 2021c) whereas, in parallel, genetic testing with FCD-specific gene panel sequencing was performed from tissue and blood samples of the very same patients. The agreement was assessed in sequential rounds of independent reviews. Histopathology review of HE stainings led to very low agreement in the first round (kappa, 0.16). Kappa increased to 0.35 in the second round, when immunohistochemical stainings were added. The third round benefited from disclosure of neuroimaging and histographs showing specific features of each lesion, and also from anonymous disclosure of all previous individual answers, i.e. the Delphi consensus method. This increased the diagnostic yield to a kappa of 0.5. In the fourth and final round, the results from genetic testing were available, i.e., pathogenic *MTOR*, *DEPDC5*, *AKT3*, *NPRL3* and *SLC35A2* mutations in 7 cases. The final agreement based on all available information was substantial with a kappa of 0.68 (Blumcke *et al.*, 2021c). This study will define the path towards an integrated genotype-phenotype diagnosis in FCD and the authors proposed a number of amendments to be recognized in an update of the 2011 ILAE classification scheme (see **Table 2**). Notwithstanding its novelty, the proposal to add the level of genetic testing to a comprehensive and reliable genotype-phenotype has already been successfully established for neuro-oncology (Blumcke *et al.*, 2021b) and is likely to be also successful for the diagnosis and classification of FCD. Genetic testing should ideally be performed from DNA extracted from a microscopically assessed surgical brain tissue and paired blood sample, to facilitate the identification of brain mosaicism that represent post-zygotic mutational events. Whether or not such genetic testing should become mandatory in clinical practice or should be reserved for scientific research remains a matter of debate and will also depend on available resources in each epilepsy surgery center.

Moreover, Jabari and coworkers presented another approach well recognized and established in the realm of neuro-oncology, i.e., DNA methylation-based classification of cortical malformations (Jabari *et al.*, 2022). This opens the avenue for an easy-to-use and objective genotype-phenotype approach also in epilepsy surgery, using routinely processed or archival formalin-fixed and paraffin-embedded (FFPE) tissue samples. This work included the most common FCD subtypes, and also polymicrogyria, hemimegalencephaly (HME), TSC, mMCD, and MOGHE specimens (**Figure 4**). Non-MCD epilepsy samples and non-epilepsy *post mortem* tissue were used as controls. The possibility to apply a DNA methylation classification for non-neoplastic lesions has been scientifically questioned, however, and remains an ongoing challenge due to the usual low content of abnormal cells with admixture of architecturally normal-appearing cortical areas. The possibility to microscopically dissect an area of the lesion which concentrates cellular abnormalities from FFPE tissue blocks is an important option to successfully apply this technology in the routine work-up of epilepsy surgery specimens in the near future.

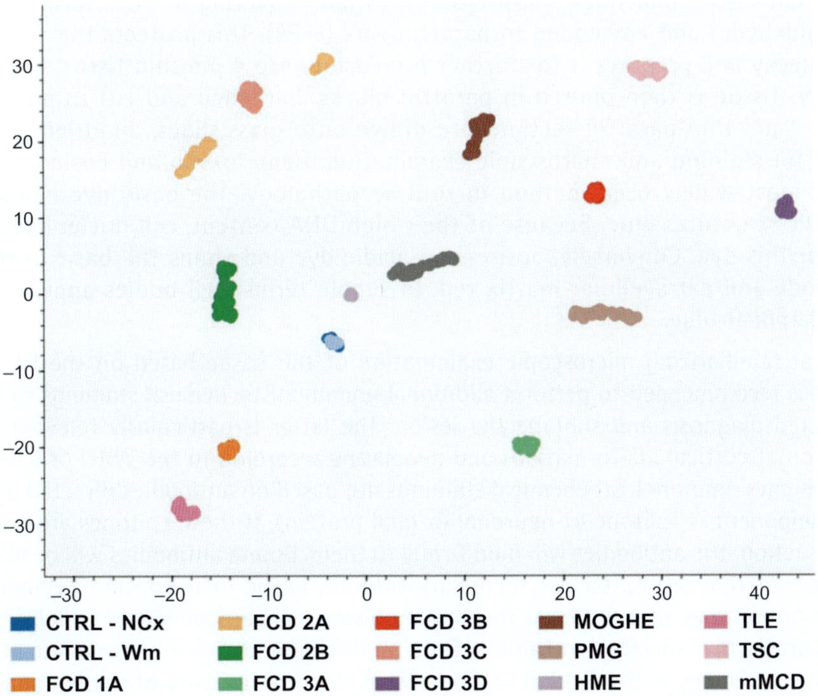

Figure 4

A novel deep learning based DNA methylation-based classifier for malformations of cortical development

Uniform Manifold Approximation and Projection of the decision boundaries of a deep learning algorithm trained to classify MCD from 308 datasets (taken from (Jabari *et al.*, 2022); this is an open access article distributed under the terms of the Creative Commons CC BY license).

CTRL: post-mortem control; NCx: neocortex; WM: white matter; FCD: Focal Cortical Dysplasia I, II and III; MOGHE: mild malformation with oligodendroglial hyperplasia in epilepsy; PMG: polymicrogyria; HME: hemimegalencephaly; TLE: temporal lobe epilepsy without cortical dysplasia; TSC: tuberous sclerosis complex; mMCD: mild malformation of cortical development.

A laboratory medicine manual for histopathology of epilepsy surgery human brain samples

It is best medical practice to submit every surgically resected human tissue sample for a systematic histopathology examination in order to obtain a scientifically sound diagnosis and provide the basis for further treatment - if necessary and applicable. It will also allow to build large enough biorepositories of well characterized human tissue samples for scientific studies. All neurosurgically resected tissues should be sent to the neuropathology laboratory to detect changes in the fine/cellular tissue structure and obtain direct information about the underlying pathomechanism. The experienced neuropathologist should also be in charge of selecting and distributing appropriate tissue samples for further research (pending approval by the institutional review board), e.g. electrophysiological intracellular recordings which require direct examination of fresh tissue or genetic research which can be performed from snap frozen tissue stored even long-term at -80°C in the biorepository. Another advantage of this protocol is that the presence and quantitative content of dysplastic tissue can be estimated by microscopy review of adjacent FFPE tissue blocks. The following laboratory manual is adapted from the ILAE recommendation for neuropathology work-up of epilepsy surgery human brain samples (Blumcke *et al.*, 2016b).

Each submitted tissue sample should be measured, weighed and documented photographically in the neuropathology laboratory. Large and anatomically coherent samples should be cut into 5 mm thick slabs, fixed in formalin overnight (10% formalin or 4% paraformaldehyde) and embedded in paraffin wax (FFPE). This protects the tissue from autolytic decay and prepares it for further processing into 4 µm thin tissue sections for microscopy. Tissue is then poured in paraffin blocks, hardened and cut using a microtome. The 4 µm thin paraffin sections are drawn onto glass slides, air-dried and made accessible for staining and microscopic examination. Hematoxylin and Eosin (HE) staining is the most widely used method in routine pathology. The basic dye hematoxylin stains acidic structures blue. Because of their high DNA content, cell nuclei have a high affinity for this dye. Conversely, eosin is an acidic dye and stains the basic proteins of the cell body and extracellular matrix red. In simple terms: cell bodies appear red and cell nuclei appear blue.

After a first familiarizing microscopic examination of the tissue based on the HE-stained sections, it is recommended to perform additional immunohistochemical stainings to confirm the suspected diagnosis and subtype the lesion. The latter is particularly relevant for the classification of cortical malformations and neoplasms according to the WHO or ILAE classification schemes. Immunohistochemical stainings are based on antibodies directed against a specific component or epitope of neuronal or glial proteins. If these epitopes are present in the tissue section, the antibodies will bind firmly to them. Bound antibodies will be visualized with a color reaction facilitated by a secondary antibody linked to an enzyme. Recommended antibodies or epitopes that are used for immunohistochemical staining of epilepsy surgery specimens are further specified in **Table 3**. Data on this Table may not be complete nor cover all available antibodies in the field. It will be always the responsibility of the histopathology laboratory to seek the necessary experience to select the appropriate antibodies and perform adjusted staining protocols. This will also allow the use of antibodies other than those recommended in **Table 3**, should similar or even more specific epitopes be recognized and scientifically confirmed by state-of-the art immunohistochemical studies, including sufficient control experiments. As mentioned above, molecular genetic testing is becoming increasingly recognized as important for an integrated neuropathological diagnosis. This involves DNA and/or RNA sequencing of selected tumor genes or the array-based examination of DNA methylation patterns. DNA or RNA extraction from microdissections of histologically selected areas is recommended to enhance the ratio of lesional to normal tissue.

Neuropathology at the operating table

In addition to the histological examination of paraffin-embedded tissue samples (as shown above), the neuropathological examination can also offer the neurosurgeon important assistance during the operation. In so-called snap frozen section examinations, a small tissue fragment from the lesion is sent intraoperatively to the neuropathologist. They will freeze the tissue in liquid nitrogen and process the hardened tissue into 10 µm thin sections using a cryostat. These sections will be thawed on a glass slide, fixed in an alcoholic solution and analyzed with a conventional HE stain using the light microscope. In this way, the neuropathologist can recognize the essential characteristics of the underlying disease and communicate these to the neurosurgeon during the operation. This can sometimes help to perform a neurosurgical procedure

Epitope	Antibody	Staining pattern	Diagnostic reasoning
CD34	QBend10	Onco-fetal marker	Ganglioglioma
CD45	LCA	Lymphocytes	Inflammation or encephalitis
CD68	KP1	Macrophages and microglia	Resorption (stroke) or Rasmussen nodules
CNPase	11-5B	Myelin sheets	Myelin architecture
GFAP	6F2	Astrocytes	Chaslin's gliosis, other astrogliosis or astroglial neoplasia
IDH1	H09	Glioma cells	IDH1 R132H mutation
Ki67	MIB1	Proliferation active nuclei	Cellular proliferation
MAP2	HM2	Neurons or neoplastically transformed glia	Heterotopic neurons or neoplastically transformed glia
NeuN	A60	Neuronal nuclei	Neocortical and hippocampal layered organization
Neurofilaments	SMI32	Dysmorphic neurons	FCD IIA and IIB
pS6	Ser 235/236	Dysmorphic neurons and balloon cells	activated mTOR in FCD IIA/IIB, TSC and HME, but also expressed in reactive astrocytes
Vimentin*	V9	Balloon cells	FCD IIB, but also expressed in reactive astrocytes
Alpha-ß-Crystallin*		Balloon cells	FCD IIB, but also expressed in reactive astrocytes

CD: cluster of differentiation; CD34: class II epitope; CNPase: cyclic nucleotide phosphodiesterase; FCD: Focal Cortical Dysplasia; GFAP: glial fibrillary acidic protein; HS: hippocampal sclerosis; IDH1: mutation-specific antibody against isocitrate dehydrogenase 1; MAP2: microtubule associated protein 2; pS6: phosphorylated S6-protein.

* suggested antibodies for the detection of balloon cells are not specific as they simultaneously stain other reactive glial cell elements.

Table 3

Panel of immunohistochemical markers to be used in the histopathology work-up of epilepsy surgery human brain samples (modified from Blumcke *et al.*, 2016b)

more precisely or to completely resect the lesion. The frozen tissue can also be preserved for many years in biorepositories and be reevaluated at a later stage when new diagnostic tools become available. In this way, we can contribute to the continuous progress in understanding of disease mechanisms and development of innovative therapies in the long term.

Outlook and conclusion

The aim of epilepsy surgery is to achieve complete freedom from seizures by resection of the brain tissue that triggers the seizures. The resected tissue removed by epilepsy surgery is sent to the neuropathological laboratory in order to detect changes in its fine structure, thus obtaining direct information about the underlying etiology and likely pathomechanism. With increasing experience and more scientifically based evidence, the neuropathological diagnosis will enhance the likelihood to predict even long-term seizure outcome (Jehi *et al.*, 2015).

During the past decade, there were considerable advances in understanding the genetic and morphogenic foundation of cortical malformations (Blumcke *et al.*, 2021a). Focal brain malformations result from somatic (post-zygotic) variants in several genes related to the mTOR pathway in FCD II, *AKT3, DEPDC5, MTOR, NPRL2/3, PIK3CA, RHEB, TSC1/2* and others, or in the galactose transporter gene *SLC35A2* in MOGHE, and which were acquired early during cortical development. The timing of the genetic event, the specific gene involved and the targeted precursor cell populations will determine the nature and size of the lesion. There is also emerging evidence of epigenetic processes underlying a 'molecular memory' in epileptogenesis (Jablonski *et al.*, 2021), and which also helped to establish a diagnostic DNA methylation classification scheme (Jabari *et al.*, 2021). This knowledge will finally accumulate and lead to a better undestanding of why and how patients with these lesions have epilepsy and to move toward precision medicine in patients with drug-resistant focal epilepsy.

These topics will be continuously addressed and discussed also at the annual ILAE summer school of Neuropathology and Epilepsy Surgery (https: //www.ilae.org/congresses). Please search the website for further information regarding next available courses and the application procedure.

References

Arena A, Zimmer T. S, Van Scheppingen J, *et al.* Oxidative Stress and inflammation in a Spectrum of Epileptogenic Cortical Malformations: Molecular insights into their interdependence. *Brain Pathol* 2019; 29: 351-65.

Avansini S. H, Torres F. R, Vieira A. S, *et al.* Dysregulation of Neurog2 Plays a Key Role in Focal Cortical Dysplasia. *Ann Neurol* 2018; 83: 623-35.

Baldassari S, Ribierre T, Marsan E, *et al.* Dissecting the Genetic Basis of Focal Cortical Dysplasia: a Large Cohort Study. *Acta Neuropathol* 2019; 138: 885-900.

Blauwblomme T, Dossi E, Pellegrino C, *et al.* Gamma-Aminobutyric Acidergic Transmission Underlies interictal Epileptogenicity in Pediatric Focal Cortical Dysplasia. *Ann Neurol* 2019; 85: 204-17.

Blumcke I, Aronica E, Becker A, *et al.* Low-Grade Epilepsy-Associated Neuroepithelial Tumours - the 2016 Who Classification. *Nat Rev Neurol* 2016a; 12: 732-40.

Blumcke I, Aronica E, Miyata, H, *et al.* international Recommendation For a Comprehensive Neuropathologic Workup of Epilepsy Surgery Brain Tissue: a Consensus Task Force Report From the Ilae Commission On Diagnostic Methods. *Epilepsia* 2016b; 57: 348-358.

Blumcke I, Budday S, Poduri A, *et al.* Neocortical Development and Epilepsy: insights From Focal Cortical Dysplasia and Brain Tumours. *Lancet Neurol* 2021a; 20: 943-55.

Blumcke I, Cendes F, Miyata, H, *et al.* Toward a Refined Genotype-Phenotype Classification Scheme For the international Consensus Classification of Focal Cortical Dysplasia. *Brain Pathol* 2021b; 31: E12956.

Blumcke I, Coras R, Busch R. M, *et al.* Toward a Better Definition of Focal Cortical Dysplasia: An Iterative Histopathological and Genetic Agreement Trial. *Epilepsia* 2021c; 62: 1416-28.

Blumcke I, Coras R, Wefers A. K, *et al.* Challenges in the Histopathological Classification of Ganglioglioma and Dnt: Microscopic Agreement Studies and a Preliminary Genotype-Phenotype Analysis. *Neuropathol Appl Neurobiol* 2019; 45: 95-107.

Blumcke I, Sarnat H. B. Somatic Mutations Rather Than Viral infection Classify Focal Cortical Dysplasia Type II As Mtoropathy. *Curr Opin Neurol, 2016;* 29: 388-95.

Blümcke I, Spreafico R, Haaker G, *et al.* Histopathological Findings in Brain Tissue Obtained During Epilepsy Surgery. *N Engl J Med,* 2017; 377: 1648-1656.

Blümcke I, Thom M, Aronica E, *et al.* The Clinico-Pathological Spectrum of Focal Cortical Dysplasias: a Consensus Classification Proposed by an Ad Hoc Task Force of the Ilae Diagnostic Methods Commission. *Epilepsia, 2011;* 52: 158-174.

Bonduelle T, Hartlieb T, Baldassari S, *et al.* Frequent Slc35a2 Brain Mosaicism in Mild Malformation of Cortical Development with Oligodendroglial Hyperplasia in Epilepsy (Moghe). *Acta Neuropathol Commun* 2021; 9: 3.

Brodmann K. 1908. Beiträge Zur Histologischen Lokalisierung Der Grosshirnrinde. Vi. Mitteilung: Die Cortexgliederung Des Menschen (in German). *J Physiol Neurol* 10: 231-246.

Capper D, Jones D. T. W, Sill M, *et al.* DNA Methylation-Based Classification of Central Nervous System Tumours. *Nature,* 2018; 555: 469-474.

Cepeda C, Andre V. M, Flores-Hernandez J, *et al.* Pediatric Cortical Dysplasia: Correlations Between Neuroimaging, Electrophysiology and Location of Cytomegalic Neurons and Balloon Cells and Glutamate/Gaba Synaptic Circuits. *Dev Neurosci,* 2005; 27: 59-76.

Chamberlain W. A, Cohen M. L, Gyure K. A, *et al.* interobserver and intraobserver Reproducibility in Focal Cortical Dysplasia (Malformations of Cortical Development). *Epilepsia* 2009, 50: 2593-8.

Chassoux F, Devaux B, Landre E, *et al.* Stereoelectroencephalography in Focal Cortical Dysplasia: a 3d Approach To Delineating the Dysplastic Cortex. *Brain* 2000, 123 (Pt 8): 1733-51.

Coras R, De Boer O. J, Armstrong D, *et al.* Good interobserver and intraobserver Agreement in the Evaluation of the New Ilae Classification of Focal Cortical Dysplasias. *Epilepsia* 2012, 53: 1341-8.

Cotter D, Honavar M, Lovestone S, *et al.* Disturbance of Notch-1 and Wnt Signalling Proteins in Neuroglial Balloon Cells and Abnormal Large Neurons in Focal Cortical Dysplasia in Human Cortex. *Acta Neuropathol (Berl) 1999,* 98: 465-72.

D'gama A. M, Woodworth Hossain A. A, *et al.* Somatic Mutations Activating the Mtor Pathway in Dorsal Telencephalic Progenitors Cause a Continuum of Cortical Dysplasias. *Cell Rep* 2017, 21: 3754-66.

Demerath T, Donkels C, Reisert M, *et al.* Gray-White Matter Blurring of the Temporal Pole Associated with Hippocampal Sclerosis: a Microstructural Study involving 3 T MRI and Ultrastructural Histopathology. *Cereb Cortex* 2021. 13: Bhab320

Emery J. A, Roper S. N, Rojiani A. M. White Matter Neuronal Heterotopia in Temporal Lobe Epilepsy: a Morphometric and Immunohistochemical Study. *J Neuropathol Exp Neurol* 1997, 56: 1276-82.

Gaballa A, Woermann F. G, Cloppenborg T, *et al.* Clinical Characteristics and Postoperative Seizure Outcome in Patients with Mild Malformation of Cortical Development and Oligodendroglial Hyperplasia. *Epilepsia* 2021; 62: 2920-2931.

Garbelli R, Milesi G, Medici V, *et al.* 2012. Blurring in Patients with Temporal Lobe Epilepsy: Clinical, High-Field Imaging and Ultrastructural Study. *Brain,* 135: 2337-49.

Hartlieb T, Winkler P, Coras R, *et al.* Age-Related Mr Characteristics in Mild Malformation of Cortical Development with Oligodendroglial Hyperplasia and Epilepsy (Moghe). *Epilepsy Behav* 2019; 91: 68-74.

Holthausen H, Coras R, Tang Y, *et al.* Multilobar Unilateral Hypoplasia with Emphasis On the Posterior Quadrant and Severe Epilepsy in Children with FCD Ilae Type 1a. *Epilepsia* 2022, 63: 42-60.

Iffland P. H, Carson V, Bordey A, Crino P. B. Gatoropathies: the Role of Amino Acid Regulatory Gene Mutations in Epilepsy and Cortical Malformations. *Epilepsia* 2019; 60: 2163-73.

Iyer A, Zurolo E, Spliet W. G, Van Rijen P. C, Baayen J. C, Gorter J. A, Aronica E. Evaluation of the innate and Adaptive Immunity in Type I and Type II Focal Cortical Dysplasias. *Epilepsia* 2010, 51: 1763-73.

Jabari S, Kobow K, Pieper T, *et al.* DNA Methylation-Based Classification of Malformations of Cortical Development in the Human Brain. *Acta Neuropathologica* 2022,; 143 (1): 93-104.

Jablonski J, Hoffmann L, Blumcke I, *et al.* Experimental Epileptogenesis in a Cell Culture Model of Primary Neurons From Rat Brain: a Temporal Multi-Scale Study. *Cells* 2021; 10 (11): 3004.

Jehi L, Yardi R, Chagin K, *et al.* Development and Validation of Nomograms To Provide individualised Predictions of Seizure Outcomes After Epilepsy Surgery: a Retrospective Analysis. *Lancet Neurol* 2015, 14: 283-90.

Lamberink H. J, Otte W. M, Blümcke I, Braun K. P. J. Seizure Outcome and Use of Antiepileptic Drugs After Epilepsy Surgery According To Histopathological Diagnosis: a Retrospective Multicentre Cohort Study. *Lancet Neurol* 2020; 19: 748-57.

Lamparello P, Baybis M, Pollard J, Hol E. M, Eisenstat D. D, Aronica E, Crino P. B. Developmental Lineage of Cell Types in Cortical Dysplasia with Balloon Cells. *Brain* 2007, 130: 2267-76.

Marin-Padilla M. Developmental Neuropathology and Impact of Perinatal Brain Damage. Iii: Gray Matter Lesions of the Neocortex. *J Neuropathol Exp Neurol* 1999, 58: 407-29.

Miyata H, Kuwashige H, Hori T, *et al.* Variable Histopathology Features of Neuronal Dyslamination in the Cerebral Neocortex Adjacent To Epilepsy-Associated Vascular Malformations Suggest Complex Pathogenesis of Focal Cortical Dysplasia Ilae Type Iiic. *Brain Patho L*2022: E13052.

Mountcastle V. B. the Columnar Organization of the Neocortex. *Brain* 1997, 120 (Pt 4): 701-22.

Muhlebner A, Coras R, Kobow K, *et al.* Neuropathologic Measurements in Focal Cortical Dysplasias: Validation of the Ilae 2011 Classification System and Diagnostic Implications For MRI. *Acta Neuropathol* 2012, 123: 259-72.

Najm I, Lal D, Vanegas MA *et al.* The ILAE consensus classification of Focal Cortical Dysplasia (FCD): an update proposed by an ad hoc Task Force of the ILAE Diagnostic Methods commission. *Epilepsia* 2022, in press.

Najm I. M, Sarnat H. B; Blümcke I. the international Consensus Classification of Focal Cortical Dysplasia - a Critical Update 2018. *Neuropathol Appl Neurobiol* 2018; 44: 18-31.

Owens G. C, Garcia A. J, Mochizuki A. Y, *et al.* Evidence For innate and Adaptive Immune Responses in a Cohort of intractable Pediatric Epilepsy Surgery Patients. *Front Immunol* 2019; 10: 121.

Palmini A, Gambardella A, Andermann F, *et al.* intrinsic Epileptogenicity of Human Dysplastic Cortex as Suggested by Corticography and Surgical Results. *Ann Neurol* 1995, 37: 476-87.

Palmini A, Najm I, Avanzini G, *et al.* Terminology and Classification of the Cortical Dysplasias. *Neurology* 2004, 62: S2-8.

Rakic, P. 1988. Specification of Cerebral Cortical Areas. *Science*, 241: 170-6.

Rampp S, Rossler K, Hamer H, *et al.* Dysmorphic Neurons As Cellular Source For Phase-Amplitude Coupling in Focal Cortical Dysplasia Type II. *Clin Neurophysiol*, 2021 132: 782-92.

Rojiani A. M, Emery J. A, Anderson K. J, Massey J. K. Distribution of Heterotopic Neurons in Normal Hemispheric White Matter: a Morphometric Analysis. *J Neuropathol Exp Neurol* 1996, 55: 178-83.

Schurr J, Coras R, Rossler K, *et al.* Mild Malformation of Cortical Development with Oligodendroglial Hyperplasia in Frontal Lobe Epilepsy: a New Clinico-Pathological Entity. *Brain Pathol* 2017, 27: 26-35.

Slegers, R. J, Blumcke, I. Low-Grade Developmental and Epilepsy Associated Brain Tumors: a Critical Update 2020. *Acta Neuropathol Commun* 2020; 8 (1): 27.

Spreafico R. 2010. Are Some Focal Cortical Dysplasias Post-Migratory Cortical Malformaitons? *Epileptic Disord*, 12: 169-71.

Tassi L, Colombo, N, Garbelli R, *et al.* Focal Cortical Dysplasia: Neuropathological Subtypes, Eeg, Neuroimaging and Surgical Outcome. *Brain* 2002, 125: 1719-32.

Taylor D. C, Falconer M. A, Bruton C. J, Corsellis J. A. Focal Dysplasia of the Cerebral Cortex in Epilepsy. *J Neurol Neurosurg Psychiatry* 1971, 34: 369-387.

Thom M, Eriksson S, Martinian L, *et al.* Temporal Lobe Sclerosis Associated with Hippocampal Sclerosis in Temporal Lobe Epilepsy: Neuropathological Features. *J Neuropathol Exp Neurol* 2009, 68: 928-38.

Urbach, H, Scheffler B; Heinrichsmeier T, *et al.* Focal Cortical Dysplasia of Taylor's Balloon Cell Type: a Clinicopathological Entity with Characteristic Neuroimaging and Histopathological Features, and Favorable Postsurgical Outcome. *Epilepsia* 2002, 43: 33-40.

Wang D, Blumcke I, Gui Q, Zhou W, Zuo H, Lin J, Luo Y. Clinico-Pathological investigations of Rasmussen Encephalitis Suggest Multifocal Disease Progression and Associated Focal Cortical Dysplasia. *Epileptic Disord* 2013a, 15: 32-43.

Wang D. D, Piao Y. S, Blumcke I, *et al.* A Distinct Clinicopathological Variant of Focal Cortical Dysplasia IIId Characterized by Loss of Layer 4 in the Occipital Lobe in 12 Children with Remote Hypoxic-Ischemic injury. *Epilepsia* 2017, 58: 1697-705.

Wang I, Bernasconi A, Bernhardt B, *et al.* MRI Essentials in Epileptology: a Review From the Ilae Imaging Taskforce. *Epileptic Disord* 2020a, 22: 421-437.

Wang I, Oh S, Blümcke I, *et al.* Value of 7t MRI and Post-Processing in Patients with Nonlesional 3T MRI Undergoing Epilepsy Presurgical Evaluation. *Epilepsia* 2020b; 61: 2509-20.

Wang Z. I, Alexopoulos A. V, Jones S. E, Jaisani Z, Najm I. M, Prayson R. A. The Pathology of Magnetic-Resonance-Imaging-Negative Epilepsy. *Mod Pathol.* 2013b.

Witters P, Tahata S, Barone R, *et al.* Clinical and Biochemical Improvement with Galactose Supplementation in Slc35a2-Cdg. *Genet Med*, 2020; 22: 1102-7.

Xu D, Robinson A. P, Ishii T, *et al.* Peripherally Derived T Regulatory and Gammadelta T Cells Have Opposing Roles in the Pathogenesis of intractable Pediatric Epilepsy. *J Exp Med* 2018; 215: 1169-86.

Zurolo E, Iyer A, Maroso M, *et al.* Activation of Toll-Like Receptor, Rage and HMGB1 Signalling in Malformations of Cortical Development. *Brain* 2011, 134: 1015-32.

Part II. FROM GENES TO CLINICAL PICTURE

CHAPTER

4. Genetics of FCD: an emerging scenario

Sara Baldassari, Stéphanie Baulac

Key points

- Post-zygotic somatic variants arising during brain development have emerged as a major cause of FCD.
- Somatic variants in the PI3K-AKT-mTOR pathway genes for FCD II: single-hit somatic gain-of-function variants in mTOR activators and two-hit germline/somatic loss-of-function variants in mTOR repressors.
- Galactose transporter *SLC35A2* loss-of-function variants account for mild MCD with oligodendroglial hyperplasia and epilepsy.
- Somatic variants are enriched in abnormal FCD II cell types, i.e. dysmorphic neurons and balloon cells.
- The size of the dysplastic lesion depends on when the mutation occurs, with mutations occurring in early progenitors causing larger lesions than late mutations.
- Genetic testing in cerebrospinal fluid is a promising tool for early genetic diagnosis.
- Advances in genetics will pinpoint novel therapeutic targets.

Introduction

FCD are malformations of brain cortical development affecting a localized brain region and manifesting with drug-resistant focal epilepsy and developmental delay (Guerrini and Dobyns, 2014). Resective neurosurgery is often required to control seizures, allowing access to dysplastic tissue for diagnostic and research purposes. In 2011, the Diagnostic Methods Commission of the International League Against Epilepsy (ILAE) released a first international consensus classification of FCD into 3 subtypes (FCD I, II, III) based on histopathological findings, when the genetic etiology was still unknown (Blumcke *et al.*, 2011). The classification was revised in 2018 (Najm *et al.*, 2018) and recently updated (Najm *et al.*, 2022, in press).

Most FCD cases are isolated (sporadic), but few familial cases have also been reported, suggesting a genetic origin of the malformations. FCD cases can be identified in families with recurrence of focal epilepsy, or co-occurrence of FCD, HME and brain tumors (ganglioglioma, dysembryoplastic neuroepithelial tumor) (Leventer *et al.*, 2014, Baulac *et al.*, 2015). In the past years, an increasingly recognized role in neurodevelopmental and neuropsychiatric diseases have been attributed to somatic variants (which occur post-zygotically in soma cells) (McConnell *et al.*, 2017). It is now well recognized that during normal human development, each dividing cell propagates mutations to its daughter cells and these mutations are considered clonal. The human brain is therefore a mosaic of cells with their own unique genome (Lodato *et al.*, 2015, Bizzotto *et al.*, 2021) (**Figure 1**). Based on the timing of the mutational event during development, a somatic variant can be present in multiple tissues (early event) or restricted to a single tissue or cell population (late event). Variants present only in neuronal cells can be identified only by accessing the mutated brain tissue.

The advent of high-coverage next-generation sequencing approaches and dedicated bioinformatic tools facilitated the identification of somatic variants in resected brain tissues from focal cortical malformations (D'Gama and Walsh, 2018, Koh and Lee, 2018, Marsan and Baulac, 2018). Recent findings have emphasized that FCD subgroups are genetically distinct: a subset of FCD I (which also includes mMCD and MOGHE) is caused by glycosylation defects as a consequence of loss-of-function *SCL35A2* somatic variants while FCD II are caused by somatic variants in the PI3K-AKT-mTOR pathway (Mirzaa *et al.*, 2016, D'Gama *et al.*, 2017, Baldassari *et al.*, 2019b, Sim *et al.*, 2019). The genetic etiology of FCD III remains unknown.

In this chapter, we review the most recent genetic findings of FCD, focusing especially on FCD II, and explore future perspectives for early genetic diagnosis and targeted therapies.

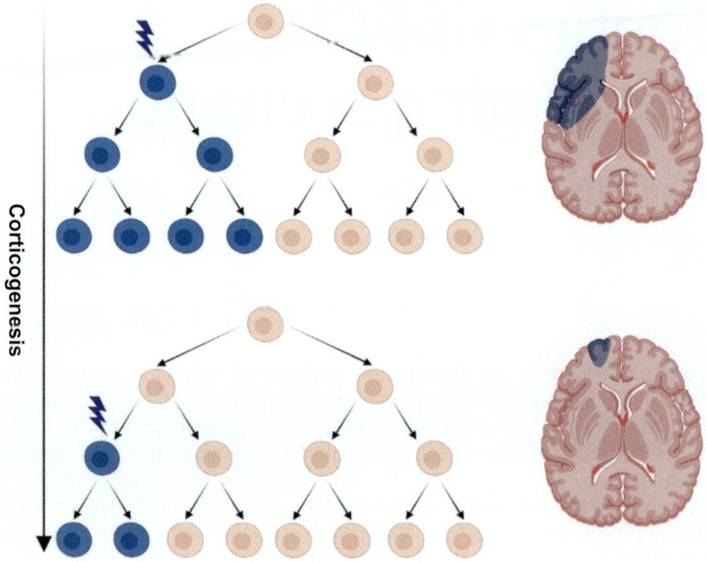

Figure 1

Somatic mosaicism in the brain

Postzygotic somatic mutations can occur in different progenitor cells during brain development (corticogenesis in particular). Somatic mutations occurring early will be shared by a larger proportion of cells derived from the initial progenitor and cause larger dysplasia (upper panel), while mutations occurring at the end of corticogenesis will be shared by fewer cells and cause a smaller dysplasia (lower panel). Mutated cells and dysplastic brain are represented in blue.

Genetics of FCD II

FCD II is histologically characterized by localized cortical disorganization and the presence of dysmorphic neurons (present in FCD IIa and FCD IIb) and balloon cells (present in FCD IIb only) (chapter 3).

The first indications pointing to mechanistic target of rapamycin complex 1 (mTORC1) pathway hyperactivation in FCD II emerged from histological comparative studies with cortical tubers found in patients with TSC. TSC is a multisystem disorder caused by germline loss-of-function variants in genes encoding components of the TSC complex (*TSC1* and *TSC2*), a repressor of the mTOR complex 1 (mTORC1). Cortical tubers, are characterized by the presence of giant cells and cytomegalic neurons, which resemble the balloon cells and dysmorphic neurons observed in FCD II. In the context of these histopathological similarities, two research groups in 2004 showed that abnormal cell types from both tubers in TSC and FCD II specimens displayed mTOR hyperactivation, as shown by increased phosphorylated-S6 (pS6) protein immunoreactivity (a standard readout of mTOR activation) (Baybis *et al.*, 2004, Miyata *et al.*, 2004) (**Figure 2**). These studies indicated that mTOR pathway hyperactivation is a hallmark common to both TSC and FCD II and may be the cause of a spectrum of developmental brain malformations with cytomegalic cells. Nonetheless, the genetic components leading to FCD II and HME remained elusive until recently (see chronological narrative review (Lee *et al.*, 2022)).

The mammalian target of rapamycin (mTOR) is an evolutionarily conserved serine/threonine kinase present in every cell of the body within two protein complexes, mTOR complex 1 (mTORC1) and mTOR complex 2 (mTORC2). The mTOR signaling cascade controls several fundamental processes, such as protein synthesis, cell growth, metabolism and autophagy (Saxton and Sabatini, 2017, Kim and Guan, 2019). mTORC1 and mTORC2 are finely regulated by several upstream factors (e.g., nutrients such as glucose and amino acids, growth factors, ATP) that signal on the energetic/metabolic state of the cell. In the brain, the mTOR signaling pathway contributes to proper neural development, synaptic transmission and plasticity and neural network activity (reviewed in (Lipton and Sahin, 2014, Lasarge and Danzer, 2014, Crino, 2016)). Given the pathway's central role in directing cell growth, it is not surprising that mTOR pathway hyperactivation leads to morphologically abnormal cells with enlarged soma size as observed in TSC and FCD II/HME specimens. A myriad of proteins, upstream effectors and substrates participate in the different branches of the mTOR pathway, to activate (e.g., in conditions of high nutrients availability), or to repress (e.g., the above cited TSC complex components, in conditions of low nutrient cellular levels) the pathway. Downstream substrates of mTORC1 signalling that modulate these pivotal cellular processes include ribosomal protein S6 kinase (S6K) and eukaryotic initiation factor 4E-binding protein, which are commonly used to monitor the activity of the pathway.

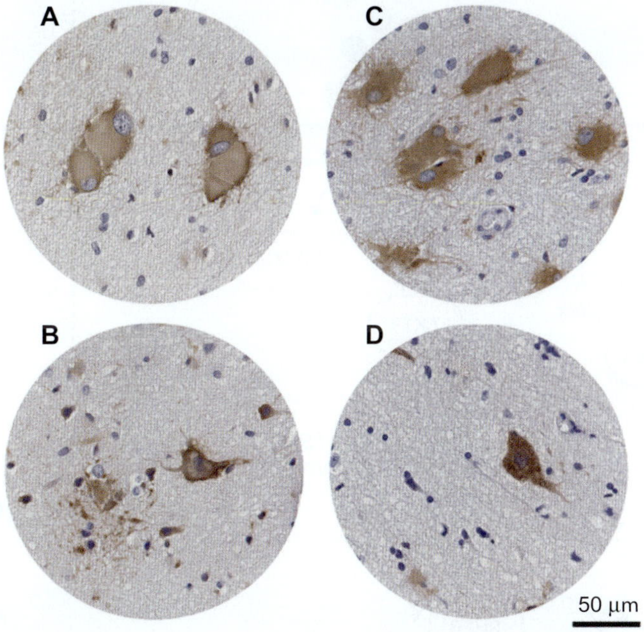

Figure 2

mTOR hyperactivation in TSC and FCD II brain tissues

Balloon cells (in A and C) and dysmorphic neurons (in B and D) in both TSC (A and B) and FCD II (C and D) tissues show strong immunoreactivity for phosphorylated S6 protein (target of mTOR kinase activity). Nuclei are stained with hematoxylin (in blue), phospho-S6 immunoreactivity is shown by DAB reactivity (in brown).

The focal nature of FCD II, combined with the mosaic pattern of mTOR hyperactivation in the resected tissues (presence of cytomegalic mTOR-hyperactivated cells intermingled with normal cells), is evocative of a possible signature of postzygotic somatic variants. This hypothesis was initially confirmed in large lesions such as megalencephaly and hemispheric dysplasia (HME), with the identification of brain somatic activating variants in the mTOR pathway components *PIK3CA, AKT3 and MTOR* genes and somatic duplication of chromosome 1q (that includes *AKT3* gene) (Lee *et al.*, 2012, Riviere *et al.*, 2012, Poduri *et al.*, 2012). Pathogenic variants were identified at high mosaic rates (or variant allele frequency (VAF), ≥ 8%). Few years later, it became clear that smaller malformations such as FCD II are also due to mutations in the PI3K-AKT-mTOR pathway genes, but are restricted to a smaller group of cells (therefore at smaller VAFs), thus requiring more sensitive sequencing techniques for their detection (e.g., high-coverage targeted gene panel or high-depth exome sequencing). Brain somatic variants in *PIK3CA, AKT3, MTOR* genes were later on discovered also in smaller FCD II malformations at lower mosaic rates (usually less than 5%) compared to those found in HME (Jansen *et al.*, 2015, Mirzaa *et al.*, 2016, D'Gama *et al.*, 2015, Baek *et al.*, 2015).

It is now well established that somatic mTOR pathway hyperactivating variants in a small set of genes account for most FCD II and HME cases (reviewed in (Blumcke *et al.*, 2021, Lee *et al.*, 2022). Two molecular mechanisms, both leading to mTOR hyperactivation are involved: 1/ single-hit gain-of-function somatic variants in an mTOR pathway activator encoding gene, and 2/ two-hit loss-of-function variants in an mTOR pathway inhibitor encoding gene. One study reported a possible cumulative effect of two mosaic variants (MTOR p.S2215F and RPS6 p.R232H) in mTOR pathway activators in a patient with HME (Pelorosso *et al.*, 2019).

Somatic single-hit mutations in mTOR pathway activators

Recent studies on large cohorts of FCD II and HME have demonstrated that somatic gain-of-function variants in activators of mTOR signaling pathway (*PIK3CA, AKT3, RHEB, MTOR*) are the most frequently encountered **(Figure 3)** (Jansen *et al.*, 2015, Baldassari *et al.*, 2019b, Sim *et al.*, 2019, D'Gama *et al.*, 2017, Lai *et al.*, 2021). These variants, usually missense variants, are brain-specific (e.g., not detected in DNA derived from blood) and are sufficient to cause the dysplastic lesion. The diagnostic rate is variable (from ~30 to ~60%) across different studies, and may depend on the sequencing approach applied (e.g., targeted panel or whole

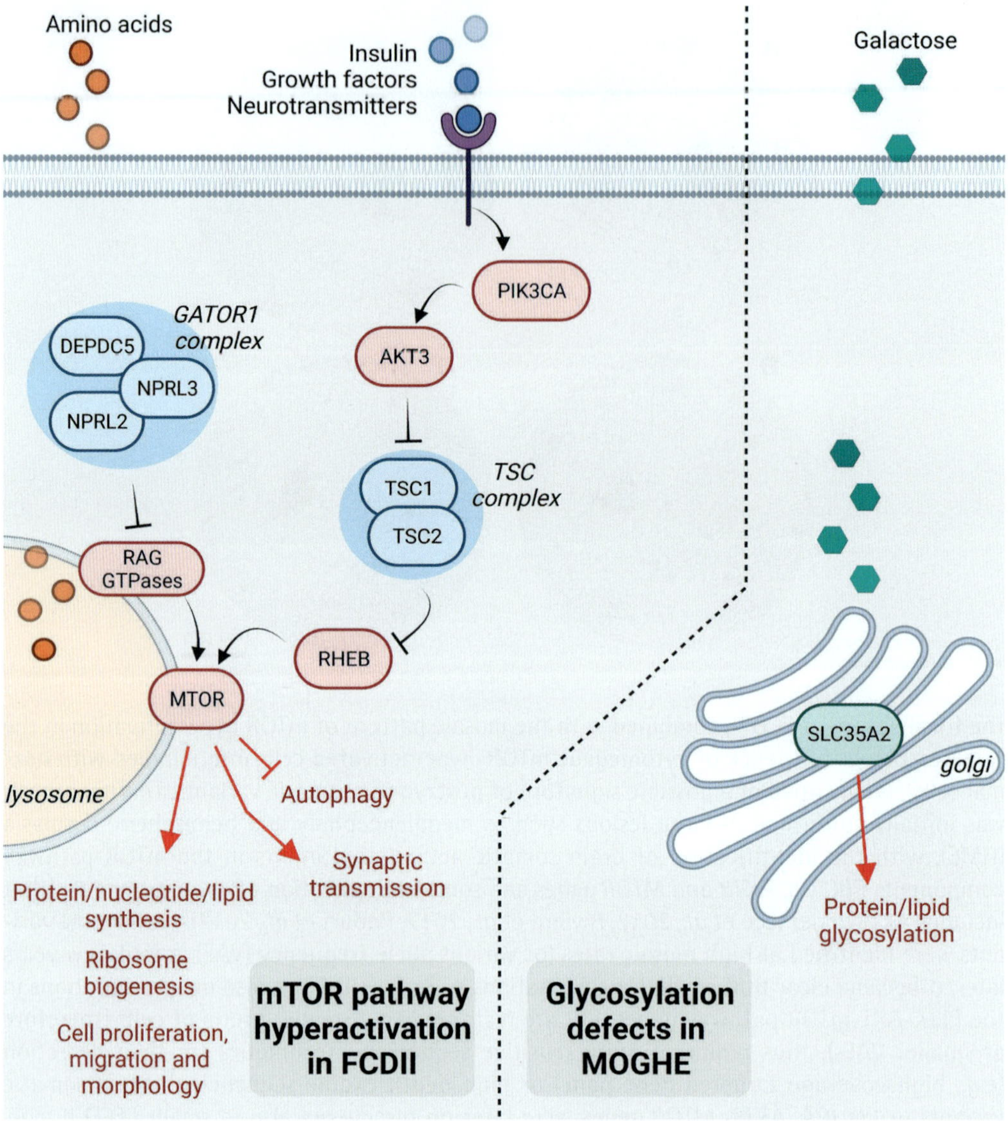

Figure 3

mTOR pathway hyperactivation and glycosylation defects cause a spectrum of focal brain malformations

On the left part of the schematic, mTOR pathway hyperactivation can be caused by somatic gain-of-function mutations in the mTOR pathway activators PIK3CA, AKT3, RHEB and MTOR (in red), or loss-of-function mutations in components of the TSC and GATOR1 complexes (in blue), that inhibit mTOR in response to different external or cellular signaling (e.g., growth factors and amino acid levels). mTOR controls several metabolic and catabolic processes in the cell, and its dysregulation has an important impact on the normal cellular functions. On the right part of the schematic, glycosylation is defective in the presence of SLC35A2 loss-of-function mutations, because of the reduced import of galactose sugars within the Golgi apparatus, where most of the glycosylation modifications occur. Mutations in different pathways lead to different histopathological entities: FCD II in the case of mTOR pathway components; MOGHE in the case of SLC35A2-mediated glycosylation.

exome sequencing), the DNA quality (whether it is extracted from formalin-fixed paraffin embedded (FFPE) or frozen tissue) or the degree of pathology of the sequenced tissue (i.e., the density of dysmorphic neurons and balloon cells in FCD II). Hotspot variants (also observed in cancer tissues) are commonly detected in *PIK3CA* (e.g. p.E545K, p.H1047R), *AKT3* (p.E17K) and *MTOR* (e.g. p.L1460P, p.T1977R, p.S2215F, p.S2215Y) gene itself, which is mutated in more than half of the FCD II cases (Baldassari *et al.*, 2019b, Sim *et al.*, 2019). A minority of FCD II/HME cases present with somatic activating variants in *RHEB* gene (Salinas *et al.*, 2018,

Baldassari *et al.*, 2019b, Zhao *et al.*, 2019). A study reported that the extent of the dysplastic malformation correlated with the somatic *RHEB* variant load, supporting the role of RHEB in a spectrum of cortical malformations from FCD to HME (Lee *et al.*, 2021).

Altogether, these studies have also highlighted that FCD II and HME represent a disease continuum, caused by somatic variants in the same genes but occurring at different developmental timepoints. Mutational events occurring during the earliest mitotic cycles of the periventricular neuroepithelial cells are present in a greater number of cells therefore causing large lesions and are present at high VAFs (above 5%). Events occurring during the latest mitotic cycles affect only few cells and are detected at low VAFs (below 5%) in small malformations restricted to one gyrus (D'Gama *et al.*, 2017, Marsan and Baulac, 2018). Mutations in upstream activators of the pathway such as *PIK3CA* and *AKT3* are preferentially found in large dysplasias and HME, while low-level *MTOR* mutations are more frequent in small FCD II.

• Two-hit mutations in mTOR pathway inhibitors

Activation of PI3K-AKT-mTOR pathway can also result from altered inhibition. The two major mTORC1 inhibitors are the TSC complex, composed of TSC1, TSC2 and TBC1D7 proteins, and the GTPase-activating protein (GAP) activity towards Rags 1 complex (GATOR1), formed by the interacting proteins DEPDC5, NPRL2 and NPRL3.

Germline heterozygous mutations in TSC1 and TSC2 cause Tuberous Sclerosis (Salussolia *et al.*, 2019, Martin *et al.*, 2017), while germline mutations in GATOR1 encoding genes, cause familial focal epilepsy (Iffland *et al.*, 2019). In the past few years, mutations in *DEPDC5, NPRL2* and *NPRL3* forming the GATOR1 complex genes have emerged as the most frequent cause of familial nonlesional focal epilepsies (Ricos *et al.*, 2016, Baldassari *et al.*, 2019a). Subsequent studies have shown that *DEPDC5* mutations are also found in individuals with FCD II (Scheffer *et al.*, 2014, Baulac *et al.*, 2015), and in a large cohort accounted for ~20% of cases diagnosed with cortical malformations, including FCD II (Baldassari *et al.*, 2019a). To explain the occurrence of FCD II cases within families with GATOR1 germline loss-of-function variants, the hypothesis of a bi-allelic somatic inactivation of *DEPDC5*, as in tumor suppressor genes according to the Knudson's two-hit hypothesis (Knudson, 1971), has been proposed. Moreover, this double-hit mechanism had already been shown for tumors and tubers development in TSC patients (Martin *et al.*, 2017). The first report of a somatic second-hit in a patient with FCD II and a *DEPDC5* germline variant was published in 2015 (Baulac *et al.*, 2015). In 2016, a somatic *de novo* frameshift deletion in *DEPDC5* with somatic copy number neutral loss of heterozygosity (LOH) on chromosome 22 was reported in an HME case (Mirzaa *et al.*, 2016). In recent years, *DEPDC5* double-hit mechanisms have been definitively proven in several FCD II cases, with either biallelic germline and somatic *DEPDC5* single nucleotide variants (SNV) or biallelic germline *DEPDC5* variants and a somatic LOH (Baldassari *et al.*, 2019b, Ribierre *et al.*, 2018, Lee *et al.*, 2019, Sim *et al.*, 2019). A subset of somatic variants in *TSC1* and *TSC2* genes have also been described in FCD II and HME cases, while none of these patients met clinical criteria for TSC, even when clinically re-assessed in light of these genetic findings (D'Gama *et al.*, 2017, Lim *et al.*, 2017, Baldassari *et al.*, 2019b, Sim *et al.*, 2019).

Overall, single-hit mutations in activators of the mTOR pathway or mTOR itself are more frequently detected than double-hit mutations in repressors.

• Link between genetics and neuropathology in FCD II and HME

Despite the evidence of the pathogenic role of somatic mTOR signaling hyperactivating variants (in both positive or negative regulators of the pathway) in FCD II and HME etiology, it was still not established if the emergence of dysmorphic neurons and balloon cells was directly due to mTOR hyperactivation, nor which cell types were mutated in the tissues.

In 2017, D'Gama and colleagues performed single-nuclei fluorescently activated nuclei sorting (FANS) of mutated brain tissues followed by sequencing, and found that in small lesions the mutations were restricted to the neuronal population, while in larger lesions the mutations were common to the neuronal and glial cell populations (D'Gama *et al.*, 2017). Subsequently, isolation of pools of dysmorphic neurons and balloon cells by laser capture microdissection proved that these cytomegalic cells carry the mTOR activating mutations, and thus emerge as a direct consequence of mTOR hyperactivation (Baldassari *et al.*, 2019b, Lee *et al.*, 2019, Lee *et al.*, 2021). The developmental origin of dysmorphic neurons and balloons cells remains enigmatic; however, the finding that both cell types harbor the same mutation in a given tissue suggests that they originate from a common progenitor cell.

According to the fact that dysmorphic neurons and balloon cells carry the mutations, their density in a given FCD II tissue has been confirmed to correlate not only with the variant mosaic rate but also with the epileptogenic activity observed by EEG (Lee *et al.*, 2019). Therefore, higher mutation mosaic rates have been reported in the center of the lesion and EZ, compared to the perilesional regions (Ribierre *et al.*, 2018, Lee *et al.*, 2019). Thus, the proportion of dysmorphic neurons and balloon cells in the surgically resected tissues will impact the successful identification of the causative variant (few mutated cells are difficult to spot with bulk DNA sequencing approaches because of very low mosaic rates), and may even predict the surgical outcome (e.g., the observation of very few abnormal cells in cases with suspected FCD II may suggest that the resection was incomplete).

SLC35A2 galactose transporter defects

While the involvement in FCD II physiopathology of the PI3K-AKT-mTOR signaling pathway is suspected since nearly two decades, years before the discovery of mTOR-activating somatic mutations, the biological mechanisms implicated in the etiology of FCD I have remained unknown until very recently. Neuronal migration defects during corticogenesis are considered to be responsible for these malformations, due to the observed disrupted cortical lamination and blurred junction between grey and white matter (Subramanian *et al.*, 2019).

In 2018, brain somatic loss-of-function variants were identified in *SLC35A2* gene by whole exome sequencing in a subset of cases with MRI-negative focal epilepsy, FCD I or mMCD, characterized by an excess of heterotopic neurons in the white matter (Winawer *et al.*, 2018, Sim *et al.*, 2018).

SLC35A2 (located on chromosome X) encodes a UDP-galactose transporter implicated in the transfer of UDP-galactose from the cytoplasm to the Golgi apparatus, which is required for N-glycosylation of proteins and sphingolipids. Germline *de novo SLC35A2* variants cause congenital disorder of glycosylation type IIm (MIM #300896), an X-linked dominant neurological disorder characterized by early onset epileptic encephalopathy manifesting with seizures, hypsarrhythmia, hypotonia, intellectual disability and brain malformations (Ng *et al.*, 2013, Kodera *et al.*, 2013). Somatic loss-of-function *SLC35A2* variants lead to aberrant N-glycosylation patterns, with particularly high degrees of N-acetylglucosamine in FCD I/mMCD brain specimens (Sim *et al.*, 2018).

Subsequently, somatic *SLC35A2* loss-of-function variants were identified by targeted gene sequencing in 30% of cases from FCD I and mMCD cohorts (Sim *et al.*, 2019, Baldassari *et al.*, 2019b). *SLC35A2* variant allele frequencies (VAF) ranged between 1.4% and 43%, with a VAF >5% in 70% of cases. In comparison, only 20% of FCD II are caused by mutations at VAF >5%. By using a targeted gene panel approach on DNA extracted from formalin-fixed paraffin embedded (FFPE) tissues, Bonduelle and colleagues reported that ~45% (9/20) of cases with the newly recognized developmental malformation MOGHE (mMCD with oligodendroglial cells hyperplasia in epilepsy) are caused by somatic *SLC35A2* variants (Bonduelle *et al.*, 2021). Subsequently, histopathological reassessment of 17 previously reported *SLC35A2* mutated cases confirmed a MOGHE diagnosis in nearly all cases (Bonduelle *et al.*, 2021). Whole exome/genome sequencing in *SLC35A2*-negative FCD I or other mMCD (including MOGHE) cases will likely allow the identification of the genetic etiology in the so far unsolved cases. The genetic elucidation of these cases will allow a better differential diagnosis and assessment of specific genotype-phenotype correlations that may potentially reveal predictors of epilepsy surgery outcome.

Disease modeling

The peculiar feature of FCD pathogenic variants is that they arise during neurodevelopment and are therefore present only in a subset of cells. *In utero* electroporation procedures in mice allow to mimic such somatic mutational events, contributing to a better understanding of the changes arising in the developing brain once the mutation occurs, and how these affect the adult brain function, structure, and circuit activity. This approach has been extensively used to investigate the pathomechanisms in FCD, particularly to understand how mTOR hyper-activation contributes to altered neuronal migration and differentiation, as well as to the establishment of proper neuronal circuits (extensively revised in Nguyen and Bordey, 2021).

Mosaic hyperactivation of the mTOR pathway in the developing mouse neocortex, through *in utero* electroporation (IUE) targeting cortical progenitors, constitutes an established model of FCD II. After the IUE procedure, only a subset of progenitors is transfected, allowing cellular mosaicism at the site of electroporation. IUE is typically performed at embryonic day (E) 14.5, a developmental timepoint that specifically targets radial glia that generate layer 2/3 pyramidal neurons. To reproduce gain-of-function effects of variants in mTOR pathway activators (e.g., Akt3, Mtor, Rheb), a plasmid containing the mutated transcript and a GFP tag can be electroporated in the brain of the developing mouse embryo, to induce the expression of the mutations in a focal region only in a limited number of neural progenitor cells, and the GFP tag will allow the recognition of the mutated cells among the surrounding wild-types (Baek *et al.*, 2015, Hsieh *et al.*, 2016, Lim *et al.*, 2015, Nakashima *et al.*, 2015, Park *et al.*, 2018). Loss-of-function mutations leading to mTOR activation can also be focally induced through a similar approach, but a CRISPR/Cas9 system is more commonly employed to delete the gene of interest (e.g., Tsc1/Tsc2 or Gator1 complex components) (Lim *et al.*, 2017, Ribierre *et al.*, 2018).

The expression of somatic mTOR-activating mutations in the mouse allows to recapitulate most of the FCD II neuropathological hallmarks: focal disorganization of the neuronal architecture, likely a consequence of delayed neuronal migration towards the cortical plate, as well as the presence of cytomegalic mTOR-activated neurons. Despite the evidence of morphological and immunoreactivity similarities between cytomegalic neurons in mice and dysmorphic neurons in human FCD II tissues (misorientation, increased dendrite thickness and arborization, accumulation of Nissl substance and neurofilament proteins), typical balloon-cells have not been reproduced in these models. Nonetheless, the induced alterations proved sufficient to induce spontaneous electroclinical postnatal seizures in all models, that can be prevented by pharmacological inhibition of the mTOR pathway by rapamycin administration (and its derivatives) to the pregnant dams or to the adult mice. Focal Mtor hyperactivation in mice has also been shown to lead to non-cell autonomous hyperexcitability of non-mutated neurons adjacent to the ones carrying the mutation, further highlighting the complex mechanisms at play in FCD pathology (Koh *et al.*, 2021).

FCD animal models have therefore provided important contributions to the field. Cellular reprogramming of human pluripotent stem cells to generate human brain organoids in 3D *in vitro* cultures has emerged as a powerful tool to study human development (Velasco *et al.*, 2020) and related diseases, including tuberous sclerosis (Blair *et al.*, 2018, Eichmuller *et al.*, 2022), and are likely to become models of choice to study FCD as well.

Promises for precision therapy

The identification of mTOR pathway activating mutations in FCD II and HME suggests that targeting the pathway may be a promising therapeutic option for these patients. The mTOR inhibitor everolimus is currently approved for the treatment of focal refractory seizures in patients with TSC and clinical trials are ongoing for FCD and HME (D'Gama and Poduri, 2021, Moloney *et al.*, 2021). A study reported on the efficacy of sirolimus treatment in a cohort of 16 FCD II patients and observed a seizure frequency reduction of 25%. Although the reduction of focal seizures did not meet the predetermined level of statistical significance, the potential for sirolimus in reducing seizures over time deserves further investigations (Kato *et al.*, 2022).

Likewise, galactose supplementation may partially restore the glycosylation defect observed in patients with *SLC35A2*-related malformations: in a cohort of 10 cases with *SLC35A2*-related congenital disorder of glycosylation, oral D-galactose supplementation resulted in clinical and biochemical improvement, with two patients becoming seizure-free (Witters *et al.*, 2020).

For a better diagnostic and therapeutic workup, early identification of the genetic etiology is essential. A pre-surgical genetic diagnosis would therefore have the potential to guide the most appropriate therapeutic approach for each patient. Studies in cancer have shown that genetic testing of cell-free DNA from liquid biopsies of cerebrospinal fluid allows for the detection of tumor DNA and for the discrimination among subtypes, based on mutational analysis (Mair and Mouliere, 2021). Two recent studies showed that brain specific somatic variants can be detected in cell-free DNA from cerebrospinal fluid samples collected from patients with refractory epilepsies subjected to neurosurgery (including ganglioglioma, FCD II, HME and MOGHE cases), thus establishing proof of concept for presurgical diagnosis from cerebrospinal fluid extracted from a lumbar puncture (Ye *et al.*, 2021, Kim *et al.*, 2021).

Conclusion

In the past decade, increasing evidence has shown that the human brain is a mosaic, with somatic variants arising during development contributing to both brain health and disease. Somatic variants, in the mTOR pathway components or altering protein and lipid glycosylation, present in only a few subsets of neurons, can have severe consequences on brain homeostasis and are sufficient to cause pediatric drug-resistant epilepsy. Understanding the pathomechanisms involved in epileptogenesis and elucidating the genetic etiology in so far unsolved FCD cases has a major importance for the development of precision medicine for these patients. While surgical resection of the EZ is a common approach to alleviate seizures, not all patients are eligible, which is why they would benefit from targeted therapeutics, developed to target specifically the underlying genetic defect.

References

Baek S. T, Copeland B, Yun E.J, *et al.* An Akt3-Foxg1-Reelin Network Underlies Defective Migration In Human Focal Malformations Of Cortical Development. *Nat Med*, 2015; 21: 1445-54.

Baldassari S, Picard F, Verbeek N. E, *et al.* The Landscape Of Epilepsy-Related Gator1 Variants. *Genet Med*, 2019a; 21: 398-408.

Baldassari S, Ribierre T, Marsan E, *et al.* Dissecting The Genetic Basis Of Focal Cortical Dysplasia: A Large Cohort Study. *Acta Neuropathol*, 2019b; 138: 885-900.

Baulac S, Ishida S, Marsan E, *et al.* Familial Focal Epilepsy With Focal Cortical Dysplasia Due To Depdc5 Mutations. *Ann Neurol*, 2015; 77: 675-83.

Baybis M, Yu J, Lee A, *et al.* Mtor Cascade Activation Distinguishes Tubers From Focal Cortical Dysplasia. *Ann Neurol*, 2004; 56: 478-87.

Bizzotto S, Dou, Y, Ganz, J,*et al.* Landmarks Of Human Embryonic Development Inscribed In Somatic Mutations. *Science*, 2021; 371: 1249-1253.

Blair J. D, Hockemeyer D, Bateup H. S. Genetically Engineered Human Cortical Spheroid Models Of Tuberous Sclerosis. *Nat Med*, 2018; 24: 1568-1578.

Blumcke I, Budday S, Poduri A, *et al.* Neocortical Development And Epilepsy: Insights From Focal Cortical Dysplasia And Brain Tumours. *Lancet Neurol*, 2021; 20: 943-955.

Blumcke I, Thom M, Aronica E, *et al.* The Clinicopathologic Spectrum Of Focal Cortical Dysplasias: A Consensus Classification Proposed By An Ad Hoc Task Force Of The Ilae Diagnostic Methods Commission. *Epilepsia*, 2011; 52: 158-74.

Bonduelle T, Hartlieb T, Baldassari S, *et al.* Frequent Slc35a2 Brain Mosaicism In Mild Malformation Of Cortical Development With Oligodendroglial Hyperplasia In Epilepsy (Moghe). *Acta Neuropathol Commun*, 2021; 9: 3.

Crino P. B. The Mtor Signalling Cascade: Paving New Roads To Cure Neurological Disease. *Nat Rev Neurol*, 2016; 12: 379-92.

D'gama A. M, Geng Y, Couto J. A, *et al.* Mammalian Target Of Rapamycin Pathway Mutations Cause Hemimegalencephaly And Focal Cortical Dysplasia. *Ann Neurol*, 2015; 77: 720-5.

D'gama A. M, Poduri A. Precision Therapy For Epilepsy Related To Brain Malformations. *Neurotherapeutics*, 2021; 18: 1548-1563.

D'gama A. M, Walsh C. A. Somatic Mosaicism And Neurodevelopmental Disease. *Nat Neurosci*, 2018; 21: 1504-1514.

D'gama A. M, Woodworth M. B, Hossain A. A, *et al.* Somatic Mutations Activating The Mtor Pathway In Dorsal Telencephalic Progenitors Cause A Continuum Of Cortical Dysplasias. *Cell Rep*, 2017; 21: 3754-3766.

Eichmuller O. L, Corsini N. S, Vertesy A, *et al.* Amplification Of Human Interneuron Progenitors Promotes Brain Tumors And Neurological Defects. *Science*, 2022; 375: eabf5546.

Guerrini R, Dobyns W. B. Malformations Of Cortical Development: Clinical Features And Genetic Causes. *Lancet Neurol*, 2014; 13: 710-26.

Hsieh L. S, Wen J. H, Claycomb K, *et al.* Convulsive Seizures From Experimental Focal Cortical Dysplasia Occur Independently Of Cell Misplacement. *Nat Commun*, 2016; 7: 11753.

Iffland P. H, 2nd, Carson V, Bordey A, Crino P. B. Gatoropathies: The Role Of Amino Acid Regulatory Gene Mutations In Epilepsy And Cortical Malformations. *Epilepsia*, 2019; 60: 2163-2173.

Jansen L. A, Mirzaa G. M, Ishak G. E, *et al.* Pi3k/Akt Pathway Mutations Cause A Spectrum Of Brain Malformations From Megalencephaly To Focal Cortical Dysplasia. *Brain,* 2015; 138: 1613-28.

Kato M, Kada A, Shiraishi, H, *et al.* Sirolimus For Epileptic Seizures Associated With Focal Cortical Dysplasia Type II. *Ann Clin Transl Neurol* 2022; 9: 181-92.

Kim J, Guan K. L. Mtor As A Central Hub Of Nutrient Signalling And Cell Growth. *Nat Cell Biol,* 2019; 21: 63-71.

Kim S, Baldassari S, Sim, N. S, *et al.* Detection Of Brain Somatic Mutations In Cerebrospinal Fluid From Refractory Epilepsy Patients. *Ann Neurol,* 2021; 89: 1248-1252.

Knudson A. G, Jr. Mutation And Cancer: Statistical Study Of Retinoblastoma. *Proc Natl Acad Sci U S A,* 1971; 68: 820-3.

Kodera H, Nakamura K, Osaka H, *et al.* De Novo Mutations In Slc35a2 Encoding A Udp-Galactose Transporter Cause Early-Onset Epileptic Encephalopathy. *Hum Mutat,* 2013; 34: 1708-14.

Koh H. Y, Jang J, Ju S. H, *et al.* 2021. Non-Cell Autonomous Epileptogenesis In Focal Cortical Dysplasia. *Ann Neurol,* 90: 285-299.

Koh H. Y., Lee J. H. Brain Somatic Mutations In Epileptic Disorders. *Mol Cells,* 2018; 41: 881-888.

Lai D, Gade M, Yang E, *et al.* Somatic Mutation Involving Diverse Genes Leads To A Spectrum Of Focal Cortical Malformations. *Medrxiv*: 2021.

Lasarge C. L., Danzer S. C. Mechanisms Regulating Neuronal Excitability And Seizure Development Following Mtor Pathway Hyperactivation. *Front Mol Neurosci,* 2014; 7: 18.

Lee J. H, Huynh M, Silhavy J. L, *et al.* De Novo Somatic Mutations In Components Of The Pi3k-Akt3-Mtor Pathway Cause Hemimegalencephaly. *Nat Genet,* 2012; 44: 941-5.

Lee W. S, Baldassari S, Chipaux M, *et al.* Gradient Of Brain Mosaic Rheb Variants Causes A Continuum Of Cortical Dysplasia. *Ann Clin Transl Neurol,* 2021; 8: 485-490.

Lee W. S, Baldassari S, Stephenson S. E. M, *et al.* Cortical Dysplasia And The Mtor Pathway: How The Study Of Human Brain Tissue Has Led To Insights Into Epileptogenesis. *International Journal Of Molecular Sciences,* 2022; 23: 1344.

Lee W. S, Stephenson S. E. M, *et al.* Second-Hit Depdc5 Mutation Is Limited To Dysmorphic Neurons In Cortical Dysplasia Type Iia. *Ann Clin Transl Neurol,* 2019; 6: 1338-1344.

Leventer R. J, Jansen F. E, Mandelstam S. A, *et al.* Is Focal Cortical Dysplasia Sporadic? Family Evidence For Genetic Susceptibility. *Epilepsia,* 2014; 55: E22-6.

Lim J. S, Gopalappa R, Kim S. H, *et al.* Somatic Mutations In Tsc1 And Tsc2 Cause Focal Cortical Dysplasia. *Am J Hum Genet,* 2017; 100: 454-472.

Lim J. S, Kim W. I, Kang H. C, *et al.* Brain Somatic Mutations In Mtor Cause Focal Cortical Dysplasia Type Ii Leading To Intractable Epilepsy. *Nat Med,* 21: 395-400.

Lipton, J. O, Sahin, M. 2014. The Neurology Of Mtor. *Neuron,* 2015; 84: 275-91.

Lodato, M. A, Woodworth M. B, Lee S, *et al.* A. Somatic Mutation In Single Human Neurons Tracks Developmental And Transcriptional History. *Science,* 2015; 350: 94-98.

Mair R, Mouliere F. Cell-Free Dna Technologies For The Analysis Of Brain Cancer. *Br J Cancer.* 2022; 126: 371-8.

Marsan E, Baulac S. Review: Mechanistic Target Of Rapamycin (Mtor) Pathway, Focal Cortical Dysplasia And Epilepsy. *Neuropathol Appl Neurobiol,* 2018; 44: 6-17.

Martin K. R, Zhou W, Bowman M. J, *et al.* The Genomic Landscape Of Tuberous Sclerosis Complex. *Nat Commun,* 2017; 8: 15816.

Mcconnell M. J, Moran J. V, Abyzov A, *et al.* Intersection Of Diverse Neuronal Genomes And Neuropsychiatric Disease: The Brain Somatic Mosaicism Network. *Science,* 2017; 356.

Mirzaa G. M, Campbell C. D, Solovieff N, *et al.* Association Of Mtor Mutations With Developmental Brain Disorders, Including Megalencephaly, Focal Cortical Dysplasia, And Pigmentary Mosaicism. *Jama Neurol,* 2016; 73: 836-845.

Miyata H, Chiang A. C, Vinters, H. V. Insulin Signaling Pathways In Cortical Dysplasia And Tsc-Tubers: Tissue Microarray Analysis. *Ann Neurol,* 2004; 56: 510-9.

Moloney P. B, Cavalleri G. L, Delanty N. Epilepsy In The Mtoropathies: Opportunities For Precision Medicine. *Brain Commun,* 2021; 3: Fcab222.

Najm I, Lal D, Vanegas MA *et al.* The ILAE consensus classification of Focal Cortical Dysplasia (FCD): an update proposed by an ad hoc Task Force of the ILAE Diagnostic Methods commission. *Epilepsia* 2022, in press.

Najm I. M, Sarnat H. B, Blumcke I. Review: The International Consensus Classification Of Focal Cortical Dysplasia - A Critical Update 2018. *Neuropathol Appl Neurobiol,* 2018; 44: 18-31.

Nakashima M, Saitsu H, Takei N, *et al.* Somatic Mutations In The Mtor Gene Cause Focal Cortical Dysplasia Type Iib. *Ann Neurol,* 2015; 78: 375-86.

Ng B. G, Buckingham K. J, Raymond K, *et al.* Mosaicism Of The Udp-Galactose Transporter Slc35a2 Causes A Congenital Disorder Of Glycosylation. *Am J Hum Genet,* 2013; 92: 632-6.

Nguyen L. H, Bordey, A. Convergent And Divergent Mechanisms Of Epileptogenesis In Mtoropathies. *Front Neuroanat,* 2021; 15: 664695.

Park S. M, Lim J. S, Ramakrishina S, *et al.* Brain Somatic Mutations In Mtor Disrupt Neuronal Ciliogenesis, Leading To Focal Cortical Dyslamination. *Neuron* 2018; 99: 83-97 E7.

Pelorosso C, Watrin F Conti, V, *et al.* Somatic Double-Hit In Mtor And Rps6 In Hemimegalencephaly With Intractable Epilepsy. *Hum Mol Genet.* 2019; 28: 3755-65.

Poduri A, Evrony G. D, Cai X,*et al.* Somatic Activation Of Akt3 Causes Hemispheric Developmental Brain Malformations. *Neuron,* 2012; 74: 41-8.

Ribierre T, Deleuze C, Bacq A, *et al.* Second-Hit Mosaic Mutation In Mtorc1 Repressor Depdc5 Causes Focal Cortical Dysplasia-Associated Epilepsy. *J Clin Invest,* 2018; 128: 2452-8.

Ricos M. G, Hodgson B. L, Pippucci T, *et al.* Mutations In The Mammalian Target Of Rapamycin Pathway Regulators Nprl2 And Nprl3 Cause Focal Epilepsy. *Ann Neurol,* 2016; 79: 120-31.

Riviere J. B, Mirzaa G. M, O'roak B. J, *et al.* De Novo Germline And Postzygotic Mutations In Akt3, Pik3r2 And Pik3ca Cause A Spectrum Of Related Megalencephaly Syndromes. *Nat Genet,* 2012; 44: 934-40.

Salinas V, Vega P, Piccirilli M. V, *et al.* Identification Of A Somatic Mutation In The Rheb Gene Through High Depth And Ultra-High Depth Next Generation Sequencing In A Patient With Hemimegalencephaly And Drug Resistant Epilepsy. *Eur J Med Genet.* 2019; 62: 103571.

Salussolia C. L, Klonowska K, Kwiatkowski D. J, Sahin, M. Genetic Etiologies, Diagnosis, And Treatment Of Tuberous Sclerosis Complex. *Annu Rev Genomics Hum Genet,* 2019; 20: 217-40.

Saxton R. A, Sabatini D. M. Mtor Signaling In Growth, Metabolism, And Disease. *Cell,* 2017; 168: 960-76.

Scheffer I. E, Heron S. E, Regan B. M, *et al.* Mutations In Mammalian Target Of Rapamycin Regulator Depdc5 Cause Focal Epilepsy With Brain Malformations. *Ann Neurol,* 2014; 75: 782-7.

Sim N. S, Ko A, Kim W. K, *et al.* Precise Detection Of Low-Level Somatic Mutation In Resected Epilepsy Brain Tissue. *Acta Neuropathol* 2019, 138: 901-12.

Sim N. S, Seo Y, Lim J. S, *et al.* Brain Somatic Mutations In Slc35a2 Cause Intractable Epilepsy With Aberrant N-Glycosylation. *Neurol Genet* 2018, 4: E294.

Subramanian L, Calcagnotto M. E, Paredes M. F. Cortical Malformations: Lessons In Human Brain Development. *Front Cell Neurosci,* 2019; 13: 576.

Velasco S, Paulsen B, Arlotta P. 3d Brain Organoids: Studying Brain Development And Disease Outside The Embryo. *Annu Rev Neurosci,* 2020; 43: 375-89.

Winawer M. R, Griffin N. G, Samanamud J, *et al.* Somatic Slc35a2 Variants In The Brain Are Associated With Intractable Neocortical Epilepsy. *Ann Neurol,* 2018; 83: 1133-46.

Witters P, Tahata S, Barone R, *et al.* Clinical And Biochemical Improvement With Galactose Supplementation In Slc35a2-Cdg. *Genet Med,* 2020; 22: 1102-7.

Ye Z, Chatterton Z, Pflueger J, *et al.* Cerebrospinal Fluid Liquid Biopsy For Detecting Somatic Mosaicism In Brain. *Brain Commun,* 2021; 3: Fcaa235.

Zhao S, Li Z, Zhang M, *et al.* A Brain Somatic Rheb Doublet Mutation Causes Focal Cortical Dysplasia Type Ii. *Exp Mol Med,* 2019; 51: 84.

CHAPTER

5. FCD and the mTORopathy spectrum

Valerio Conti, Carmen Barba, Renzo Guerrini

Key points

- The mTOR pathway is a crucial cellular hub.
- mTOR pathway regulates many cellular functions, from gene expression to cytoskeleton organization, cell cycle progression, and cell growth and survival.
- Germline and somatic mutations of genes in this pathway have been associated with a phenotypic continuum of MCD, ranging from FCDII to megalencephaly/dysplastic megalencephaly.
- Germline, somatic and somatic two-hit-variant can be demonstrated in up to 59% cases of FCDII.
- Everolimus, an mTOR inhibitor, was successfully tested as adjunct therapy for drug-resistant focal seizures associated with Tuberous Sclerosis Complex (TSC).
- Because of the possible common genetic background of TSC and FCD type II, mTOR inhibitors are being tested in clinical trials in patients with refractory seizures and FCD II and might represent an example of personalized treatment of epilepsy based on the known mechanisms of disease.

Introduction

The mechanistic (or 'mammalian') target of rapamycin (mTOR) pathway is a crucial cellular hub that integrates internal and external cues to regulate many cellular functions including gene expression, transcription, macromolecules biosynthesis, metabolic balance, autophagy, metabolism, organelle biogenesis and maintenance, cytoskeleton organization, cell cycle progression, and cell growth and survival.

Germline and somatic mutations of genes in this pathway have been associated with a phenotypic continuum of MCD, ranging from FCD II to megalencephaly (MEG)/dysplastic megalencephaly (DMEG). Germline, somatic and somatic two-hit-variants can be demonstrated in up to 59% of FCD II. A large experience has been gathered for the surgical treatment of epilepsy associated with FCD or larger hemispheric dysplasias and with tuberous sclerosis. Following multiple preclinical studies and early small clinical trials, everolimus, an mTOR inhibitor, was successfully tested as an adjunct therapy for drug-resistant focal seizures associated with TSC. Owing to the possible common genetic background of TSC and FCD type II, mTOR inhibitors are being tested in clinical trials in patients with refractory seizures and FCD II and might represent an example of personalized treatment of epilepsy based on the known mechanisms of disease.

The physiology of the mTOR pathway

Mammalian target of rapamycin (mTOR) is a serine/threonine kinase belonging to the phosphatidylinositol 3-kinase (PI3K)-related kinase family (Budanov and Karin, 2008). mTOR associates with several proteins to form two large biochemical complexes, mTOR Complex 1 (mTORC1) and 2 (mTORC2) (**Figures 1 and 2**).

mTORC1 responds to inputs from intracellular and extracellular cues (**Figure 1**). In response to growth factors, the kinases AKT/PKB (protein kinase B), ERK1/2 (extracellular-signal-regulated kinase 1/2) and RSK1 (ribosomal S6 kinase) phosphorylate and inactivate TSC1/2, maintaining mTORC1 active. AKT can also directly activate mTORC1 by phosphorylating PRAS40. Growth factors indirectly activate mTORC1 via the WNT pathway, which inhibits glycogen synthase kinase-3 (GSK3), a TSC2 activator (Bockaert and Marin, 2015).

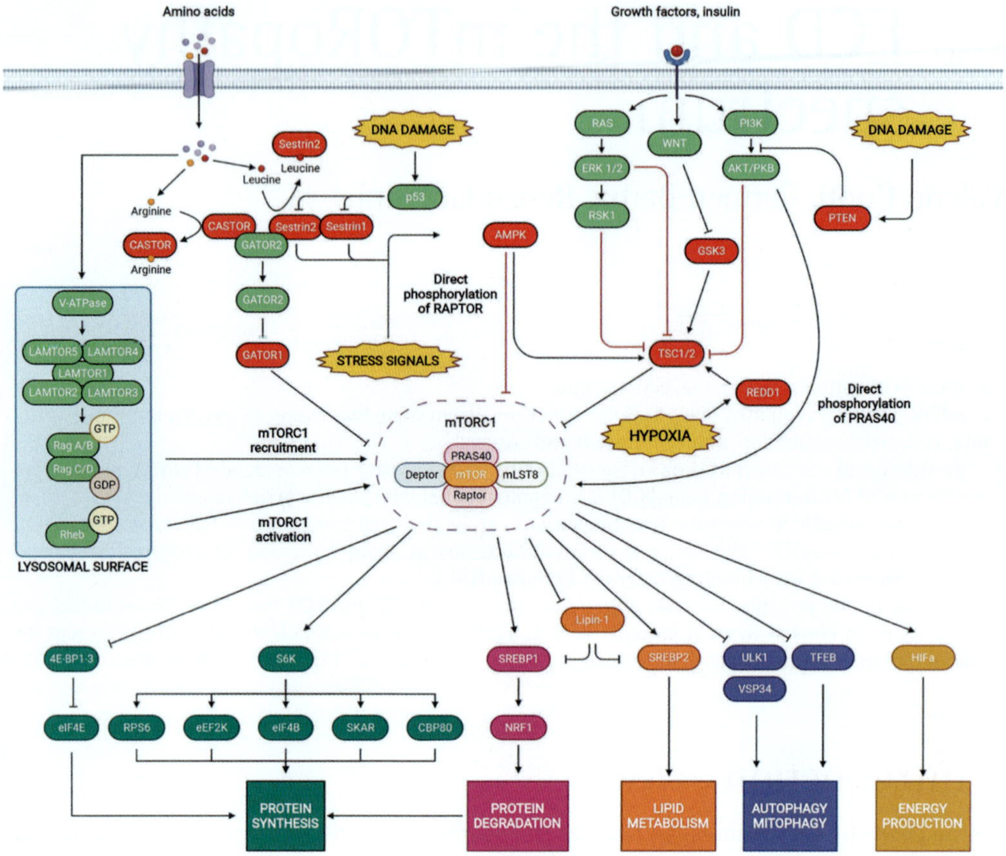

Figure 1

The mTORC1 signaling pathway.

mTORC1 is composed by MTOR, Mammalian lethal with sec13 protein 8 (mLST8), inhibitory DEP domain containing mTOR-interacting protein (DEPTOR), the regulator-associated protein of the mammalian target of rapamycin (RAPTOR) and the proline-rich Akt substrate of 40 kDa (PRAS40). mTORC1 is mainly involved in the regulation of protein synthesis and degradation, lipid metabolism, autophagy/mitophagy, and energy production. Proteins with activating effects on mTORC1 are depicted in green while those with inhibiting effects are in red. Polygons in yellow indicate stress signals. mTORC1 downstream proteins are colored according to the downstream pathways they regulate. Figure 1 was created with BioRender.com.

Amino acids-dependent mTORC1 activation is mediated by a large lysosomal protein complex comprising RAGULATOR (a pentameric complex formed by LAMTOR1-5), RagA-D GTPases, and vacuolar H^+-ATPase (V-ATPase). V-ATPase activates RAGULATOR, which acts as a guanine nucleotide exchange factor for RagA/B GTPases. The GTP-loaded RagA/B heterodimerizes with the GDP-loaded RagC/D and recruits inactive mTORC1 to the lysosomal surface, where it is activated by RheB (Kim and Guan, 2019). Several amino acids can regulate mTORC1 signaling, but arginine and leucine are best characterized. Leucine activates mTORC1 through the phosphoprotein Sestrin2. Binding of leucine causes Sestrin2 dephosphorylation and its dissociation from the GAP protein complex activity towards Rags 2 (GATOR2). Free GATOR2 positively regulates mTORC1 by inhibiting its repressor GATOR1 (Switon *et al.*, 2017). Arginine exerts its action on mTORC1 through the cellular arginine sensor for mTORC1 (CASTOR1). Homodimers of CASTOR1, or heterodimers of CASTOR1/CASTOR2, bind to and regulate GATOR2 through a mechanism analogous to leucine sensing. The CASTOR dimers bind to GATOR2 at distinct sites from the Sestrins, permitting a non-redundant and independent regulation of this complex by arginine and leucine (Hallett and Manning, 2016).

In response to low energy or hypoxia, the Adenosine Monophosphate-activated Protein Kinase (AMPK) phosphorylates TSC2, increasing its repressing activity on mTORC1. AMPK can also inhibit mTORC1 phosphorylating RAPTOR. Phospho-RAPTOR binds with 14-3-3 proteins and causes the allosteric inhibition of mTORC1 (Bockaert and Marin, 2015). Hypoxia induces mTORC1 repression also enhancing the expression of REDD1 (regulated in development and DNA damage responses 1). When expressed, REDD1 promotes the dissociation of TSC2 from 14-3-3 proteins and the inhibition of mTORC1. (DeYoung *et al.*, 2008). DNA damage signals to mTORC1 through multiple p53-dependent mechanisms acting on Sestrin1 and Sestrin2. Sestrin1/2 activate AMPK, which in turn phosphorylates TSC2, stimulating its activity (Kim and Guan, 2019). DNA damage also promotes the expression of PTEN (phosphatase and tensin homolog), causing the downregulation of the entire mTORC1 axis (Switon *et al.*, 2017).

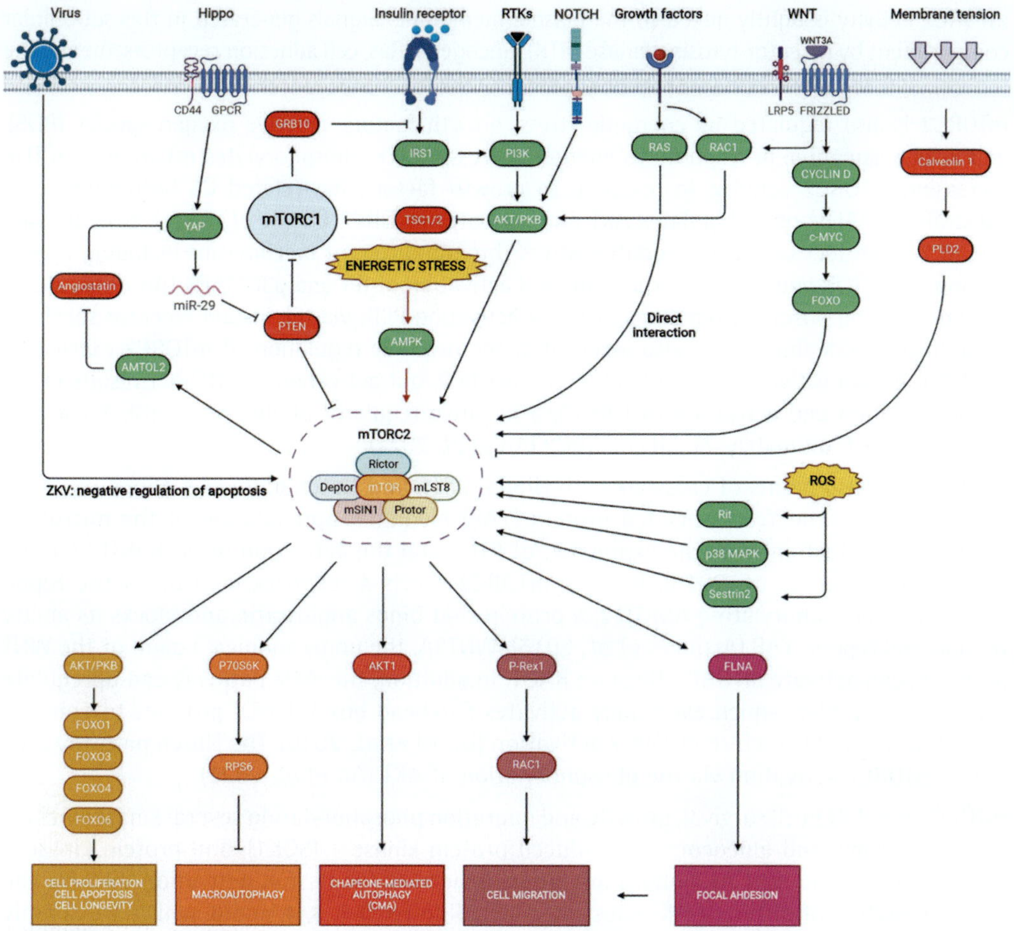

Figure 2

The mTORC2 signaling pathway.

mTORC2 is composed by MTOR, Mammalian lethal with sec13 protein 8 (mLST8), inhibitory DEP domain containing mTOR-interacting protein (DEPTOR), rapamycin-insensitive companion of mTOR (RICTOR), mammalian stress-activated MAP kinase-interacting protein 1 (mSIN1), and the protein observed with RICTOR 1 and 2 (PROTOR1/2). mTORC2 is mainly involved in the regulation of cell proliferation and apoptosis, autophagy, and cell migration. Proteins with activating effects on the mTORC2 are depicted in green while those with inhibiting effects are depicted in red. Yellow polygons indicate stress signals. mTORC2 downstream genes are colored according to the downstream pathways they regulate. Figure 2 was created with BioRender.com.

mTORC1 controls protein synthesis phosphorylating eukaryotic translation initiation factor 4E (eIF4E)-binding proteins (4E-BP) 1, 2, and 3 and the p70 ribosomal S6 kinase (S6K) 1 and 2 (Laplante and Sabatini, 2012). 4E-BPs bind to eIF4E and inhibit the formation of the eIF4F complex that is required for the initiation of cap-dependent translation of mRNAs, but their mTORC1-mediated phosphorylation inhibits this binding (Laplante and Sabatini, 2012). S6K1 phosphorylates different proteins including the ribosomal protein S6 (RPS6), eukaryotic elongation factor-2 kinase (eEF2K), eIF4B, cell growth regulator (SKAR)-like substrate, and cap-binding protein 80 (CBP80) to positively regulate translation (Zoncu *et al.*, 2011). mTORC1 is also involved in protein degradation by regulating the activity of sterol regulatory element-binding protein 1 (SREBP1) and its downstream effector nuclear factor erythroid-derived 2-related factor 1 (NRF1) (Bockaert and Marin, 2015). By promoting SREBP1/2 phosphorylation and activation, as well as the phosphorylation of Lipin-1, which suppress its inhibitory effects on SREBP1/2 transcription, it also participates to lipid metabolism (Bockaert and Marin, 2015). mTORC1 controls autophagy and mitophagy inhibiting the ULK1 and VPS34 complexes. Activation of both ULK1 and VPS34 leads to autophagosome formation. mTORC1 can inactivate this process phosphorylating ULK1 or the Autophagy And Beclin 1 Regulator 1 (AMBRA1). AMBRA1 phosphorylation blocks ULK1 ubiquitination and enhances its activity (Bockaert and Marin, 2015). A second mechanism of autophagy regulation involves the phosphorylation of the transcription factor EB (TFEB), which inhibits its nuclear translocation and, consequently, the expression of some genes implicated in lysosome and autophagosomes biogenesis (Laplante and Sabatini, 2012). Finally, mTORC1 is involved in energy production by increasing the transcription/translation ratio of hypoxia inducible factor 1 ? (HIF1?) (Düvel *et al.*, 2010), as well as by positively regulating the mitochondrial biogenesis and oxidative function via the transcription factor yin-yang 1 (YY1) (Bockaert and Marin, 2015).

mTORC2 activity is tightly linked to the plasma membrane. Signals generated in this subcellular compartment by receptor tyrosine kinase (RTK), oncogenic Ras, cell adhesion receptors, membrane tension, and viruses or viral proteins modulate its activity (**Figure 2**) (An *et al.*, 2021).

mTORC2 is also regulated by energetic stress, growth factors, reactive oxygen species (ROS), and insulin signaling. In response to energetic stress, AMPK phosphorylates mTOR and RICTOR increasing mTORC2 activity. In response to growth factors, Ras-related C3 botulinum toxin substrate 1 (RAC1) phosphorylates AKT and activates mTORC2 (An *et al.*, 2021). ROS activate mTORC2 to protect cells from oxidative stress through different mechanisms including upregulation of RICTOR and Sestrin2 expression and activation of Rit and p38MAPK (An *et al.*, 2021). Insulin signaling positively regulates mTORC2 activating PI3K via the insulin receptor substrate (IRS). Insulin/PI3K signaling is also involved in the negative regulation of mTORC2 exerted by mTORC1. Insulin activates both mTORC1 and mTORC2, but activation of mTORC1 results in the phosphorylation and activation of GRB10, a negative regulator of the insulin/IGF-1 receptor signaling, which ultimately inhibits mTORC2 (An *et al.*, 2021).

mTORC2 has also points of crosstalk with Hippo, WNT, and Notch pathways. Hippo inactivation determines the Yes-associated protein (YAP)-mediated upregulation of the microRNA 29 (miR-29), which inhibits the expression of PTEN and the activation of both mTORC1 and mTORC2 (Artinian *et al.*, 2015). In turn, mTORC2 exerts a feedback control on the Hippo pathway by phosphorylating AMOTL2, a protein that binds angiostatin and blocks its ability to bind and repress YAP (Artinian *et al.*, 2015). WNT3A, the non-canonical ligand of the WNT pathway, can activate mTORC2 through RAC1. In addition, the WNT pathway can upregulate cyclin D and c-Myc, which eventually activates Forkhead boxO (FoxO) proteins to enhance RICTOR levels and therefore mTORC2 activation (Düvel *et al.*, 2010). The Notch pathway promotes mTORC2 activation via the phosphorylation of AKT (An *et al.*, 2021).

mTORC2 regulates cell survival, growth, and migration phosphorylating several kinases including AKT, serum- and glucocorticoid-induced protein kinase 1 (SGK1), and protein kinase C (PKC). mTORC2-induced AKT phosphorylation is needed for its full activation and for the phosphorylation of different AKT substrates including FoxO 1, 3, 4, and 6, which are directly implicated in regulating cell proliferation and apoptosis. AKT-mediated phosphorylation of FoxO proteins blocks their export from the nucleus and thereby abrogates their function (Bockaert and Marin, 2015). mTORC2 negatively regulates macroautophagy phosphorylating p70S6 kinase (p70S6K), which through RPS6 induces protein synthesis at the ribosome (Datan *et al.*, 2014). In addition, it regulates chaperone-mediated autophagy (CMA), which contributes to the cellular adaptation to stress. This specific mTORC2 function is mediated by AKT1 activation (Arias *et al.*, 2015).

mTORC2 regulates cell migration through its association with the guanine nucleotide exchange factor P-Rex1, one of the major effectors linking mTORC2 to RAC1. RAC1 activation promotes actin polymerization, lamellipodia formation, and eventually cell migration (Hernández-Negrete *et al.*, 2007). mTORC2 promotes cell migration also by phosphorylating Filamin A (FLNA). FLNA cross-links actin filaments by forming dimers and binds to β-integrin linking actin filaments to extracellular matrices, thereby regulating focal adhesion. mTORC2-mediated phosphorylation of FLNA strengthens its interaction with β-integrin and may stabilize focal adhesion. However, wound healing assays have demonstrated that the stabilization of focal adhesion is not sufficient to promote cell migration, suggesting that mTORC2 phosphorylates other regulatory molecules of actin dynamics to regulate Filamin A-induced cell migration (Sato *et al.*, 2016).

mTOR pathway alterations in human malformations of cortical development

Previous inferences suggested that FCD arose from cellular and/or architectural abnormalities mainly occurring during *in utero* brain development but that perinatal and postnatal insults, including severe prematurity, asphyxia, shaking injury, bleeding, hydrocephalus, and stroke could also play a role in some specific cases (Barkovich *et al.*, 2012; Krsek *et al.*, 2010).

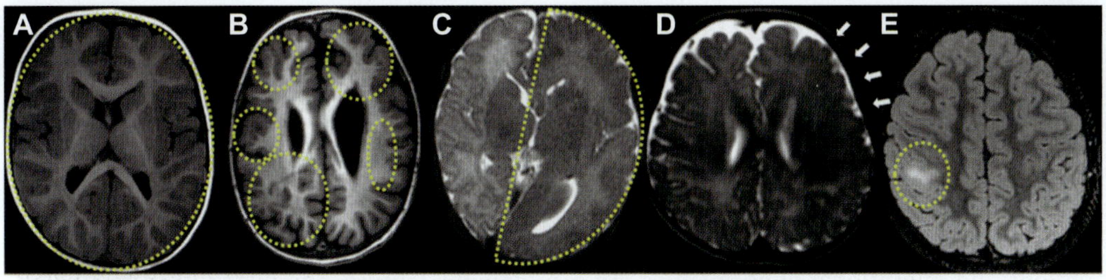

Figure 3

Different possible combinations between mutant cells distribution, malformations of cortical development and epileptogenesis. Yellow markers indicate the localization and extent of the different epileptogenic malformations of cortical development.

It is now well established that FCD II can result from mutations in genes in mTOR pathway (Baldassari *et al.*, 2019b) and that germline, somatic and somatic two-hits variants can be demonstrated in up to 59% of the cases as extensively presented by S. Baldassari and S. Baulac in chapter 4. Germline and somatic mutations of genes within this pathway, including *AKT1*, *AKT3*, *DEPDC5*, *MTOR*, *NPRL2/3*, *PIK3CA*, *PIK3R2*, and *TSC1/2* have been associated with a phenotypic continuum of MCD, ranging from FCD II to megalencephaly (MEG)/dysplastic megalencephaly (DMEG) (Baldassari *et al.*, 2019b; Mirzaa *et al.*, 2016) (**Figure 3**). mTOR hyperactivation during neurodevelopment may cause the cellular hypertrophy that characterizes dysmorphic neurons and balloon cells (Baldassari *et al.*, 2019b). Mirzaa and colleagues observed that cultured neurons carrying *mTOR* mutations exhibited significant increases in cell size that could be reversed by 7 days of mTOR inhibition with a rapamycin analogue, thus demonstrating a causal link between *mTOR* mutations and induction of elevated mTORC1 activity and neuronal hypertrophy (Mirzaa *et al.*, 2016). Alternative allele fraction (AAF) and somatic distribution of mosaicism influence the phenotype. Low-level mosaic mutations have mainly been associated with FCD II, while intermediate-level mosaic mutations affecting a single hemisphere result in larger brain malformations such as hemimegalencephaly (HME), and high-level mosaic mutations affecting multiple organs (systemic mosaic) and germline mutations cause megalencephaly/dysplastic megalencephaly (D'Gama *et al.*, 2017). About 79% of mutated FCD II patients exhibit brain mosaic rates lower than 5% (Baldassari *et al.*, 2019b). Of the remaining patients in whom a mutation is found in the dysplastic tissue, 50% exhibit mosaic rates ranging from 6.5% to 18.6% and 50% carry germline mutations. It has been suggested that bottom-of-sulcus FCD IIB and somatic *MTOR* variants may show a 'mutation gradient,' with higher mutation load at the bottom of the sulcus compared to the gyral crown (Lee *et al.*, 2020) and that the hyperactivating properties of each specific variant may influence the severity of epileptogenicity (Guerrini *et al.*, 2021) (**Figure 4**). Disclosing somatic mosaicism in surgically removed tissue specimens does not reveal whether mosaicism is present in remote, homolateral or contralateral, brain areas that are normal looking but may still harbor somatic mosaicism at levels that are not sufficient to cause a visible dysplasia (Guerrini *et al.*, 2021). Around 62% of patients carrying constitutional mutations in negative regulators of the mTORC1 pathway *DEPDC5*, *NPRL2* or *NPRL3* have a normal brain MRI (Baldassari *et al.*, 2019a). A possible 'two-hit' mechanism combining somatic and germline mutations in the same gene, according to the Knudson's two-hit model, has been demonstrated in patients with a somatic variant in *DEPDC5* in the dysplastic cortex and a constitutional variant in the other allele, to cause biallelic inactivation of the gene (Baldassari *et al.*, 2019a; Ribierre *et al.*, 2018). Pelorosso and collaborators (Pelorosso *et al.*, 2019) and Bennet and collaborators (Bennett *et al.*, 2022) identified variants affecting two different genes (*MTOR* plus *RPS6* and *NPRL3* plus *WNT2*) in single patients with HME or FCD. These two studies uncovered a possible novel double-hit mechanism for the pathogenesis of FCD and HME, resulting from two independent activating somatic variants, each affecting a single allele of a positive regulator of the mTOR pathway.

Shared histopathological and genetic features between different mTORopathies: different facets of a neurobiological continuum or truly distinct diseases?

TSC is a genetic disorder affecting multiple organs including the brain, where cortical malformations and migrational abnormalities are a prominent feature. The histopathological characteristics of tubers and radial migration lines are similar, if not identical, to the phenotypic continuum of MCD including FCD II, HME, MEG, and DMEG (Aronica *et al.*, 2012). Although it has long been recognized that TSC is caused by loss-of-function mutations in *TSC1* or *TSC2* (European Chromosome 16 Tuberous Sclerosis Consortium, 1993; Slegtenhorst *et al.*, 1997) and associated with abnormal activation of the mTOR pathway, the causative role of activating mutations in mTOR pathway genes in the FCD-DMEG spectrum has been demonstrated only recently (D'Gama *et al.*, 2017; Guerrini *et al.*, 2021; Mirzaa *et al.*, 2016). As they are all caused by pathogenic variants affecting mTOR pathway genes, these conditions are included in the so called mTORopathies. All mTORopathies are associated with hyperactivation of the mTOR signaling (Nguyen and Bordey, 2021) and studies performed in a mouse model of TSC and FCD have demonstrated that mTOR hyperactivity levels appear to correlate with the severity of epilepsy and associated neuropathology (Nguyen *et al.*, 2019). The tight correlation between TSC and FCD is also corroborated by the observation that TSC mutations can cause isolated FCD or HME without hamartomas (D'Gama *et al.*, 2017). In addition, D'Gama and collaborators (D'Gama *et al.*, 2017) have demonstrated that both lesions likely reflect mutations in dorsal telencephalic progenitors that normally give rise to excitatory neurons. Both the degree of mosaicism and the radiographic extent of these two lesions suggest that FCD, HME and the other mTORopathies represent a phenotypic continuum rather than truly distinct diseases. In this continuum, the different extent the lesions would reflect the time and place of origin of the somatic mutations.

Studies on cellular and animal models of TSC have led to the clinical use of rapamycin, a pharmacological inhibitor of the mTOR pathway. Previous studies on *in vivo* maintained slices of resected human tissue demonstrated that rapamycin may reduce the amplitude

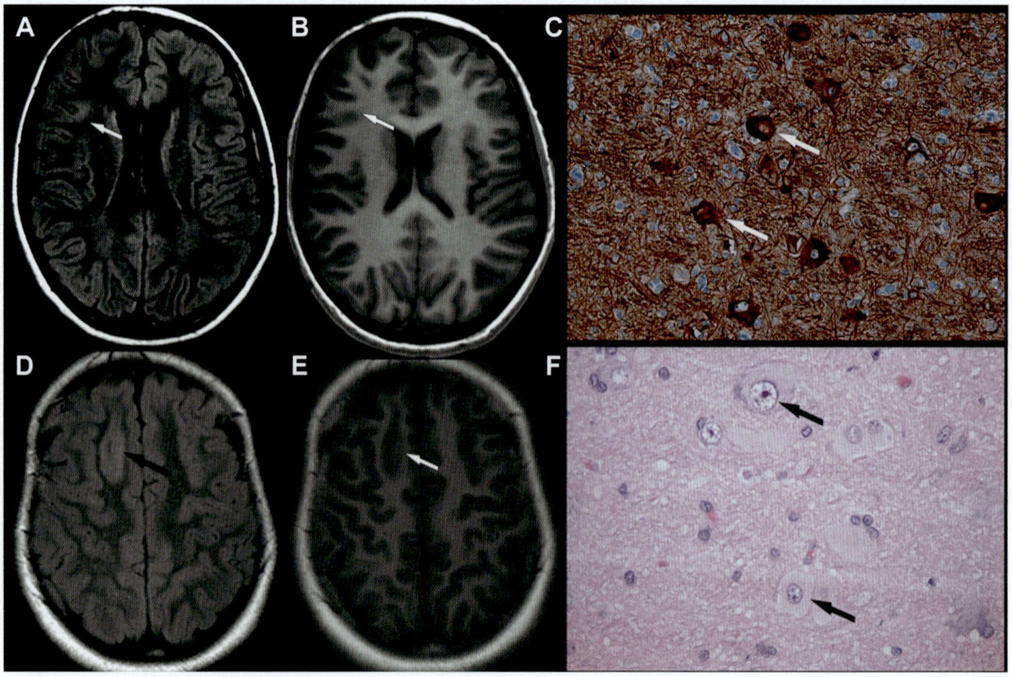

Figure 4

(A-C) 9-year-old boy with drug-resistant seizures and FCD IIA. Axial 3 T FLAIR (A) and T1-weighted (B) brain MRI images showing an area of abnormal thickening and mild gray-white blurring in the right frontal area (white arrows). Histological slice revealing dyslamination and dysmorphic cells (C, white arrows). (D-F) 5-year-old boy with drug-resistant seizures and FCD IIB.

and frequency of 4-AP-induced paroxysmal discharges (Cepeda *et al.*, 2018), spontaneous excitatory postsynaptic activity, and burst discharges induced by blockade of γ-aminobutyric acid A (GABAA) receptors (Cepeda *et al.*, 2018).

Mechanisms of epileptogenesis: opening the way to personalized therapies

Excessive mTORC1 activation appears to be implicated in epileptogenesis by altering established neural networks. However, it remains unclear whether seizures are a direct consequence of mTORC1 hyperactivation or of the network disruption resulting from co-occurring brain structural abnormalities. In a rodent model of biallelic Tsc1 deletion, mice developed early epileptic seizures, without significant alteration of the brain structure, suggesting that excessive mTOR activation alone is sufficient to generate seizures (Abs *et al.*, 2013). On the other hand, FCD and HME can show spontaneous pacemaker γ-aminobutyric acid (GABA) receptor-mediated synaptic activity (PGA) that might contribute to epileptogenesis in malformed postnatal cortex by facilitating pyramidal neuron synchrony (Cepeda *et al.*, 2014). Advanced signal processing techniques during stereoelectroencephalography (SEEG) procedures provide corroborative evidence of the role of FCD in generating and propagating ictal activity (Panzica *et al.*, 2013). The intrinsic epileptogenicity of FCD II is further confirmed by its sensitivity to electrical stimulation which reliably reproduces electrographic seizure patterns in human cortical areas with typical interictal patterns (Chassoux *et al.*, 2012).

Following multiple preclinical studies, case series, and early human clinical trials (Krueger *et al.*, 2016, 2013, 2010), everolimus, an mTOR inhibitor, was tested as an adjunct and targeted therapy for drug-resistant focal seizures associated with TSC in a randomized, placebo-controlled, double-blind trial (EXIST-3; clinicaltrials.gov #NCT01713946). The overall response rate (>50% seizure reduction from baseline) in the high-exposure add-on everolimus treatment arm was 40.0%, compared to 15.1% in the placebo arm, and the median seizure reduction was 39.6 vs 14.9% (French *et al.*, 2016). In the post-hoc analysis performed in the 299 children included in the study (Curatolo *et al.*, 2018), the response rate in the subgroup <6 years of age was as high as 60% compared to the 30% observed in the older subgroup. Data from the 2-year open-label extension phase suggested long-term seizure reduction and a safety profile comparable with the results from the core phase of the EXIST-3 trial (Franz *et al.*, 2018). Based on these results, MTOR inhibitors are now used as an adjunctive treatment option for epilepsy in TSC patients. Recent lines of evidence suggest that the highest efficacy of mTOR inhibitors occurs in younger patients and with sustained use (Overwater *et al.*, 2019; van der Poest Clement *et al.*, 2020). More recently, it has been suggested that the use of mTOR inhibitors prior to epilepsy might delay seizure onset and relieve their severity (Shen, 2022).

The significance of these findings is important not only for the treatment of epilepsy in TSC, but has possible therapeutic implications for FCD (Jeong and Wong, 2016). Local cortical expression of mTOR mutant p.Leu2427Pro by *in utero* electroporation in mice was sufficient to disrupt neuronal migration and cause spontaneous seizures and cytomegalic neurons. Inhibition of mTOR with rapamycin suppressed cytomegalic neurons and epileptic seizures (Lim *et al.*, 2015). Some single case reports or small series assessed mTOR inhibitors in non-TSC epilepsy. One open-label prospective study (Parker *et al.*, 2013) enrolled five children with Pretzel syndrome, a rare neurodevelopmental disorder characterized by polyhydramnios, MEG, and symptomatic epilepsy syndrome (PMSE) and caused by a homozygous deletion of exons 9 to 13 of the LYK5/STRADA gene, which encodes the pseudokinase STRADA, an upstream inhibitor of mTORC1. The five children were treated with daily rapamycin (blood concentration between 5 and 15 ng/ml) with subsequent 1-year seizure freedom in four and improvement in receptive language in all. Xu and collaborators (Xu *et al.*, 2019) reported >50% reduction in seizures in a single patient with HME after one week of treatment with rapamycin. However, everolimus was ineffective in a further patient with *mTOR* mosaic mutation (Hadouiri *et al.*, 2020). Owing to the possible common genetic background of TSC and FCD II, three ongoing trials are evaluating the effects of everolimus in patients with TSC and FCD undergoing epilepsy surgery (https: //clinicaltrials.gov/ct2/ show/NCT02451696) and in patients with refractory seizures who have FCD II (https: //clinicaltrials.gov/ct2/show/NCT03198949).

Conclusion

Improved knowledge of the genetic causes of FCD-DMEG spectrum offers promising new avenues for personalized treatment. Epilepsy surgery is a form of personalized treatment but is usually performed before molecular neuropathology is known and is therefore based on individual phenotypic anatomoelectroclinical features. However, FCD II results from mutations in genes in the mTOR pathway, a key regulator of many cellular functions and mTOR inhibitors are currently used as an adjunctive treatment option for epilepsy in TSC patients and tested in FCD II-associated epilepsy. There is growing evidence that combined surgical and medical treatment approaches enhance the chances of success in the treatment of epilepsy associated with FCD-DMEG spectrum disorders.

References

Abs, E, Goorden, S.M.I, Schreiber, J, *et al.* TORC1-dependent epilepsy caused by acute biallelic *Tsc1* deletion in adult mice: Epilepsy upon *Tsc1* Deletion. *Ann Neurol.* 2013; 74, 569–79.

An, P, Xu, W, Luo, J, Luo, Y. Expanding TOR Complex 2 Signaling: Emerging Regulators and New Connections. *Front. Cell Dev. Biol.* 2021; 9, 713806.

Arias, E, Koga, H, Diaz, A, Mocholi, E, Patel, B, Cuervo, A.M. Lysosomal mTORC2/PHLPP1/Akt Regulate Chaperone-Mediated Autophagy. *Molecular Cell* 2015; 59, 270–84.

Aronica, E, Becker, A.J, Spreafico, R. Malformations of Cortical Development: Malformations. *Brain Pathology* 2012; 22, 380–401.

Artinian, N, Cloninger, C, Holmes, B, Benavides-Serrato, A, Bashir, T, Gera, J. Phosphorylation of the Hippo Pathway Component AMOTL2 by the mTORC2 Kinase Promotes YAP Signaling, Resulting in Enhanced Glioblastoma Growth and Invasiveness. *Journal of Biological Chemistry* 2015; 290, 19387-401.

Baldassari, S, Picard, F, Verbeek, N.E, *et al.* The landscape of epilepsy-related GATOR1 variants. *Genetics in Medicine* 2019a; 21, 398–408.

Baldassari, S, Ribierre, T, Marsan, E, *et al.* Dissecting the genetic basis of focal cortical dysplasia: a large cohort study. *Acta Neuropathologica* 2019b; 138, 885–900.

Barkovich, A.J, Guerrini, R, Kuzniecky, R.I, Jackson, G.D, Dobyns, W.B, 2012. A developmental and genetic classification for malformations of cortical development: update 2012. *Brain* 135, 1348–69.

Bennett, M.F, Hildebrand, M.S, Kayumi, S, *et al.* 2022. Evidence for a Dual-Pathway, 2-Hit Genetic Model for Focal Cortical Dysplasia and Epilepsy. *Neurol Genet* 8, e0652.

Bockaert, J, Marin, P. mTOR in Brain Physiology and Pathologies. *Physiological Reviews* 2015; 95, 1157–87.

Budanov, A.V, Karin, M. p53 Target Genes Sestrin1 and Sestrin2 Connect Genotoxic Stress and mTOR Signaling. *Cell* 2008; 134, 451–60.

Cepeda, C, Chen, J.Y, Wu, J.Y, *et al.* Pacemaker GABA synaptic activity may contribute to network synchronization in pediatric cortical dysplasia. *Neurobiology of Disease* 2014; 62, 208–17.

Cepeda, C, Levinson, S, Yazon, V.W, *et al.* Cellular anti-seizure mechanisms of everolimus in pediatric tuberous sclerosis complex, cortical dysplasia, and non-mTOR-mediated etiologies. *Epilepsia Open* 2018; 3, 180–90.

Chassoux, F, Landré, E, Mellerio, C, *et al.* Type II focal cortical dysplasia: Electroclinical phenotype and surgical outcome related to imaging: Phenotype and Imaging in TTFCD. *Epilepsia* 2012; 53, 349-358.

Curatolo, P, Franz, D.N, Lawson, J.A, *et al.* Adjunctive everolimus for children and adolescents with treatment-refractory seizures associated with tuberous sclerosis complex: post-hoc analysis of the phase 3 EXIST-3 trial. *The Lancet Child and Adolescent Health* 2018; 2, 495–504.

Datan, E, Shirazian, A, Benjamin, S, *et al.* mTOR/p70S6K signaling distinguishes routine, maintenance-level autophagy from autophagic cell death during influenza A infection. *Virology* 2014; 452–453, 175–190.

DeYoung, M.P, Horak, P, Sofer, A, Sgroi, D, Ellisen, L.W. Hypoxia regulates TSC1/2-mTOR signaling and tumor suppression through REDD1-mediated 14-3-3 shuttling. *Genes Dev* 2008; 22, 239–251.

D'Gama, A.M, Woodworth, M.B, Hossain, A.A, *et al.* Somatic Mutations Activating the mTOR Pathway in Dorsal Telencephalic Progenitors Cause a Continuum of Cortical Dysplasias. *Cell Reports* 2017; 21, 3754–66.

Düvel, K, Yecies, J.L, Menon, S, *et al.* Activation of a Metabolic Gene Regulatory Network Downstream of mTOR Complex 1. *Molecular Cell* 2010; 39, 171–83.

European Chromosome 16 Tuberous Sclerosis Consortium,. Identification and characterization of the tuberous sclerosis gene on chromosome 16. *Cell* 1993; 75, 1305–15.

Franz, D.N, Lawson, J.A, Yapici, Z, *et al.* Everolimus for treatment-refractory seizures in TSC: Extension of a randomized controlled trial. *Neurology: Clinical Practice* 2018; 8, 412–20.

French, J.A, Lawson, J.A, Yapici, Z, *et al.* Adjunctive everolimus therapy for treatment-resistant focal-onset seizures associated with tuberous sclerosis (EXIST-3): a phase 3, randomised, double-blind, placebo-controlled study. *The Lancet* 2016; 388, 2153–63.

Guerrini, R, Cavallin, M, Pippucci, T, *et al.* Is Focal Cortical Dysplasia/Epilepsy Caused by Somatic MTOR Mutations Always a Unilateral Disorder? *Neurology Genetics* 2021; 7, e540.

Hadouiri, N, Darmency, V, Guibaud, L, *et al.* Compassionate use of everolimus for refractory epilepsy in a patient with MTOR mosaic mutation. *Eur J Med Genet.* 2020; 63, 104036.

Hallett, J.E.H, Manning, B.D. CASTORing New Light on Amino Acid Sensing. Cell 2016; 165, 15–17.

Hernández-Negrete, I, Carretero-Ortega, J, Rosenfeldt, H, *et al.* P-Rex1 Links Mammalian Target of Rapamycin Signaling to Rac Activation and Cell Migration. *Journal of Biological Chemistry* 2007; 282, 23708–15.

Jeong, A, Wong, M. Tuberous sclerosis complex as a model disease for developing new therapeutics for epilepsy. *Expert Review of Neurotherapeutics* 2016; 16, 437–47.

Kim, J, Guan, K.-L. mTOR as a central hub of nutrient signalling and cell growth. *Nat Cell Biol* 2019; 21, 63–71.

Krsek, P, Jahodova, A, Maton, B, *et al.* 2010. Low-grade focal cortical dysplasia is associated with prenatal and perinatal brain injury: Perinatal Injury and Cortical Dysplasia. *Epilepsia* 51, 2440–8.

Krueger, D.A, Care, M.M, Holland, K, *et al.* Everolimus for Subependymal Giant-Cell Astrocytomas in Tuberous Sclerosis. *New England Journal of Medicine* 2010; 363, 1801–11.

Krueger, D.A, Wilfong, A.A, Holland-Bouley, K, *et al.* Everolimus treatment of refractory epilepsy in tuberous sclerosis complex. *Annals of neurology* 2013; 74, 679–87.

Krueger, D.A, Wilfong, A.A, Mays, M, *et al.* Long-term treatment of epilepsy with everolimus in tuberous sclerosis. *Neurology* 2016; 87, 2408–15.

Laplante, M, Sabatini, D.M. mTOR Signaling in Growth Control and Disease. *Cell* 2012; 149, 274–293.

Lee, W.S, Stephenson, S.E.M, Pope, K, *et al.* Genetic characterization identifies bottom-of-sulcus dysplasia as an mTORopathy. *Neurology* 2020; 95, e2542–51.

Lim, J.S, Kim, W. il, Kang, H.C, *et al.* Brain somatic mutations in MTOR cause focal cortical dysplasia type II leading to intractable epilepsy. *Nature medicine* 2015; 21, 395–400.

Mirzaa, G.M, Campbell, C.D, Solovieff, N, *et al.* Association of MTOR Mutations With Developmental Brain Disorders, Including Megalencephaly, Focal Cortical Dysplasia, and Pigmentary Mosaicism. *JAMA neurology* 2016; 73, 836–45.

Nguyen, L.H, Bordey, A. Convergent and Divergent Mechanisms of Epileptogenesis in mTORopathies. *Front. Neuroanat.* 2021; 15, 664695.

Nguyen, L.H, Mahadeo, T, Bordey, A. mTOR hyperactivity levels influence the severity of epilepsy and associated neuropathology in an experimental model of tuberous sclerosis complex and focal cortical dysplasia. *Journal of Neuroscience* 2019; 39, 2762–73.

Overwater, I, Rietman, A, van Eeghen, A, de Wit, M. Everolimus for the treatment of refractory seizures associated with tuberous sclerosis complex (TSC): current perspectives. *TCRM* 2019; 15, 951–5.

Panzica, F, Varotto, G, Rotondi, F, Spreafico, R, Franceschetti, S. Identification of the Epileptogenic Zone from Stereo-EEG Signals: A Connectivity-Graph Theory Approach. *Front. Neurol* 2013; 4.

Parker, W.E, Orlova, K.A, Parker, W.H, *et al.* Rapamycin Prevents Seizures After Depletion of STRADA in a Rare Neurodevelopmental Disorder. *Sci Transl Med* 2013. 5, 1–22.

Pelorosso, C, Watrin, F, Conti, V, *et al.* Somatic double-hit in MTOR and RPS6 in hemimegalencephaly with intractable epilepsy. *Human Molecular Genetics* 2019; 28, 3755–65.

Ribierre, T, Deleuze, C, Bacq, A, *et al.* Second-hit mosaic mutation in mTORC1 repressor DEPDC5 causes focal cortical dysplasia-associated epilepsy. *Journal of Clinical Investigation* 2018; 128, 2452–8.

Sato, T, Ishii, J, Ota, Y, Sasaki, E, Shibagaki, Y, Hattori, S. Mammalian target of rapamycin (mTOR) complex 2 regulates filamin A-dependent focal adhesion dynamics and cell migration. *Genes Cells* 2016; 21, 579–93.

Shen, Y.-W. Sirolimus treatment for tuberous sclerosis complex prior to epilepsy: Evidence from a registry-based real-world study. *Seizure* 2022; 97: 23-31.

Slegtenhorst, M. van, Hoogt, R. de, Hermans, C, *et al.* Identification of the Tuberous Sclerosis Gene *TSC1* on Chromosome 9q34. *Science* 1997; 277, 805–8.

Switon, K, Kotulska, K, Janusz-Kaminska, A, Zmorzynska, J, Jaworski, J. Molecular neurobiology of mTOR. *Neuroscience* 2017; 341, 112–53.

van der Poest Clement, E, Jansen, F.E, Braun, K.P.J, Peters, J.M. Update on Drug Management of Refractory Epilepsy in Tuberous Sclerosis Complex. *Pediatr Drugs* 2020; 22, 73–84.

Xu, Q, Uliel-Sibony, S, Dunham, C, *et al.* mTOR Inhibitors as a New Therapeutic Strategy in Treatment Resistant Epilepsy in Hemimegalencephaly: A Case Report. *J Child Neurol* 2019. 34, 132-138.

Zoncu, R, Efeyan, A, Sabatini, D.M. mTOR: from growth signal integration to cancer, diabetes and ageing. *Nat Rev Mol Cell Biol* 2011; 12, 21–35.

CHAPTER

6. Drug therapies in FCD: are they specific and why?

Sarah Buts, J. Helen Cross

Key points

- The natural course of epilepsy due to FCD is mainly known from surgical centres and therefore limited to drug resistant patients.
- No anti-seizure drug has proven to be superior to others, although carbamazepine appears to be relatively more frequently reported in patients who are seizure-free.
- Ketogenic diet may have specific efficacy in children, possibly related to changes of DNA methylation and also modulation of mTOR pathways.
- mTOR inhibitors used in Tuberous Sclerosis remain under investigation in FCD.

Introduction

FCD remains the most common pathology in paediatric epilepsy surgical series, leading to the presumption that many of the epilepsies associated with cortical dysplasia remain pharmacoresistant. As most series are reported from surgical centres, little is reported on response to antiepileptic medication. It may therefore be presumed that little specific response may be seen, and surgical referral remains inevitable (Ben Zvi *et al.*, 2022).

In this chapter, we will discuss the effect of standard anti-seizure medication in the course of epilepsy due to FCD and the potential efficacy of more specific therapies such as ketogenic diet and drugs influencing the mammalian target of rapamycin (mTOR) pathway.

Effect of standard anti-seizure medication

Fauser *et al.* reported on the natural history of a series of 120 patients with FCD presenting to a surgical unit; 17% reported a history of a transient response to pharmacotherapy, defined as a seizure free period of at least one year, that could last up to 9-12 years - 28 years in one case (Fauser *et al.*, 2006). The medications utilised to achieve this were highly variable with no specific medication appearing to be responsible more than another - either monotherapy with carbamazepine, valproate, phenobarbital, topiramate and phenytoin, or combination therapy with phenytoin and phenobarbital, valproate and gabapentin and carbamazepine with phenytoin. Three remained seizure-free without medication. The fact that this period of seizure freedom could be achieved early or late in the disease course suggests direct response to anti-seizure medications may not have been responsible.

Although there appears a relative higher proportion reported on carbamazepine or oxcarbazepine, this may not reflect specific responsiveness, but moreover the likelihood of these medications being utilised in focal onset seizures. There is little evidence that any anti-seizure medication is superior in efficacy in FCD. A further series reported Level 4 evidence that valproate and benzodiazepines were the most promising therapies (Bast *et al.*, 2006), whilst other authors have noted relative insensitivity to benzodiazepine treatment (Talos *et al.*, 2012) or raised concern that drugs targeting the GABAA receptor may be poorly effective or even detrimental (Guerrini *et al.*, 2015).

Ketogenic diet: specific efficacy through specific mechanisms?

The ketogenic diet (KD) is a high fat, adequate protein and low carbohydrate diet, used in the treatment of the epilepsies. It has been proven to be effective in several randomised trials in childhood epilepsies (Neal *et al.*, 2008; Neal *et al.*, 2009; Sharma *et al.*, 2013), with a meta-analysis of four studies within a Cochrane systematic review demonstrating efficacy in favour of the ketogenic diet over care as usual in children with drug resistant epilepsy (Martin-McGill *et al.*, 2020). There is little data in adults, but available evidence suggests it can also be beneficial if tolerated and compliance is good. A particularly favourable response has been demonstrated in children with FCD: in a study of 42 children with intractable epilepsy due to FCD who started the diet, 61.7% had a more than 50% reduction in seizure frequency and 44.7% became seizure-free at three months. 76.2% of the seizure-free group stayed on the diet for the next two years without relapse and 42.9% remained seizure free after weaning of the diet over a mean follow-up period of 3 years and 10 months (Jung *et al.*, 2008). A subsequent study of response according to aetiology has also suggested a favourable response in epilepsies due to FCD; seizure freedom seen in 15% with a further 30% having a seizure reduction of 90-95% (Breu *et al.*, 2021).

• Why should there be a specifically favourable effect on epilepsy associated with FCD?

When considering possible mechanisms of action many effects on cell metabolism have been proposed, although this would not appear to be specific to FCD (Lutas *et al.*, 2013). Further, tantalising is the lasting effect that is apparent, even when the KD is weaned, suggesting a degree of disease modification. In vitro studies in a rat model of epilepsy have shown that the KD attenuates epigenetic chromatin modifications induced by seizures, and therefore may impact epigenetic regulation (Kobow *et al.*, 2013a). Epigenetic regulation is a mechanism defining the versatile activity states of a gene, whereby a set of chromatin-modifying actions leads to a change in genetic activity, without affecting DNA sequence itself. Such modifications may include DNA methylation, posttranslational histone tail modifications (e.g., acetylation, methylation, phosphorylation, ubiquitination, or SUMOylation), incorporation of histone variants (e.g., macroH2A, H2A.X,H2A.Z, H3.3, CENP-A), nucleosome and higher order chromatin remodeling processes, as well as nuclear localization and the action of noncoding RNAs (ncRNAs) (Kobow *et al.*, 2013b). Such processes have been shown to play a role in treatment response and manifestations in various pathological conditions, including cancer and response to treatment. Epigenetic mechanisms could be seen to be responsible for many aspects of epilepsy, not least pharmaco-responsiveness and comorbidities. Utilising a pilocarpine rat model of temporal lobe epilepsy, Kobow and colleagues demonstrated an increase in DNA methylation changes in the brain in the chronic epilepsy model when compared to controls. Aberrant methylation patterns were inversely correlated with gene expression changes using mRNA sequencing from animals and tissue specimens (Kobow *et al.*, 2013a). Administration of a ketogenic, high-fat, low-carbohydrate diet to the rats attenuated seizure progression and ameliorated DNA methylation mediated changes in gene expression, suggesting the KD protected from the same degree of change. Utilising 15 surgical specimens of FCD, matched with 5 epilepsy and 6 non-epilepsy controls, differential hierarchical cluster analysis of DNA methylation distinguished major FCD subtypes (i.e., IA, IIA, and IIB) from patients with temporal lobe epilepsy and non-epileptic controls suggesting aetiology dependent patterns (Kobow *et al.*, 2019). This said, further study has shown evidence that such changes may be a general pathomechanism associated with epileptogenesis and epilepsy, but that the broad pathophysiological differences between models assessed are reflected in distinct aetiology-dependent DNA methylation patterns (Dębski *et al.*, 2016).

• Effect on the mTor pathway

There is also the hypothesis however, that the KD has an action on the mTOR pathway. Limited clinical data suggest a favourable response of epilepsy associated with Tuberous Sclerosis to treatment with the KD (Kossoff *et al.*, 2005; Coppola *et al.*, 2006), with 92% achieving a

>50% reduction in seizures at 6m in one retrospective series (Kossoff *et al.*, 2005). In a further study, 21 of 31 (67.7%) children commenced on a KD for treatment of epilepsy associated with Tuberous Sclerosis had >50% reduction in seizures at 3 months after initiating the KD. Thirteen of the 31 patients (41.9%) were seizure-free for at least 3 months, but 10/13 (76.9%) experienced seizure recurrence during the 24-month follow-up period (Youna *et al.*, 2020). At 24 months of the KD observational period, however, there was >50% response in 10/31 patients (32.3%), including 6 (19.4%) seizure-free patients. In vitro data suggest inhibition of the mammalian target of rapamycin (mTOR) pathway by the ketogenic diet. Utilising a kainate model of epilepsy, rats that had been fed a ketogenic diet had decreased markers for the activation of mTOR complex 1 (mTORC1) (decreased expression levels in the hippocampus and liver of phosphorylated S6 (pS6)) and and mTOR complex 2 (phosphorylated AKT (pAKT)) (McDaniel *et al.*, 2020). In a further clinical study, 25 patients with pathologically confirmed FCD, who were screened for the presence of detectable somatic mTOR pathway mutations had received a sufficient KD prior to surgery for evaluation (Ko *et al.*, 2022). Twelve of these patients (48.0%) had germline or somatic detectable mTOR pathway mutations. A response to KD was defined as a ≥50% reduction in seizure frequency. The efficacy of the KD after 3 months of dietary therapy was superior in patients with detectable mTOR pathway mutations than in patients without detectable mTOR pathway mutations, although the difference was not statistically significant (responder rates of 58.3% vs 38.5%, p=0.434).

Role of mTOR inhibitors

As highlighted elsewhere, low-level mosaic somatic mutations in mTOR pathway activating genes (MTOR, AKT3, PIK3CA, RHEB) are a major cause of FCD II and Germline TSC1, TSC2, DEPDC5, NPRL2 and NPRL3 variants are also associated with FCD II. The relationship between abnormalities in the mTOR pathway and pathogenesis of FCD therefore leads to the question as to a possible role of mTOR inhibitors in the management of epilepsy associated with this pathology. Efficacy has been demonstrated in the treatment of epilepsy associated with Tuberous Sclerosis with mTOR inhibitors both in open label studies (evirolimus (Krueger *et al.*, 2013), sirolimus (rapamycin) (Cardamone *et al.*, 2014) and metformin (Amin *et al.*, 2020) as well as a randomised controlled trial utilising everolimus (French *et al.*, 2016). In the latter, although primary outcome was determined at 3 months, a steady increment in benefit was noted both in the high and low dose group, suggesting a degree of disease modification. Rapamycin has been demonstrated to reduce seizures in rodent models of FCD (Lim *et al.*, 2015, Hsich *et al.*, 2016).

The outcome of a multicentre clinical trial of sirolimus (rapamycin) has recently been reported from Japan (Kato *et al.*, 2022). This involved an initial exploratory study involving 16 patients to review pharmacokinetics and efficacy. Patients were included aged 6–65 years who were diagnosed with FCD II via brain MRI in accordance with radiological criteria or histopathological findings. All patients had focal onset seizures, including focal to bilateral tonic-clonic seizures, at a frequency of more than twice in a 28-day baseline phase. All had a treatment history of more than two antiepileptic drugs for at least 52 weeks after epilepsy diagnosis and were receiving one to four concomitant anti-seizure medications. None dropped out during baseline, but one dropped out during the phase of dose adjustment due to concomitant utilisation of drugs contraindicated for status epilepticus. A further 2 patients were excluded from the final analysis due to non-compliance and use of prohibited drugs. The median reduction rate of focal seizure frequency per 28 days during the maintenance therapy period was 25% (range: -89% to 100%), which was not determined to be significant. The response rate was 33% (5/15, 90% CI: 14–58%). One patient was seizure free during the maintenance therapy period (7%, 90% CI: 0.3–28%). The authors noted that the reduction in focal seizures did not meet the predetermined level of statistical significance, but did note that seizure frequency reduced over time on treatment and the efficacy response rate was comparable to that seen with everolimus, albeit this being an open label study. It was also noted that all patients experienced adverse events, particularly stomatitis, the most frequent adverse event also seen in the everolimus trials. This was a very limited trial, but results and safety profile suggest further study is warranted. A prospective, placebo-controlled clinical trial of everolimus is underway for patients with drug resistant epilepsy due to FCD II previously treated with surgery (NCT03198949).

Conclusion

Epilepsy associated with FCD has traditionally proven resistant to standard anti-seizure medications, although periods of remission may be seen. No specific anti-seizure medication has been shown to be effective. This said, the ketogenic diet, has been shown to be selectively effective, with persistence of efficacy beyond weaning of the diet. Changes to DNA methylation have been postulated to be a possible mechanism of action in this effect. Further the KD has been suggested to have effects on the mTOR pathway, abnormalities of which have been associated with the pathogenesis of FCD. MToR inhibitors, shown to be effective in the treatment of epilepsy associated with Tuberous Sclerosis characterised by tubers indistinguishable pathologically from FCD, are now being explored with regard to the treatment of FCD associated epilepsy and may be an option for medical treatment in the future.

References

Amin S, Mallick AA, Edward H, *et al.* The metformin in tuberous sclerosis (MiTS) study: A randomised double blind placebo-controlled trial. *EClinicalMedicine* 2020; 100715.

Bast T, Ramantani G, Seitz A, Rating D. Focal cortical dysplasia: prevalence, clinical presentation and epilepsy in children and adults. *Acta Neurol Scand* 2006: 113: 72-81.

Ben Zvi I, Enright N, D'arco F *et al.* Children with seizures and radiological diagnosis of focal cortical dysplasia: can drug resistant epilepsy be predicted earlier? *Epileptic Disorders* 2022.

Breu M, Häfele C Trimmel-Schwahofer P, *et al.* The relation of etiology based on the 2017 ILAE classification to the effectiveness of the ketogenic diet in drug-resistant epilepsy in childhood. *Epilepsia* 2021; 62: 2814-25.

Cardamone M, Flanagan D, Mowat D, *et al.* Mammalian target of rapamycin inhibitors for intractable epilepsy and subependymal giant cell astrocytomas in tuberous sclerosis complex. *Journal of Pediatrics.* 2014; 164: 1195-200.

Coppola G, Klepper J, Ammendola E, *et al.* The effects of the ketogenic diet in refractory partial seizures with reference to tuberous sclerosis. *European Journal Paediatric Neurology* 2006; 10: 148-51.

Dębski KJ, Pitkanen A, Puhakka N, *et al.* Etiology matters - Genomic DNA Methylation Patterns in Three Rat Models of Acquired Epilepsy. *Sci Rep.* 2016 May 9; 6: 25668.

Fauser S, Huppertz HJ, Bast T, *et al.* Clinical characteristics in focal cortical dysplasia: a retrospective evaluation in a series of 120 patients. *Brain* 2006; 129: 1907-16.

French JA, Lawson JA, Yapici Z, *et al.* Adjunctive everolimus therapy for treatment-resistant focal-onset seizures associated with tuberous sclerosis (EXIST-3): a phase 3, randomised, double-blind, placebo-controlled study. *Lancet* 2016; 388: 2153-63.

Guerrini R, Duchowny M, Jayakar P *et al.* Diagnostic methods and treatment options for focal cortical dysplasia. *Epilepsia* 2015; 56(11): 1669-86.

Hsieh LS, Wen JH, Claycomb K, *et al.* Convulsive seizures from experimental focal cortical dysplasia occur independently of cell misplacement. *Nature Communications.* 2016; 7: 11753.

Jung DE, Kang HC, Kim HD. Long-term outcome of the ketogenic diet for intractable childhood epilepsy with focal cortical malformation of cortical development. *Pediatrics* 2008; 122: e330-3.

Kato M, Kada A, Shiraishi H *et al.* Sirolimus for epileptic seizures associated with focal cortical dysplasia type II. *Annals of Clinical and Translational Neurology* 2022; 9(2): 181-92.

Ko A, Sim NS, Choi HS, *et al.* Efficacy of the ketogenic diet for pediatric epilepsy according to the presence of detectable somatic mTOR pathway mutations in the brain. *J Clin Neurol* 2022 18(1): 71-8.

Kobow K, Kaspi A, Harikrishnan KN, *et al.* Deep sequencing reveals increased DNA methylation in chronic rat epilepsy. *Acta Neuropathol* 2013a; 126: 741-56.

Kobow K, El-Osta A, Blümcke I. The methylation hypothesis of pharmacoresistance in epilepsy. *Epilepsia* 2013b 54 Suppl 2: 41-47.

Kobow K, Ziemann M, Kaipananickal H, *et al.* Genomic DNA methylation distinguishes subtypes of human focal cortical dysplasia. *Epilepsia.* 2019; 60(6): 1091-103.

Kossoff EH, Thiele EA, Pfeifer HH, *et al.* Tuberous sclerosis complex and the ketogenic diet. *Epilepsia* 2005; 46: 1684-6.

Krueger D, Wilfong AA, Holland-Bouley K, *et al.* Everolimus treatment of refractory epilepsy in tuberous sclerosis complex. *Annals of Neurology* 2013; 74: 679-87.

Lim JS, Kim WI, Kang HC, *et al.* Brain somatic mutations in MTOR cause focal cortical dysplasia type II leading to intractable epilepsy. *Nature Medicine.* 2015; 21: 395-400.

Lutas A, Yellen G. The ketogenic diet: metabolic influences on brain excitability and epilepsy. *Trends in Neurosciences* 2013; 36, (1) 40.

Martin-McGill KJ, Bresnahan R, Levy RG, Cooper PN. Ketogenic diets for drug resistant epilepsy. *Cochrane Database of Systematic Reviews* 2020, Issue 6. Art. No.: CD001903.

McDaniel SS, Rensing NR, Thio LL, Yamada KA, Wong M. The ketogenic diet inhibits the mammalian target of rapamycin (mTOR) pathway. *Epilepsia* 2011; 52: e7-e11.

Neal EG, Chaffe HM, Edwards N, *et al.* The ketogenic diet in the treatment of epilepsy in children: a randomised, controlled trial (NCT00564915). *Lancet Neurol* 2008; 7: 500-6.

Neal EG, Chaffe HM, Schwartz RH, *et al.* A randomised trial of classical and medium chain triglyceride ketogenic diets in the treatment of childhood epilepsy. *Epilepsia* 2009; 50: 1109-17.

Sharma S, Sankhyan N, Gulati S, *et al.* Use of the modified Atkins diet for treatment of refractory childhood epilepsy: a randomised controlled trial. *Epilepsia* 2013; 54: 481-6.

Talos DM, Sun H, Kosaras B, *et al.* Altered inhibition in tuberous sclerosis and type IIb cortical dysplasia. *Annals of Neurology* 2012; 71(4): 539-51.

Youna SE, Park S, Kima SH, *et al.* Long-term outcomes of ketogenic diet in patients with tuberous sclerosis complex-derived epilepsy. *Epilepsy Research* 2020; 164: 106348.

CHAPTER

7. Electroclinical phenotypes in FCD

Francine Chassoux, Andre Palmini, Laura Tassi

Key points

- FCD II are characterized by early epilepsy onset, high seizure frequency, focal seizures pointing to a well localized brain area and sleep related epilepsy.
- They are mainly located in extratemporal areas, especially in the frontal lobes and usually affects children with normal development.
- A stormy course with explosive onset followed by a relatively long remission may be observed. Anti-seizure drug withdrawal during remission may induce relapses, including status epilepticus and mark the onset of intractable seizures.
- Interictal EEG is pathognomonic in about half of the cases, showing continuous rhythmic or pseudorhythmic spikes, increasing during sleep.
- FCD I are associated with heterogeneous electroclinical features and non-specific imaging, but can be suspected in children with severe epilepsy, early onset, mental retardation, posterior location and lobar hypotrophy.
- FCD III have no specific features but behave like the major associated lesions (hippocampal sclerosis, glioneuronal tumors, vascular malformations, scars).

Introduction

Correct diagnosis and treatment planning in epilepsy begin with the identification of electroclinical phenotypes that raise suspicion of the underlying pathology. Beyond sheer choice of anti-seizure medications according to seizure types, pathology is crucial to decide on level of dosages and anticipate prognosis regarding seizure control. Therefore, because early referral for presurgical evaluation is key to foster development and improve prognosis in children with recurrent seizures, knowing what disease is causing the epilepsy is crucial.

As detailed in previous chapters, cumulative data indicated that FCD II was a singular pathological entity with specific properties, especially strikingly focal and high epileptogenicity, first identified by a clinician from the charts in a small surgical series (Taylor *et al.*, 1971). The same approach achieved the same results at the same time when looking at patients in the Montreal and Sainte-Anne groups 25 years ago. Clinical and EEG features were so similar that it couldn't be haphazard. From the initial descriptions, the clinical picture was rapidly drawn (Palmini *et al.*, 1991, 1995; Chassoux *et al.*, 2000; Tassi *et al.*, 2002), and later confirmed in all further studies focusing on FCD II (Fauser *et al.*, 2006; Chassoux *et al.*, 2012; Tassi *et al.*, 2012; Guerrini 2015). On the other hand, electroclinical features in FCD I are less reliable, probably related to its heterogeneity.

This chapter describes how clinical data has been collected according to the evolution of concepts and how they were integrated into the current knowledge, providing the key clinical features that should prompt suspicion of an FCD, and particularly FCD II. Furthermore, we highlight aspects that must be taken into account in the management of patients with FCD both to prevent serious complications, such as flurries of seizures or status epilepticus, and to streamline surgical referral.

Historical overview: from clinical phenotypes to classifications and vice-versa

FCD are considered one of the most frequent epileptogenic brain malformations, and because of their propensity to be cured with surgical treatment, a specific classification was needed. Based upon a combination of imaging, electroclinical, and neuropathological findings, a first classification of FCD was proposed (Tassi *et al.*, 2002; Colombo *et al.*, 2003), and further refined by Palmini *et al.* (2004) then the ILAE (Blumcke *et al.*, 2011). As discussed in the previous chapters by Palmini and Blümcke, neuropathological characteristics were depicted and classified in 3 subtypes, in which Type II corresponded to the initial description by Taylor *et al* (1971). Clinical pictures followed the course of these classification updates but also influenced their validation.

The first detailed electroclinical description of patients suffering from drug-resistant focal epilepsy, with typical EEG pattern, both surface and intracerebral, was provided by Palmini *et al* (1995) who wrote: "Intractable partial epilepsy is often associated with structural lesions of the cerebral cortex. Among the different types of structural epileptogenic abnormalities, cortical dysplastic lesions (CDyL) have generated a great deal of interest lately, since many can now be reliably detected during life by magnetic resonance imaging (MRI)". In this initial report, the mean age of epilepsy onset was 5 years, there was a close correlation between the anatomic lesion site and EEG abnormalities, the ECoG epileptiform pattern was continuous or nearly continuous, and from a surgical point of view an incomplete resection of the dysplastic lesion was the more significant finding associated with an unfavorable outcome.

A few years later, Chassoux *et al* (2000) suggested that FCD were an increasingly recognized cause of focal intractable epilepsy necessitating a complete removal to obtain a good surgical outcome. The neurophysiological pattern with the support of Stereo-EEG was characterized by interictal rhythmic or pseudorhythmic spiking and low epileptogenic threshold. At the time, FCD accounted for 3 -7% of all histological diagnosis in epilepsy surgery series. However, most patients were operated before the era of imaging, and in others detection of the lesion with MRI was difficult, especially small FCD. In addition, defining the boundaries of the lesion on neuroimaging and macroscopic appearance during surgery was challenging. Most patients had frontal localization, early onset and high seizure frequency with multi-daily focal seizures, rarely generalizing. SEEG seizures showed a characteristic pattern with low voltage fast activity or rhythmic spikes.

Other attempts at neurophysiological and histopathological correlations were carried out (Boonyapisit *et al.*, 2003) with the purpose to match cellular patterns of MCD with focal cortical epileptogenicity, as assessed by direct extraoperative electrocorticographic recordings using subdural grids. That study highlighted that within a single dysplastic lesion, areas containing balloon cells (BC) were less epileptogenic than those without BC, suggesting for the first time a different "neurophysiological behavior" in different parts of an FCD lesion and a possible protective effect of BC - or a disruption within the neuronal networks in BC-containing dysplastic tissue. Moreover, patients with BC-containing FCD had an earlier age at seizure onset, more frequent seizures, and worse postoperative outcome, a data not confirmed in recent studies.

One of the major difficulties in the classification of FCD, that currently prevents a firm association of typical phenotypes with each FCD subtype, is the lack of agreement between neuropathologists, who should provide a final diagnosis. In fact, it was demonstrated that interobserver concordance was at best moderate (Chamberlain *et al.*, 2009). The higher concordance was obtained in FCD IIA/B, and the lower for mild MCD and FCD IA/B (chapter 2). In addition, the main difficulties were differentiating mild MCD and FCD I from normal and/or gliotic tissue. Based on this assumption, anatomo-electroclinical correlations can be validated only in FCD II. Importantly, it must be therefore considered that studies grouping all FCD subtypes are no longer suitable, because mixing completely different pathologies, whose relevance have yet to be confirmed from the etiopathogenetic standpoint, may lead to confusing results.

According to these views, the clinical picture of FCD II was refined from studies based on homogeneous groups of patients. This was well illustrated by the identification of a relationship between seizures during sleep-time and FCD II (Nobili *et al.*, 2007, 2009). Analysis of patients undergoing surgery with both frontal and extrafrontal sleep-related epilepsy (SRE) demonstrates a high proportion of FCD II as an etiologic factor, suggesting that this histologic substrate could be an important determinant of sleep-related seizures. This high prevalence could reflect the sleep-induced modification of the pattern of epileptic activity: during slow-wave sleep, interictal activity is mainly organized in pseudo-periodically recurrent short bursts of fast discharges (between 14 and 18 Hz) that could spread over the surrounding non-lesional areas and develop into a seizure. Notably, in those studies, despite a significantly higher proportion of FCD II into the frontal lobe (67% in the frontal, 33% and 37% in the temporal lobe and posterior quadrant, respectively), one in two patients suffered from SRE, regardless of location. This data confirmed the effect of FCD II as an independent risk factor for the correlation between sleep and seizures, thus suggesting the presence of FCD II as an etiologic factor in drug-resistant patients with SRE (Nobili *et al* 2009, Losurdo *et al.*, 2014).

Subsequently, Chassoux *et al* (2012) reported the first suggestive clinical picture to identify FCD II in epileptic patients: a severe partial epilepsy beginning in childhood, with high seizure frequency including status epilepticus, stereotyped seizures, extratemporal location, pseudorhythmic activity on EEG and typical Stereo-EEG pattern. Furthermore, some fundamental points were highlighted: in about one third of patients MR remains negative despite optimal imaging, and FDG-PET can be very useful having a localization value in 84% in MRI-negative cases and helping to delineate the dysplastic cortex in 65% of the MRI-positive cases and the clear correlation between FCD II and SRE was confirmed. For the first time it was also emphasized that cognitive deficit was mostly observed in children with large dysplastic lesions and early onset of epilepsy, whereas no or mild impairment was observed in adults with small FCD.

At the same time, Tassi *et al.* (2012), analyzing a series of 100 patients operated for intractable epilepsy due to FCD II, found no significant differences in gender, age at epilepsy onset, duration of epilepsy, age at surgery or seizure frequency between those with and those without BC. However, patients with FCD IIB more frequently presented with SRE. The peculiar Stereo-EEG pattern was characterized by rhythmic or pseudo-rhythmic spikes or polyspikes ("brushes") in 76% of the patients with FCD IIB, ie, with BC ($p < 0.001$). Type IIA also differed from IIB in the higher probability of having a negative MRI and a less good surgical outcome.

A very important issue is how relevant clinical data may guide basic research. Based on homogeneous electroclinical phenotypes rapidly identified and disseminated among epilepsy centers, the first reports supporting a possible genetic origin of FCD arose almost simultaneously at both ends of the world (Scheffer *et al.*, 2014; Baulac *et al.*, 2015), showing that DEPDC5 mutations may be associated with FCD II in individuals with familial epilepsy. This innovative concept that a single gene mutation may generate non-lesional epilepsy in a family member and FCD in another challenges previous notions based on the distinction between genetic malformations and "non-lesional" epilepsy syndromes. Further exponential progress in the genetics of FCD is detailed by Baulac and Baldassari (chapter 4).

Over the following years, the neuropathological, neuroradiological and clinical knowledge has been refined: FCD II are assumed to be due to cellular and/or architectural abnormalities occurring during early brain development *in utero*, while other subtypes may be related to peri-postnatal causes (Najm *et al.*, 2014). The growing incidence of FCD in surgical series was attributed to better identification of the lesions through improved MRI, as well as better understanding of the electroclinical variant of various FCD subtypes and consequently more favorable surgical outcomes depending on completeness of surgical resection of the epileptic tissue.

In addition to the well delineated clinical picture of FCD II, a number of studies focused specifically in the distinction between FCD II from FCD I and other MCD (Krsek *et al.*, 2009; Lerner *et al.*, 2009; Tassi *et al.*, 2010; Hauptman and Mathern, 2012). These studies showed that patients with FCD II generally have a younger age at seizure onset (usually pre-school) and at surgery, as well as higher seizure frequency than isolated FCD I and other etiologies. FCD II are most often located in extratemporal areas or may be hemispheric, whereas FCD I is most often encountered in the temporal lobe. FCD I may be multilobar in about 30% of cases, and in these cases, epilepsy start at a younger age, and may present with focal seizures evolving to an epileptic encephalopathy, with epileptic spasms, although encephalopathy may be a feature of either FCD I or II.

Full electroclinical data are detailed in the second part of this chapter.

Typical presentation of FCD II: red flags that should not be missed

As previously indicated, the main location of FCD II in extratemporal regions and frontal lobe, observed in the pioneer's series, has been confirmed in more recent collective studies (Blumcke *et al.*, 2017, Wagstyl *et al.*, 2021). This must be kept in mind when searching for FCD II.

• Early epilepsy onset: a childhood disease

The first remarkable clinical feature is the early onset of seizures, with a median age at onset of 2 years (mean 5.6 ± 6.9), probably the earliest for focal lesional epilepsy. This was found in monocentric studies and confirmed in a multicentric collection of data (Blumcke *et al.*, 2017). Epilepsy onset in infancy or young children in preschool age is indeed more frequent than in epilepsy due to other lesions such hippocampal sclerosis (11.3 ± 10.1), gangliogliomas (12.1±10.3) and other malformations of cortical development (9.6 ± 10.0) such heterotopias and polymicrogyrias. Notably the age at seizure onset has been related to the size of the dysplastic lesion, the larger the earliest, as shown in pediatric series (chapter 8). However, later onset in teenagers or adults may also be observed and does not preclude the diagnosis.

• High seizure frequency and stormy course

The second striking feature is the very high seizure frequency, usually several per day including clusters (10- 80 seizures per day), that may be particularly explosive at the beginning of the disease, but sometimes dramatically resolves with anti-seizure monotherapy (frequently a sodium channel blocker). Epilepsy may also be refractory from onset, at times with status epilepticus and associated with severe disability. This stormy course in a developmentally normal child is indeed very suggestive of FCD II and can be retrospectively found in the history of patients investigated at adulthood with a "non-lesional" focal epilepsy.

Another possible course is a seizure-free period under medication, yet with unexpected return of seizures after a number of years, that then become medically refractory (Fauser *et al*, 2006, Chassoux *et al.*, 2012). Importantly, long silent period, lasting 2 years or more (up to 20 years in our experience), encouraging the patient and the neurologist to discontinue medication, may be followed by severe relapse including status epilepticus. These possible trajectories must be considered from a decision-making standpoint when a FCD II is suspected or identified.

• Strikingly focal semiology

Listening to the patient is probably the best way to find the lesion. Nowadays, with all the available investigative technology, it is a rare enough situation in clinical practice that it needs to be emphasized. Stereotyped seizures pointing very accurately to a brain area (a well localized pain in a finger, a funny feeling in a hemiface, a loss of control of a limb, a bad taste on the tongue...), continuing with a fixed scenario suggestive of a brain region, allow to determine the location of the lesion with a high confidence. Of note, focal aware is the main seizure type in most patients while bilateral tonic-clonic seizures are rare, despite the high frequency of attacks. One of the most demonstrative examples is the "Chapeau de gendarme" sign, also described under the term "ictal pouting", reported in a series of FCD patients in whom ictal networks included the anterior cingulate gyrus (Souirti *et al.*, 2014). This rare but peculiar finding immediately induced a clinical enthusiasm and led to a myriad of case reports coming from everywhere in the word with various European, Turkish, American, Japanese and Chinese "chapeaux", including pediatric cases and mostly related to FCD as underlying pathology (Tan *et al.*, 2016, Koc *et al.*, 2017, Hayakawa *et al.*, 2018, Wiwchar *et al.*, 2019, Cebeci *et al.*, 2020, Rusch *et al.*, 2021, Lu *et al.*, 2021). Interestingly, more recent reports postulated that such sign was highly suggestive of FCD because it was not observed in other epileptogenic lesions associated with more diffuse epileptic networks. Another example are insular epilepsies, whose specific semiology is usually associated with FCD pathology and helps distinguish different networks originating from the insula (Mullati *et al.*, 2019, Martinez-Lizana, 2021). Finally, precise semiology reported in patients with FCD located in the central region allows accurate navigation in each part of these eloquent anatomo-functional areas (Chassoux *et al.*, 2022). This clinical information, the sole basis for location of FCD before the era of modern imaging, is unique in the field of lesional focal epilepsy and must be emphasized as probably underused in the clinical practice.

• Sleep induced seizures: a specific hallmark

Sleep related epilepsy (SRE), characterized by at least 70% of seizures occurring during sleep, is frequently found in epilepsy due to FCD II, comprising up to 50% of cases in our and others' experience (Nobili *et al.*, 2009, Chassoux *et al.*, 2012, Tassi *et al.*, 2012, Eltze *et al.*, 2020). Seizures mostly occur during NREM sleep (stage II) especially in extratemporal areas, while in the temporal lobe they often occur after a waking period (Eltze *et al.*, 2020). Of note, the strong relationship between FCD II and SRE became obvious relatively late, firstly reported by the Milano group (Nobili *et al.*, 2007, 2009) and then in other centers such as ours (Chassoux *et al.*, 2012, Jin *et al.*, 2018, Eltze *et al.*, 2020). This delay was probably due to the time it took to recruit large cohorts and also the need for a dissemination of epilepsy centres able to provide continuous recordings including during sleep. There was also some confusion because nocturnal seizures were initially associated with the frontal lobe, without a knowledge of the underlying pathology. The propensity to have seizures during sleep in epilepsy due to FCD II was secondarily demonstrated, proving to be an independent factor for SRE whatever the location (Nobili *et al.*, 2009). Moreover, FCD II proved to be the most common histopathological substrate of drug-resistant sleep related hypermotor seizures, regardless of its location inside the brain (Gibbs and al, 2016, 2018). However, as FCD II are mainly located in the frontal lobe, both factors may be cumulative for the risk of SRE.

SRE has been found significantly more frequent in FCD IIB than in FCD IIA in a single series (Tassi *et al.*, 2012). On the other hand, it was also significantly more frequent in MRI-negative FCD II (Chassoux *et al.*, 2012), which are reported to be more often associated with FCD IIA.

In a recent series, we still found a high proportion of patients with negative or doubtful MRI despite better imaging (54% in the whole series, 45% with 3T MRI), in line with our previous observations (Eltze *et al.*, 2020). These findings suggest a relationship between the lesion size and SRE, as smaller FCD can be more difficult to detect on MRI. This hypothesis has been corroborated by a recent study based on volumetric analysis, showing a significant relationship between small FCD II and SRE (Jin *et al.*, 2018). A possible explanation is that smaller FCD II might not be able to recruit sufficient non-dysplastic cortex for seizure initiation and propagation during wakefulness due to a low critical mass of neurons and therefore "need sleep to seize".

To summarize, for any intractable epilepsy of early onset with high seizure frequency, focal seizures, mainly occurring during sleep, and well localizing ictal semiology, the causal lesion is FCD II until proven otherwise. Negative imaging can be considered as additional evidence, since FCD is the only epileptogenic lesion than can correspond to this picture with a normal MRI.

• Neurological and cognitive status

In addition to the characteristics of epilepsy, clinical examination may provide some complementary information. Neurological examination and cognitive functions are usually normal. However, specific deficits have been reported correlating with FCD location, such as sensorimotor deficits in the central region or visual field abnormalities in the occipital lobe. Such deficits are rare and mainly reported in the most severely disabled patients or after status epilepticus. They may also fluctuate according to the frequency of seizures (Chassoux *et al.*, 2022). Intellectual deficiency was not observed except in patients with neonatal onset, and mainly in pediatric series (chapter 8). Psychiatric disorders may be observed in temporal, insular and frontal locations.

• Peculiar patterns

Besides the typical clinical picture, misleading features must be known to avoid a regrettable loss of time to make the diagnosis and refer to surgical consideration. In some patients, the difficult-to-treat epilepsy may have a malignant course, mimicking a progressive disease such Rasmussen encephalitis or other catastrophic encephalopathies. This is particularly true for large FCD with early onset as described by Holthausen and Krsek, in the pediatric chapter. This may also occur in central location, in which epilepsy may present as epilepsia partialis continua (EPC) and progressive motor deficit. We observed such scenario in 3/60 patients in a recent series of central FCD, the myoclonus being associated with a permanent spastic deficit and limb atrophy in 2 (Chassoux *et al.*, 2022). In these patients, the diagnosis of FCD was significantly delayed, and motor disability was irreversible despite surgical cure of the epilepsy. Even not being common in this situation, searching for FCD is mandatory to avoid harmful mismanagement.

• Interictal EEG

As detailed in chapters dedicated to neurophysiologic features, scalp-EEG recordings show a peculiar electrographic pattern rarely observed in other epileptogenic lesions, characterized by rhythmic or pseudo-rhythmic spikes and polyspikes, continuous during the recordings and replacing the background activity. This striking activity may be found during the wakefulness or only during sleep in around 40-50% of patients depending on the location of the FCD and, when seen, has high localizing value (**Figure 1**). Since the first description by Palmini *et al* (1995) and Gambardella *et al* (1996), it has been further emphasized by other teams taking care of patients with FCD (Chassoux *et al.*, 2000, 2012, Tassi *et al.*, 2002, 2012, Epitashvili *et al.*, 2018). When associated with the clinical features described above, this EEG pattern can be considered pathognomonic of FCD II.

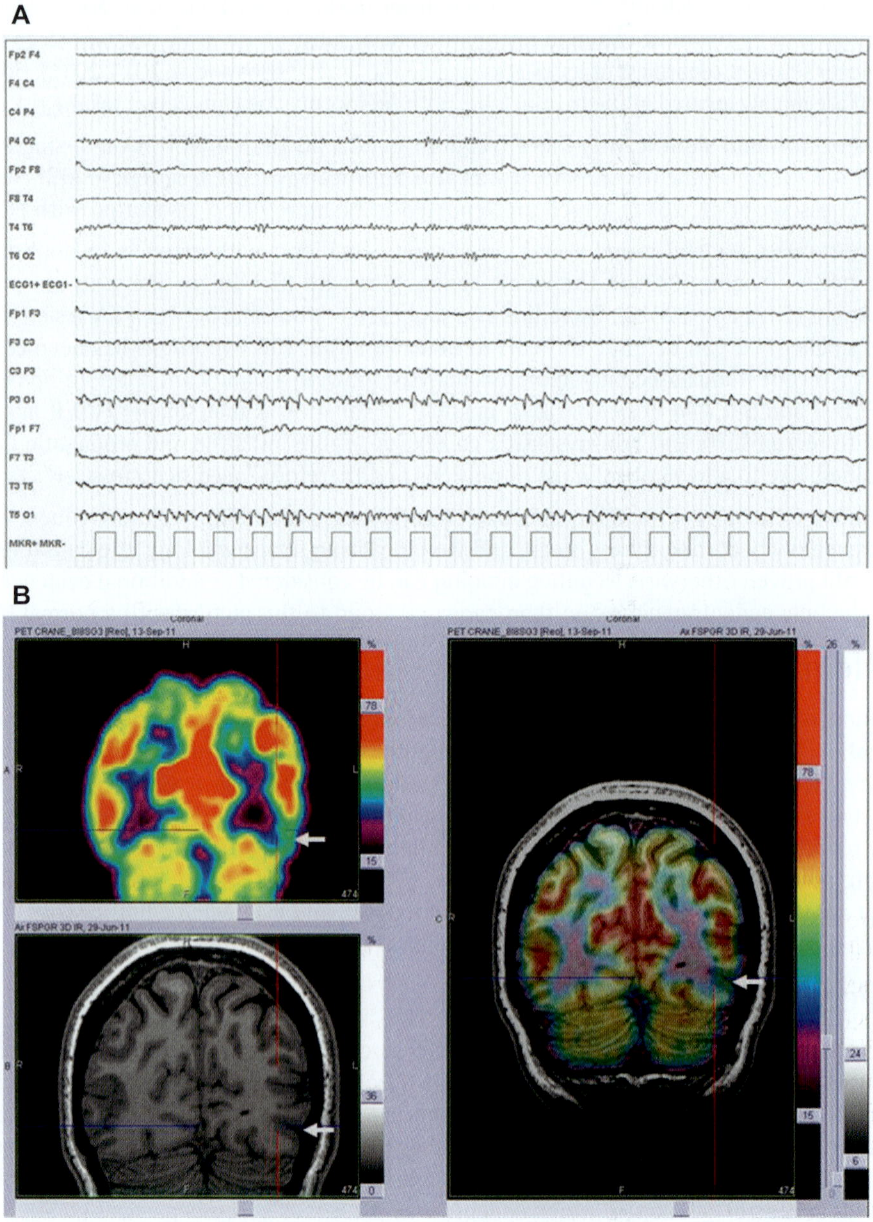

Figure 1

Electroclinical features in a left occipital FCD II.

35 year-old female, epilepsy onset at 7 years. Several seizures per day, blurred vision with impairment of reading from childhood without treatment, nocturnal seizures with loss of consciousness and confusion from the age of 25 years. A. Interictal EEG showing continuous rhythmic spiking on the left occipital region. B. MRI considered normal, FDG-PET allowing detection of a single hypometabolic gyrus in the left lateral occipital region, for which a blurring of the grey-white matter interface was retrospectively found on MRI (MRI-negative becoming positive after coregistration with PET). PET-MRI guided resection, histology FCD II B, seizure-free since surgery; anti-seizure drug withdrawal (follow-up 5 years).

Other FCD subtypes: are there suggestive features?

Less typical and relevant electroclinical features have been associated with other FCD subtypes, except for FCD I for which specific pictures have been identified due to careful analysis of homogeneous cohorts. The best example is provided by the recent description by Holthausen *et al* (2021) for MUSEC ILAE FCD IA, as detailed in this volume (chapter 8).

In a previous study focusing on isolated FCD I, Tassi *et al.*, (2010) have reported 66 patients with a wide variable age at onset (0-53 years, mean: 8, SD: 10) and seizure frequency (1-1,000/month, mean: 115, SD: 200). This large variability initially suggested that different pathologies were mixed under the apparently similar histologic diagnosis. Interestingly, a clear distinction was done at that time between isolated FCD I and those associated with other lesions (hippocampal sclerosis, glioneuronal tumors and others), currently classified as FCD III, who shared the same characteristics as than the main lesion. For instance, median monthly seizure frequency in patients with isolated FCD I was 115 versus 10 in those with FCD associated with hippocampal sclerosis (currently classified as FCD IIIA).

In the series reported by Tassi *et al* (2012), no specific EEG or imaging findings were found to be associated with isolated FCD I. Location was frontal in a third of the cases, temporal or multilobar in the others. Despite SEEG performed in about half of the patients, surgical outcome was poor when compared with FCD II or other lesional epilepsies (46% of seizure-free patients vs 80% for other lesions). We reported our personal experience based on a small series of 15 patients among 111 operated on for intractable epilepsy due to FCD, including 96 FCD II (Chassoux, 2013). We observed the same range of onset age than in the Tassi *et al*'s series (0.5-46 years), but when including only the posterior location - temporal and occipital lobes (7 patients), the clinical picture appeared more homogeneous: epilepsy onset before 4 years, infantile spasms in 2, developmental delay in 3, neurological deficit in 3 and high seizure frequency (several per day, up to 30/day). The surgical outcome was similar to that reported by Tassi *et al* (2012): 47% seizure free patients versus 90% for FCD II.

Considering the clinical features identified by Holthausen *et al* (2021), similarities in the clinical picture may indicate that our posterior cases correspond to relatively focal forms of what is now described as MUSEC-ILAE FCD IA, including lobar hypotrophy and blurring of the grey-white matter interface on MRI (**Figure 2**). The identification of this new entity highlights the need of integration of electroclinical and anatomical data with histopathological findings to improve the relevance of FCD classifications.

As a conclusion, some tips

The natural history of FCD II is of drug resistant epilepsy, without prolonged seizure free periods, although these may occasionally occur in some patients. Moreover, FCD II is a common pathology in refractory SRE.

Taken together, some features are characteristic of FCD II and may help define this as an emerging syndrome, or constellation, of clinical, electrographic and imaging features. Hence, clinicians must strongly consider whatever the patient's age if he or she has refractory focal epilepsy with a normal or apparently normal MRI, especially if seizures started during childhood, have high frequency, are predominantly during sleep, ictal semiology points accurately to a focal brain area, cognition is normal or relatively normal and the scalp EEG shows strikingly focal continuous epileptiform abnormalities (**Figure 3**). These clinical features are characteristic to a point that if a patient presents with this electroclinical phenotype, imaging evidence of FCD II (including FDG-PET) should be vigorously pursued. In this scenario, as well in the more common situation in which a localized dysplastic lesion is seen, management has to be very clear: robust dosages of the chosen anti-seizure medication in mono or polytherapy must be adjusted, reduction of dosages or discontinuation of treatment in the uncommon event that seizures are controlled should not be considered or only in exceptional circumstances, and surgical referral should be streamlined as soon as it becomes clear that seizures are not controlled by drugs. There is no point in repeated medication trials, particularly when the FCD is seen. Also, patients with EPC, normal cognition and normal MRI must be considered as having a FCD in the central lesion, unless evolution over a few months point to, for instance, Rasmussen's encephalitis. Finally, FCD I should be strongly suspected when a child has very frequent seizures of apparently unilateral onset, cognitive deterioration, very frequent, posterior-predominant multifocal EEG discharges and mild lobar or quadrant hypotrophy, especially reduced white matter volume.

Other suggestive phenotypes will be certainly described in the future, taking advantage of careful correlations with imaging and genetics.

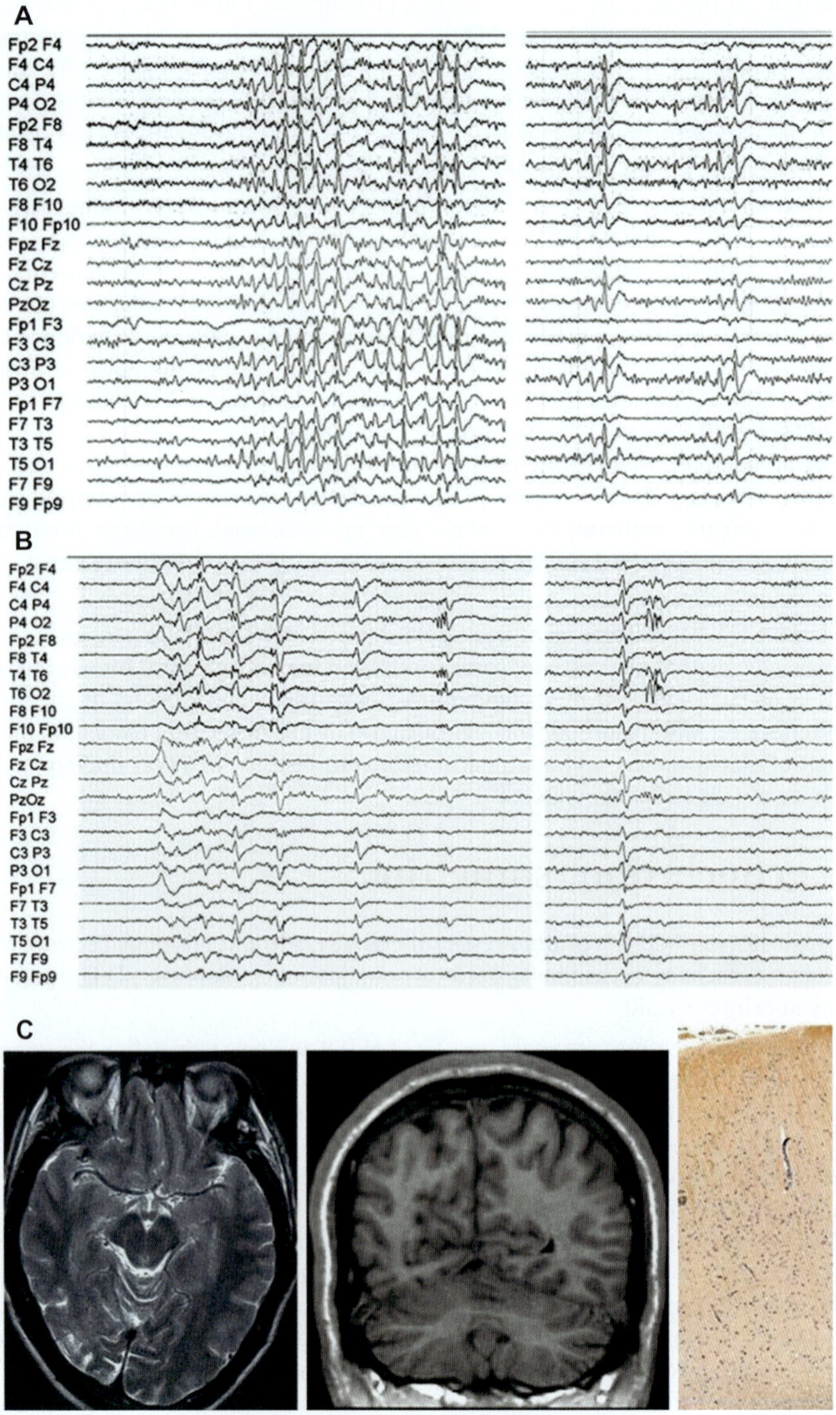

Figure 2

Electroclinical features in a right temporo-occipital FCD I.

26 year-old male, infantile spasms at 10 months, mild cognitive impairment, several seizures per day (2-15) from the age of 9 years. Vertigo, nausea, blurred vision, eyes and head deviation on the left, partial loss of contact, gestural automatisms, no post-ictal deficit. A. Interictal EEG showing discontinuous rhythmic spikes on the right posterior region, propagating to the right hemisphere and to the left side. B. More localized spikes during sleep on the right posterior region. C. MRI (axial T2 and coronal T1 showing a right posterior hypotrophy with a blurring of the grey-white interface; surgery after SEEG, pathological specimen with cortical dyslamination (NeuN). Post-operative improvement with few disabling seizures but monthly focal aware seizures, and still on anti-seizure drugs (follow -up 20 years).

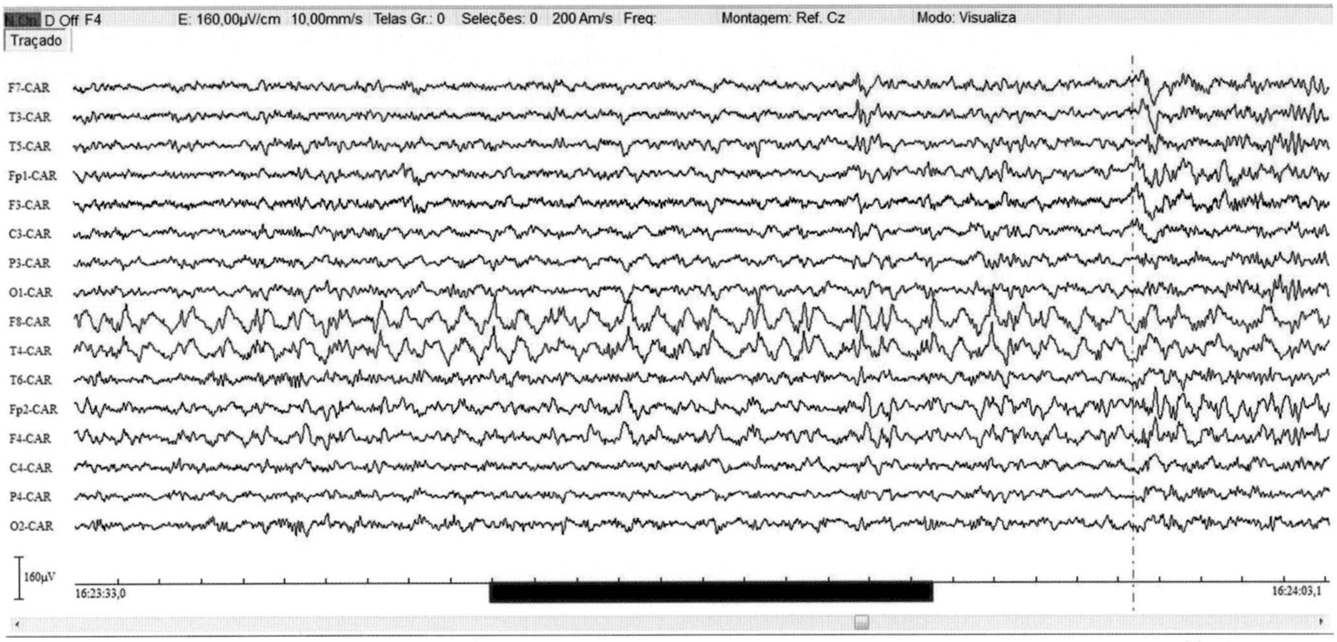

Figure 3

Scalp EEG in a 34-year old man with daily seizures which started at age 14. Right fronto-temporal rhythmic spikes on EEG, blurring and increased cortical thickness in the MRI. Pathology showed FCD IIA. The continuous EEG pattern cannot be missed and undoubtedly points to the pathology.

References

Baulac S, Ishida S, Marsan E, *et al.* Familial focal epilepsy with focal cortical dysplasia due to DEPDC5 mutations. *Ann Neurol.* 2015; 77: 675-83.

Blumcke I, Spreafico R, Haaker G, *et al.* Histopathological findings in brain tissue obtained during epilepsy surgery. *N Engl J Med.* 2017; 377: 1648-56.

Blümcke I, Thom M, Aronica E, *et al.* The clinico-pathological spectrum of Focal Cortical Dysplasias: a consensus classification proposed by an ad hoc Task Force of the ILAE Diagnostic Methods Commission *Epilepsia.* 2011; 52: 158-74.

Boonyapisit K, Najm I, Klem G, *et al.* Epileptogenicity of focal malformations due to abnormal cortical development: direct electrocorticographic-histopathologic correlations. *Epilepsia.* 2003; 44: 69-76.

Cebeci D, Arhan E, Hirfanoglu T, *et al.* Ictal pouting ('Chapeau de gendarme') in three pediatric cases with cortical dysplasia. *Eur J Paediatr Neurol.* 2020; 26: 82-8.

Chamberlain WA, Cohen ML, Gyure KA, *et al.* Interobserver and intraobserver reproducibility in focal cortical dysplasia (malformations of cortical development). *Epilepsia.* 2009; 50: 2593-8.

Chassoux F, Devaux B, Landre E, *et al.* Stereoelectroencephalography in focal cortical dysplasia: a 3D approach to delineating the dysplastic cortex. *Brain* 2000; 123: 1733-51.

Chassoux F, Landre E, Mellerio C, *et al.* Type II focal cortical dysplasia: electroclinical phenotype and surgical outcome related to imaging. *Epilepsia* 2012; 53: 349-58.

Chassoux F. Presurgical evaluation in FCD type I: When you know and when you suspect that is the villain. 22nd International Epilepsy Surgery Symposium. Malformations of cortical development: The biology, the identification, the epilepsy and the pragmatic approaches to treatment. *J Epilepsy Clin Neurophysiol* 2013; 19 (Suppl 1): 11-27.

Chassoux F, Mellerio C, Laurent A, *et al.* Benefits and risks of epilepsy surgery in patients with focal cortical dysplasia type 2 in the central region. *Neurology* 2022.

Colombo N, Citterio A, Galli C, *et al.* Neuroimaging of focal cortical dysplasia: neuropathological correlations. Epileptic Disord. 2003; 5 Suppl 2: S67-72.

Eltze CM, Landre E, Soufflet C, Chassoux F. Sleep related epilepsy in focal cortical dysplasia type 2: Insights from sleep recordings in presurgical evaluation. *Clin Neurophysiol.* 2020; 131: 609-15.

Epitashvili N, San Antonio-Arce V, Brandt A, Schulze-Bonhage A. Scalp electroencephalographic biomarkers in epilepsy patients with focal cortical dysplasia. *Ann Neurol* 2018; 84: 564–75.

Fauser S, Huppertz HJ, Bast T, *et al.* Clinical characteristics in focal cortical dysplasia: a retrospective evaluation in a series of 120 patients. *Brain* 2006; 129: 1907-16.

Gambardella A, Palmini A, Andermann F, *et al.* Usefulness of focal rhythmic discharges on scalp EEG of patients with focal cortical dysplasia and intractable epilepsy. *Electroencephalogr Clin Neurophysiol* 1996; 98(4): 243–9.

Gibbs SA, Proserpio P, Terzaghi M, *et al.* Sleep related epileptic behaviors and non-REM-related parasomnias: Insights from stereo-EEG. *Sleep Med Rev* 2016; 25: 4-20.

Gibbs SA, Proserpio P, Francione S, *et al.* Seizure duration and latency of hypermotor manifestations distinguish frontal from extrafrontal onset in sleep-related hypermotor epilepsy. *Epilepsia* 2018; 59(9): e130-4.

Guerrini R, Duchowny M, Jayakar P, *et al.* Diagnostic methods and treatment options for focal cortical dysplasia. *Epilepsia* 2015; 56: 1669-86.

Hauptman JS, Mathern GW. Surgical treatment of epilepsy associated with cortical dysplasia: 2012 update. *Epilepsia.* 2012; 53 Suppl 4: 98-104.

Hayakawa I, Kubota M. Ictal pouting: kabuki visage or chapeau de gendarme? *Pract Neurol.* 2018; 18: 410-2.

Holthausen H, Coras R, Tang Y, *et al.* Multilobar unilateral hypoplasia with emphasis on the posterior quadrant and severe epilepsy in children with FCD ILAE Type 1A. *Epilepsia* 2021.

Jin B, Hu W, Ye L, *et al.* Small lesion size is associated with sleep-related epilepsy in focal cortical dysplasia type II. *Front Neurol* 2018; 9: 106.

Koc G, Bek S, Gokcil Z *et al.* Localization of ictal pouting in frontal lobe epilepsy: a case report. *Epilepsy Behav Case Rep.* 2017; 8: 27-30.

Krsek P, Pieper T, Karlmeier A, *et al.* Different presurgical characteristics and seizure outcomes in children with focal cortical dysplasia type I or II. *Epilepsia.* 2009; 50: 125-37.

Lerner JT, Salamon N, Hauptman JS, *et al.* Assessment and surgical outcomes for mild type I and severe type II cortical dysplasia: a critical review and the UCLA experience. *Epilepsia.* 2009; 50: 1310-35.

Losurdo A, Proserpio P, Cardinale F, *et al.* Drug-resistant focal sleep related epilepsy: results and predictors of surgical outcome. *Epilepsy Res.* 2014; 108: 953-62.

Lu H, Zhang W, Long Q, *et al.* Semiological marker of emotional insulo-cingulate network activation in epileptic human brain. *Epilepsy and behavior* 2021; 120: 107970.

Martinez-Lizana E, Brandt A, Foit NA, Urbach H, Schulze-Bonhage A. Ictal semiology of epileptic seizures with insulo-opercular genesis. *Journal of Neurology* 2021.

Mullatti N, Landré E, Mellerio C, *et al.* Stereotactic thermocoagulation for insular epilepsy: lessons from successes and failures. *Epilepsia* 2019; 60: 1565-79.

Najm IM, Tassi L, Sarnat HB, Holthausen H, Russo GL. Epilepsies associated with focal cortical dysplasias (FCDs). *Acta Neuropathol.* 2014; 128: 5-19.

Nobili L, Francione S, Mai R, *et al.* Surgical treatment of drug-resistant nocturnal frontal lobe epilepsy. *Brain* 2007; 130: 561-73.

Nobili L, Cardinale F, Magliola U, *et al.* Taylor's focal cortical dysplasia increases the risk of sleep-related epilepsy. *Epilepsia* 2009; 50: 2599-2604.

Palmini A, Andermann F, Olivier A, *et al.* Focal neuronal migration disorders and intractable partial epilepsy: a study of 30 patients. *Ann Neurol* 1991; 30: 741-9.

Palmini A, Gambardella A, Andermann F, *et al.* Intrinsic epileptogenicity of human dysplastic cortex as suggested by corticography and surgical results. *Ann Neurol.* 1995; 37: 476-87.

Palmini A, Najm I, Avanzini G, *et al.* Terminology and classification of the cortical dysplasias *Neurology.* 2004; 62: S2-8.

Rüsch C, Bölsterli BK, Carosio C, Ramantani G. *Chapeau de gendarme* in a toddler points to focal epilepsy originating from the subcentral gyrus. *Epileptic Disorders.* 2021; 23: 412-418.

Scheffer I[c], Heron SE, Regan BM, *et al.* Mutations in mammalian target of rapamycin regulator DEPDC5 cause focal epilepsy with brain malformations. *Ann Neurol.* 2014; 75: 782-7.

Souirti Z, Landré E, Mellerio C, Devaux B, Chassoux F. Neural network underlying ictal pouting ("chapeau de gendarme") in frontal lobe epilepsy. *Epilepsy Behav.* 2014; 37: 249-57.

Tan YL, Muhlhofer W, Knowlton R. Pearls and Oy-sters: the sign and other localizing gems in frontal lobe epilepsy. *Neurology.* 2016; 87: e103-5.

Tassi L, Colombo N, Garbelli R, *et al.* Focal cortical dysplasia: neuropathological subtypes, EEG, neuroimaging and surgical outcome. *Brain* 2002; 125: 1719-732.

Tassi L, Rita Garbelli R, Colombo N, *et al.* Type I focal cortical dysplasia: surgical outcome is related to histopathology. *Epileptic Disord* 2010; 12: 181-91.

Tassi L, Garbelli R, Colombo N, *et al.* Electroclinical, MRI and surgical outcomes in 100 epileptic patients with type II FCD. *Epileptic Disord* 2012; 14: 257-66.

Taylor DC, Falconer MA, Bruton CJ, Corsellis JA. Focal dysplasia of the cerebral cortex in epilepsy. *J Neurol Neurosurg Psychiatry.*1971; 34: 369-87.

Wagstyl K, Whitaker K, Raznahan A, *et al.* Atlas of lesion locations and post-surgical seizure freedom in focal cortical dysplasia: a MELD study. *Epilepsia,* 2022; 63: 61-74.

Wiwchar LD, Hader W, Pauranik A, Joseph JT, Appendino JP. Focal seizures associated with the chapeau de gendarme sign or ictal pouting of insular origin. *Epilepsy Behav Rep.* 2019; 12: 100347.

CHAPTER 8. FCD in children: specific clinical findings and management

Pavel Kršek, Hans Holthausen

Key points

- FCD represents the most frequent etiology of focal drug-resistant epilepsy in pediatric surgical series.
- Recent studies show that pathogenic variants in genes encoding for mTOR and other signaling cascades disrupt normal cortical development and lead to FCD.
- Clinical presentation of FCD in children reflects its genetic-developmental origin: patients tend to manifest epilepsy in the first months or years of life, often accompanied by developmental delay and cognitive disability.
- Whereas in older children we observe focal electrophysiological abnormalities, infants may display generalized EEG abnormalities despite unequivocal focal disease.
- MRI findings vary in extent and visibility from small but obvious and well-circumscribed FCD IIB, to extensive, barely discernable FCD IA.
- The progress of myelination affects MRI findings of FCD in infants
- A number age-specific clinical, electrophysiological and neuroimaging characteristics differ between infants, children and adults.

Introduction

FCD represents the most frequent etiology of focal drug-resistant epilepsy in pediatric surgical series. Since the first description by Taylor and colleagues in 1971, we have seen major progress in the understanding of FCD neurobiology, diagnostic processes and patient management. In the past, FCD was considered a developmental pathology, caused by *in utero* or perinatal insults. However, recent studies show that pathogenic variants in genes encoding for mTOR and other signaling cascades disrupt normal cortical development and lead to FCD. Clinical presentation of FCD in children reflects its genetic-developmental origin: patients tend to manifest epilepsy in the first months or years of life, often accompanied by developmental delay and cognitive disability. Whereas in older children we observe focal electrophysiological abnormalities, infants may display generalized EEG abnormalities despite unequivocal focal disease. MRI findings vary in extent and visibility from small but obvious and well-circumscribed FCD IIB, to extensive, barely discernable FCD IA. In addition, the progress of myelination also affects MRI (dis) appearance of FCD in infants. The ensuing chapter summarizes key clinical, electrophysiological, neuroimaging and genetic features of FCD in children and highlights age-specific characteristics that differ between infants, children and adults.

Prevalence of FCD in children

The exact prevalence of FCD in children is difficult to ascertain. The best data currently available in surgical series come from the European Epilepsy Brain Bank (EEBB) consortium that has collected specimen from epilepsy surgery centers around Europe for the past 25 years. Two major studies based on EEBB data (Blümcke *et al.*, 2019; Lamberink *et al.*, 2020) have shown that FCD specimen (FCD I, II, mMCD and FCD not otherwise specified) constitute 17 – 20% of all samples. Among children, FCD represented the most frequent finding, accounting to 31% of all samples. Notwithstanding, the prevalence of FCD in the general population of children with epilepsy remains unknown. Bast *et al.* (2006) suggested it might be around 5 to 10 %, based on an extensive review of the literature; more recent data are not available.

FCD II in children

• Clinical features

Some clinical features that could distinguish this entity from FCD I and other types of MCD have been identified (Tassi *et al.*, 2002; Widdess-Walsh *et al.*, 2005; Krsek *et al.*, 2008, 2009; Lerner *et al.*, 2009; Guerrini *et al.*, 2015). It must however be emphasized that clinical presentation differs even among patients with the same histopathological type of FCD. There are significant differences between patients with truly focal dysplasias such as "bottom of sulcus" FCD IIB and extensive – multilobar or hemispheric – malformations; yet, they occasionally may share the same histopathological characteristics.

Smaller FCD II typically manifests in preschool age in previously healthy children of normal intelligence, without focal neurological signs. There are typically no obvious precipitating factors at seizure onset, although some parents report a temporal association with nonspecific provoking factors, such as febrile illness. Seizure onset is often "explosive" with a rapid increase in seizure frequency; seizures tend to occur daily. Most frequently we see highly stereotyped focal seizures and focal-to-bilateral tonic-clonic seizures (FBTCS) are relatively rare. Frontal, central and opercular-insular location of the EZ is reported more often than temporal location; FCD II however, can occur in any location. In many children, high seizure frequency warrants inpatient treatment with intravenous administration of anti-seizure medication (ASM). No ASM proved to be specifically effective in FCD II although some reports favor sodium voltage-gated channel blockers, such as carbamazepine or lacosamide. Following an initial explosive period, we sometimes encounter prolonged seizure remission that can lead to ASM tapering, especially in patients whose MRI was reported as normal. Seizures, however, generally return after some time and eventual drug-resistance is almost invariable – permanently seizure-free patients with unequivocal MRI findings of FCD II are only scarcely reported (Chassoux *et al.*, 2012; Kršek *et al.*, 2008; Lerner *et al.*, 2009; Guerrini *et al.*, 2015; Wang *et al.*, 2020).

On the other hand, children with extensive FCD II frequently exhibit different phenotypes. They are younger at seizure onset, and in many cases, seizures occur in the first two or three years of life. In infants and toddlers, seizure semiology as well as scalp EEG findings are in general more characteristic of the age than of the etiology or location of the EZ; despite focal EZ and focal or lateralized lesions, patients may manifest generalized seizure types and generalized EEG abnormality. Consequently, in young children presenting with an epileptic encephalopathy, it is more challenging to distinguish FCD II from type I and even from other etiologies (both structural and genetic), based solely on clinical presentation and initial EEG findings. MRI often (but not always!) holds the key to the correct diagnosis. Young children frequently present with spasms and other features of epileptic encephalopathy. Subtle localizing features indicating focal seizure onset are easy to miss, and therefore some patients receive an initial misdiagnosis of diffuse epileptic encephalopathy. Indeed, the disease severely impacts psychomotor development and often results in marked developmental regression. Due to the more prominent neuropathological changes in FCD II we more frequently encounter lateralized neurological deficits (such as hemiparesis) in children with extensive lesions, depending on the location of the dysplastic cortex. In children suffering from epileptic encephalopathy, we may also see non-lateralized deficits such as hypotonia and ataxia (Kršek *et al.*, 2008, 2009; Holthausen *et al.*, 2014; Wang *et al.*, 2020).

It is very important to recognize these clinical features suggestive of FCD II (abrupt onset of frequent highly stereotyped focal seizures in a previously healthy child, no precipitating factors, possible seizure remission after an initial explosive period, eventual drug-resistance) since auxiliary diagnostic tests frequently fail in the timely detection of this pathology. Initial scalp EEG abnormalities could be nonspecific or affected by the patient's age (see below). The structural pathology may not be visible on MRI or is frequently overlooked if subtle abnormalities are not correctly interpreted. Typical clusters of clinical features thus represent the best clue for early identification of children with FCD who can significantly benefit from timely epilepsy surgery. In general, except for extensive lesions and very young children, distinct clinical manifestations of FCD II allow for early recognition, in contrast to FCD I or III that manifests with less clear-cut symptoms.

• Scalp EEG features

Similar to clinical presentation, EEG characteristics in children with FCD II are determined not only by the histopathological subtype but also by the patient's age, extent and location of the lesion. Prominent localized rhythmic epileptiform discharges are seen in some, especially older children, with more superficially located dysplastic cortex. Different terms have been used for these peculiar epileptiform patterns: continuous epileptiform discharges (CED), frequent epileptiform discharges on irregular slow (FEDOIS), ictal-like bursting pattern or brushes (Gambardella *et al.*, 1996; Holthausen *et al.*, 1997; Tassi *et al.*, 2012). Although they are not pathognomonic, in combination with typical clinical features they represent an invaluable aid in presurgical identification and non-invasive localization of FCD II. Their recognition is crucial especially in children with initially "normal" MRI findings since they can guide reevaluation of anatomical and functional neuroimaging.

In patients with smaller FCD lesions in deep cortical areas, these characteristic epileptiform patterns may remain undetected by scalp EEG and only identified by invasive monitoring (either intraoperative electrocorticography or long-term intracranial EEG). In some cases, they may appear only in NREM sleep. Increase in interictal rhythmic/pseudorhythmic spike rate and frequent ictal seizure patterns in NREM sleep has been observed in both children and adults with FCD II and sleep-related epilepsy (Eltze *et al.*, 2020).

EEG findings in infants and toddlers presenting with typically larger EZ and features of epileptic encephalopathy are much less localized and pathology-specific. FCD II, similarly to other focal lesions at this age, frequently manifests with generalized scalp EEG patterns such as hypsarrythmia and burst-suppression. It is necessary to specifically search for localized or at least unilateral EEG abnormalities suggestive of the EZ location. It is crucial to stress that young children with localized dysplastic lesions warrant detailed investigation in centers for epilepsy surgery, as they represent suitable epilepsy surgery candidates, despite generalized/bilateral synchronous epileptiform scalp EEG abnormalities (Wyllie *et al.*, 2007).

• Neuroimaging (Figures 1 and 2)

High-quality MRI is essential in the evaluation of patients with clinical suspicion of FCD. First, MRI enables pre-surgical identification of the structural lesion, prediction of its histopathological type, and delineation of the extent of the dysplastic cortex for the purposes of surgical planning (Bernasconi *et al.*, 2019). MRI features of FCD II in older children and adults are well-defined: increased cortical thickness, abnormal gyral/sulcal patterns, blurring of the cortical-white matter junction, increased signal on T2/FLAIR images, often at the bottom of a single sulcus and, occasionally, a radially-oriented linear or conical stripe of T2 hyperintensity extending to the ventricle surface, the so called „transmantle" sign (Widdess-Wals *et al.*, 2006; Kršek *et al.*, 2008; Colombo *et al.*, 2012; Wang *et al.*, 2013). These changes may be subtle and, regrettably, are easily missed when the MRI is performed outside specialized centers with well-designed acquisition protocols and/or on MRI machines with low resolution. In contrast, visual analysis of MRI scans by experienced neuroradiologists revealed dysplastic lesions in up to 90% of patients with histopathologically proven FCD IIB and in up to 50% of type IIA (Colombo *et al.*, 2012). Reliable distinction of types IIA and IIB is not always possible, even though the transmantle sign appears to be more frequently associated with FCD IIB. In fact, two distinct radiological subtypes of MRI-detectable lesions are strongly suggestive of FCD IIB: a tuber-like "crown of gyrus" dysplasia and a more subtle "bottom of sulcus" dysplasia, often associated with the transmantle sign (Wang *et al.*, 2013; Guerrini *et al.*, 2015).

Identification of the dysplastic cortex can be much more challenging in young children in whom brain myelination is still ongoing. In contrast to older children and adults, FCD II lesions are hypointense on T2-weighted sequences ("black hole lesion") in infants younger than 10 months. Eltze and colleagues have shown that some FCD II lesions may temporarily "disappear" on MRI due to the ongoing maturation of myelination. In addition, it is practically impossible to recognize the transmantle sign on T2w sequences of incompletely myelinated white matter (Eltze *et al.*, 2005). Therefore, we strongly recommend repeating high-resolution MRI in young children with ongoing myelination and clinical/electroencephalographic suspicion of FCD (any type). On the other hand, this "wait and see" approach must be balanced against the risk of permanent cognitive deficits. One needs to bear in mind that FCD is the most likely pathology in MRI-negative cases of children with signs of focal epilepsy and developmental delay, especially after other possible etiologies were excluded and the results of modern genetic testing shown to be negative (see below).

• Genetic testing in pediatric patients with suspected FCD II

Genetic testing by methods of next-generation sequencing (targeted gene panel testing – TGPT, whole-exome sequencing – WES, whole-genome sequencing – WGS) has become a standard diagnostic tool for patients with MCD (Oegema *et al.*, 2020), and somatic gene

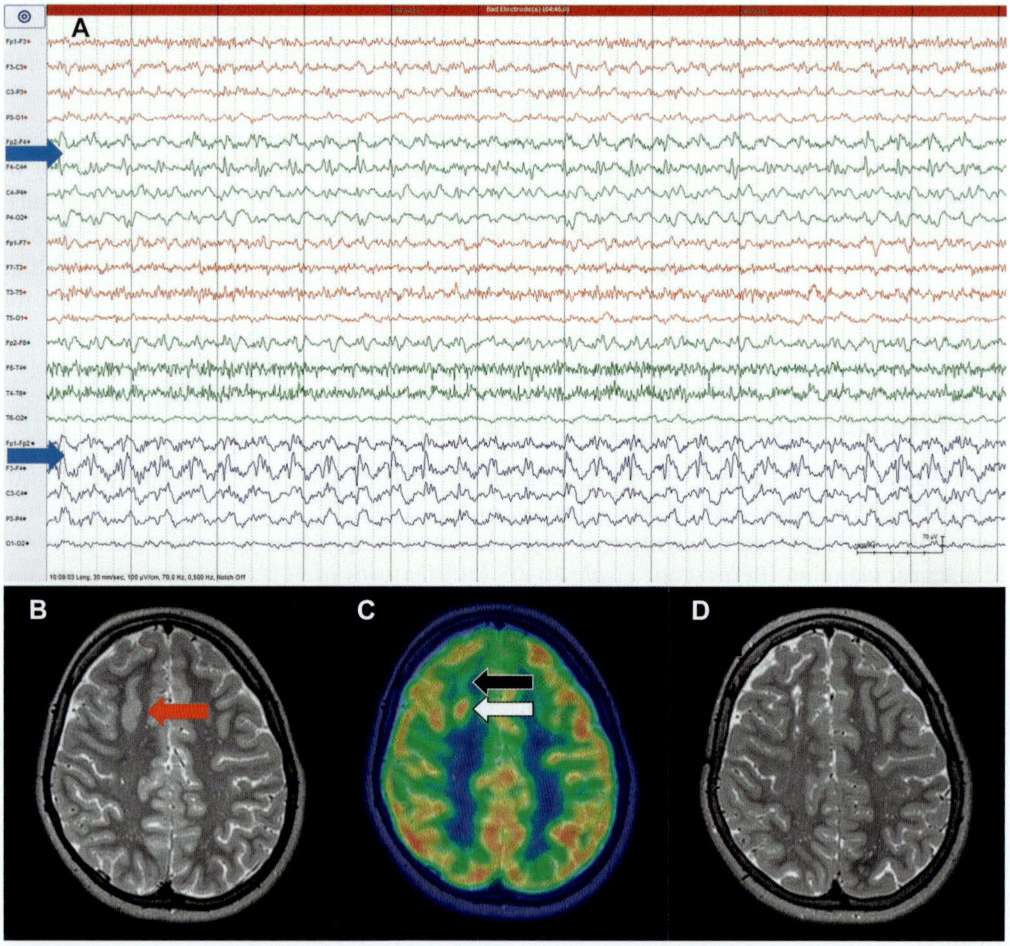

Figure 1

Nine year-old previously healthy girl presented with multiple daily focal seizures (feeling of dizziness, deviation of the eyes and head to the left, asymmetric tonic posture prevailing on the left, vocalisations, sometimes laughing, no impaired awareness). Scalp EEG displayed focal continuous epileptiform discharges (CED) over the right frontal mesial region (A, blue arrows, phase reversal to F4 electrode, double-banana bipolar montage). Initial MRI was evaluated as normal, high-resolution epilepsy protocol revealed bottom-of-sulcus FCD, most likely type IIB (later confirmed by histopathology) – B, red arrow. FDG-PET co-registered with MRI showed posterior hypermetabolic (C, white arrow) and anterior hypometabolic (C, black arrow) parts of the dysplastic lesion. One-stage resection guided by multimodal neuroimaging and intraoperative electrocorticography performed 6 months after the epilepsy onset resulted in complete removal of the lesion (D). Three years after the surgery the girl is seizure-free and drug-free, with normal cognitive functions in all domains.

testing is gradually finding its way in the neuropathological diagnostic process of FCD (Blümcke *et al.*, 2021). However, in many countries, genetic testing for surgical candidates with suspected FCD has not yet been established as part of pre-surgical evaluation, despite growing body of evidence that genetic diagnosis may influence surgical planning and post-surgical prognosis (Stevelink *et al.*, 2018, Sanders *et al.*, 2019, Beňová *et al.*, 2021).

The reasons for including genetic testing in pre- and post-surgical evaluation are threefold. First, multiple studies have proven that pathogenic variants in mTOR pathway genes cause FCD II and HME (Baldassari *et al.*, 2019), and genetic testing of brain tissue samples are gradually becoming standard part of neuropathological work-up (Blümcke *et al.*, 2021). However, given the yet limited data available, we currently cannot conclude whether post-surgical prognosis is associated with the genetic origin of FCD. The second reason is that individual cases and small series clearly show that patients with mutations in ion channels and synaptic proteins achieve far less favourable outcomes than those with pathogenic variants in mTOR complex genes (Stevelink *et al.*, 2018). Finally, yet importantly, genetic testing may reveal the diagnosis of genetic focal epilepsy in patients with negative MRI, and therefore spare unnecessary invasive procedures such as stereo-electroencephalography (SEEG) studies. In our Centre in Prague (PK), we investigated a patient with mild cognitive disability initially referred for MRI-negative focal epilepsy with suspected FCD who was later diagnosed with *STXBP1*-related focal epilepsy. Another patient underwent SEEG study with inconclusive results for drug-resistant focal epilepsy, and WES later revealed two variants in *SZT2* – a gene associated with epileptic encephalopathy. Also, genetic testing may uncover the cause of familial epilepsy, even in families with a variable severity of epilepsy phenotype from focal epilepsy to FCD (Beňová *et al.*, 2021).

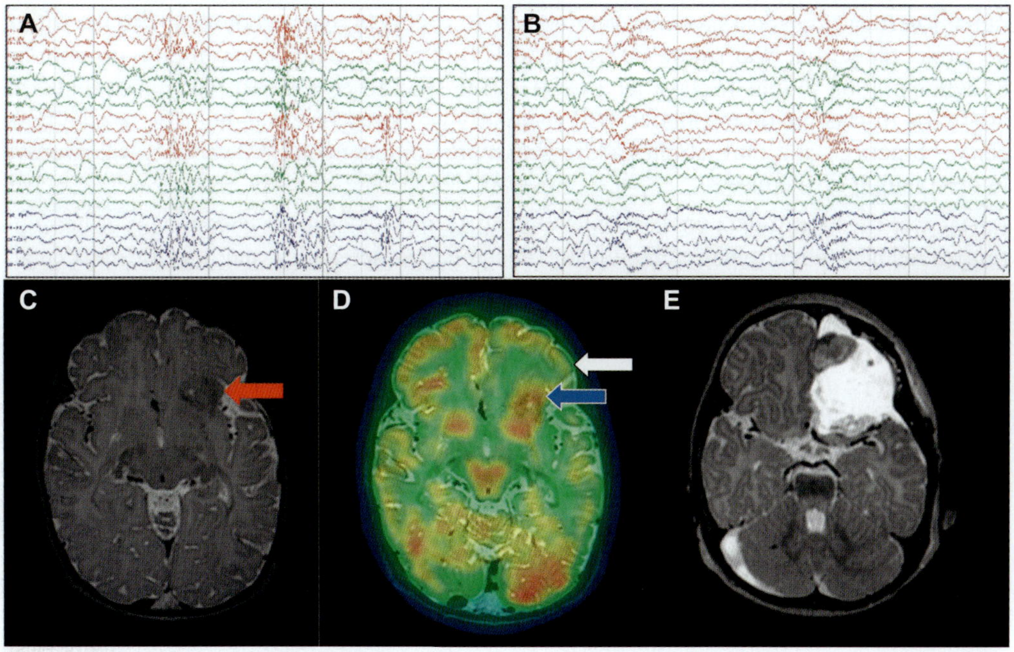

Figure 2

Three month-old girl with no pre-/perinatal adverse events presented with frequent daily seizures (initially behavior arrests with autonomic signs, at 4 months evolving to bilateral spasms only occasionally prevailing on the right). Scalp EEG displayed frequent bilateral symmetric polyspike activity more prominent over the left hemisphere (A, double-banana bipolar montage). Ictal EEG consisted of generalized fast rhythmic activity more pronounced on the left (B). MRI showed T2-hypointense calcified dysplastic lesion localized in the dorsal orbitofrontal, frontal opercular and anterior insular regions of the left hemisphere – C, red arrow. FDG-PET co-registered with MRI revealed hypermetabolic dysplastic lesion (D, blue arrow) with anterior hypometabolic rim (white arrow). One-stage resection guided by multimodal neuroimaging and intraoperative electrocorticography (ECoG) was performed 4 months after the epilepsy onset; ECoG finding prompted anterior extension of the resection (D). Histopathology confirmed FCD IIB. Seven months after the surgery the girl is seizure-free with normal neurological finding and psychomotor development, we have just started tapering-down anti-seizure medication.

The disadvantages of genetic testing in the pre-surgical setting include a possible diagnostic delay, difficulties in interpretation of variants of unknown significance, and a potential loss of motivation for surgery even when indicated for structural genetic epilepsy (e.g. GATOR1 cases). Diagnostic delay and uncertain variant interpretation represent an especially pertinent issue in children with developmental arrest/regression in whom we aim for the earliest surgical intervention.

In summary, genetic testing and counselling represent novel valuable tools in pre- and post-surgical evaluation, especially in patients with MRI-negative focal epilepsy and those with positive family history of epilepsy.

FCD I in children

• Classification issues in FCD I

Epilepsies caused by FCD I cannot be discussed without addressing still persisting uncertainties in the neuropathological classification of the milder focal cortical changes, which are restricted to cortical dyslaminations and which are to be classified as one or the other subtype of FCD I. Rather vague definitions of the pathological changes labeled as FCD I in the Palmini Classification of the FCD (Palmini *et al.*, 2004) and major discrepancies in the classification of these changes by an international panel of neuropathologists (Chamberlain *et al.*, 2009) was one of the reasons for a revision of the classification by an ad-hoc ILAE TASK-force for the classification of the FCD in 2011 (Blümcke *et al.*, 2011). As detailed in chapters 2 and 3 by A. Palmini and I. Blümcke, a three-tiered classification scheme was proposed for changes to be labeled as FCD I: cortical dyslamination restricted to an abnormal radial ("vertical") cortical layering were classified as FCD IA, cortical dyslamination with an abnormal tangential ("horizontal") layering as FCD IB and a combination of both orientation of dyslamination should be classified as FCD IC. The TASK force however recognized that "the approach to classify three isolated FCD I variants will need re-evaluation for feasibility in clinical practice", and that "studies addressing more homogeneous FCD variants will improve understanding of the disease".

A review of the literature in 2018 revealed that FCD I are still lacking a comprehensive description of clinical phenotypes, reproducible imaging characteristics and specific molecular/genetic biomarkers" (Najm *et al.*, 2018). With the exception of the very recent characterization of the entity with *Multilobar Unilateral Hypoplasia with emphasis in the posterior quadrant and Severe Epilepsy in Children with ILAE FCD IA,* for which the acronym MUSEC is proposed (Holthausen *et al.*, 2021), there are still no further comprehensive descriptions of epilepsies associated with FCD I subtypes. One reason for this could be that isolated (pure) ILAE FCD I have become rare since the introduction of the ILAE FCD classification (Muehlebner *et al.*, 2014; Mrelashvili *et al.*, 2015; Kwon *et al.*, 2016; Huang *et al.* 2017; Veersma *et al.*, 2018; Holthausen *et al.*, 2021), most likely because changes within the temporal lobe, often in association with hippocampal sclerosis, previously classified as FCD I, have turned out to be of degenerative nature (Garbelli *et al.*, 2012) and are no longer classified by most centres as dysplastic (see discussion by Ingmar Blümcke in chapter 3). The introduction of FCD classes IIIa – IIId in the ILAE classification of the FCD is very likely the other reason for that the number of reported cases with FCD I has gone down.

Even in publications in which FCD I is not that rare, FCD II cases are still far more frequent (Fauser *et al.*, 2015; Lagarde *et al.*, 2016; Choi *et al.*, 2018; Chen *et al.*, 2019). This might explain why authors tend to lump the three FCD I subtypes together when clinical and electro-encephalographic features are reported and when MRI characteristics are described. The three FCD I subtypes, however, may have different underlying pathophysiology, distinct neuroimaging, clinical and electro-encephalographic presentations as well as pose different diagnostic challenges and perspectives with respect to epilepsy surgery outcomes. Mild multilobar unilateral hypoplastic changes in MUSEC-ILAE FCD IA suggest interference with cortical development around mid-gestation (Blümcke *et al.*, 2010; Holthausen *et al.*, 2021). In FCD IB with horizontal dyslamination due to loss of cortical neurons in layer 4, one must always think of the possibility of a milder form of hypoxia/ischemia, with changes not clearly visible on MRI. The correct classification in these cases would then be FCD IIID instead, as this is also the correct classification of pathological microcolumns post hypoxic-ischemic events (Marin-Padilla, 1999, 2000). No pathophysiological hypotheses exist for FCD IC. There is reason to assume that FCD IC may serve as a kind of basket when things are not so clear (Najm *et al.*, 2018; Coras *et al.*, 2021).

Clinical features (Figure 3)

Children with MUSEC-ILAE FCD IA (Holthausen *et al.*, 2021) tend to have an explosive onset of frequent seizures, not responding to ASM from the beginning. The onset of epilepsy is most often in the first year of life, yet not in the neonatal period and not in the first 2-3 months of life, which can be a helpful guiding feature in the differential diagnosis between FCD I and epileptic encephalopathies caused by channelopathies, the latter often presenting seizure onset soon after birth or shortly thereafter. Tonic seizures, both asymmetric and symmetric, are the most prominent seizure type, although most children have several types of attacks. Subclinical seizures occurring in sleep is another frequent finding. Boys are two times more affected than girls. All patients in the published series had severe developmental delay, yet parents claimed that development was normal prior to the onset of the epilepsy. There was no overrepresentation of pre-/perinatal adverse events and affected children did not have severe neurological deficits such as spastic hemiparesis. Not a single patient had febrile convulsions and a family history for epilepsy was documented in one patient only.

Data regarding clinical features (and other variables) of FCD I are scarce. Not only are data from FCD I subtypes lumped together, but very often data from FCD II and FCD I are described together when clinical features are reported. Few figures are worth mentioning. In contrast to figures in the MUSEC study, others did find almost equal numbers of boys and girls in their cohorts with FCD I (Mata-Mbemba *et al.*, 2018; Veersma *et al.*, 2018; Isler *et al.*, 2014).

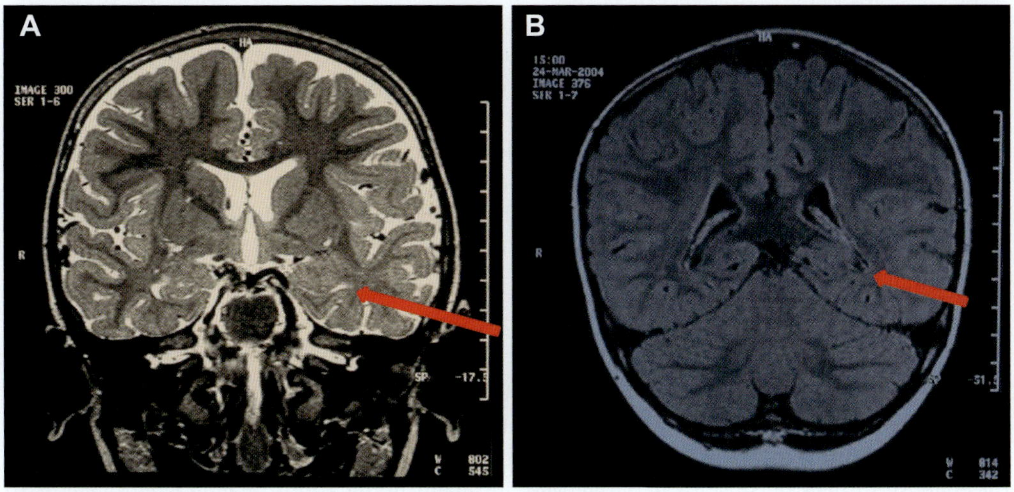

Figure 3

MRI in 2 patients with MUSEC ILAE FCD IA

A. Coronal T2 showing an increased signal of the white matter of the left (somewhat smaller) temporal lobe.

B. Coronal FLAIR showing the extension of the area with increased signal of the white matter and a reduction of the volume of the white matter towards posterior temporal and to the mesial temporo-occipital junction. This patient with age at onset of epilepsy at 20 months had multifocal sharp-waves left fronto-temporal, frontal medial and right fronto-temporal and a EEG-seizure pattern fronto-centro-parietal medial, tonic seizures, hyperkinetic seizures and epileptic negative myoclonus. He did not become seizure free after a left temporo-partial-parietal-occipital resection but is seizure free for more than 10 years after resection of remaining parietal cortex, posterior from the parietal sulcus and a corticectomy inferior from the somato-sensory foot area, including a portion of the cingulate gyrus.

There are also no reports anymore about the association of FCD I with pre-/perinatal complications and their neurological sequalae, as this was the case prior to the introduction of FCD IIID subclass in the 2011 ILAE FCD classification (Krsek *et al.*, 2008, 2010). Average age at onset of epilepsy in FCD I in recently published pediatric series ranges from 4,6 years to 8,1 years (Isler at al., 2017; Choi *et al.* 2018; Mata-Mbemba, 2018; Veersma *et al.*, 2019), which is markedly different from the situation in MUSEC–ILAE FCD IA (average onset of epilepsy 0,9 years). Two thirds of patients were younger than 2 years in the series from Seoul (Kwon *et al.*, 2016). Seizure onset before the age of 3 months is reported in a few children only (Kudr. *et al.*, 2016; Mata-Mbemba *et al.*, 2018; Veersma *et al.*, 2019).

Data about cognitive function in patients with FCD I are hard to find in the newer literature: 6/11 children (54,5 % vs 17,2 % in FCD II and III in the publication by Kwon *et al.*, 2016); 3/6 in the series from the Netherlands (Veersma *et al.*, 2019) had severe intellectual disability.In these studies, the majority of children with FCD I had daily seizures, but lower frequency – weekly or monthly – of seizures were also reported (Wu *et al.*, 2014; Choi *et al.*, 2018; Mata-Mbemba *et al.*, 2018). Reports about seizure semiology in FCD I are also scarce: 81% of the children from the Toronto-cohort had focal seizures, 19% non-focal seizures. In a series from Seoul, patients with FCD I had more often EEG and clinical signs of Lennox-Gastaut syndrome or West syndrome than patients with FCD II (Kwon *et al.*, 2016). There are no reports about a possible association of epilepsies caused by FCD I with febrile convulsions or positive family history of epilepsy.

• Scalp EEG features

EEG features in ILAE FCD I are also rarely reported. There are no hallmarks in the EEG as in FCD II (see above). Eighty-three per cent of children with FCD I in the Toronto cohort had epileptiform activity during video/EEG recording. Choi *et al.* (2018) found more localizing interictal and ictal EEG in FCD II than in FCD I. In a report about epilepsy surgery in children with FCD focusing on mental development, encephalopathic EEG patterns of either Lennox-Gastaut syndrome or West syndrome were seen in 63,6% of children with FCD I, 41,2% of those with FCD IIA and only in 10, 5% in patients with FCD IIB (Kwon *et al.*, 2016). The publication about MUSEC – ILAE FCD IA (Holthausen *et al.*, 2021) contains very detailed descriptions of the EEGs in each of the 19 patients. 18/19 children had abundant epileptiform activity in their EEG, escalating to an EEG status epilepticus in 9/19, mainly during sleep. Very frequent subclinical EEG seizure patterns were documented in 11/19. Diffuse and bilateral IED and EEG seizure onsets over multiple brain regions were not rare. The multifocal and diffuse EEG findings may lead to under-recognition of children with FCD IA as epilepsy surgery candidates. A clue in this direction may come from the presence of regional non-epileptiform abnormalities such as (uni-) regional pathological continuous irregular slow, most often over the posterior quadrant. Of note, despite very abnormal EEGs, posterior background activity was normal in 16/19 of cases.

• Neuroimaging (Figure 4)

In the past, it has often been said that MRI in FCD I would be normal in most patients affected with these mild cortical changes. But this is not true anymore in children with FCD I undergoing epilepsy surgery. Nevertheless, a considerable number of children with FCD I may be rejected for epilepsy surgery because of negative MRI. In recent publications dealing exclusively or to a large extent with children in which it is claimed that the ILAE 2011 FCD classification was applied, percentages of MRI positive cases in FCD I were in the range of 22% – 100%, more often positive in around half the cases (Fauser *et al.*, 2015; Kudr. *et al.* 2016; Kwon *et al.*,2016; Isler *et al.*, 2017; Mata-Mbemba *et al.*, 2018, Veersma *et al.*, 2018, Holthausen *et al.* 2021). In the Toronto series of 21 children with FCD IA (Mata-Mbemba *et al.*, 2018), the following MRI features were evaluated: 0% increased cortical thickness, 6% abnormal sulcation/ gyration, 28% high T1 signal in the cortex,11% high T2/FLAIR in the cortex, 72% high T2/FLAIR/PD signal in white matter, 17% gray/white matter blurring. The MRI was normal in 5 patients. In the series from Freiburg with the exceptionally high number of 67 patients with FCD I (both adults and children; 10 FCD IA, 49 FCD IB, and 8 with FCD IC), gyral abnormalities were seen in

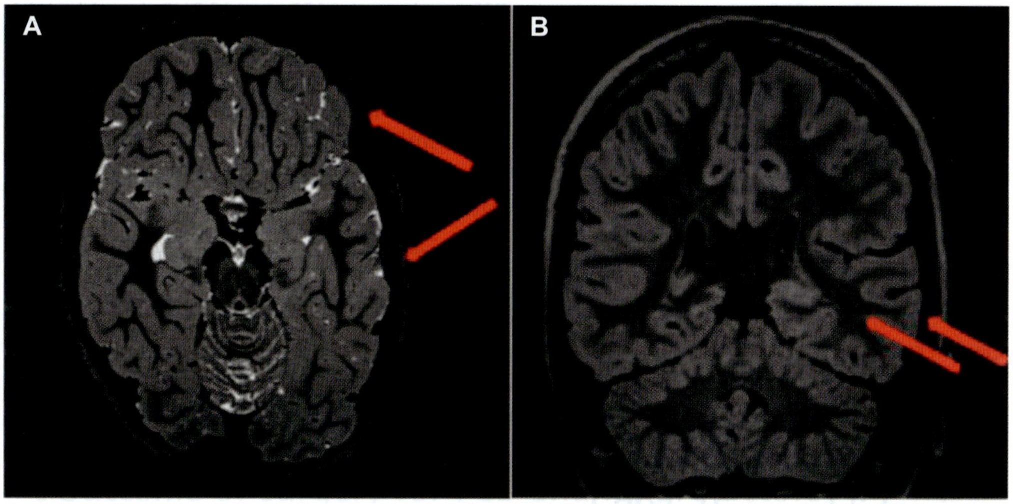

Figure 4

A. Axial T2 showing a marked reduction of the volume of the white matter left frontal and left temporal.
B. Coronal FLAIR showing subtle increased signals of the white matter of the left temporal lobe. This patient was already 11 years old at surgery and severely mentally impaired; functional language tests could not be done. Based on the EEG during presurgical evaluation, which revealed, that the majority of epileptiform discharges were located over frontal and temporal areas, a palliative fronto-temporal resection was tried by sparing "Wernicke`s area" and the visual tract – with a very disappointing result (seizure outcome Engel 4b).

33% and subcortical increased signal in 28% of the cases (Fauser *et al.*, 2015). In a publication from Marseille, MRI changes were localized in most patients to frontal and temporal regions and in a few to the parietal lobe; 32% were MRI negative (Lagarde *et al.* 2016). The localization of the changes on MRI in a small series of four infants with FCD I was temporo-occipital in two, parieto-occipital plus contralateral central in one, and frontal in one (Kudr *et al.*, 2016). Others described resection sites which might or might not have been identical with the sites of abnormalities on MRI. The MRI was abnormal in 18/19 children with MUSEC-ILAE FCD IA (Holthausen *et al.*, 2021). Diagnostic hallmarks for the recognition of the disease were subtle unilateral reductions of the volume and subtle increased signal of the white matter on T2 and FLAIR images, with emphasis of the posterior quadrant,but with extension to the frontal lobe in 8/19 patients (**figures 3, 4**). Quite characteristic are changes at the posterior-temporo-(parieto-) occipital junctions. Of note, no involvement of the frontal lobe was found without involvement of posterior areas! There were no gyral or sulcal abnormalities. Cortical changes were not seen on visual inspection, yet solely by MRI postprocessing analysis.

Genetic testing in children with suspected FCD I

Genetic testing is highly recommended, often even mandatory, in patients in whom FCD I is discussed as the underlying pathology, because epilepsies caused by FCD do not present with features on the MRI or in the EEG, which are pathognomonic or almost pathognomonic (as is the case in many patients with FCD II). In patients with FCD II, genetic testing may be wanted for several reasons, but is otherwise not that decisive in management plan. In a child with an epileptic encephalopathy, the differential diagnosis of the underlying cause of the severe epileptic condition between FCD I and a channelopathy due to a genetic mutation (almost always an exclusion criterium for epilepsy surgery; Stevelink *et al.* 2018; Sanders *et al.*, 2019) can be challenging. Furthermore, there are also early-onset epilepsies caused by genetic mutations or chromosomal abnormalities which do not present as epileptic encephalopathies, yet in whom epilepsy surgery is also not an option, such as children with milder forms of Dravet syndrome or with a ring chromosome 20. Due to the peculiar underlying genetics in this condition, a few children with mutations in the PCDH19 gene may however benefit from epilepsy surgery (Kurian *et al.*, 2018). New insights in the genetics of mild forms of cortical dysplasias has been gained from postsurgical genetic investigation of specimen of operated patients. So far,

Part III. NEUROPHYSIOLOGY OF FCD: THE PACEMAKER PATTERN

CHAPTER

9. In search of the epileptogenic neuron in FCD

Carlos Cepeda, Daphne Marina, Harry V. Vinters, Gary W. Mathern

Keypoints

- *In vitro* studies of tissue samples resected from children with FCD have provided new mechanistic insights on epileptogenesis.
- Abnormal cells, including dysmorphic cytomegalic neurons and balloon cells, have been characterized and their epileptogenic potential is now known.
- With the exception of balloon cells, different abnormal cell types in FCD can become epileptogenic.
- More than a single cell type, it is a circuit with dysmature intrinsic and synaptic properties that causes epileptic discharges in FCD.
- *In vitro* studies have opened up new potential therapeutic avenues targeting GABA receptors, the mTOR pathway, and ketone bodies in FCD.

Introduction

Throughout the history of epilepsy research, investigators frequently ask the following questions: which are the morphological and electrophysiological properties of epileptogenic neurons? Is there a distinctive feature that separates them from normal-appearing neurons? Morphologically, are they larger, smaller? Do they have less or more dendritic spines? Does the axon have more branches? Functionally, are they more excitable, e.g., higher input resistance? Do they have increased excitatory and/or reduced inhibitory inputs? Do they express more Na^+ and Ca^{2+} channels, and/or diminished K^+ channels?

In the late 1960's, David Prince, with his investigation of the depolarizing shift in penicillin-induced epileptic foci using animal models, unknowingly set off the search for the epileptogenic neuron. His conclusions led to the hypothesis that the epileptogenic agent *per se* does not alter cell membrane properties but, instead, the depolarizing shift is caused by synchronous firing and excessive excitatory drive, i.e., summation of multiple excitatory postsynaptic potentials (EPSPs) from a group of neurons (Prince, 1968).

In 1976, the first intracellular and extracellular recordings of neurons in slices from human cortex were made by Schwartzkroin and Prince. They also suggested that the slice technique would be useful for investigating the electrophysiology of cortical cells and their abnormalities in epilepsy (Schwartzkroin and Prince, 1976). A few years later, Prince and Wong began *in vitro* studies of neocortical brain tissue resected from epileptic patients with a variety of etiologies compared with non-epileptic tissue. They found that slightly less than 50% of pyramidal neurons from epileptic tissue generated membrane depolarizations and bursts of action potentials after orthodromic electrical stimulation, whereas no neurons from non-epileptic tissue generated such discharges. However, no spontaneous bursts or epileptiform membrane depolarizations were seen, making it difficult to ascertain if those discharges truly related to epileptogenesis (Prince and Wong, 1981). Nonetheless, the authors concluded that epileptogenic neurons retain abnormal properties *in vitro.*

In the late 1980's, the pediatric epilepsy program at the University of California Los Angeles, under the direction of Don Shields, assembled a group of clinical and basic scientists to study morphological and functional properties of cortical tissue resected from children with brain malformations, with at least 50% identified histopathologically as FCD cases. *In vitro* electrophysiological intracellular recordings of cortical pyramidal neurons in 10 patients with intractable epilepsy (ages 8 mo-13 yr) demonstrated membrane properties similar to those found in animal models (Wuarin *et al.*, 1990). Further, although spontaneous epileptiform activity was not recorded, addition of bicuculline, a $GABA_A$ receptor antagonist, induced spontaneous depolarizing shifts and bursts of action potentials. However, the morphological properties of pyramidal neurons stained with a fluorescent dye, Lucifer yellow (LY), appeared normal and potentially epileptogenic neurons could not be identified. Interestingly, in a follow-up study with a larger cohort (n=25 patients, ages 3 mo-14 yr), an age-dependent decline in gap junctional coupling was observed (Cepeda *et al.*, 1993). Increased dye-coupling in younger brains could explain their higher susceptibility to generate synchronous activity. However, the incidence of dye-coupling did not appear to correlate with the degree of epileptogenicity of the tissue sample, i.e., most versus least abnormal. Importantly in the present context, intracellular injections of LY uncovered the presence of abnormal-looking neurons, including dysmorphic cytomegalic pyramidal neurons. However, identification of abnormal cells could only be done *a posteriori*, i.e., after histological processing of the slice. Blind electrophysiological intracellular recordings did not allow for an active search of potentially abnormal cells before electrode impalement.

Two technological advances in the 1980's and 1990's, namely infrared (IR) illumination combined with differential interference contrast (DIC) optics and the development of the whole-cell patch clamp recording technique, allowed for the first time a more detailed characterization of morphological and electrophysiological intrinsic and synaptic properties of living neurons maintained *in vitro* (Dodt and Zieglgansberger, 1990). One of the limitations of IR-DIC videomicroscopy is that visualization is better in younger tissue, with less myelination. In collaboration with pediatric neurosurgeon Gary Mathern, one of our co-authors, we were fortunate to obtain tissue samples from very young patients undergoing epilepsy surgery for FCD and other brain malformations. Visualization of single cells was optimal, particularly in children under 5 yr of age. The youngest cases were just a few months old. It was also noted that the viability and good health of these cells for long periods of time were greater in the younger tissue samples. Studies in dissociated cells after enzymatic treatment of slices also were possible.

The seminal paper by Taylor and associates describing their histopathological observations in FCD (Taylor *et al.*, 1971), renewed interest in finding the culprit(s) of epileptic activity. Two abnormal-looking cell types caught the attention of epileptologists; cytomegalic pyramidal neurons and "grotesque", glial-like cells, now termed as balloon cells. Importantly, the authors noticed a close histopathological similarity between FCD and TSC. Tubers also contain cytomegalic neurons and giant glial-like cells, reminiscent of those found in subependymal giant cell astrocytomas, also present in a small percentage of TSC cases.

Based on electrophysiological recordings, both *in vivo* and *in vitro*, it had been known for a long time that FCD tissue is intrinsically epileptogenic (Mattia *et al.*, 1995, Palmini *et al.*, 1995). However, which cell type was more prone to generate epileptiform activity remained unknown. Thanks to the introduction of IR-DIC videomicroscopy and whole-cell patch clamp electrophysiology, a more in-depth morphological and functional characterization of the two main abnormal cell types in FCD, balloon cells and dysmorphic cytomegalic pyramidal neurons, became feasible. Another conceptual advancement was the introduction of new classifications of FCD, categorizing different types depending on the severity of histopathological changes and the presence or absence of abnormal cells (Blumcke *et al.*, 2011, Palmini *et al.*, 2004, Mischel *et al.*, 1995). According to the International League Against Epilepsy, FCD IA, IB and IC, are characterized by architectural abnormalities (dyslamination). In addition, small, immature-looking pyramidal neurons, as well as hypertrophic and misoriented pyramidal neurons can be observed. In FCD II, in addition to dyslamination, dysmorphic cytomegalic pyramidal neurons (FCD IIA) and balloon cells (FCD IIB) are typically found (Blumcke *et al.*, 2011, Najm *et al.*, 2018).

As research on FCD began to grow and stratify into different classifications, hallmark features of each cell type were scrutinized for their possible role in epileptogenesis. Next, we will describe the main morphological and electrophysiological properties of abnormal cells in FCD, as well as their epileptogenic potential (**Figure 1**).

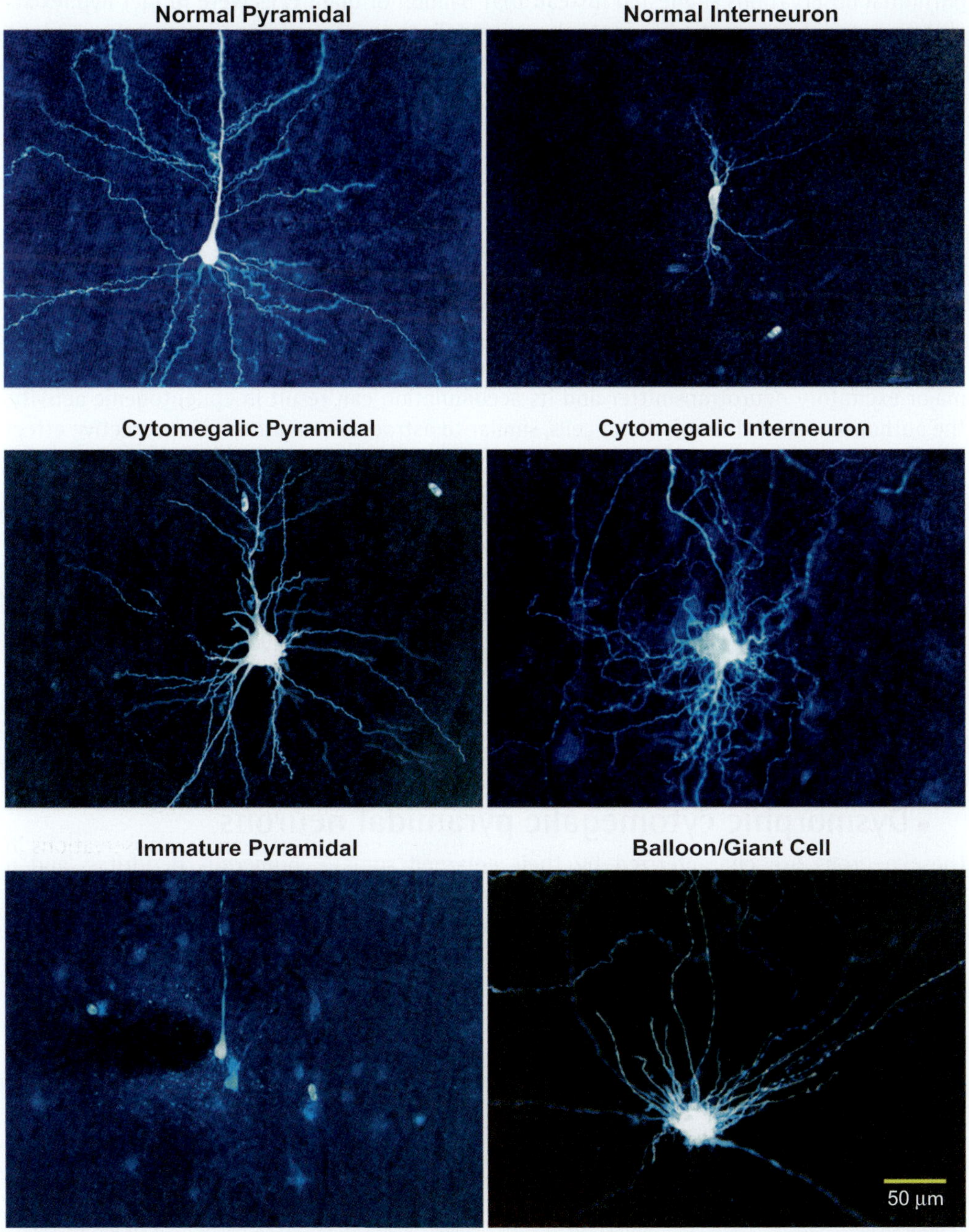

Figure 1
Morphological properties of abnormal cell types in FCD compared with normal-appearing pyramidal neurons and interneurons. Cells were recorded in slices from resected surgical tissue and filled with biocytin. Dysmorphic cytomegalic pyramidal neurons had enlarged somata. Immature pyramidal neurons had small somata and primitive dendrites with very few spines. Balloon/giant cells had large somata, abundant branches, but no discernible axon. The normal pyramidal neuron is from the temporal lobe of a tumor case (8.93 yr old). The normal interneuron is from the frontal lobe of a CD I case (9.65 yr). The dysmorphic cytomegalic pyramidal neuron and the cytomegalic interneuron are from the temporal lobe of a FCD IIB case (4 mo old). The immature pyramidal neuron is from the frontal lobe of a FCD IIB (11 mo old). The giant cell is from the frontal lobe of a TSC case (3.27 yr old).

Abnormal cell types in FCD

• Balloon cells

These cells are reminiscent of astrocytes and are characteristic of FCD IIB. Similar cells are also prominent in TSC cases, and are called giant cells. Although similar, there are differences in terms of cortical localization, expression of specific markers, and others. Some balloon cells have morphological features of both neurons and glia. Their neuronal-like features include large somata and large dendritic fields. However, balloon cells show no discernable axon and secondary branching is rare, properties more typical of glia. At first, based on morphological observations (Spreafico *et al.*, 1998), balloon cells were thought to be the epileptogenic neuron due to their abnormal morphology, abundant processes (potentially innervating a large number of pyramidal neurons), and enlarged somata (Schwartzkroin and Walsh, 2000). However, our initial observations suggested instead that balloon or giant cells were in fact hypoexcitable as they did not respond to iontophoretic application of excitatory amino acids, and did not display inward Na^+ and Ca^{2+}currents, hence could not generate action potentials, even though some of them expressed neuronal markers (Mathern *et al.*, 2000). Compared to normal-appearing pyramidal neurons, balloon cells have a significantly higher input resistance. Moreover, these cells do not seem to receive synaptic inputs (Cepeda *et al.*, 2005, Cepeda *et al.*, 2003). Because axon terminals slated to innervate cortical areas now occupied by balloon cells are unable to form synaptic connections, there might be aberrant synaptic organization in adjacent areas that could lead to hyperexcitability and epileptogenesis (Cepeda *et al.*, 2003, Abdijadid *et al.*, 2015). In contrast, the areas with larger accumulation of balloon cells do not appear to be epileptogenic, in fact they display less paroxysmal activity than adjacent areas (Boonyapisit *et al.*, 2003). In a subsequent study, balloon cells outside of ictal onset areas were found to have an increased expression of glial glutamate transporters. As glutamate is the major excitatory neurotransmitter and its accumulation can result in epileptogenic activity, the authors concluded that balloon cells, similar to astrocytes, might have a protective effect by buffering glutamate and K^+ from the extracellular milieu (Gonzalez-Martinez *et al.*, 2011). Increased neuronal glutamate transporters also were found in cortical tubers (White *et al.*, 2001). On the down side, recent studies indicate that expression of innate immune markers is elevated in areas with high concentration of balloon cells in FCD IIB, particularly in the white matter (Zimmer *et al.*, 2021). Thus, therapies targeting inflammation could be beneficial in FCD IIB. Similar to balloon/giant cells are intermediate cells, which display both neuronal and glial markers (Blumcke *et al.*, 2011, Talos *et al.*, 2008). These cells have somata similar to pyramidal neurons, but with processes typical of balloon/giant cells (Cepeda, *et al.*, 2012). They, too, lack the ability to generate action potentials and display no inward currents. As a general conclusion, while balloon/giant and intermediate cells do not appear to participate actively in epileptogenic processes, they could instead dampen epileptic activity.

• Dysmorphic cytomegalic pyramidal neurons

These neurons are characterized by their enlarged somata, numerous dendrites, and a very thick axon initial segment. Such characteristics reflect a capacity for dense innervation with surrounding neurons, potentially leading to cortical synchronization. However, these neurons have reduced dendritic fields and spine density. Because of increased membrane area, cell capacitance and time constant are also increased while input resistance is decreased when compared with normal-appearing pyramidal neurons (Cepeda *et al.*, 2003)

Table 1

Morphological and electrophysiological properties of abnormal cells relative to normal-appearing pyramidal neurons in FCD

	Basic Membrane Properties						
	Cm (pF)	R_i (MΩ)	Tau (ms)	Morphology	Excitability	Glutamate Transmission	GABA Transmission
Dysmorphic Cytomegalic Pyramidal	↑	↓	↑	Enlarged soma, numerous dendrites, reduced dendritic field	↑ due to repetitive, slowly inactivating Ca^{2+} spikes	Reduced Mg^{2+} sensitivity of NMDA channel	Formation of PV- baskets around the soma
Cytomegalic Interneuron	↑	↓	↑	Enlarged soma, increase in primary dendrites, thick axon hillock	↑ due to spontaneous depolarizing shifts and action potential bursts	Variable	Variable
Immature Pyramidal	↓	↑	↓	Small soma, rudimentary dendrites, few spines	↑ due to depolarizing GABAergic inputs	Reduced Mg^{2+} sensitivity	Increased GABA synaptic activity, PGA
Balloon/ Giant Cells	-	↑	-	Glassy and large soma, large dendritic field, no axon	↓ due to lack of inward currents	No inputs or response to EAAs	No synaptic inputs

Cm: cell membrane capacitance; Ri: cell membrane input resistance; Tau: decay time constant; pF: picofarads; MΩ: megaohms; ms: milliseconds; ↑: increased; ↓: decreased; -: no significant change; EAA: excitatory amino acids; PV: parvalbumin; PGA: pacemaker GABA synaptic activity.

(Table 1). Furthermore, cytomegalic pyramidal neurons show signs of hyperexcitability due to the appearance of repetitive, slowly inactivating Ca^{2+} spikes when held at depolarized membrane potentials. Although these cells were a popular candidate for the instigation of epileptic activity, they occur typically in FCD II but not in FCD I, thus they cannot be the sole culprit of epileptogenic activity. On the other hand, due to their relatively hyperpolarized resting membrane potential and low input resistance, in order to reach firing threshold a strong, coordinated excitatory input is required. However, once voltage threshold is reached, cytomegalic pyramidal neurons could sustain epileptic activity for long periods of time. An interesting feature of cytomegalic pyramidal neurons is the presence of baskets formed by GABAergic terminals enveloping their somata (Spreafico *et al.*, 1998, André *et al.*, 2008). The possible role of these baskets surrounding cytomegalic neurons will be discussed later.

• Cytomegalic interneurons

As more cytomegalic neurons in FCD II cases were studied, a new cell type emerged, cytomegalic interneurons (André *et al.*, 2007). This cell type had not been described in the literature, probably because of the lack of correlation between morphological and electrophysiological findings. When compared to normal-appearing interneurons, these cells have a significantly larger somatic area and an increase in primary dendrites. Unlike cytomegalic pyramidal neurons, their dendritic field is more complex and display more branching. This suggested cytomegalic interneurons could receive a large amount of synaptic inputs. In the case of normal-appearing interneurons, they have a higher input resistance when compared to pyramidal neurons. However, their cytomegalic counterparts have a low input resistance similar to cytomegalic pyramidal neurons. Also similar is the large membrane capacitance and long time constant. Cytomegalic interneurons generally lack inward Ca^{2+} currents, akin to their normal counterparts. Their hyperexcitability is demonstrated by the occurrence of spontaneous membrane depolarizations and bursts, reminiscent of the depolarizing shifts described by Prince. They also display non-inactivating Na^{+} spikes without proconvulsant drugs, and an increased firing rate compared to normal interneurons. This suggests that cytomegalic interneurons participate actively in the epileptogenic process.

• Immature pyramidal neurons

Another cell type of interest are the immature pyramidal neurons, frequently found in FCD I. Because of possible developmental delays, these cells have a small soma and rudimentary dendrites. Mature dendritic spines are rarely present (Cepeda *et al.*, 2007, Cepeda *et al.*, 2003). Their main intrinsic properties are a low membrane capacitance, high input resistance and fast time constant; all of these characteristics are expected of a developing neuron and are significantly different from mature neurons. While their Na^{+} currents are comparable to normal-appearing pyramidal neurons, their Ca^{2+} currents are significantly smaller. An interesting feature of these cells is the occurrence of abundant, sometimes rhythmic GABAergic synaptic inputs (Cepeda *et al.*, 2007, Cepeda *et al.*, 2003). Although it seems unlikely that immature pyramidal neurons can generate paroxysmal activity, their high input resistance, abundance of depolarizing GABAergic inputs, increased gap junctional connectivity, and clustering could effectively lead to network synchronization (Cepeda *et al.*, 2007).

Epileptogenic cells or circuits?

Based on intrinsic membrane properties of abnormal cell types in FCD we can conclude that, except for the balloon/giant cells, the other cell types can potentially become epileptogenic provided some conditions are fulfilled. Thus, with not one cell type recognized as the unique epileptogenic culprit, the lens of focus has to be shifted onto epileptogenic circuits instead. The balance excitation/inhibition has long been postulated as the critical tipping point for epileptic activity. Too much excitation or reduced inhibition can potentially induce paroxysmal discharges. Thus far, the main focus has been on glutamate N-methyl-D-aspartate (NMDA) receptors and $GABA_A$ type receptors.

• NMDA receptors

Excessive glutamatergic excitatory transmission, particularly that mediated by NMDA receptors, has been suggested as a primary driver of epileptogenic activity. In a landmark paper (Spreafico *et al.*, 1998), excess GluA2/3 AMPA and GluN1 NMDA receptor subunits were observed in 3 adult cases of FCD. Importantly, dysmorphic cytomegalic and some balloon cells expressed these subunits, suggesting increased excitatory elements. Other studies demonstrated selective expression of GluN2A/B subunits co-assembled with GluN1 subunits in FCD but not in non-dysplastic cortex (Ying *et al.*, 1998, Kerfoot *et al.*, 1999), which could result in increased excitability and epileptic activity. GluN2B also was increased in cortical tubers (White *et al.*, 2001). Further supporting an important role of GluN2B subunits in epileptogenesis, ifenprodil, a selective antagonist of NMDA receptor-containing GluN2B subunits, reduced epileptiform activity in dysplastic tissue but had no effect in non-dysplastic slices (Moddel *et al.*, 2005). In contrast, our own studies using single-cell RT-PCR showed reduced expression of GluN2B mRNA and less sensitivity to ifenprodil in a subset of pyramidal neurons from pediatric dysplastic tissue (André *et al.*, 2004). In addition, immunohistochemistry also showed reduced GluN2B immunoreactivity in a subpopulation of neurons in cortical areas containing cytomegalic neurons. The reason for this discrepancy remains unknown but age of the FCD patients in our study, around 4 yr on average, and fixation protocols could be important factors. Another possibility is the existence of neuronal subpopulations expressing different levels of GluN2B subunits. Assuming GluN2B is indeed increased in FCD, the mechanism by virtue of which increased expression of this receptor subunit leads to paroxysmal activity is less evident. For example, GluN2B expression measured by Western blotting was found to be upregulated in dysplastic tissue but downregulated in heterotopic neurons, yet both malformations lead to epileptic activity (Finardi *et al.*, 2006). Notably, NR2B upregulation in FCD cases was greater in the total homogenate than the post-synaptic membrane fraction, suggesting extrasynaptic mechanisms of hyperexcitability or deficient subunit trafficking onto the membrane surface, which could explain our finding that balloon cells do not respond to excitatory amino acids despite expressing some glutamate receptor subunits. The possibility that the GluN2B increase observed in FCD samples could be the result of recurrent epileptic activity was entertained by these authors. Interestingly, in an animal model of FCD no widespread alterations in NMDA receptor subunit expression could be detected by immunohistochemistry, again suggesting other mechanisms of epileptogenicity (Hagemann *et al.*, 2003). Importantly, in our studies on NMDA receptor alterations in pediatric FCD, we also demonstrated reduced Mg^{2+} sensitivity in most cytomegalic and about 30% of normal-appearing pyramidal neurons from FCD tissue compared with neurons from non-CD tissue (André *et al.*, 2004). Reduced Mg^{2+} block of NMDA receptors suggests an alternative mechanism of hyperexcitability in FCD.

• GABA receptors

There are two main types of GABA receptors in the brain, ionotropic type A and metabotropic type B receptors. $GABA_A$ receptors are predominantly inhibitory and there is substantial evidence for reduced GABA inhibition in FCD. Studies have described reduced expression of Ca^{2+} binding proteins in GABAergic neurons in cortical tissue samples from adult patients with intractable epilepsy due to FCD or TSC (Spreafico *et al.*, 1998, White *et al.*, 2001). There was an overall decrease in neurons immunoreactive to Ca^{2+} binding proteins, such as parvalbumin (PV), calbindin (CB), and calretinin (CR). These proteins are known to label subpopulations of GABAergic interneurons. The decrease in GABAergic interneurons, in particular those expressing PV, would lead to a reduction of the inhibitory mechanisms in a normal cortex, thus, promoting hyperexcitability. However, as commonly occurs in science, simple explanations are not the norm. Altered GABA receptors may differ among FCD types. For example, our studies found fewer GAD-positive interneurons in FCD II but not in FCD I. In addition, sensitivity to selective $GABA_A$ receptor subunit agonists or antagonists also was different in both FCD types with dysmorphic cytomegalic pyramidal neurons showing responses similar to those of immature neurons (André *et al.*, 2008). Another study showed impaired PV expression in FCD I but not in FCD II, where only the cortical distribution of PV interneurons was altered (Medici *et al.*, 2016). Further, reduced PV expression occurred in the absence of a significant reduction in the total number of GABAergic interneurons. In FCD II, a profound rearrangement in the distribution of PV-positive cells and terminals was detected instead (Medici *et al.*, 2016). This brings us back to the observation of a paradoxical increase in GABA terminals preferentially on dysmorphic cytomegalic pyramidal neurons (Spreafico *et al.*, 1998, André *et al.*, 2008). This could be interpreted as a compensatory mechanism to reduce hyperexcitability of these neurons. However, these terminals could also support depolarizing GABA responses and trigger epileptic activity. Thus, influx of negative chloride ions hyperpolarizes the membrane and reduces its membrane input resistance. However, GABA can also be depolarizing and potentially excitatory depending on the presence or absence in postsynaptic neurons of the two main types of chloride transporters, NKCC1 and KCC2, which determine the net influx or outflux of Cl^- ions respectively (Rivera *et al.*, 1999, Ben-Ari, 2014). For example, in immature pyramidal neurons NKCC1 is predominant, thus facilitating depolarization of the cell membrane. In some neurological conditions including epilepsy resulting from FCD, there is reduced expression of KCC2 (Shimizu-Okabe *et al.*, 2011), which favors depolarizing actions of GABA and the occurrence of interictal discharges (Blauwblomme *et al.*, 2019). Also, in TSC and FCD IIB cases increased NKCC1 and decreased KCC2 levels have been reported (Talos *et al.*, 2012). Notably, excitatory $GABA_A$ receptor-mediated responses recorded in slices from these patients were significantly attenuated by the NKCC1 inhibitor bumetanide, suggesting a possible therapeutic avenue for FCD.

In contrast to $GABA_A$ receptors, metabotropic $GABA_B$ receptors, coupled with K^+ channels, are always inhibitory. These receptors have been understudied in epilepsy research, particularly in FCD, but they may play a critical role in the transition from interictal to ictal activity (Levinson *et al.*, 2020) and also could be a target for therapeutic development, as discussed later.

• Pacemaker GABA synaptic activity (PGA)

In FCD II, one of the most striking observations at the stereo EEG level is the occurrence of continuous rhythmic spikes and poly-spikes within the dysplastic cortex (Chassoux *et al.*, 2000, Guerrini *et al.*, 2015). In fact, continuous and rhythmic epileptiform discharges have proven to be of diagnostic value in FCD II, as they are not found in FCD I nor in other epileptogenic lesions (Gambardella *et al.*, 1996, Tassi *et al.*, 2002). In our original studies characterizing the basic and synaptic properties of abnormal cells in pediatric FCD, we first observed the existence of highly rhythmic GABA synaptic activity (Cepeda *et al.*, 2007, Cepeda *et al.*, 2003), later called PGA due to its clockwise regularity with a frequency of 5-10 Hz (Cepeda *et al.*, 2014).

PGA is action potential dependent, mediated by $GABA_A$ receptors, and unaffected by blockade of glutamate receptors. Cells displaying PGA are found more frequently in cases of FCD compared with non-CD etiologies, and generally occur in the most epileptogenic samples. It was observed in different cells types including normal-like, dysmorphic cytomegalic, and immature pyramidal neurons. As FCD tissue demonstrates signs of immaturity, GABA can depolarize these types of pyramidal neurons. Indeed, we found that subthreshold, rhythmic GABA depolarizations can induce action potentials by rising cytosolic Ca^{2+}. Furthermore, when PGA activity was blocked with bicuculline action potentials also stopped (Cepeda *et al.*, 2007). We thus hypothesized that PGA represents the cellular substrate of rhythmic EEG paroxysmal discharges, particularly in FCD II, and could contribute to network synchronization. As for the potential generator of PGA, we narrowed down the source to the bitufted or double-bouquet interneuron subtypes (**Figure 2**).

• GABA synaptic activity and HFO

High frequency oscillations (HFO), most notably fast ripples (FRs) in the 250-500 Hz range, have been detected in infants with epilepsy using intracranial ECoG and scalp EEG recordings. A few clinical studies have suggested that complete resection of areas that present with FRs lead to a higher probability of postoperative seizure freedom (van 't Klooster *et al.*, 2015, Wu *et al.*, 2010). Hence, FRs recorded intraoperatively are considered a superior diagnostic measure in terms of

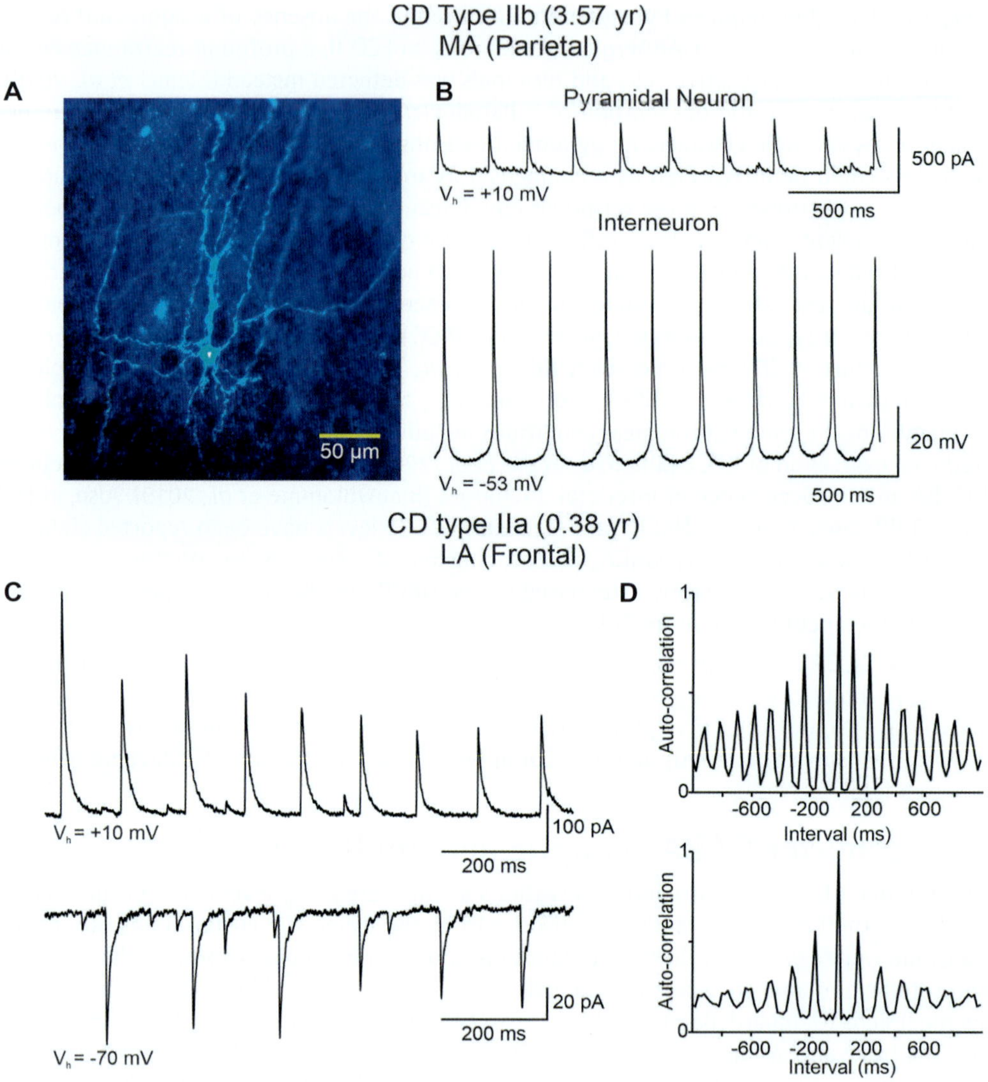

Figure 2

A. Interneuron, possibly bitufted or double-bouquet, recorded and filled with biocytin. B. In current clamp mode this cell generated rhythmic action potentials with a frequency similar to the PGA (5 Hz) recorded from a pyramidal neuron in the same slice, suggesting this type of interneuron could be a potential generator of PGA. C. PGA recorded from a pyramidal neuron in voltage clamp mode at two holding potentials. D. In both cases, a high degree of autocorrelation was observed, suggesting high degree of rhythmicity.

localization of EZ. In a recent paper we showed that, across FCD pathologies, the frequency of spontaneous inhibitory postsynaptic currents (sIPSCs) was higher in HFO+ areas when compared to HFO- areas. In fact, a recent study reported that regions of FCD are associated with increased levels of GABA compared with contralateral cortical regions or cortex from healthy controls (Gong *et al.*, 2021). There also was a close association between PGA and pathological HFO (Cepeda *et al.*, 2020). Furthermore, HFO+ areas containing GABAergic interneurons, mostly PV-expressing fast-spiking interneurons (FSIs), showed increased firing frequencies, ictal-like discharges, and slowly- or non-inactivating Na^+ "spikelets"; all of which are signs of hyperexcitability. Hence, PV-expressing FSIs were proposed as another potential generator of HFO. Because of the presence of HFO in multiple etiologies, this suggests that there is a common functional abnormality in the GABAergic circuitry. However, increased excitability of pyramidal neurons can also contribute to the generation of pathological HFO.

Therapies based on knowledge acquired from slice electrophysiology

Because of depolarizing and potentially excitatory actions of GABA in immature and epileptic brains, due primarily to reduced KCC2 levels and predominant NKCC1 presence, it was proposed that blocking NKCC1 with bumetanide or furosemide could have antiepileptic effects, particularly for neonatal seizures (Dzhala *et al.*, 2005). *In vitro* recordings of dysplastic neurons from a young TSC patient confirmed depolarizing $GABA_A$ receptor-mediated responses that were significantly attenuated by bumetanide (Talos *et al.*, 2012). Similarly, in FCD cases, blockade of NKCC1 led to a reduction of interictal discharges (Blauwblomme *et al.*, 2019). Unfortunately, clinical trials to treat neonatal seizures with bumetanide have been inconclusive (Pressler *et al.*, 2015). On the other hand, depolarizing actions of GABA during brain development are critical as blocking GABA depolarization with bumetanide results in permanent alterations in cortical circuits (Wang and Kriegstein, 2011). Nonetheless, continuing studies on the effects of bumetanide are still warranted and in a pilot clinical trial, it was reported that this NKCC1 blocker enhances antiepileptic effects of phenobarbital (Soul *et al.*, 2021), similar to early studies in animal models (Dzhala *et al.*, 2008). However, in a different animal model of neonatal seizures bumetanide was ineffective (Johne *et al.*, 2021).

While $GABA_A$ receptors have occupied most of the research on AED, the role of $GABA_B$ receptors has been largely neglected. This is unfortunate as, in contrast to bidirectional effects of $GABA_A$ receptors, activation of metabotropic $GABA_B$ receptors is always hyperpolarizing due to activation of inwardly rectifying K^+ channels. In a recent study, we demonstrated that antagonism of $GABA_B$ receptors facilitates the transition from interictal to ictal activity in pyramidal neurons and interneurons of pediatric FCD patients (Levinson *et al.*, 2020). This finding agrees with a previous study using FCD tissue from teenage and adult patients demonstrating that baclofen, a $GABA_B$ receptor agonist, reduces seizure activity and proposed that these receptors can be a target of AED (D'Antuono *et al.*, 2004). However, use of baclofen in the clinic is not recommended as it may also precipitate seizures.

In pediatric epilepsy, the ketogenic diet has demonstrated beneficial effects but its antiepileptic mechanisms remain ill-defined (Rho, 2017). Artificial cerebrospinal fluid enriched with β-hydoxybutyrate (BHB), the main ketone body, and pyruvate (eACSF), can reduce the depolarizing actions of GABA in early development (Holmgren *et al.*, 2010). We tested the effects of eACSF on paroxysmal activity induced by 4-aminopyridine (4-AP), a proconvulsant agent, in FCD cases. This eACSF solution quickly reduced the frequency and amplitude of paroxysmal discharges, suggesting that addition of these energy substrates has antiepileptic effects (Levinson *et al.*, 2020). In support, a prospective study found a strong correlation between seizure frequency and blood concentrations of BHB (Buchhalter *et al.*, 2017).

Finally, it is known that in FCD II and in TSC, there is hyperactivation of the mTOR pathway, which could explain cellular hypertrophy. Thus, blocking this pathway could help seizure control (Galanopoulou *et al.*, 2012). We found that prolonged bath application of everolimus reduced spontaneous excitatory postsynaptic activity and paroxysmal discharges induced by 4-AP (Levinson *et al.*, 2020). The anti-seizure effects were more pronounced in TSC and FCD cases, whereas in non-mTOR-mediated pathologies, the effects were subtle at best. These results support further clinical trials of everolimus in mTOR pathway-mediated pathologies.

Conclusions, limitations, and future studies

Based on our *in vitro* studies of pediatric epilepsy surgery tissue samples, spanning more than 30 years and including more than 300 patients, we proposed a potential mechanism for the generation of epileptic activity in FCD I and II (**Figure 3**). Considering the different histopathological and ontogenetic factors underlying these FCD types, it can also be expected that epileptogenic mechanisms are different. Thus, compared with FCD I, FCD II is more severe, occurs earlier during brain development, shows typical rhythmic EEG activity patterns, the EZ is easier to define, and has a better surgical outcome (Lerner *et al.*, 2009, Guerrini *et al.*, 2015, Krsek *et al.*, 2009, Tassi *et al.*, 2002). In FCD IIB and TSC, we know now that balloon/giant cells are not epileptogenic. Instead, they may prevent the spread of epileptic activity by buffering glutamate and K^+ ions. However, the suggestion that cytomegalic neurons alone are the triggers of epileptic activity in FCD II would be a risky proposition due to the presence of other cell types with high epileptogenic potential. Thus, we can propose that, in FCD II and probably also in TSC, dysmorphic cytomegalic pyramidal neurons, cytomegalic interneurons, and immature pyramidal neurons can be or become epileptogenic. In addition, pyramidal

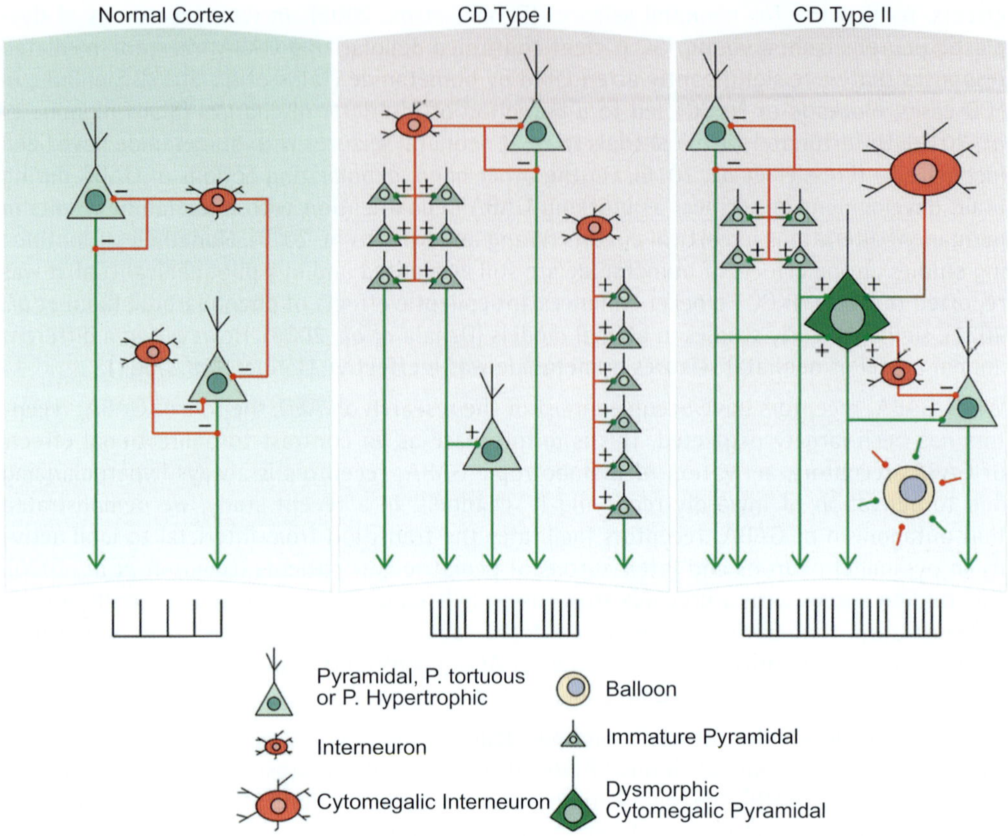

Figure 3
Simplified diagram of possible mechanisms of hyperexcitability in FCD I and II compared with normal cortex. In normal cortex, pyramidal neuron output is tightly regulated by inhibitory GABAergic interneurons. In FCD I, neuronal disorganization and microcolumns or clusters of immature pyramidal neurons contribute to hyperexcitability due to depolarizing actions of GABA on these neurons. In FCD II, in addition to increased excitation caused by immature pyramidal neurons, cytomegalic pyramidal neurons and cytomegalic interneurons intensify the generation and propagation of epileptic discharges. In contrast, balloon cells, which lack synaptic inputs and are unable to fire action potentials, are probably not involved in epileptogenesis, but could play an antiepileptic role by buffering glutamate and K^+ (reproduced from Abdijadid *et al.*, 2015, with permission from John Wiley and Sons).

neurons undergoing degenerative changes, i.e., regressing to an immature state, can also become epileptogenic (Cepeda *et al.*, 2006). FCD I tissue is also highly epileptogenic, yet no dysmorphic cytomegalic neurons are found histopathologically. Instead, a disorganized cortical architecture and the presence of clusters of immature pyramidal neurons, as well as depolarizing GABA actions seem sufficient to induce epileptic activity. In addition, the occurrence of misoriented and hypertrophic pyramidal neurons could also play a role.

Based on our findings at the single-cell level, we can conclude that probably there is no true epileptic neuron but an epileptogenic circuit. In fact, any neuron displaying increased excitability by virtue of high membrane input resistance, increased Ca^{2+} channels, depolarizing GABA actions, or increased glutamatergic inputs, has the potential of generating paroxysmal discharges. Needless to say, subtle morphological changes are likely associated with changes in electrophysiological properties, e.g., loss of dendritic spines could make the cell more excitable. Thus, a combination of altered intrinsic membrane properties and synaptic inputs can make a neuron hyperexcitable. Intrinsic changes in membrane properties in combination with PGA can explain the tendency of FCD networks to produce a hypersynchronous, epileptic state.

We have to acknowledge that studying epileptic activity in a dish has important limitations including severance of subcortical excitatory inputs, damage of dendritic and axonal processes, different external milieu than in human brains, dependence on internal recording solution in whole-cell patch clamp recordings, and so forth. In addition, the reader has to realize that our findings are applicable mainly to pediatric populations and adults with childhood epilepsy onset due to FCD. Morphological and electrophysiological alterations could be at variance in adult populations with FCD, due to developmental changes (e.g., differences in receptor subunit expression) and longer duration of epileptic activity, which may trigger activity-dependent compensatory mechanisms (Finardi *et al.*, 2006).

In spite of these limitations, a close collaboration between clinicians, neurosurgeons, and basic scientists has proven very fruitful in revealing some intrinsic and synaptic mechanisms of epileptogenicity in FCD. There are still many unanswered questions that need to be addressed, for example; how can we improve the definition of the EZ in FCD I, particularly if we consider the existence of different subtypes? What is the role of misoriented and hypertrophic pyramidal neurons present in FCD I in the generation of epileptic discharges? More studies on the electrophysiological and morphological characteristics of balloon/giant cells compared with normal astrocytes also are warranted. The role of other glutamate receptor subtypes, e.g., AMPA and kainate, should be examined. Specifically, studies on Ca^{2+}-permeable AMPA receptors in FCD could open new therapeutic avenues. Finally, from a clinical point of view, how can we explain the striking property of the epileptogenic network in FCD II to remain focalized, whereas it is much more diffuse in FCD I, which could help explain the poorer surgical outcome? Could balloon/giant cells prevent the spread of epileptic activity in FCD IIB? The future will tell.

Acknowledgments

This work was supported by previous NIH grant NS 38992 (GWM, CC). Pharmacological studies on the effects of Everolimus were supported by Novartis (Joyce Wu and CC as Co-PIs). We would like to thank Pr. Michael S. Levine for his unwavering support, the late Pr. Robin S. Fisher for his anatomical insights, as well as a number of post-doctoral fellows, in particular Drs. John P. Walsh, Raymond S. Hurst, Gloria J. Klapstein, Jorge Flores-Hernández, Véronique M. André, and Elizabeth Hernández-Echeagaray for their contributions. Immunohistochemical processing of tissue slices was performed by My Huynh, Julia Chang, Jan Asai, and Irene Yamazaki. A special thanks to the parents of pediatric patients undergoing surgery for the treatment of intractable epilepsy, who graciously agreed the use of resected tissue samples for experimental purposes. Needless to say, these samples were part of the planned resection.

References

Abdijadid S, Mathern G. W, Levine M. S, Cepeda C. Basic mechanisms of epileptogenesis in pediatric cortical dysplasia. *Cns Neurosci Ther* 2015; 21: 92-103.

André V. M, Cepeda C, Vinters H. V, Huynh M, Mathern G. W, Levine M. S. Pyramidal cell responses to gamma-aminobutyric acid differ in type I and type II cortical dysplasia. *J Neurosci Res* 2008; 86: 3151-62.

André V. M, Flores-Hernández J, Cepeda C, *et al.* NMDA receptor alterations in neurons from pediatric cortical dysplasia tissue. *Cereb Cortex* 2004; 14: 634-46.

André V. M, Wu N, Yamazaki I, *et al.* Cytomegalic interneurons: a new abnormal cell type in severe pediatric cortical dysplasia. *J Neuropathol Exp Neurol* 2007; 66: 491-504.

Ben-Ari Y. The GABA excitatory/inhibitory developmental sequence: a personal journey. *Neuroscience* 2014; 279: 187-219.

Blauwblomme T, Dossi E, Pellegrino C, *et al.* Gamma-Aminobutyric acidergic transmission underlies interictal epileptogenicity in pediatric Focal Cortical Dysplasia. *Ann Neurol* 2019; 85: 204-17.

Blumcke I, Thom M, Aronica E, *et al.* The clinicopathologic spectrum of Focal Cortical Dysplasias: a consensus classification proposed by an ad hoc task force of the ilae diagnostic methods commission. *Epilepsia* 2011; 52: 158-74.

Boonyapisit K, Najm I, Klem G, *et al.* Epileptogenicity of focal malformations due to abnormal cortical development: direct electrocorticographic-histopathologic correlations. *Epilepsia* 2003; 44: 69-76.

Buchhalter J. R, D'alfonso S, Connolly M, *et al.* The relationship between d-beta-hydroxybutyrate blood concentrations and seizure control in children treated with the ketogenic diet for medically intractable epilepsy. *Epilepsia Open* 2017; 2: 317-21.

Cepeda C, André V. M, Levine M. S, *et al.* Epileptogenesis in pediatric cortical dysplasia: the dysmature cerebral developmental hypothesis. *Epilepsy Behav* 2006; 9: 219-35.

Cepeda C, André V. M, Vinters H. V, Levine M. S, Mathern G. W. Are cytomegalic neurons and balloon cells generators of epileptic activity in pediatric cortical dysplasia? *Epilepsia* 2005; 46 Suppl 5: 82-8.

Cepeda C, André V. M, Wu N, *et al.* Immature neurons and GABA networks may contribute to epileptogenesis in pediatric cortical dysplasia. *Epilepsia* 2007; 48 Suppl 5: 79-85.

Cepeda C, Chen J. Y, Wu J. Y, *et al.* Pacemaker GABA synaptic activity may contribute to network synchronization in pediatric cortical dysplasia. *Neurobiol Dis* 2014; 62: 208-17.

Cepeda C, Hurst R. S, Flores-Hernández J, *et al.* Morphological and electrophysiological characterization of abnormal cell types in pediatric cortical dysplasia. *J Neurosci Res* 2003; 72: 472-86.

Cepeda C, Levinson S, Nariai H, *et al.* Pathological high frequency oscillations associate with increased GABA synaptic activity in pediatric epilepsy surgery patients. *Neurobiol Dis* 2020; 134: 104618.

Cepeda C, Walsh J. P, Peacock W, Buchwald N. A, Levine M. S. Dye-coupling in human neocortical tissue resected from children with intractable epilepsy. *Cereb Cortex* 1993; 3: 95-107.

Chassoux F, Devaux B, Landré E, *et al.* Stereoelectroencephalography in Focal Cortical Dysplasia: a 3D approach to delineating the dysplastic cortex. *Brain* 2000; 123 (Pt 8): 1733-51.

D'antuono M, Louvel J, Kohling R, *et al.* GABAa receptor-dependent synchronization leads to ictogenesis in the human dysplastic cortex. *Brain* 2004; 127: 1626-40.

Dodt H. U, Zieglgansberger W. Visualizing unstained neurons in living brain slices by infrared dic-videomicroscopy. *Brain Res* 1990; 537: 333-6.

Dzhala, V. I, Brumback, A. C, Staley, K. J. Bumetanide Enhances phenobarbital efficacy in a neonatal seizure model. *Ann Neurol* 2008; 63: 222-35.

Dzhala V. I, Talos D. M, Sdrulla D. A, *et al.* Nkcc1 transporter facilitates seizures in the developing brain. *Nat Med* 2005; 11: 1205-13.

Finardi A, Gardoni F, Bassanini S, *et al.* NMDA receptor composition differs among anatomically diverse malformations of cortical development. *J Neuropathol Exp Neurol* 2006; 65: 883-93.

Galanopoulou A. S, Gorter J. A, Cepeda C. Finding a better drug for epilepsy: the mtor pathway as an antiepileptogenic target. *Epilepsia* 2012; 53: 1119-30.

Gambardella A, Palmini A, Andermann F, *et al.* Usefulness of focal rhythmic discharges on scalp eeg of patients with Focal Cortical Dysplasia and intractable epilepsy. *Electroencephalogr Clin Neurophysiol* 1996; 98: 243-9.

Gong T, Liu Y, Chen Y, Lin L, Lin Y, Wang G. Focal corticarl dysplasia in epilepsy is associated with GABA increase. *NeuroImage Clin* 2021; 31: 102763.

Gonzalez-Martinez J. A, Ying Z, Prayson R, Bingaman W, Najm I. Glutamate clearance mechanisms in resected cortical dysplasia. *J Neurosurg* 2011; 114: 1195-202.

Guerrini R, Duchowny M, Jayakar P, *et al.* Diagnostic methods and treatment options for Focal Cortical Dysplasia. *Epilepsia* 2015; 56: 1669-86.

Hagemann G, Kluska M. M, Redecker C, Luhmann H. J, Witte O. W. Distribution of glutamate receptor subunits in experimentally induced cortical malformations. *Neuroscience* 2003; 117: 991-1002.

Holmgren C. D, Mukhtarov M, Malkov A. E, Popova I. Y, Bregestovski P, Zilberter Y. Energy substrate availability as a determinant of neuronal resting potential, GABA signaling and spontaneous network activity in the neonatal cortex in vitro. *J Neurochem* 2010; 112: 900-12.

Johne M, Romermann K, Hampel P, *et al.* Phenobarbital and midazolam suppress neonatal seizures in a noninvasive rat model of birth asphyxia, whereas bumetanide is ineffective. *Epilepsia* 2021; 62: 920-34.

Kerfoot C, Vinters H. V, Mathern G. W. Cerebral cortical dysplasia: giant neurons show potential for increased excitation and axonal plasticity. *Dev Neurosci* 1999; 21: 260-70.

Krsek P, Pieper T, Karlmeier A, *et al.* Different presurgical characteristics and seizure outcomes in children with Focal Cortical Dysplasia type I or II. *Epilepsia* 2009; 50: 125-37.

Lerner J. T, Salamon N, Hauptman J. S, *et al.* Assessment And surgical outcomes for mild type I and severe type II cortical dysplasia: a critical review and the UCLA experience. *Epilepsia* 2009; 50: 1310-35.

Levinson S, Tran C. H, Barry J, *et al.* Paroxysmal Discharges in tissue slices from pediatric epilepsy surgery patients: critical role of GABAb receptors in the generation of ictal activity. *Front Cell Neurosci* 2020; 14: 54.

Mathern G. W, Cepeda C, Hurst R. S, Flores-Hernandez J, Mendoza D, Levine M. S. Neurons recorded from pediatric epilepsy surgery patients with cortical dysplasia. *Epilepsia* 2000, 41 Suppl 6: S162-7.

Mattia D, Olivier A, Avoli M. Seizure-like discharges recorded in human dysplastic neocortex maintained in vitro. *Neurology* 1995; 45: 1391-5.

Medici V, Rossini L, Deleo F, *et al.* Different parvalbumin and GABA expression in human epileptogenic Focal Cortical Dysplasia. *Epilepsia* 2016; 57: 1109-19.

Mischel P. S, Nguyen L. P, Vinters H. V. Cerebral cortical dysplasia associated with pediatric epilepsy. review of neuropathologic features and proposal for a grading system. *J Neuropathol Exp Neurol* 1995; 54: 137-53.

Moddel G, Jacobson B, Ying Z, *et al.* The NMDA receptor nr2b subunit contributes to epileptogenesis in human cortical dysplasia. *Brain Res* 2005; 1046: 10-23.

Najm I. M, Sarnat H. B, Blumcke I. Review: The International Consensus Classification Of Focal Cortical Dysplasia - A Critical Update 2018. *Neuropathol Appl Neurobiol* 2018; 44: 18-31.

Palmini A, Gambardella A, Andermann F, *et al.* Intrinsic epileptogenicity of human dysplastic cortex as suggested by corticography and surgical results. *Ann Neurol* 1995; 37: 476-87.

Palmini A, Najm I, Avanzini G, *et al.* Terminology and classification of the cortical dysplasias. *Neurology* 2004; 62: S2-8.

Pressler R. M, Boylan G. B, Marlow N, *et al.* Bumetanide for the treatment of seizures in newborn babies with hypoxic ischaemic encephalopathy (nemo): an open-label, dose finding, and feasibility phase 1/2 trial. *Lancet Neurol* 2015; 14: 469-77.

Prince D. A. The depolarization shift in "epileptic" neurons. *Exp Neurol* 1968; 21: 467-85.

Prince D. A, Wong R. K. Human epileptic neurons studied in vitro. *Brain Res* 1981; 210: 323-33.

Rho J. M. How does the ketogenic diet induce anti-seizure effects? *Neurosci Lett* 2017; 637: 4-10.

Rivera C, Voipio J, Payne J. A, *et al.* The K+/Cl- Co-Transporter Kcc2 renders GABA hyperpolarizing during neuronal maturation. *Nature* 1999; 397: 251-5.

Schwartzkroin P. A, Prince D. A. Microphysiology of human cerebral cortex studied in vitro. *Brain Res* 1976; 115: 497-500.

Schwartzkroin P. A, Walsh C. A. Cortical malformations and epilepsy. *Ment Retard Dev Disabil Res Rev* 2000; 6: 268-80.

Shimizu-Okabe C, Tanaka M, Matsuda K, *et al.* Kcc2 was downregulated in small neurons localized in epileptogenic human Focal Cortical Dysplasia. *Epilepsy Res* 2011; 93: 177-84.

Soul J. S, Bergin A. M, Stopp C, *et al.* A pilot randomized, controlled, double-blind trial of bumetanide to treat neonatal seizures. *Ann Neurol* 2021; 89: 327-40.

Spreafico R, Battaglia G, Arcelli P, *et al.* Cortical dysplasia: an immunocytochemical study of three patients. *Neurology* 1998; 50: 27-36.

Talos D. M, Kwiatkowski D. J, Cordero K, Black P. M, Jensen F. E. Cell-specific alterations of glutamate receptor expression in tuberous sclerosis complex cortical tubers. *Ann Neurol* 2008; 63: 454-65.

Talos D. M, Sun H, Kosaras B, *et al.* Altered inhibition in tuberous sclerosis and type iib cortical dysplasia. *Ann Neurol* 2012; 71: 539-51.

Tassi L, Colombo N, Garbelli R, *et al.* Focal Cortical Dysplasia: neuropathological subtypes, eeg, neuroimaging and surgical outcome. *Brain* 2002; 125: 1719-32.

Taylor D. C, Falconer M. A, Bruton C. J, Corsellis J. A. Focal dysplasia of the cerebral cortex in epilepsy. *J Neurol Neurosurg Psychiatry* 1971; 34: 369-87.

Van 'T Klooster M. A, Van Klink N. E, Leijten F. S, *et al.* Residual fast ripples in the intraoperative corticogram predict epilepsy surgery outcome. *Neurology* 2015; 85: 120-8.

Wang D. D, Kriegstein A. R. Blocking early GABA depolarization with bumetanide results in permanent alterations in cortical circuits and sensorimotor gating deficits. *Cereb Cortex* 2011; 21: 574-87.

White R, Hua Y, Scheithauer B, Lynch D. R, Henske E. P, Crino P. B. Selective alterations in glutamate and GABA receptor subunit mRNA expression in dysplastic neurons and giant cells of cortical tubers. *Ann Neurol* 2001; 49: 67-78.

Wu J. Y, Sankar R, Lerner J. T, Matsumoto J. H, Vinters H. V, Mathern G. W. Removing interictal fast ripples on electrocorticography linked with seizure freedom in children. *Neurology* 2010; 75: 1686-94.

Wuarin J. P, Kim Y. I, Cepeda C, *et al.* Synaptic transmission in human neocortex removed for treatment of intractable epilepsy in children. *Ann Neurol* 1990; 28: 503-11.

Ying Z, Babb T. L, Comair Y. G, Bingaman W, Bushey M, Touhalisky K. Induced expression of NMDAr2 proteins and differential expression of NMDAr1 splice variants in dysplastic neurons of human epileptic neocortex. *J Neuropathol Exp Neurol* 1998; 57: 47-62.

Zimmer T. S, Broekaart D. W. M, Luinenburg M, *et al.* Balloon cells promote immune system activation in Focal Cortical Dysplasia type 2b. *Neuropathol Appl Neurobiol* 2021; 47: 826-39.

CHAPTER

10. Intrinsic epileptogenicity of FCD: insights from electrocorticography

Andre Palmini, Eliseu Paglioli

Key points

- Acute electrocorticography (ECoG) can identify highly epileptogenic patterns of electrical activity that blur the boundaries between interictal and ictal states.
- Such ictal-like or continuous epileptiform discharges (I/CED) on ECoG takes one of three forms: recurrent electrographic seizures, recurrent bursts of high frequency spikes or the even more typical pacemaker-like, virtually rhythmic, continuous discharges.
- I/CEDs not only often colocalizes with the region of ictal onset identified on chronic invasive recordings, but also may index relevant epileptogenic tissue that extends beyond that area and, although having a higher ictal threshold at the time of current evaluation, may prove relevant for seizure generation.
- Crucially, flexible ball-pointed electrodes that can be freely moved to explore the exposed cortical surface, thus allowing sequential exploration of potentially epileptogenic cortical regions, must be used.

A historical account

The history behind the now widely accepted concept of the intrinsic epileptogenicity of the dysplastic cortex is, as a personal account (AP), both a demonstration that novelty has preferential access to memory and a tribute both to mentorship and the luck of being surrounded by smart, competent people. I had the privilege of observing and discussing dozens of acute ECoG recordings performed by Pierre Gloor at the Montreal Neurological Institute in the early 90's. He was a fantastic, very methodical neurophysiologist and I recall his examination of two patients over several months whose ECoG displayed continuous spiking and recurrent electrographic seizures. He was impressed by the striking epileptogenicity represented by those particular patterns but the connection with dysplasia was not initially made. Nevertheless, those patterns were new to me and stuck in my mind.

A couple of years later, already in Porto Alegre, a patient with rolandic dysplasia was being operated by Eliseu Paglioli, my coauthor in this chapter, and the acute ECoG over the lesion looked like an EKG. Spikes were continuous, recurring at about 2 per second, and suggested a focal pacemaker, to the point that we were in doubt of whether that simply represented an EKG artifact or a pacemaker-like pattern of epileptogenic brain activity. Jaderson Costa, with us at the operating room, suggested we did a concomitant EKG, and that was crucial to show that that was not an artifact, but a truly epileptic focal pacemaker in the central region (*figure 4 in* Palmini *et al.*, 1995).

I immediately made the connection between this observation and the cases seen with Gloor in Montreal and realized all 3 cases had cortical dysplasia as the underlying pathology. I then presented this observation at the next American Epilepsy Society Meeting and was greeted with a big encouragement from Professor Olivier Dulac, who told me that he had never seen that before and that I should pursue that further. From there, I organized with my mentor Frederick Andermann a full review of all ECoG recordings of the patients with neuronal migration disorders from the MNI series that we had published a few years before (Palmini *et al.*, 1991), and also the cases operated in Porto Alegre. Lo and behold, almost 70% of those with Taylor type FCD had one of three exquisitely epileptogenic patterns (the third being recurrent focal bursts of very high frequency spikes, as detailed below). Review of the involved electrodes showed that those patterns were recorded directly from dysplastic regions, and the surgical outcome regarding seizure control was related to the complete resection of the cortical regions displaying them. That led to the proposal that the dysplastic tissue was 'intrinsically epileptogenic' (Palmini *et al.*, 1995).

In the years that followed, the finding was confirmed by distinct methods of recording (scalp EEG (Gambardella *et al.*, 1996), magnetoencephalography (Morioka *et al.*, 1999) and subdural chronic direct recordings (Widess-Walsh *et al.*, 2007)). However, the best confirmation of the intrinsic epileptogenicity came from recordings directly from within the dysplastic lesions through stereoelectrencephalography (SEEG). For the anecdote, the story began informally in a tavern in Nuremberg during a symposium on brain plasticity in epilepsy in 1996, where the issue was brought to the table and discussed with doctors Francine Chassoux and Frank Morrell. At the time, Francine mentioned the series from Bancaud and Talairach with SEEG electrodes implanted in tissue before the era of imaging that proved to be Taylor type FCD and showed a very similar, if not the same, continuous, pacemaker-like pattern published the year before (Palmini *et al.*, 1995). She went on to mention that that historical series was being complemented by new patients whose SEEG evaluation she was personally conducting at Saint-Anne, with MRI-positive Taylor-type FCD, with the exact same pattern. We discussed that those findings should be published as a clear advance on the understanding of the intrinsic epileptogenicity of those lesions and a marker of the relevant tissue to be resected. The material appeared in the Brain paper of 2000 (Chassoux *et al.*, 2000), confirming that the pacemaker pattern was recorded only from regions harboring dysplastic neurons. Moreover, that study set the stage for the realization that interictal pacemaker discharges were the best biomarker of the EZ in dysplasia, a finding replicated by the Milano group – which not only confirmed the findings but showed that such epileptogenic patterns were seen exclusively in Taylor-type FCD, (i. e., FCD II; Tassi *et al.*, 2002). Furthermore, basic scientists set to study the biological bases of the highly epileptogenic patterns in FCD (Avoli *et al.*, 1999; Cepeda *et al.*, 2006; Cepeda, this volume). Because of the virtual uniqueness of mainly the pacemaker pattern as a fingerprint of FCD II, several chapters of this book will touch upon this issue of highly epileptogenic electrographic patterns associated with refractory seizures in FCD, providing up-to-date accounts of the underlying mechanisms and the role their identification play in delineating the resection.

In this chapter we will detail the morphology of the highly epileptogenic patterns as they are seen in acute ECoG, how frequent these are and the relation with the type of FCD. We will then discuss how these ECoG patterns relate to the ictal onset zones as determined by chronic subdural recordings and SEEG. Finally, we will explore the concept of that in some types of FCD relevant epileptogenic tissue may extend beyond the EZ as defined at the time of the evaluation, and that acute ECoG may be one of the methods that contribute to the localization of such tissue (Palmini and Paglioli, 2019).

Intrinsic epileptogenicity of FCD: characterization of acute ECoG patterns

• What's in a name? A word about acute ECoG

Essentially, acute ECoG is a recording method of the irritative zone. It explores the cortical areas exposed by the craniotomy and allows conclusions to be drawn from several features of the recorded spikes. Unquestionably, the risks, costs, and technology involved in acute ECoG recordings are much less impressive in comparison with other invasive methods, which is an important asset from the perspective of sustainable epilepsy surgery. However, the usefulness of acute ECoG depends upon a priori knowledge of at least the quadrant of the brain where the EZ is contained and, in our view, on the type of electrodes used for recording. The main premise is that the epilepsy team have taken the best possible advantage of data collected on the noninvasive presurgical evaluation. While this is obviously the case for the correct use of all recording methods, it is crucial for acute ECoG because, unlike chronic recordings with intracranial electrodes, acute ECoG cannot rely on ictal data. The a priori knowledge of the brain quadrant where the EZ is contained should be the topographical synthesis of localizing data gathered from semiology, interictal and ictal scalp EEG, neuropsychology and imaging, both structural MRI and PET. Careful integration of these data often allows a target craniotomy, with further refinement of the epileptogenic zone from acute ECoG.

Such refinement depends upon interpretation of the amplitude, frequency and rhythmicity of the spikes, and the associated background abnormalities (Palmini and Paglioli, 2019). However, as important as these spike features is the possibility of both direct exploration of various subregions within the exposed cortex and sequential, stepwise recordings following each stage of the resection. This demands ECoG electrodes that can be moved easily over the cortex and record from the depth of gyri (crucial in FCD surgery). Thus, we believe of utmost importance that acute ECoG be recorded with ballpoint electrodes attached to flexible, long-reaching arms, allowing comprehensive exploration as traditionally performed by the Montreal school (Feindel, 1998; **Figure 1**). On the other hand, no special type of anesthetic is needed to elicit the epileptogenic patterns, although it is important to lower the pCO2 to around 27-28 mmHg at the time of the recording. In our Center, anesthesia is induced with propofol and maintained with isoflurane.

Finally, we believe that acute recordings with grids or strips make it difficult to customize the stepwise exploration of superficial and deep portions of the cortex at each stage of the resection, thus falling short of providing truly reliable information – particularly in lesions such as FCD that may extend deeper into the cortical banks. Therefore, not all ECoG recordings are the same, and that is why it is important to know what is meant by ECoG in different studies.

• Highly epileptogenic acute ECoG patterns indicative of intrinsic epileptogenicity of FCD

In our original publication we used the denomination ictal or continuous epileptogenic discharges (I/CEDs) to describe the highly epileptogenic patterns seen in FCD (Palmini *et al.*, 1995). 'Ictal' because one of the patterns is the acute recording of recurrent electrographic seizures, manifested as recruiting/derecruiting prolonged trains of rhythmic activity (**Figure 1**) and a second pattern are repetitive bursts of fast spiking discharges of variable duration (**Figure 2**). The third pattern is the 'pacemaker', ie, continuous or quasicontinuous rhythmic spikes or sharp waves at 1-8 Hz, for very prolonged periods (**Figures 3 and 4**). At least one of these 3 patterns was present in 70% of the patients with dysplastic neurons and/ or balloon cells, ie, Taylor-type or FCD II in our original series and in 58 of 66 (87%) in a recent series (Palmini *et al.*, in preparation).

Repetitive electrographic seizures (recruiting/derecruiting pattern)

This is characterized by activity that progressively increased in frequency and rhythmicity for several seconds reaching a rhythmic plateau around 12 to 16 Hz and followed by slowing or attenuation of the recording. These recurrent electrographic seizures are seen in between 25 to 30% of the patients.

Repetitive bursting patterns

This pattern was observed in about 20% of the patients and characterized by high-frequency bursts of polyspikes that appeared suddenly, lasted for 5 to 10 seconds, and abruptly disappeared. Frequency varied from 10 to 20 Hz, or faster. There was no change in background rhythms after the bursts.

Continuous or quasicontinuous rhythmic spiking lasting for the whole duration of the recording or recurring frequently: The 'pacemaker'

Forty to 45% of patients had prolonged, virtually continuous trains of rhythmic 2- to 8-Hz spikes or sharp waves. In most cases they were present over dysplastic lesions throughout the duration of the ECoG recording. Occasionally, these were slower in frequency, however with almost fixed periodicity.

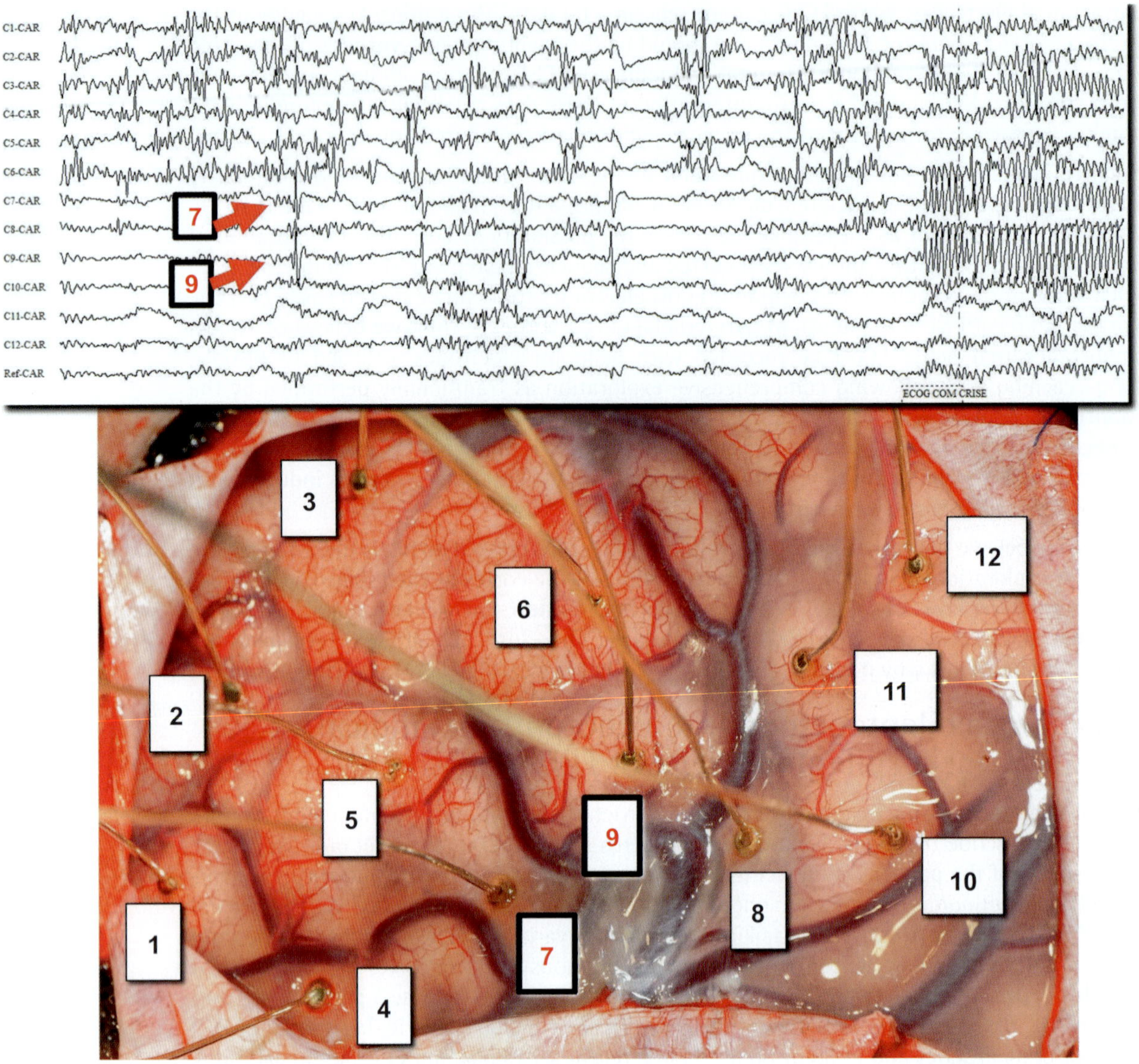

Figure 1

The 'Montreal Neurological Institute (MNI)' ECoG apparatus.

Note that it resembles a 'spider', with multiple flexible 'limbs', allowing free exploration of the cortical surface. The customized 'limbs' and points are made of metal and the ball-pointed ends bathed in gold. An electrographic seizure is recorded mostly in channels '7'and '9', where repetitive high amplitude spikes were also seen throughout the recording, exactly where the structural lesion was located. Note involvement of channels 3 and 8, at seizure onset. Repetitive spikes were not recorded over these electrodes.

Figure 2

ECoG bursting pattern on cortical electrodes exploring a dysplastic region shown to have FCD IIA histopathology.

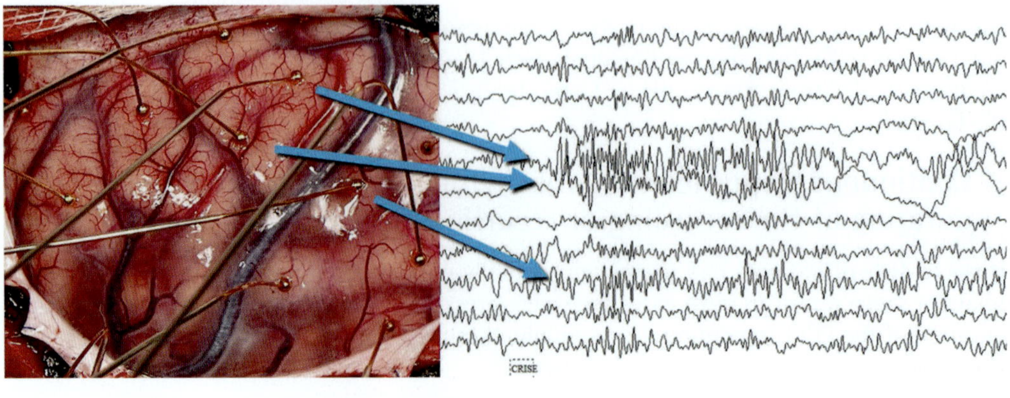

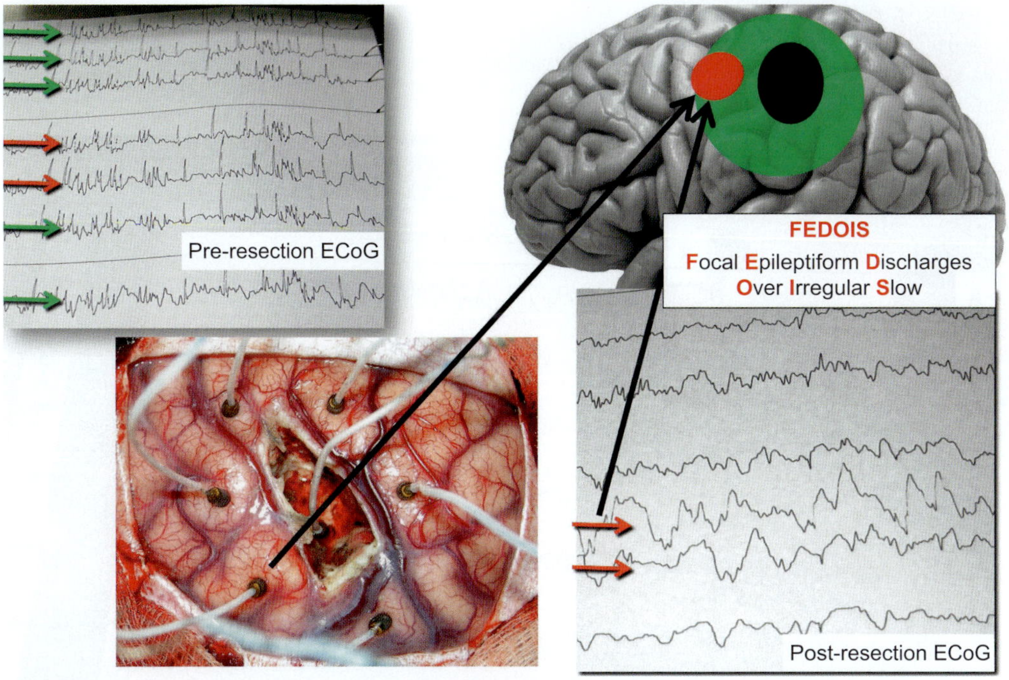

Figure 3

Acute ECoG exploration of a patient with an FCD IIA over the rolandic region.

On the upper left, note samples showing recurrent bursts of discharges and continuous spiking over a large area, schematically pictured in the upper right of the figure. Following initial resection (lower left), a pattern characterized by focal epileptiform discharges over irregular slow waves (FEDOIS) was recorded in the 'hand knob' (lower right).

Finally, Teixeira and colleagues have presented in abstract form an interesting interictal pattern recorded in the ECoG of some patients with FCD, combining focal hyperexcitability and neuronal dysfunction (Teixeira *et al.*, 1997). They named that as FEDOIS – Focal Epileptiform Discharges Over Irregular Slowing. We found this pattern in the ECoG of 3 of 60 patients in whom highly epileptogenic patterns were seen, all with FCD II, and always combined with the pacemaker pattern is adjacent regions. Interestingly, in one of these patients FEDOIS were recorded as the sole pattern over the hand area (**Figure 3**). Resection included adjacent peri-rolandic regions displaying the pacemaker pattern but did not include this primary motor cortex region with FEDOIS – and seizures continued unabated. More research is needed into this pattern, although it seems a marker of neuronal dysfunction rather than another indication of intrinsic epileptogenicity. However, the presence of FEDOIS may point to a degree of dysfunction with epileptogenic potential and the regions displaying this pattern should perhaps be resected, if functionally feasible.

Highly epileptogenic acute ECoG patterns in other types of FCD

In a recent analysis of 24 patients with either FCD I or mild malformations of cortical development (mMCD, including MOGHE) who had surgery and acute ECoG, around 20% had a pacemaker-like pattern (Palmini and Paglioli, 2019, personal communication, presented at the 2019 Cleveland Clinic Neurological Institute Summit on Focal Cortical Dysplasia). However, in contrast to the continuous pacemaker (ie, continuous, rhythmic or semi-rhythmic spikes) lasting throughout all the ECoG examination seen in FCD II, this pattern was discontinuous in those with FCD I/mMCD (**Figure 5**). Moreover, it is interesting to mention that patients with gliotic lesions have also been reported as occasionally presenting continuous epileptogenic discharges. However, is unclear whether these discharges were recorded for long periods of time, suggesting a true pacemaker (Guerreiro *et al.*, 2003).

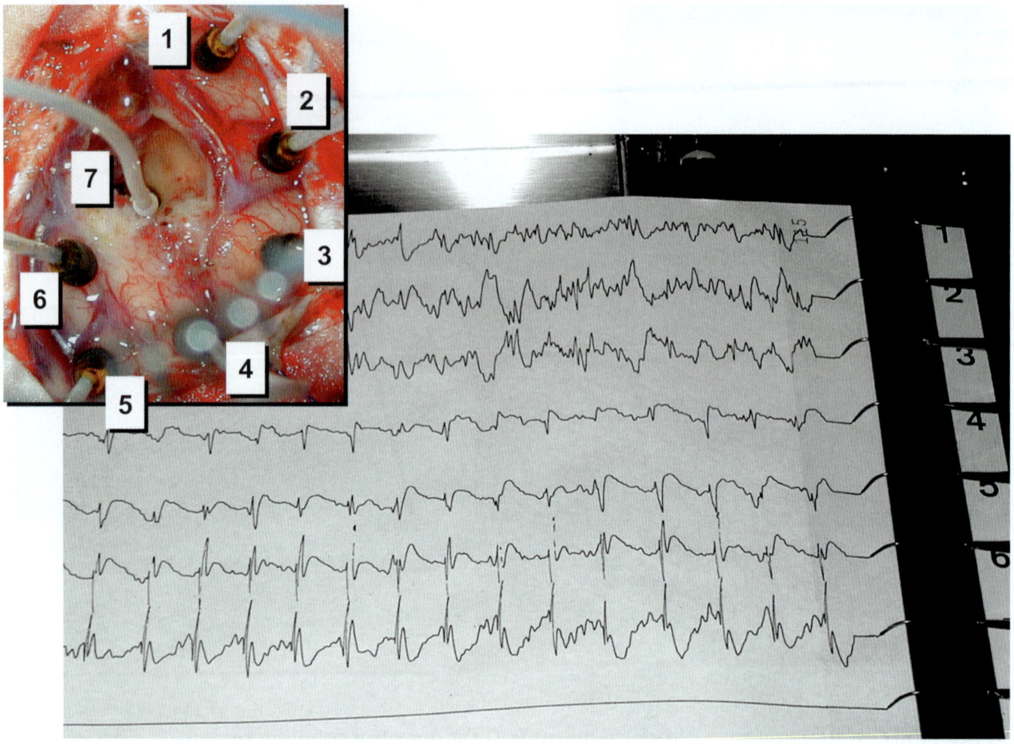

Figure 4

Continuous, 'pacemaker-like' epileptiform discharges recorded in the surface and banks of the gyri being explored with flexible ECoG electrodes. This interictal pattern strongly co-localizes with the zone of ictal onset. Note the previous version of the apparatus, with carbon-ball electrodes, currently changed to metal.

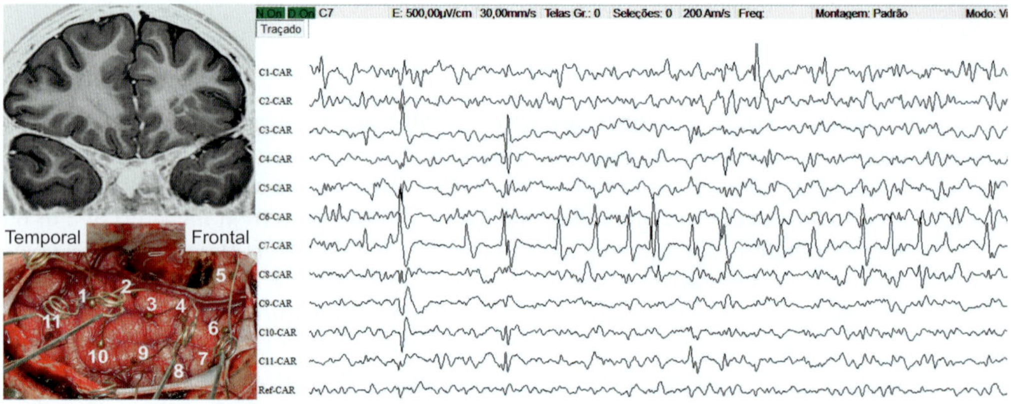

Figure 5

Discontinuous ECoG discharges over a large cortical region shown to harbor FCD IA pathology. In the upper left, note dysplastic lesion in the basal part of the left anterior frontal lobe.

ECoG 'dysplastic patterns': topographical relation to the ictal onset zone as determined by chronic subdural recordings and SEEG

• A conceptual first word

Epilepsy surgery is a paradigmatic subspecialty. People tend to stick to methods for presurgical evaluation with which they are familiar. This inevitably leads to accumulated experience with some approaches in detriment of others – and has animated heated debates on which is the best approach. Perhaps there is no best approach, or at least one that has empirically been proven as better than others. There is, on the one hand, the experience with one method of evaluation and, on the other, broadly accepted concepts of epileptogenesis and resective strategies. A successful approach is one that matches method, concept and strategy, in the hands of experienced people – and leads to seizure control.

This debate is relevant in the presurgical evaluation of patients with FCD, because in this pathology surgical outcome regarding seizure control is directly related to complete resection of dysplastic tissue. Thus, whichever method is used should provide a precise delineation of the extent of tissue to be resected. This issue, naturally, intersects with the surgical strategies to patients with FCD, directly related to each pre-resection method of localizing the EZ, discussed in specific chapters of this volume by experienced surgeons.

• 'Interictal' ECoG patterns in relation to the ictal onset zone in FCD

Because highly epileptogenic, virtually specific, interictal patterns are seen in FCD II, it is reasonable to ask whether ictal recordings of the habitual clinical seizures are needed to plan the resection. In other words, the question is whether this 'special' or 'dysplastic' irritative zone may define the extent of the EZ and dispense with ictal recordings directly from cortical tissue. If ictal recordings are not needed, then the next question is whether chronic recordings with intracranial electrodes are needed to define this 'dysplastic' irritative zone or if acute ECoG would suffice.

Because acute ECoG provides essentially *interictal* data, the crucial question is how frequently the *ictal* onset zone identified by chronic intracranial recordings *colocalize with interictal continuous epileptogenic discharges.* Interestingly, this number is quite consistent and revolves around 75% (Chassoux *et al.*, 2000, Tassi *et al.*, 2002, Bartolomei *et al.*, 2016; Widess-Walsh *et al.*, 2007), both with SEEG and subdural grids. In other words, in 3 out of 4 patients, the interictal pattern defines the ictal zone, probably dispensing with costly ictal recordings. Careful studies with SEEG (Chassoux *et al.*, 2000) have shown that when electrode contacts are within the lesion, the pacemaker pattern is virtually always seen and define the extent of the resection. Taking these figures in a broader perspective, it is interesting to hypothesize that the boundaries between interictal and ictal states are blurred in FCD II (Palmini 2010). This issue of the transition between the interictal and ictal state in FCD II is discussed in detail by Chassoux in this volume (chapter 11), through the analysis of dynamic electrographic patterns recorded with intracerebral SEEG electrodes. These point to a build up toward the ictal state.

Acute ECoG in the delineation of potentially relevant epileptogenic tissue extending beyond the EZ in FCD

A final point concerning the intrinsic epileptogenicity of the dysplastic cortex as identified by acute ECoG is the possibility that persistence of epileptogenic abnormalities recorded acutely during surgery may help understand the not uncommon observation that in some types of FCD seizures may recur despite apparently complete resection of the EZ (Najm *et al.*, 2013; Fauser *et al.*, 2015; Sacino *et al.*, 2017). If one takes at face value the essential definition of the EZ, seizure recurrence is paradoxical because, by definition, the EZ is the region that if completely resected should lead to seizure freedom. Consequently, if seizures recur despite complete resection of a correctly delineated EZ, this indicates the EZ is a more dynamic concept than previously thought.

That possibility was advanced by Rosenow and Ludders, coining the terminology 'potential EZ' (Rosenow and Luders, 2002) to account for cortical regions that have covert (latent) epileptogenicity at initial evaluation, but may lead to seizure relapse assuming the role of a previously unsuspected EZ in the long term. In this respect, epileptogenic patterns recorded during acute ECoG, particularly in a 'post-resection recording' following the initially planned resection of dysplastic tissue, may help anticipate cortical regions that could harbor a 'potential EZ'.

This issue had already been raised decades earlier by the historical MNI group of Penfield, Jasper and Rasmussen, who proposed that within an area of epileptogenic cortex, seizures could originate in more than one subregion and propagate through facilitated pathways (Jasper *et al.*, 1961; Penfield 1956; Penfield 1958; Rasmussen, 1983). These are scenarios in which the EZ (or the 'potential' EZ) is more extensive than the seizure onset zone, justifying the individualization of these concepts. It is possible that incomplete resection of a 'potential' EZ, ie, leaving intact epileptogenic cortical tissue with potential to generate seizures but higher ictal threshold at the time of the initial evaluation/resection may facilitate seizure recurrence after resection of the lowest threshold EZ (Hemb *et al.*, 2013). The relevant issue is how to identify the complete extent of epileptogenic cortical tissue with potential to generate seizures, either at the time of evaluation or some time following the initial resection. In a recent publication, we have discussed how acute ECoG could contribute to localize such relevant epileptogenic tissue with variable ictal thresholds (Palmini and Paglioli, 2019).

In summary, the exact localization of the EZ at a given point in time may not hold in the longer term. Therefore, epileptologists should struggle to localize not only the current EZ, but also the additional amount of tissue that could become clinically (ie, ictally) relevant over the years due to some epileptogenic mechanism – and ultimately lead to seizure recurrence (Rasmussen, 1983). We speculate that epileptogenic patterns of spikes recorded during intraoperative acute ECoG may prove valuable for the localization of such tissue, ie, the cortical regions encompassing both the current EZ and additional epileptogenic tissue with the potential to represent a 'latent EZ' (**Figure 6**). This possibility is supported by our observations that incomplete resection of cortical tissue displaying interictal highly epileptogenic patterns on ECoG lead to seizure recurrence, at times several years after protracted periods of post-operative seizure freedom (Palmini *et al* in preparation; Ferrier *et al.*, 2001; Fauser *et al*, 2015).

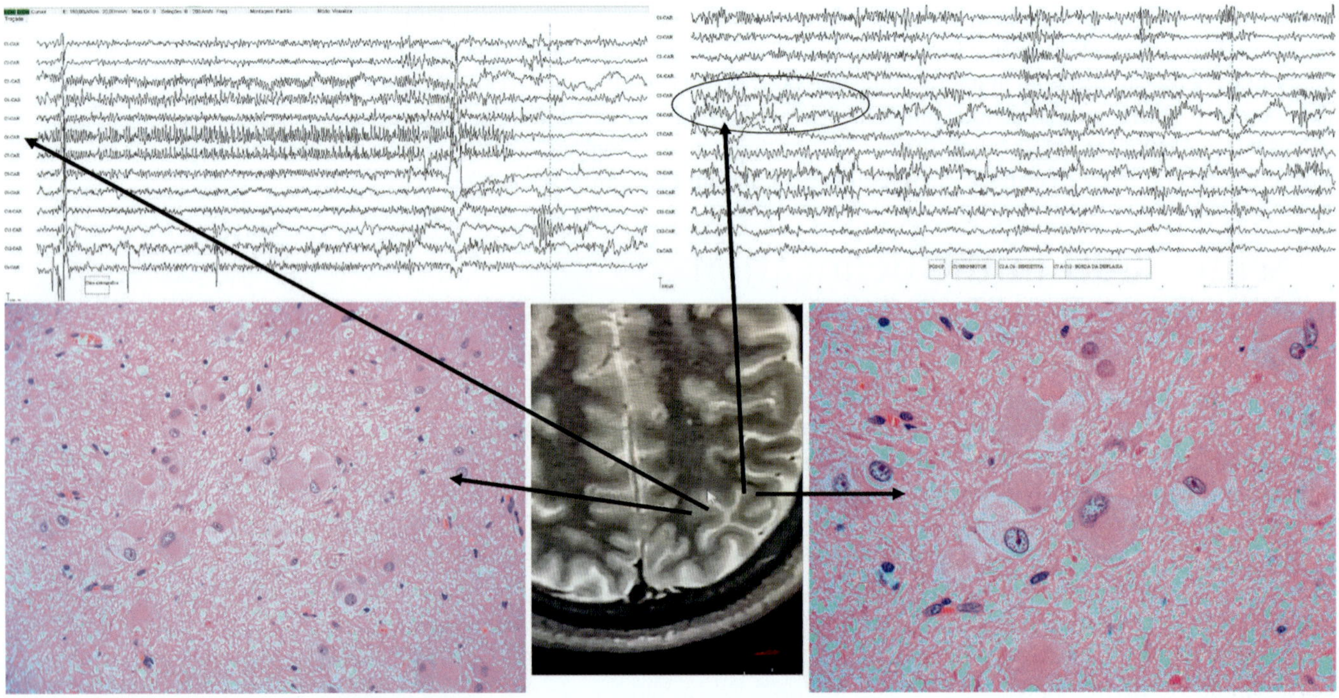

Figure 6

Epileptiform patterns in the acute ECoG.

The left upper panel shows an electrographic seizure recorded over a dysplastic lesion (lower center) before resection. Note cortical thickening and underlying FCD II histopathology (lower left). The right upper panel shows remaining active spiking in an adjacent cortical region after resection of the visible lesion. Note that histopathology was the same, despite normal appearance of the cortex.

Conclusion

Intraoperative acute ECoG may find itself in the middle of an apparent paradox: as technology advances and high-resolution imaging of epileptogenic lesions gets traction, a traditional, time-honored method of the early 1950's may re-emerge as a valid tool to refine the delineation and resection of the EZ. Highly epileptogenic patterns can be identifiable by ECoG and guide resection of the dysplastic lesion and of additional cortical tissue that may have lower ictal threshold at the time of the evaluation, but lead to recurrent seizures months or years after the initial resection of the EZ. Because the apparatus championed at the MNI with ballpoint electrodes attached to flexible, long-reaching arms has been replaced by subdural grids and strips in most, if not all, Centers, the method lost some of its appeal. Clearly, the possibility to freely explore superficial and (most importantly) deep portions of the exposed cortical surface at sequential stages during the resection is crucial, as also shown by Cardinale in this volume (chapter 19) – and somewhat lost with the use of grids and strips. Therefore, it may be high time to revive the traditional ECoG apparatus and put it to use more widely in the surgery of FCD.

References

Avoli M, Bernasconi A, Mattia D, Olivier A, Hwa GG. Epileptiform discharges in the human dysplastic neocortex: in vitro physiology and pharmacology. *Ann Neurol.* 1999; 46: 816-26.

Bartolomei F, Trébuchon A, Bonini F, *et al.* What is the concordance between the seizure onset zone and the irritative zone? A SEEG quantified study. *Clin Neurophysiol.* 2016; 127: 1157-62.

Cepeda C, André VM, Levine MS, *et al.* Epileptogenesis in pediatric cortical dysplasia: the dysmature cerebral developmental hypothesis. *Epilepsy Behav.* 2006; 9: 219-35.

Chassoux F, Devaux B, Landré E, *et al.* Stereoelectroencephalography in focal cortical dysplasia. A 3D approach to delineating the dysplastic cortex. *Brain* 2000; 123: 1733-55.

Fauser S, Essang C, Altenmüller DM, *et al.* Long-term seizure outcome in 211 patients with focal cortical dysplasia. *Epilepsia.* 2015; 56: 66-76.

Feindel W. Brain stimulation combined with electrocorticography in the surgery of epilepsy: Historical highlights. Electrocorticography: Current trends and future perspectives. *Electroencephalogr Clin Neurophysiol* 1998; 48: 1–8.

Ferrier CH, Alarcon G, Engelsman J, *et al.* Relevance of residual histologic and electrocorticographic abnormalities for surgical outcome in frontal lobe epilepsies. *Epilepsia* 2001; 42: 363-71.

Gambardella A, Palmini A, Andermann F, *et al.* Usefulness of focal rhythmic discharges on scalp EEG of patients with focal cortical dysplasia and intractable epilepsy. *Electroencephalogr Clin Neurophysiol.* 1996; 98: 243-9.

Guerreiro MM, Quesney LF, Salanova V, Snipes GJ. Continuous electrocorticogram epileptiform discharges due to brain gliosis. *J Clin Neurophysiol* 2003; 20: 239-42.

Hemb M, Paglioli E, Dubeau F, *et al.* "Mirror EPC": epilepsia partialis continua shifting sides after rolandic resection in dysplasia. *Neurology.* 2014 Oct 14; 83(16): 1439-43.

Jasper HH, Arfel-Capdeveille G, Rasmussen T. Evaluation of EEG and cortical electrographic studies for prognosis of seizures following surgical excision of epileptogenic lesions. *Epilepsia.* 1961; 2: 130-7.

Morioka T, Nishio S, Ishibashi H, *et al.* Intrinsic epileptogenicity of focal cortical dysplasia as revealed by magnetoencephalography and electrocorticography. *Epilepsy Res* 1999; 33: 177-187.

Najm I, Jehi L, Palmini A, Paglioli E. Temporal patterns and mechanisms of epilepsy surgery failure. *Epilepsia*, 2013; 54: 772–82.

Palmini A, Andermann F, Olivier A, Tampieri D, Robitaille Y. Focal neuronal migration disorders and intractable partial epilepsy: results of surgical treatment. *Ann Neurol.* 1991; 30: 750-7.

Palmini A, Gambardella A, Andermann F, *et al.* Intrinsic epileptogenicity of human dysplastic cortex as suggested by corticography and surgical results. *Ann Neurol.* 1995; 37: 476-87.

Palmini A. Electrophysiology of the focal cortical dysplasias. *Epilepsia.* 2010; 51 Suppl 1: 23-6.

Palmini A, Paglioli E. The irritative zone and seizure onset zone in acute ECoG: the quest for the relevant epileptogenic tissue. In: Lhatoo SD, Kahane P, Luders H (eds*). Invasive Studies of the Human Epileptic Brain: Principles and Practice.* New York: Oxford University Press, 2019.

Penfield W. Epileptogenic lesions. *Acta Neurol Psychiatr Belg.*1956; 56: 75-88.

Penfield W. Pitfalls and successes in the surgical treatment of focal epilepsies. *Br Med J.* 1958 45: 669-72.

Rasmussen T. Characteristics of a pure culture of frontal lobe epilepsy. *Epilepsia.* 1983; 24: 482-93.

Rosenow F, Lüders H. Presurgical evaluation of epilepsy. *Brain* 2002; 124: 1683-700.

Sacino MF, Ho CY, Whitehead MT, *et al.* Repeat surgery for focal cortical dysplasias in children: indications and outcomes. *J Neurosurg Pediatr.* 2017; 19: 174-81.

Tassi L, Colombo N, Garbelli R, *et al.* Focal cortical dysplasia: neuropathological subtypes, EEG, neuroimaging and surgical outcome. *Brain.* 2002; 125: 1719-32.

Teixeira, WA, Holthausen, H, Pannek, H, *et al.* Abstractband, 4. Symposium "Epilepsiechirurgie in Deutschland" Bielefeld,1997.

Widdess-Walsh P, Jeha L, Nair D, *et al.* Subdural electrode analysis in focal cortical dysplasia: predictors of surgical outcome. *Neurology.* 2007; 69: 660-7.

CHAPTER 11. Intrinsic epileptogenicity of FCD: insights from SEEG to scalp EEG

Francine Chassoux

Key points

- Intrinsic epileptogenicity of FCD has been demonstrated by intracranial recordings, showing intralesional interictal continuous epileptiform activity and ictal onset with recognizable discharge patterns.
- A specific pattern characterized by a rhythmic or pseudo-rhythmic spike activity is highly suggestive of FCD II, identified on SEEG, acute electrocorticography and scalp EEG.
- This FCD EEG pattern is not found in other FCD subtypes and therefore refers to FCD II only.
- Sleep recordings may increase the sensitivity of EEG for the detection of this peculiar activity.
- Knowledge of intralesional interictal and ictal activities demonstrated by SEEG and corresponding features on scalp EEG may help to identify and to localize FCD II in MRI-negative cases.

Introduction

Intrinsic epileptogenicity of FCD has been first demonstrated by Palmini and colleagues in 1995, who found that a peculiar activity recorded by ECoG, characterized by continuous epileptiform discharges, was specific of brain areas harboring Taylor-type FCD, later classified as FCD II (Palmini *et al.*, 1995). A complementary study has shown that rhythmic epileptiform discharges (REDs) corresponding to CEDs may be recorded on scalp EEG in 44% of the patients with FCD, but none in patients having nondysplastic structural lesions (Gambardella *et al.*, 1996). The authors concluded that this EEG pattern was useful for the diagnosis of FCD. Similar findings were found in patients investigated by SEEG for intractable epilepsy due to FCD II, demonstrating a clear concordance between the continuous rhythmic spiking recorded from the dysplastic tissue and the related pattern recorded on scalp EEG (Chassoux *et al.*, 2000). Moreover, sleep recordings have been shown to increase the sensitivity of the EEG to identify the electrographic FCD pattern (Tassi *et al.*, 2012; Gibbs *et al.*, 2016; Eltze *et al.*, 2020).

In this chapter, we will describe the correspondence between intracranial and scalp EEG and the role of sleep recordings for FCD localization. Overall, we will describe an attempt at refining the interpretation of the scalp EEG in light of neurophysiological data provided by SEEG. The final goal is to recognize the typical FCD II signature on scalp EEG without invasive monitoring, whenever possible.

Interictal FCD patterns: best criteria for delineating the dysplastic cortex

The initial description of FCD patterns recorded by ECoG consisted in ictal or continuous epileptogenic discharges (I/CEDs) with one of the following three patterns:

- repetitive electrographic seizures,
- repetitive bursting discharges,
- or continuous or quasi-continuous rhythmic spiking.

These activities tended to colocalize with MRI lesions and the resection of areas displaying them correlated with favorable outcome (Palmini *et al.*, 1995). These striking patterns were also identified by SEEG recordings, consisting in a continuous or sub-continuous spiking within the dysplastic cortex, interrupted by seizures and reappearing immediately at the end of the ictal discharge (Chassoux *et al.*, 2000). Of relevance, our original SEEG publication pointed out that this activity was observed in all patients in whom an electrode was implanted within the FCD, whereas it was less continuous, attenuated or not identified when the electrodes were in the vicinity of the lesion. This neurophysiological scenario has been confirmed ever since. The typical activity consisted of rhythmic or pseudo-rhythmic spikes discharges (RSD), ranging from 0.5 to 10 Hz – more often from 1 to 3 Hz – or pseudo-periodic activity made of burst of spikes interrupted by the suppression of background activity. RSD were restricted to the FCD during wakefulness but recorded over areas larger than the FCD during NREM sleep and after ictal discharges. Early reappearance of RSD after post-ictal depression of activity was reliable for localizing the dysplastic areas. In addition, this rhythmic activity was not suppressed by IV Diazepam, whereas this drug led to fast rhythms over non-dysplastic areas. This interictal pattern is now considered a marker of the dysplastic cortex, with a clear limit between dysplastic and non-dysplastic areas. Furthermore, it is not found in other FCD subtypes (Tassi *et al.*, 2002), making it an electrical signature for FCD II. Therefore, we will refer to FCD II when using the term "FCD pattern" in the following part of the chapter. Importantly, this peculiar pattern has been simultaneously recorded on scalp EEG during SEEG, and found synchronous with the intracranial spiking, despite some distortion or attenuation due to the intervening skull (**Figure 1**). It was retrospectively found on scalp EEG in 50% of the cases during wakefulness in our historical series (Chassoux *et al.*, 2000), and in up to 65% during sleep in other studies (Eltze *et al.*, 2020).

More recently, other EEG biomarkers have been described in FCD I or II, or even in some other types of MCD. Although 12 patterns came to be described, they clearly overlap and revolve around continuity, rhythmicity and bursting features (Epitashvili *et al.*, 2018):

- stereotyped, rhythmic sequences of repetitive sharp waves or spikes lasting >1 second (REDs); RED type 1: trains of repetitive, rhythmic 4–10 Hz spikes/sharp waves lasting 1–4 seconds,
- RED type 2: slower, rhythmic 2–7 Hz sharp waves,
- isolated intermittent sharp waves,
- positive quasi-continuous epileptiform discharges,
- focal, fast, continuous spikes,
- focal fast REDs (FREDs),

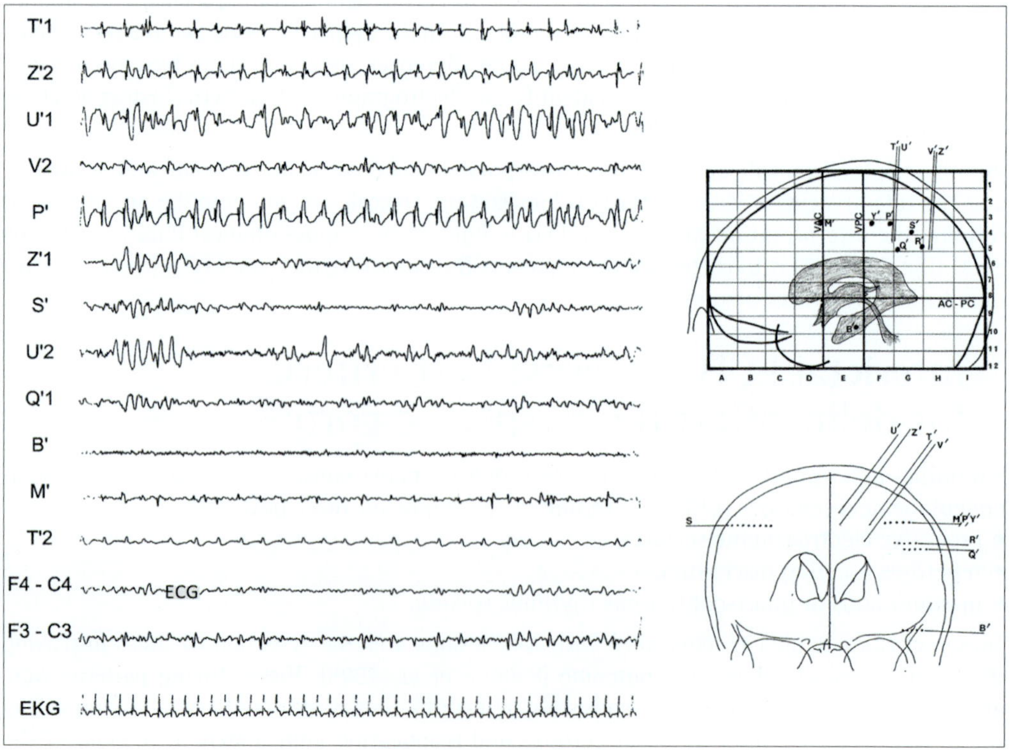

Figure 1
SEEG recording, interictal FCD II pattern
Typical FCD II pattern characterized by rhythmic spiking within a FCD II involving the left parietal convexity and delineated by four oblique electrodes (T'1, Z'2, U'1, V'2) and one orthogonal electrode (P'). Note that a similar activity was identified on scalp EEG (F3-C3), which was recorded simultaneously to intracranial EEG.

- frequent rhythmic bursting epileptiform activity (FRBEA),
- repetitive discharges lasting ≥5 seconds,
- CED occupying >80% of the recording,
- polyspikes,
- continuous irregular slowing,
- brushes.

Most distinguishing features in that publication relate to the duration of sequences of spikes or spiking frequency, without reference to the recording conditions (wakefulness or sleep, seizure frequency and time from the last seizure in particular). Considering the skull-related attenuation of intralesional spiking when recorded on scalp EEG – as demonstrated by simultaneous SEEG/scalp recordings – we postulate that the major characteristic which should be considered is the rhythmicity of the epileptiform activity. Other features (including the morphology of the spikes and waves) are rather due to the location and extent of FCD, and the orientation of the spike generator according to the placement of scalp electrodes. Deeply located FCD (i.e. at the bottom of the sulcus) may be totally silent on scalp EEG, whereas others may be easily detected despite a small size, especially when located near the midline (**Figure 2**). However, some locations such as the insula or cingulate gyrus may be very difficult for scalp EEG identification, as discussed latter.

• Transition between interictal and ictal activity: a second step for FCD identification

The relationship between interictal and ictal activity has proved to be complex in most models of epileptogenic networks. However, FCD II represents the prototype of epileptogenic lesion in which the interictal activity may have the same value than ictal discharges for determining the EZ. On SEEG, seizure onset is usually characterized by a pattern of low voltage fast activity (LVFA) ranging from beta/low gamma (15-30 Hz) to higher frequencies (gamma range, 30-100 Hz) (Isnard *et al.*, 2018; Bartolomei *et al.*, 2018). In FCD lesions, when depth electrodes are adequately placed, the faster activity at seizure onset is found within the dysplastic tissue. However, fast activity may also be recorded in surrounding areas, especially in extratemporal locations, leading to a perception that the EZ is larger than the FCD II lesions in most instances. Thus, to accurately delineate the extent of the FCD II, it may be useful to consider the transition between interictal and ictal states, consisting of the sudden interruption of the rhythmic spiking preceding LVFA (**Figure 3**). Another frequent pre-ictal pattern consists in a brief increase of spike frequency or bursts of polyspikes evolving into high-voltage fast-spike discharge before LVFA (**Figure 4**). In the post-ictal phase, a focal depression of activity combined with an early reappearance of the rhythmic spikes is observed in FCD II areas generating seizures (Chassoux *et al.*, 2000). All these criteria allow to accurately delineate the dysplastic tissue, helping to restrict the areas that need to be resected, a crucial issue when FCD II involves functional areas.

Sleep patterns

The last condition to keep in mind is the role of sleep on FCD EEG patterns. There is indeed a high rate of sleep related epilepsy (SRE), defined as at least 70% of seizures occurring during sleep, in epilepsy due to FCD II. This was especially true in small FCD II and in MRI-negative cases, where SRE was seen in 50- 60% of cases in our series (Chassoux *et al.*, 2012; Eltze *et al.*, 2020). Moreover, different stages of sleep may influence the interictal activity (Nobili *et al.*, 2009; Tassi *et al.*, 2012; Gibbs *et al.*, 2016).

Importantly, FCD EEG patterns may be recorded during sleep over large areas, encompassing both the dysplastic lesion and surrounding regions. These spiking patterns can vary in amplitude, frequency and rhythmicity, and may evolve into periodic activity during NREM sleep, whereas spikes are reduced during the REM stage (Tassi *et al.*, 2012, Gibbs *et al.*, 2016). These findings may explain why FCD patterns may be more easily detected on scalp EEG during sleep, whatever the FCD location, including in the temporal lobe for which the typical pattern is rarely observed during wakefulness. Accordingly, the frequency of identifiable FCD patterns increases from 40% during wakefulness to 65% during sleep (Eltze *et al.*, 2020).

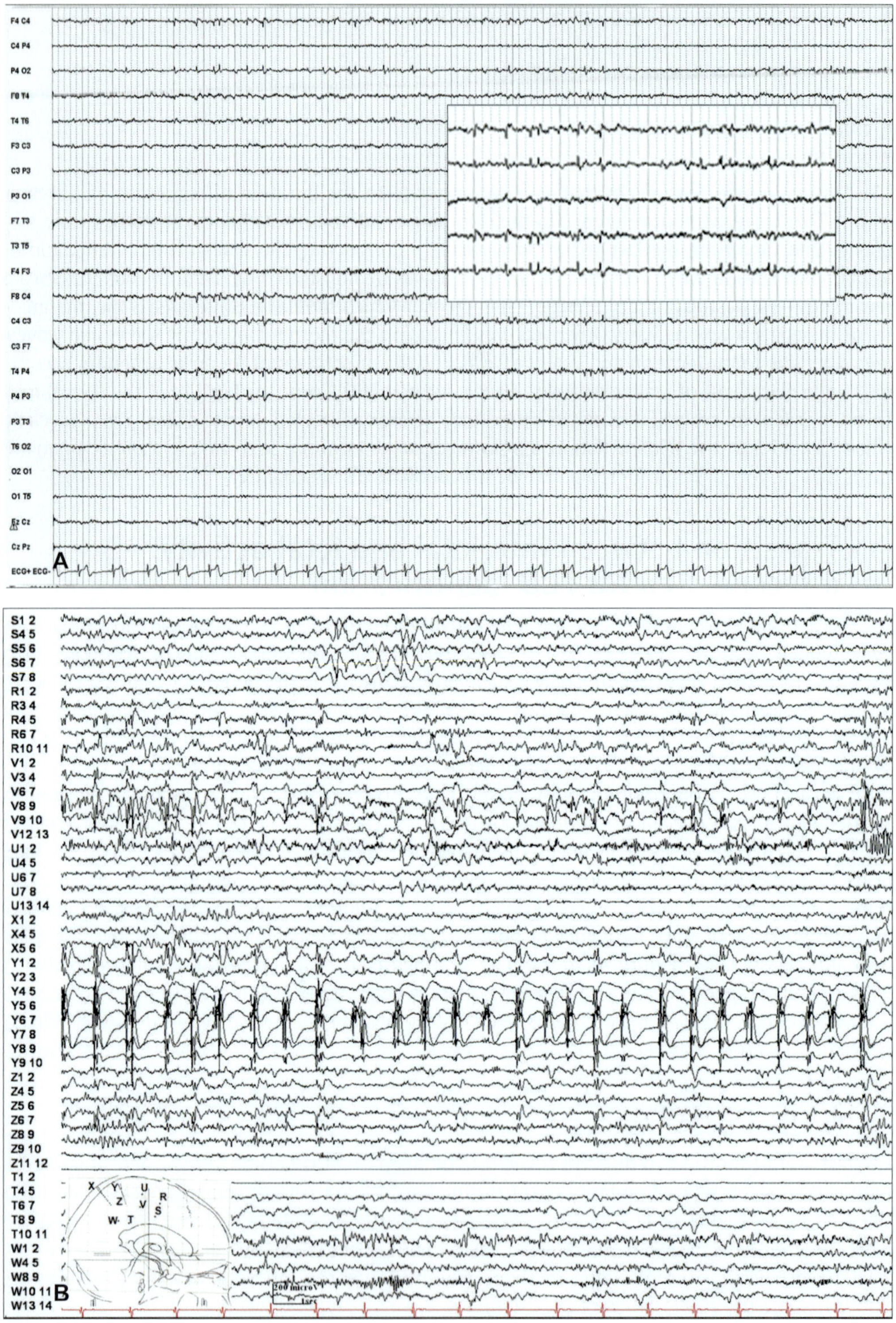

Figure 2

Comparison between EEG and SEEG

A. Scalp EEG, typical FCD pattern, sub-continuous well localized low amplitude spikes in a right parietal MRI-negative case. Magnification of EEG showing the rhythmic spikes (P4). B. SEEG showing the corresponding continuous rhythmic spikes and polyspikes without background activity. This activity was limited to 2 contacts of a single electrode (Y 5-6 and 6-7), allowing the localization of a small mesial FCD II, near the parietal convexity.

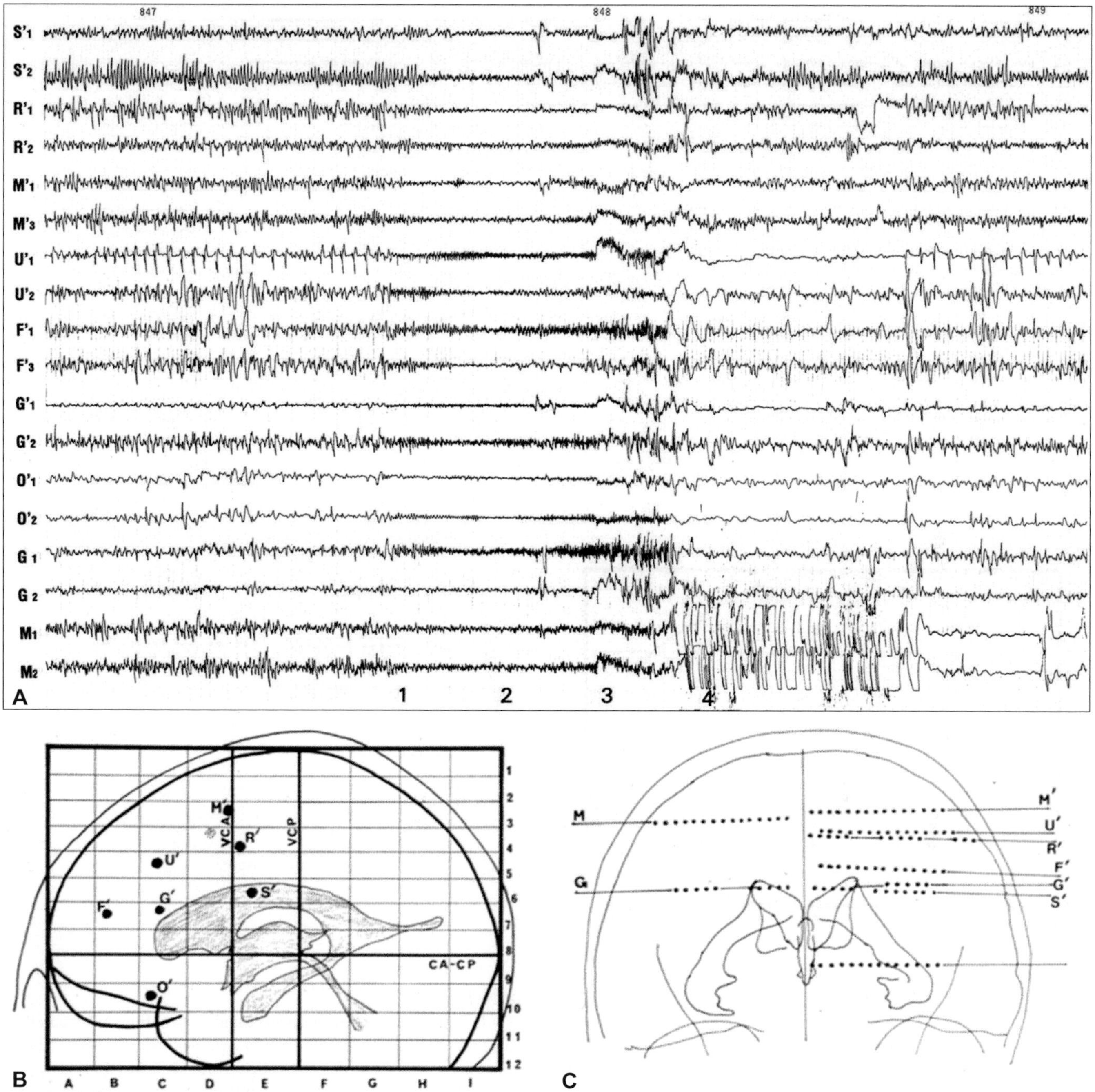

Figure 3

Transition between interictal and ictal state

Interictal and ictal SEEG pattern in a MRI-negative FCD II located in the left mesial frontal lobe involving the anterior cingulate gyrus (ACG). Note the continuous spiking interrupted by the low voltage fast activity (LVFA) and the early recurrence of spikes on the same derivation (U'_1) after a brief depression of activity. This transitional pattern between the interictal and ictal state, and the post-ictal pattern allow together to restrict the FCD II to the part of ACG around the mesial contact of the electrode U'_1, whereas the LVFA was also recorded in a large territory on the left side, including the mesial aspect of the prefrontal cortex (F'_1), the lateral convexity (middle frontal gyrus: U'2), inferior frontal gyrus: G'2), the orbitofrontal cortex (O'_2) and the contralateral ACG (G_1). The large involvement by LVFA corresponds to early spread to strongly connected areas from the FCD generator, corresponding to non-dysplastic areas. The discrepancy between FCD pattern and the areas involved by LVFA explains the controversial interpretation for determining the epileptogenic zone and its relationship with the dysplastic cortex. Comparison with histology proved than the dysplastic cortex was limited to the areas displaying the FCD pattern.

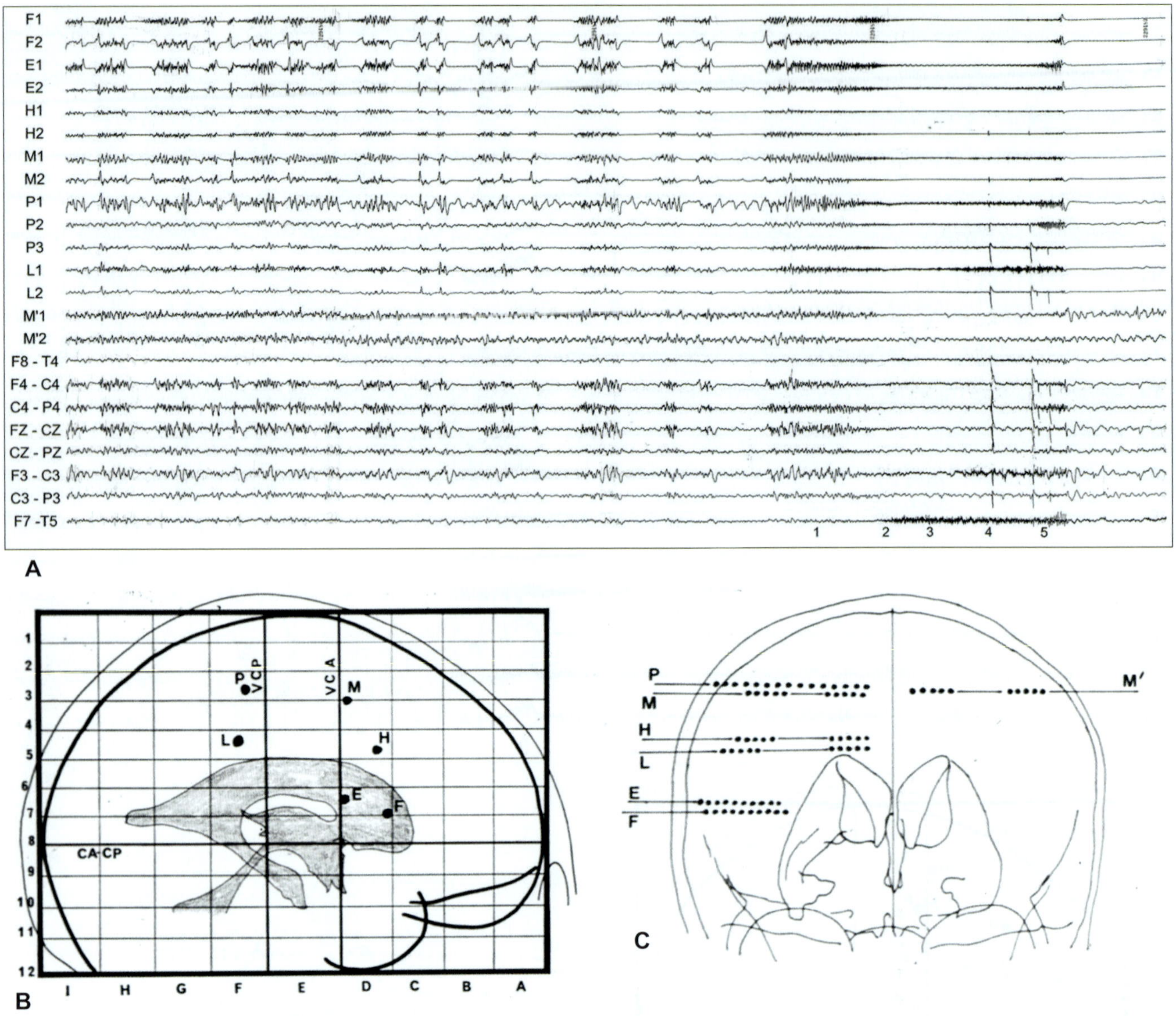

Figure 4

SEEG and scalp EEG correspondence of interictal and ictal FCD II pattern

Simultaneous SEEG and scalp EEG recordings in a large right fronto-central FCD II. Repetitive burst of polyspikes and fast rhythms interrupted by the suppression of background activity during the interictal state, high amplitude fast discharge preceding the low voltage fast activity at seizure onset, post-ictal suppression of activity on the same territory. FCD pattern is predominant in the precentral area (electrodes F, E, M, H) with a spread of ictal discharge to the post central region (P and L). Note the similarity with scalp EEG including the interictal, preictal, ictal and post-ictal phases (F4-C4, C4-P4 and FZ-CZ).

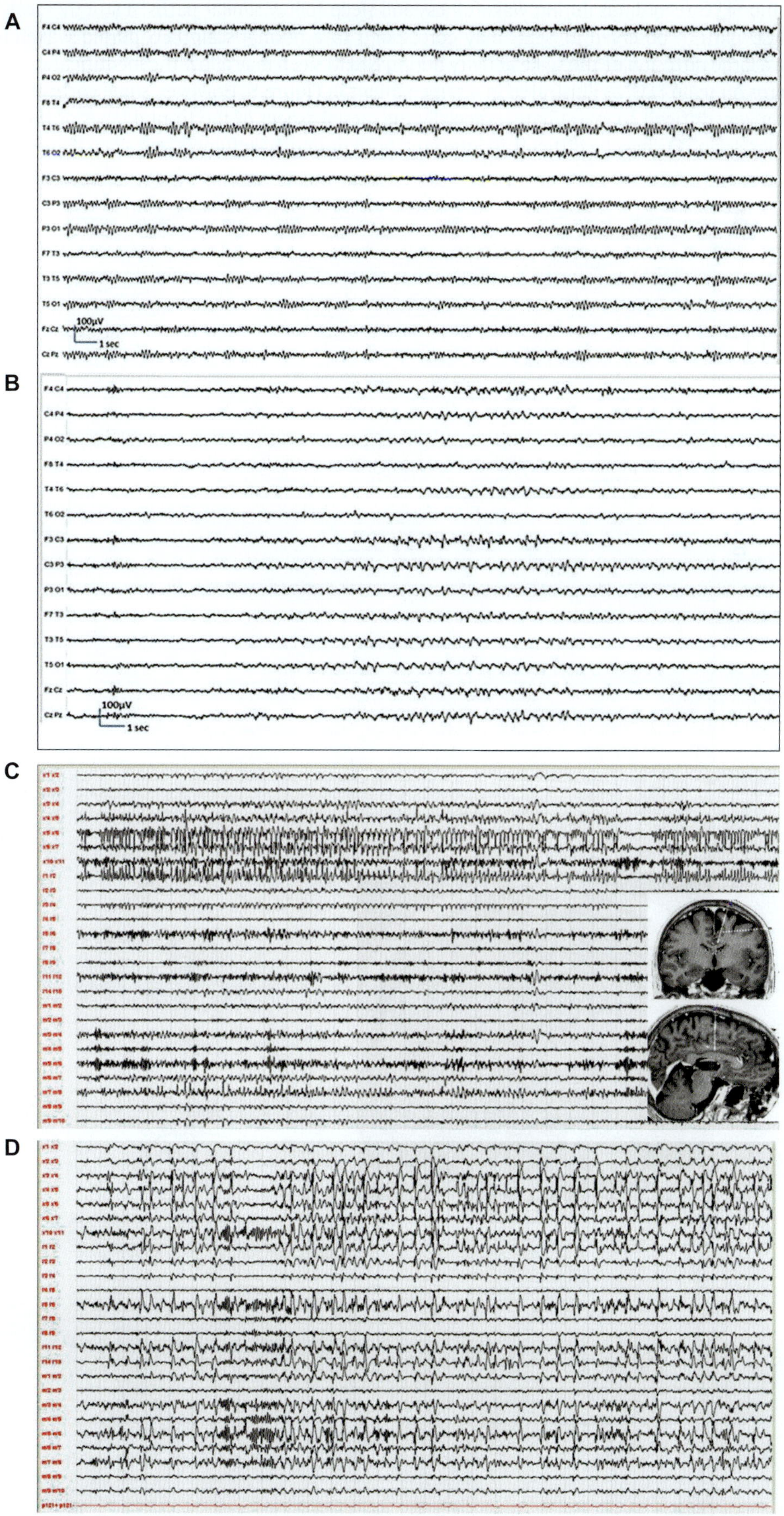

Figure 5

Sleep recordings

Scalp EEG and SEEG recordings during wakefulness and sleep. Left frontal mesial FCD II, located in the supplementary motor area (MRI-negative). A. Normal scalp EEG during wakefulness; B. During NREM stage sleep, repetitive sequences of rhythmic spikes and slow waves on the left frontocentral region; C. SEEG, well localized rhythmic spiking, recorded by two closed electrodes L' (L'1-2) (X'5-6 - X'6-7); D. Diffusion of the spiking activity to surrounding areas during sleep. Note the change of spike frequency and the occurrence on fast rhythms (spindles) visible on non-dysplastic areas only.

EEG and SEEG recordings during wakefulness and sleep follow similar paths: a strictly focal, typical FCD pattern observed in SEEG may correspond to a normal scalp EEG during wakefulness, while a large diffusion of the spike activity during NREM sleep may allow the identification of FCD patterns on scalp EEG, as illustrated in a same patient in **Figure 5**. However, some cortical regions remain very difficult to investigate, especially the mesial aspect of the frontal lobes or the insula, in which scalp EEG may be difficult to interpret, both during wakefulness and sleep (**Figures 6-7**).

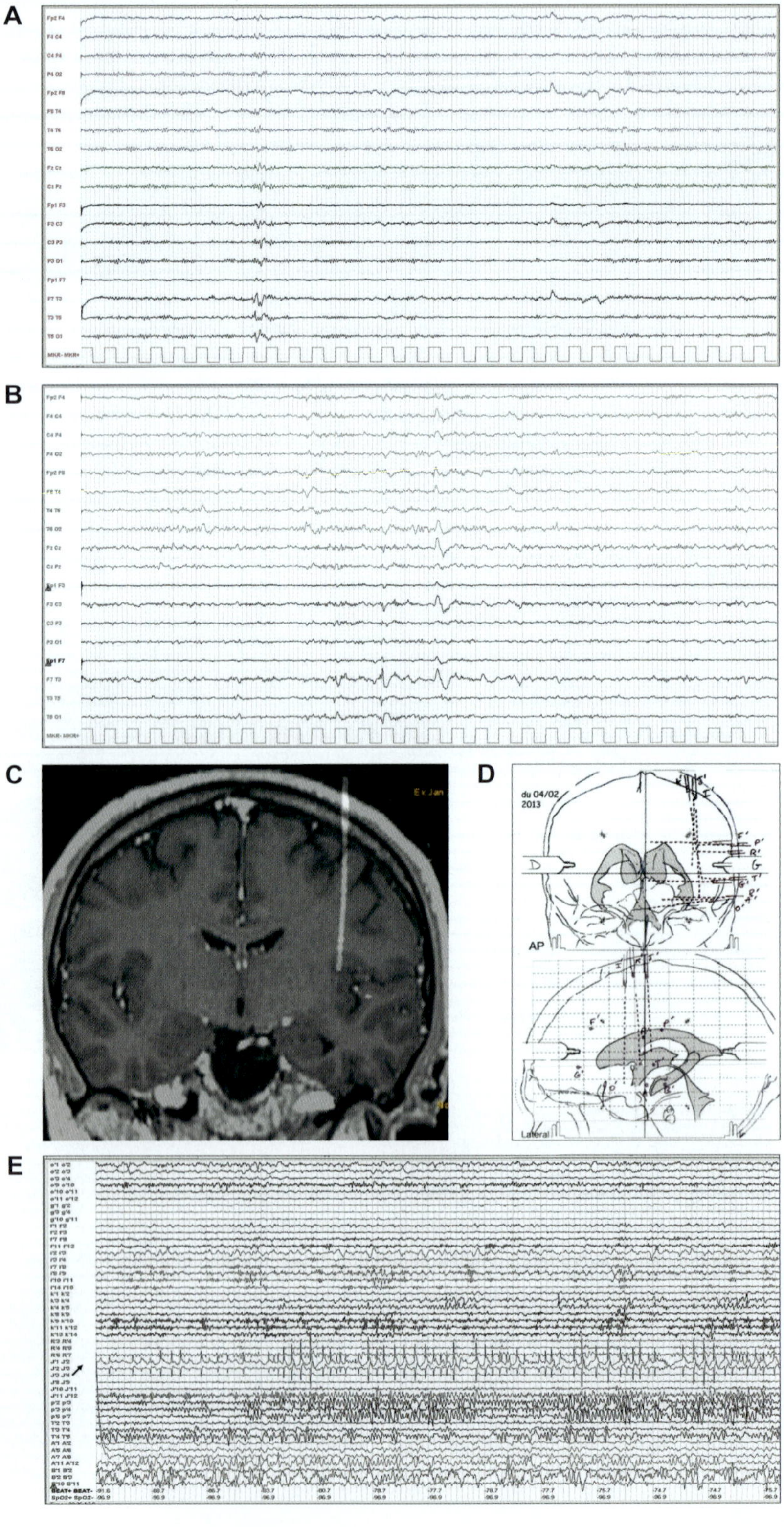

Figure 6

Difficult to localize pattern: Insular FCD II

A. Scalp EEG showing few or non-specific interictal abnormalities projecting on the left temporal region, either during wakefulness (rare spikes) or sleep (repetitive spikes and slow waves associated with K complexes). B. In contrast, SEEG recordings demonstrate a continuous rhythmic spiking well localized on the deep contacts of a single electrode (J'_{1-2}, J'_{2-3}) located in the superior and middle part of the left insula. This case illustrates the discrepancy between scalp EEG and SEEG in deep FCD II location like the insula.

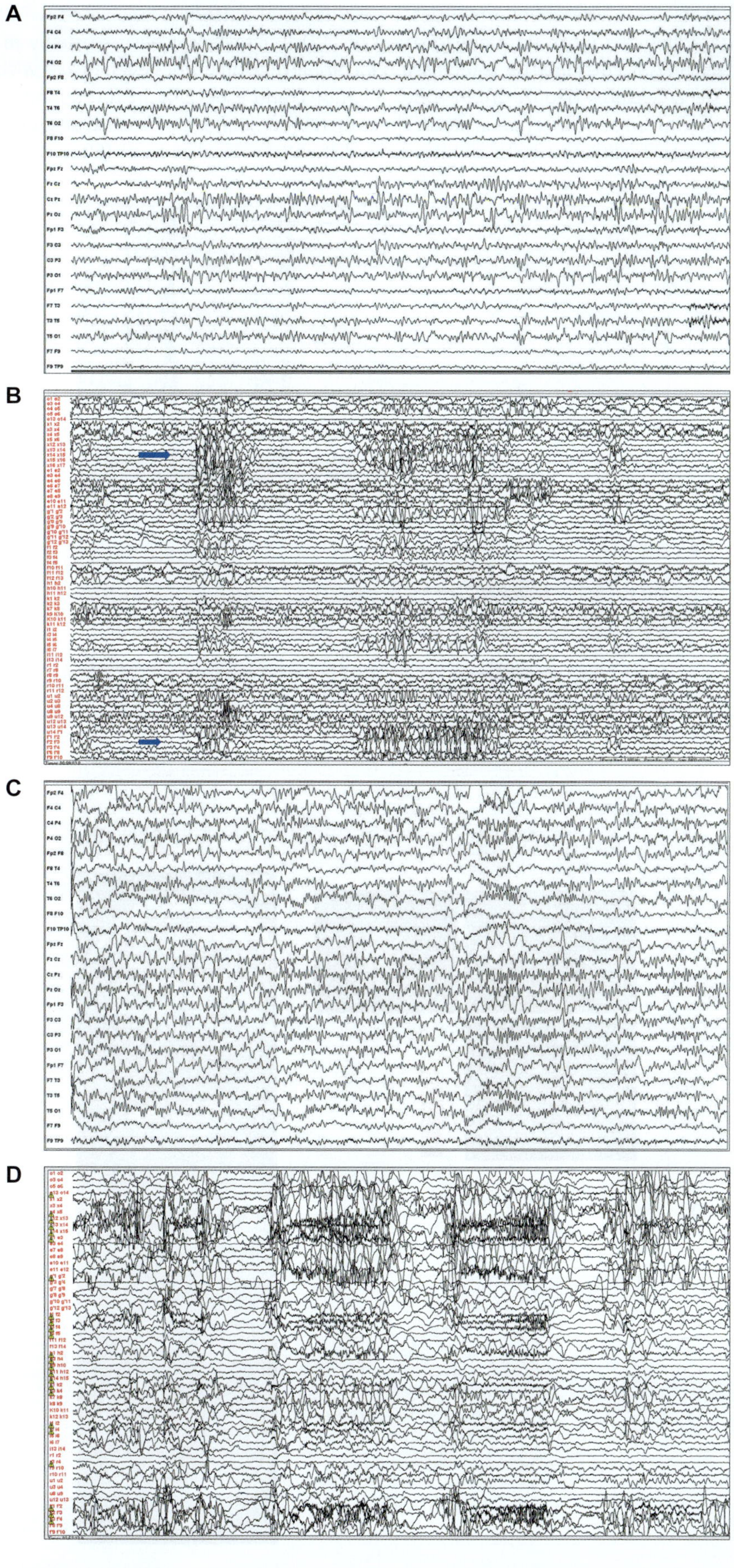

Figure 7

Difficult to localize FCD II: mesial frontal lobe

A. Scalp EEG in a small MRI-negative FCD II located in the right anterior cingulate gyrus (ACG) showing no specific abnormalities (few sharp waves on the right frontal lobe) during wakefulness; physiological bilateral posterior slow waves in a 14-year-old patient. B. SEEG showing repetitive bursts of polyspikes localized within the right ACG (large arrow) with a diffusion to the contralateral side (thin arrow). C. During sleep EEG, repetitive sequences of slow spikes and rapid rhythms on the right frontal lobe. D. SEEG recordings showing bursts of polyspikes mixed with fast rhythm discharges on the right frontal mesial region, involving the contralateral side. In this location, FCD pattern remains difficult to identify on scalp EEG despite major abnormalities found by SEEG.

In addition to the interictal abnormalities, a peculiar ictal pattern is associated with SRE. In the frontal lobes, the more frequent location of FCD II, ictal onset occurs usually in NREM stage 2, the LVFA occurring after spindles and K complexes, sometimes even mixed with physiological sleep features (**Figure 8**). In other locations, and especially in the temporal lobes, seizures more often start after an arousal. These distinct modalities of seizure onset in frontal and extrafrontal locations may be of interest in difficult-to-localize cases (Eltze *et al.*, 2020).

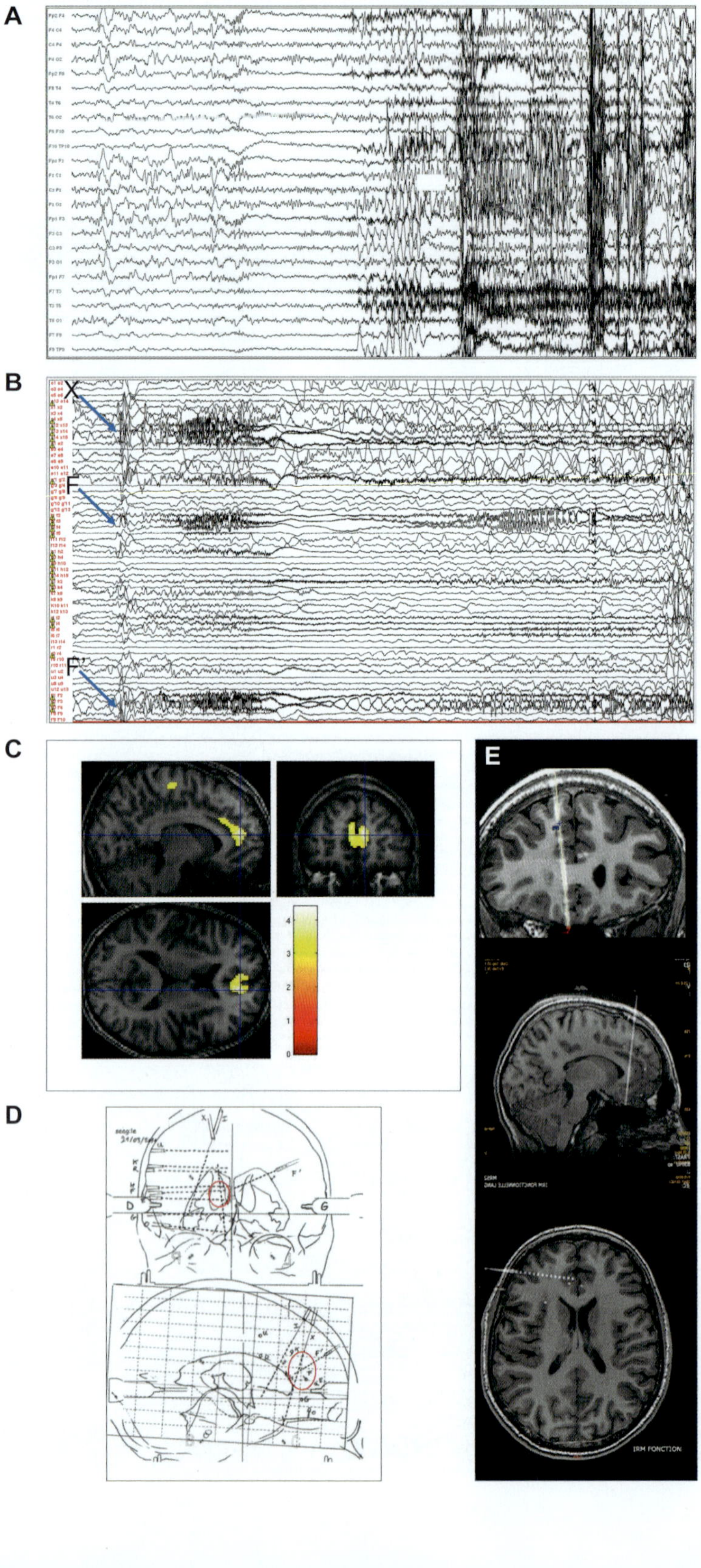

Figure 8

Ictal pattern in mesial frontal lobe

Same patient than in figure 7. A. Right frontal seizure onset after repetitive sikes and high amplitude fast discharge preceding the low voltage fast activity (LVFA) that appears bilateral on scalp EEG but predominating on the right side (FP2-F4 and FP2-F8). B. SEEG recordings demonstrated the ictal onset (electrodes X and F) with the same preictal and ictal patterns and an immediate propagation to the contralateral side (F'). This location explains the difficult to lateralize seizure onset in some FCD II cases. C. FDG-PET SPM maps showing a bilateral ACG involvement. D. Scheme of SEEG planning, electrodes X and F are located within the ACG and FCD II (cercle). E. Depth electrodes fusion with MRI showing the precise location of oblique (X) and orthogonal (F) electrodes.

Correspondence between SEEG and scalp EEG: from inside to outside and vice-versa

A thoughtful interpretation of typical FCD patterns assessed by SEEG needs combined consideration of electrographic features observed during interictal, ictal and post-ictal phases. Despite skull-related attenuation, the same sequences may be identified on scalp EEG and, according to the location of the generator, specific combinations of pathological and physiological features may be seen. For example, intralesional continuous spiking in deeply located FCD II may appear as rhythmic slow waves on scalp EEG. Other times, a similar SEEG pattern may be missed in scalp recordings or represented only by isolated spikes, corresponding to propagated activity. Ictal patterns may be difficult to recognize when generated in the mesial aspect of the brain or in the insula, causing false localization and lateralization on scalp EEG (**Figure 8**). Extrapolating from intracranial recordings to scalp EEG may be useful to understand these apparently discordant data.

In contrast, in large FCD II involving the lateral convexity, intracranial and scalp recordings may be impressively similar, in interictal, ictal and post-ictal phases (**Figure 4**). Of note, the post-ictal depression of activity observed in SEEG corresponds to a focal slowing (delta range, 1-3 Hz) on scalp EEG. Analyzing the post-ictal activity may be helpful because post-ictal depression of activity and focal slowing are usually more restricted. This is especially important when ictal onset is difficult to determine, especially in extratemporal regions, where the LVFA may be found in over large territories that include but extend beyond the FCD, suggesting connections with nondysplastic areas. Combined with early reappearance of rhythmic spikes, these post-ictal features may be used as FCD II markers in difficult cases.

Conversely, scalp EEG findings may help determine the placement of depth electrodes and the planning of SEEG, especially in MRI-negative cases. Importantly, if typical FCD patterns are found on scalp EEG but not on intracranial recordings, SEEG sampling should be reconsidered.

Interpretation of scalp EEG in light of SEEG data: implication for localizing the FCD

We know from SEEG data that RSD are a marker of the dysplastic tissue. Considering the patterns described with SEEG, the corresponding patterns on the surface may refine the interpretation of scalp EEG when searching for a FCD lesion. The following are key points to be kept in mind:

- Recording rhythmic spike activity on scalp EEG indicates FCD until proven otherwise. Repeated imaging including high field MRI and FDG-PET should be considered in MRI-negative cases.
- FCD patterns are recorded on scalp EEG in 30-50% of patients during wakefulness. Sleep recordings increase the sensitivity to 65% and should be obtained when FCD is suspected. NREM sleep is the best stage to look for a FCD pattern, a condition that can be obtained with short recordings, including naps.
- Seizure recordings may help to identify a FCD pattern in previously normal scalp EEGs, particularly the appearance of rhythmic spiking post-ictally.
- Transitional activity between interictal and ictal state (high-voltage fast spike discharge) can be identified on scalp EEG and helps to localize the ictal onset.
- Post-ictal pattern combining focal slowing and rhythmic spikes is reliable for FCD localization.
- FCD patterns found on scalp EEG usually correspond to a dorsolateral location. On the parasagittal convexity, it is predominantly recorded on the midline electrodes (FZ, CZ, PZ).
- Atypical patterns despite strong suspicion of FCD suggests a deep lesion location. Rhythmic slow waves on scalp EEG may correspond to intracranial rhythmic spikes.
- FCD patterns can be missed or misleading in mesial frontal and insular cortex. Normal or non-specific EEG do not rule out an underlying FCD.
- In SRE, ictal onset patterns may differ according to FCD location.
- In frontal lobe FCD lesions, seizure onset mainly occurs in NREM sleep (stage 2). In extra-frontal FCD (especially in temporal lobe), seizure onset occurs after an arousal. These different modalities may be helpful in difficult-to-localize FCD cases.

SEEG has obviously a lot to teach in terms of consistent scalp EEG interpretation of patients with refractory seizures. Accumulated knowledge of the correspondence between intracranial and scalp patterns should be integrated in the scalp EEG interpretation and often helps to identify and localize a FCD lesion. When concordant with clinical and imaging data, recognition of typical patterns may obviate the need of intracranial recordings. In other cases, these patterns are helpful for the SEEG planning.

References

Bartolomei F, Nica A, Valenti-Hirsch MP, Adam C, Denuelle M. Interpretation of SEEG recordings. *Neurophysiol Clin.* 2018; 48: 53-7.

Chassoux F, Devaux B, Landré E, *et al.* Stereoelectroencephalography in Focal Cortical Dysplasia: a 3D approach to delineating the dysplastic cortex. *Brain* 2000; 123: 1733-51.

Chassoux F, Landré E, Mellerio C, *et al.* Type II Focal Cortical Dysplasia: electro-clinical phenotype and surgical outcome related to imaging. *Epilepsia.* 2012; 53: 349-58.

Gambardella A, Palmini A, Andermann F, *et al.* Usefulness of focal rhythmic discharges on scalp EEG of patients with Focal Cortical Dysplasia and intractable epilepsy. *Electroencephalogr Clin Neurophysiol.* 1996; 98: 243-9.

Gibbs SA, Proserpio P, Terzaghi M, *et al.* Sleep-related epileptic behaviors and non-REM-related parasomnias: Insights from stereo-EEG. *Sleep Med Rev.* 2016; 25: 4-20.

Eltze CM, Landre E, Soufflet C, Chassoux F. Sleep related epilepsy in Focal Cortical Dysplasia type 2: Insights from sleep recordings in presurgical evaluation. *Clin Neurophysiol.* 2020; 131: 609-15.

Epitashvili N, San Antonio-Arce V, Brandt A, Schulze-Bonhage A. Scalp electroencephalographic biomarkers in epilepsy patients with Focal Cortical Dysplasia. *Ann Neurol.* 2018; 84: 564-75.

Isnard J, Taussig D, Bartolomei F, *et al.* French guidelines on stereoelectroencephalography (SEEG). *Neurophysiol Clin.* 2018; 48: 5-13.

Nobili L, Cardinale F, Magliola U, *et al.* Taylor's Focal Cortical Dysplasia increases the risk of sleep-related epilepsy. *Epilepsia.* 2009; 50: 2599-604.

Palmini A, Gambardella A, Andermann F, *et al.* Intrinsic epileptogenicity of human dysplastic cortex as suggested by corticography and surgical results. *Ann Neurol.* 1995; 37: 476-87.

Tassi L, Colombo N, Garbelli R, *et al.* Focal Cortical Dysplasia: neuropathological subtypes, EEG, neuroimaging and surgical outcome. *Brain.* 2002; 125: 1719-32.

Tassi L, Garbelli R, Colombo N, *et al.* Electroclinical, MRI and surgical outcomes in 100 epileptic patients with type II FCD. *Epileptic Disord.* 2012; 14: 257-66.

CHAPTER

12. The epileptogenic zone in FCD: SEEG patterns in FCD subtypes

Fabrice Bartolomei

Key points

- The EZ (defined here as the brain region(s) generating the seizures) has historically been studied in FCD using invasive EEG recordings. They have revealed important features in these pathologies:
  - they are lesions intrinsically capable of generating epileptic discharges
  - several patterns of seizure onset can be observed with a majority of patterns including a rapid discharge
  - there are differences in the electrical behavior of the two main forms of FCD (I and II)
  - the spatial extension of the epileptic discharge can in a significant number of cases affect not only the lesion site but also remotely connected regions.
- These data are correlated with the surgical prognosis (better if focal onset and with a pattern including a rapid discharge)

Introduction

Epilepsy surgery is an effective treatment for achieving seizure freedom in patients with FCD. Approximately 65% of patients are Engel class I after FCD II surgery and 50% after FCD I surgery (Guerrini *et al.*, 2015; Lamberink *et al.*, 2020). In the presurgical evaluation of FCD, SEEG may be necessary to precisely define the EZ (Kahane *et al.*, 2006), guiding the delineation of the area to be resected (Isnard *et al.*, 2018). Data from intracranial EEG, including SEEG and ECoG, have confirmed that FCD are intrinsically epileptogenic (Chassoux, 2000; Palmini *et al.*, 1995; Tassi, 2002). However, in a proportion of cases, it is established that the EZ extends beyond the structural lesion seen on MRI (Aubert *et al.*, 2009; Varotto *et al.*, 2012). It is not our purpose in this chapter to discuss in detail the indication for SEEG in the context of FCD. In particular, for FCD II, in many cases, non-invasive approaches are sufficient to determine the surgical strategy. In some cases, however, the use of SEEG is required.

Invasive recordings should be considered when clinical semiology and/or EEG findings show discrepancies with the location, type, or extent of the lesion, suggesting that the EZ is not limited to the lesion. In such cases, the purpose of invasive recordings will be to define the relationship between the EZ and the lesion and to establish the limits of surgical resection (Minotti *et al.*, 2018). Other indications include cases with negative MRI. In a recent study (Lagarde *et al.*, 2019b) of 59 patients with SEEG in focal epilepsy with negative MRI who underwent subsequent surgery, histopathology revealed FCD I in 13% and FCD II in 17% of cases. In this context, SEEG can record suggestive electrophysiological patterns that will be confirmed by histopathological analysis. FCD I have less characteristic MRI lesion boundaries and are often more extensive (Review in Guerrini *et al.*, 2015). Apart from cases limited to the anterior temporal regions (that could benefit from a standard resection), the use of SEEG is often necessary. This is all the more relevant since the epileptogenic networks are often more complex and extended in these lesions (Lagarde *et al.*, 2016).

SEEG patterns and characteristics of the epileptogenic zone network

In SEEG, the onset of focal seizures must be analyzed both in terms of seizure onset patterns (SOP) (Lagarde *et al.*, 2016; Perucca *et al.*, 2014; Singh *et al.*, 2015) and in terms of spatial extent (Bartolomei *et al.*, 2018). Various SOP can be observed during SEEG recordings but most include LVFA (Singh *et al.*, 2015). LVFA may be preceded by SEEG changes in the form of preictal spikes, spike trains, or slow wave complexes (Lagarde *et al.*, 2019a). The frequencies involved in LVFA range from beta/low gamma ranges (15-30 Hz) (e.g., in mesial temporal seizures), to higher frequencies (gamma range, 30-100 Hz, typically seen in neocortical seizures (Lagarde *et al.*, 2019a; Wendling *et al.*, 2003)

The spatial extent is also an important parameter. The EZ can be very focal but more often it is distributed in several interconnected anatomical regions, reflecting the concept of EZ network (Bartolomei *et al.*, 2017).

Importantly, in some cases, seizures may begin with patterns involving lower frequencies. These "slow" SOP are observed in 15-25% of cases (Lagarde *et al.*, 2016). These patterns include frequencies in the alpha and theta range or patterns with spike waves (Lagarde *et al.*, 2016). However, interpretation must remain cautious in these cases, as this aspect may only reflect a propagation pattern and an inadequate sampling of the EZ.

Seizure onset patterns in Focal Cortical Dysplasia

In a study focusing on FCD and neurodevelopmental tumours investigated by SEEG, we described 6 main SOP (Lagarde *et al.*, 2016). **Figure 1** shows the different patterns of seizure onset:

- LVFA, with rhythmic fast oscillations > 14 Hz and low amplitude < 30 µV (**Figure 1A**). This was the most prevalent pattern (32%);
- pre-ictal spiking with rhythmic spikes of low frequency (median = 1,5 Hz; SD = 0,7), high amplitude and prolonged duration (median = 20 s) followed by LVFA (**Figure 1B**). It was observed in 17% of cases;
- burst of polyspikes of high frequency and amplitude (median frequency = 19.3 Hz; SD = 3.7) and short duration (median = 3.3) followed by LVFA (**Figure 2C**). It was observed in 19% of cases:
- slow wave or baseline shift followed by LVFA (median frequency = 31 Hz; SD = 11) (**Figure 2D** and occurring in 15% of cases;
- rhythmic spikes or spike-waves, at lower frequency (median = 3.5 Hz; SD = 0.8) and with high amplitude (**Figure 1E**). This pattern was rarely observed (5% of cases):
- theta/alpha sharp activity (median = 9.5 Hz; SD = 0.8) with progressive increasing amplitude (**Figure 1F**) that was observed in 11% of cases.

It is interesting to note that in about 80% of cases there is a rapid discharge in the SOP. In 20% of the cases, however, the SOP does not contain a fast discharge ("slow pattern").

Seizure onset pattern and histological type

In our previous study (Lagarde *et al.*, 2016), we observed that the majority of seizure onset patterns were common to all histological types, with the exception of pattern 5 (rhythmic spikes/spike-waves) not found in FCD II. There were some differences, however, according to the subtype of FCD. In FCD I, the most prevalent were pattern 1 (LVFA; 23.1%) and pattern 4 (slow wave or baseline shift followed by LVFA; 15.4%). In FCD II, the most prevalent were pattern 3 (burst of polyspikes followed by LVFA; 31%) (**Figure 2**), pattern 1 (LVFA; 27.6%), and pattern 2 (pre-ictal spiking followed by LVFA; 27.6%). Slow patterns were most prevalent in FCD I and were exceptionally or never observed in FCD II (**Figure 3**).

A more recent study from our group (Lagarde *et al.*, 2019b), including patients from two centers, investigated SOP on SEEG in MRI-negative patients and was able to confirm the previous data. SOP featuring LVFA were the most common in FCD II (80%) and histologically normal (76%) groups, whereas they were encountered in only 50% of patients with FCD I.

More specifically, however, the pattern of bursts of multiple spikes before LVFA was not only the most frequent SOP in FCD II (as already found by Francione *et al.*, 2003) but was seen only in patients with FCD (type I and II). On the other hand, slow-wave/DC shift prior to LVFA was mostly found in normal histology and not found in FCD I.

Interestingly, this study has shown that some common seizure onset patterns such as LVFA from the start, not preceded by rhythmic spikes or bursts of polyspikes can be observed in EZ either with normal histology or with confirmed FCD (type I and II).

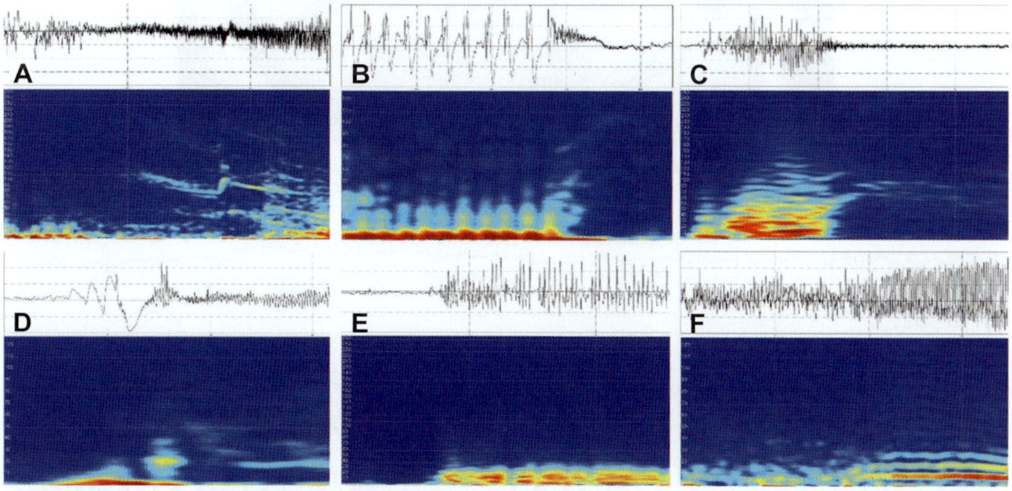

Figure 1

The six patterns of seizure onset according to the time-frequency representation from SEEG trace.
A. Low voltage fast activity (LVFA); B. Pre-ictal spiking with rhythmic spikes of low frequency followed by LVFA; C. Burst of polyspikes of high frequency and amplitude followed by LVFA; D. Slow wave or baseline shift followed by LVFA; E. Rhythmic spikes or spike-waves, at low frequency and with high amplitude; F. Theta/alpha sharp activity with progressive increasing amplitude. (from Lagarde *et al.*, 2016, with authorization)

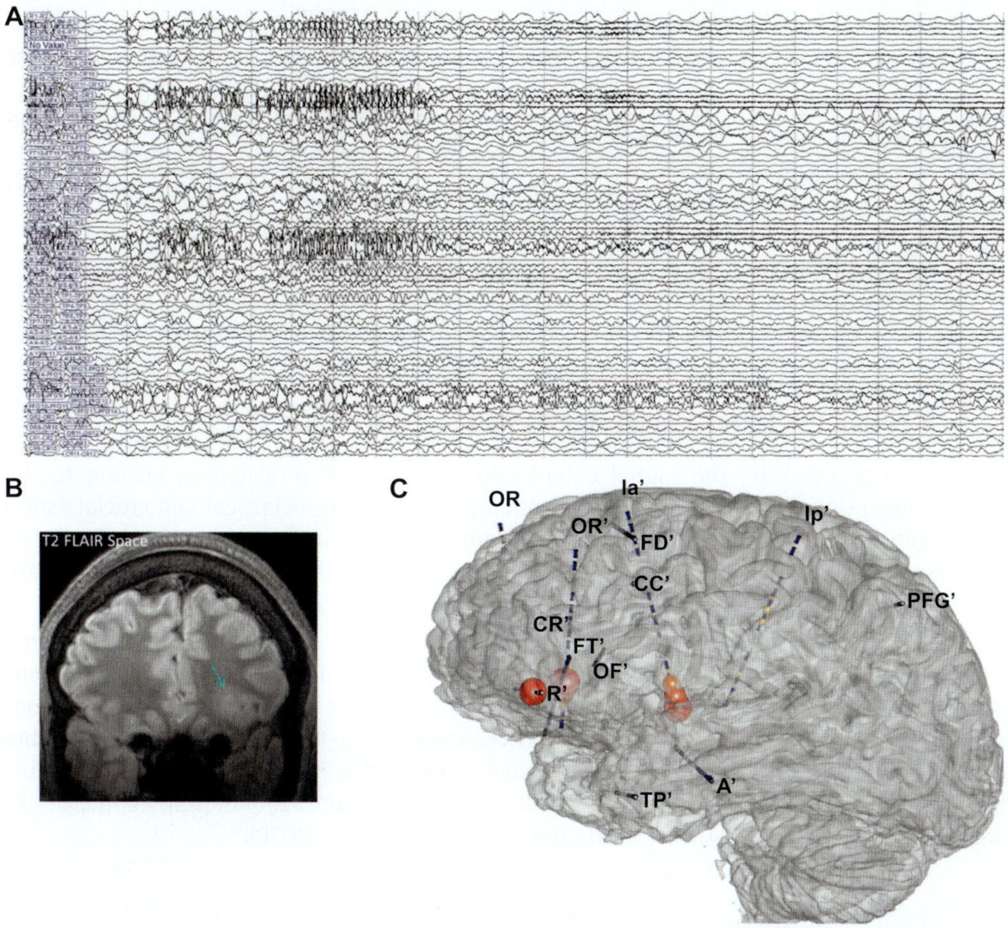

Figure 2

SEEG recorded seizure in a case of a FCD II located in the orbitofrontal cortex.
A. SEEG traces showing a pattern of high amplitude polyspike followed by a fast discharge and affecting simultaneously the orbitofrontal cortex (OR'1-4, R'4-5; 5-6, 6-7) and the insular cortex (Ia'4-5, 6-7, 7-8) B. 3T MRI. Flair sequence showing a blurring of the gray-white maters interface in the left orbitofrontal cortex C. Epileptogenicity Index values projected into a 3D MESH of the patient's brain with electrodes. Note the involvement of both orbitofrontal cortex and insular cortex. The surgery in this case removed the orbitofrontal region (histology FCD IIA) and the anterior insular region (normal histology). Unfortunately, the patient is not seizure free. A postoperative MEG shows a residual interictal activity in the operculo-insular region and a more extensive surgery of this region is planned.

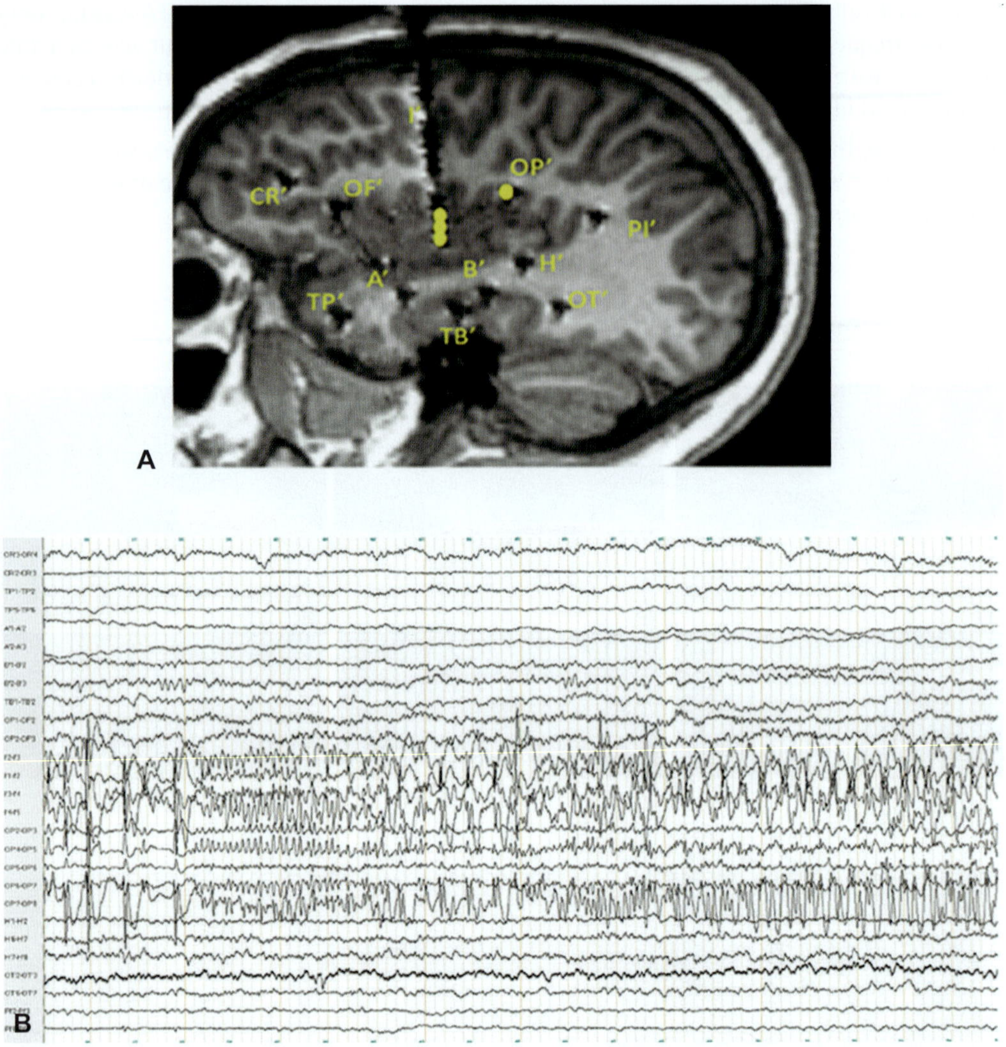

Figure 3

Example of a SEEG recorded seizure in a patient with FCD I (normal MRI, histopathological confirmation).
A. MRI with electrodes showing the main site of onset in the insular cortex (yellow dots) B. SEEG recordings, showing a slow onset pattern (theta/alpha sharp activity) in the insular and opercular contacts (I and OP contacts).

Spatial extent and network approaches

In addition to the SOP, the spatial extent and the speed of propagation leading to this broader extension ("early spread") of the epileptic discharge is a classical and crucial aspect of the spatio-temporal dynamics of seizures in the brain (Bartolomei *et al.*, 2020). These two aspects can be quantified by the epileptogenicity index method (Bartolomei *et al.*, 2008) which measures on the one hand the amount of rapid activity produced per region and on the other hand the speed of involvement of each region.

The EI shows that some regions can be considered as highly epileptogenic nodes (EZ network) especially above a certain threshold of the normalized index value (>0.4). There is a good correlation between surgical prognosis and resection of high value nodes. Other regions (nodes) of the epileptogenic networks are called "propagation networks" and show AR values between 0.1 and 0.4. Some of these nodes have epileptogenic capabilities and could be the cause of surgical failures (Aubert *et al.*, 2009; Balatskaya *et al.*, 2020).

Applied to FCD (types I and II), this method showed that in patients explored with SEEG, nearly 2/3 showed a spatial extension of the discharge with epileptogenicity values extending beyond the lesion itself (Aubert *et al.*, 2009). The surgical prognosis was better when the epileptogenicity values were limited to the lesion site ("focal cases") and worse when the EZ was formed by a network with epileptogenicity values distant from the lesion ("network cases").

These data were confirmed by functional connectivity studies showing that not only the lesion but also distant sites can be involved in the networks of the EZ (Janca *et al.*, 2021; Varotto *et al.*, 2012). Again, the surgical prognosis is related to the non-resection of the most epileptogenic nodes (Janca *et al.*, 2021). **Figure 2** shows an example of FCD II visible in the orbitofrontal cortex but associated with a more extended EZ (orbitofrontal cortex and insular cortex).

Interestingly, alterations of functional connectivity have been described in the interictal period (Lagarde *et al.*, 2018; Varotto *et al.*, 2012) mainly in the networks of the EZ but also in the propagation zone. The surgical prognosis was related to these distant alterations of functional connectivity (Lagarde *et al.*, 2018).

Link with surgical outcome

Despite its intrinsic epileptogenicity, epilepsy surgery in FCD is associated with a significant number of failures. The reasons for this are probably multiple including poor definition of the EZ, insufficient surgery, histological and genetic factors, and the networked organization of the EZ (Guerrini *et al.*, 2015).

SEEG analysis can provide prognostic information. Indeed, some seizure onset patterns are associated with a worse surgical prognosis (slow onset patterns, slow-wave DC shift). (Lagarde *et al.*, 2019a, 2016). Similarly, the spatial extension of the discharge and the networked nature of the EZ is a factor in effective focal surgery (Aubert *et al.*, 2009; Janca *et al.*, 2021).

Finally, the following points may contribute to a larger EZ than the lesion visible on MRI:
- the histology, as the networks tend to be larger in FCD I
- the SEEG pattern: slow patterns and slow wave-fast activity patterns have larger networks

The role of genetic factors and the duration of the disease are still to be better determined but probably play an important role in the final configuration of an EZ associated with FCD.

Conclusion

There is a limited repertoire of seizure onset patterns in FCD. They are characterized by a variable transition pattern from the interictal period and by a discharge frequency that most often includes high-frequency activities. Slow patterns of onset are however observable, especially in FCD I. The spatial extension of the ictal discharge at its onset is an important factor to recognize and may be broader than the lesion itself. It is important to know these aspects which are determinant for the surgical prognosis.

References

Aubert S, Wendling F, Regis J, *et al.* Local and remote epileptogenicity in Focal Cortical Dysplasias and neurodevelopmental tumours. Brain 2009; 132, 3072-86.

Balatskaya A, Roehri N, Lagarde S, *et al.* The "Connectivity Epileptogenicity Index" (cEI), a method for mapping the different seizure onset patterns in StereoElectroEncephalography recorded seizures. Clinical neurophysiology : official journal of the International Federation of Clinical Neurophysiology 2020; 131, 1947-55.

Bartolomei F, Chauvel, P, Wendling F. Epileptogenicity of brain structures in human temporal lobe epilepsy: A quantified study from intracerebral EEG. Brain 2008; 131, 1818-30.

Bartolomei F, Lagarde S, Wendling F, *et al.* Defining epileptogenic networks: Contribution of SEEG and signal analysis. Epilepsia 2017; 48(1): 53-7.

Bartolomei F, Nica A, Valenti-Hirsch M.P, Adam C, Denuelle M. Interpretation of SEEG recordings. Neurophysiologie Clinique 2018; 48(1): 53-7.

Bartolomei F, Scholly J, Lagarde S. Ictal Activity, in: A Practical Approach to Stereo EEG. Springer Publishing Company 2020; 27: 339-50.

Chassoux, F. Stereoelectroencephalography in Focal Cortical Dysplasia: A 3D approach to delineating the dysplastic cortex. Brain 2000; 123, 1733-51.

Francione S, Nobili L, Cardinale F, Citterio A, Galli C, Tassi L. Intra-lesional stereo-EEG activity in Taylor's Focal Cortical Dysplasia. Epileptic disorders : international epilepsy journal with videotape 2003; 5 Suppl 2, S105-14.

Guerrini R, Duchowny M, Jayakar P, *et al.* Diagnostic methods and treatment options for Focal Cortical Dysplasia. Epilepsia 2015; 56, 1669-86.

Isnard J, Taussig D, Bartolomei F, *et al.* French guidelines on stereoelectroencephalography (SEEG). Neurophysiologie Clinique 2018; 48: 5-13.

Janca R, Jahodova A, Hlinka J, *et al.* Ictal gamma-band interactions localize ictogenic nodes of the epileptic network in Focal Cortical Dysplasia. Clinical Neurophysiology 2021; 132, 1927-36.

Kahane P, Landré E, Minotti L, Francione S, Ryvlin P. The Bancaud and Talairach view on the epileptogenic zone: A working hypothesis. Epileptic Disorders 2006.

Lagarde S, Bonini F, McGonigal A, *et al.* Seizure-onset patterns in Focal Cortical Dysplasia and neurodevelopmental tumors: Relationship with surgical prognosis and neuropathologic subtypes. Epilepsia 2016; 57, 1426-35.

Lagarde S, Buzori S, Trebuchon A, *et al.* The repertoire of seizure onset patterns in human focal epilepsies: Determinants and prognostic values. Epilepsia 2019[a]; 60, 85-95.

Lagarde S, Roehri N, Lambert I, *et al.* Interictal stereotactic-EEG functional connectivity in refractory focal epilepsies. Brain 2018; 141, 2966-80.

Lagarde S, Scholly J, Popa I, *et al.* Can histologically normal epileptogenic zone share common electrophysiological phenotypes with Focal Cortical Dysplasia? SEEG-based study in MRI-negative epileptic patients. Journal of Neurology 2019b; 266, 1907-18.

Lamberink H.J, Otte, W.M, Blümcke I, *et al.* Seizure outcome and use of antiepileptic drugs after epilepsy surgery according to histopathological diagnosis: a retrospective multicentre cohort study. The Lancet Neurology 2020; 19, 748-57.

Minotti L, Montavont A, Scholly J, Tyvaert L, Taussig D. Indications and limits of stereoelectroencephalography (SEEG). Neurophysiologie clinique 2018; 48, 15-24.

Palmini A, Gambardella A, Andermann F, *et al.* Intrinsic epileptogenicity of human dysplastic cortex as suggested by corticography and surgical results. Annals of Neurology 1995; 37, 476-87.

Perucca P, Dubeau F, Gotman J. Intracranial electroencephalographic seizure-onset patterns: effect of underlying pathology. Brain 2014; 137, 183-96.

Singh S, Sandy S, Wiebe S. Ictal onset on intracranial EEG: Do we know it when we see it? State of the evidence. Epilepsia 2015; 56, 1629-38.

Tassi L, Colombo N, Garbelli R. Focal Cortical Dysplasia: neuropathological subtypes, EEG, neuroimaging and surgical outcome. Brain 2002; 125, 1719-32.

Varotto G, Tassi L, Franceschetti S, Spreafico R, Panzica F. Epileptogenic networks of type II Focal Cortical Dysplasia: a stereo-EEG study. NeuroImage 2012; 61, 591-8.

Wendling F, Bartolomei F, Bellanger J.J, Bourien J, Chauvel P. Epileptic fast intracerebral EEG activity: Evidence for spatial decorrelation at seizure onset. Brain 2003; 126, 1449-59.

CHAPTER

13. MEG and HR-EEG in FCD: non-invasive localization of the epileptogenic zone

Francesca Bonini, Jean-Michel Badier, Martine Gavaret

Key points

- The relevance of source analysis is maximal in cases with suspected FCD and negative structural MRI.
- HR EEG and MEG yield significant additional data during the presurgical evaluation whatever the patient's standard EEG characteristics. In case of sub-continuous interictal activities, HR EEG and MEG do aid in the localization of the sources. In case of negative EEG, HR EEG and MEG may highlight some discrete interictal epileptiform activity.
- Very few MEG studies detailed neurophysiological data according to anatomopathological characteristics.
- Closed-field effects due to the random orientation of neurons within the FCD, low density of neural cells and small size of especially bottom-of-sulcus FCDs are suggested as potential reasons for low amplitude spikes.
- HR-EEG and MEG can be complementary in terms of sensitivity for spike detections, since HR-EEG can be negative while MEG is not, and vice-versa.

Introduction

Magnetoencephalography (MEG) and EEG measure the weak electromagnetic fields induced by post-synaptic neural currents in a non-invasive fashion. Hence, they can be performed in children and adults and are particularly useful in patients with FCD, because interictal and ictal onset zones are closely related (Bast *et al.*, 2004; Ishii *et al.*, 2008; Bartolomei *et al.*, 2016; Kasper *et al.*, 2018).

MEG and HR-EEG in focal lesional epilepsies: research or clinical tools?

MEG and HR EEG are work intensive processes that demand both clinical and procedural expertise. There are few MEG devices due to their high purchase and maintenance costs, and given this limited availability, the experience in MEG analysis and interpretation remains relatively constrained to selected institutions and their experienced personnel (Laohathai *et al.*, 2020). Given the low cost and high flexibility of EEG devices even with high channel counts, HR EEG - electric source imaging (ESI) - is more widely used than MEG in pre-surgical epilepsy evaluation.

In clinical practice both MEG and EEG recordings are visually analysed by trained neurophysiologists to detect epileptiform activities. Quantitative analyses have also been implemented, allowing the inspection of multiple aspects of electromagnetic signals not visible for human eyes: besides interictal HFO, which will be discussed later, further perspectives arise from functional connectivity analysis. This estimates statistical associations between physiologic signals recorded from different brain regions, describing how these regions (defining a cerebral network) coordinate their electrical activities. Estimates of intracerebral connectivity can be used to study the synchrony of epileptogenic networks, which drastically change during seizures (decrease synchrony among structures) and propagation (increased synchrony within the network). Moreover, cerebral connectivity can be also be modified during the interictal period: alteration of regional (ie, close to the EZ) and widespread connectivity has been demonstrated in focal epilepsies using functional-MRI, intracerebral recordings (particularly of patients with MCD, Lagarde *et al.*, 2018) as well as with MEG (Englot *et al.*, 2015).

The respective contribution of MEG and HR-EEG for localizing FCD

MEG captures a more selective set of brain sources with greater spectral and spatial definition than EEG (Ahlfors *et al.*, 2010). EEG senses dipolar electrical activity in all three directions with an increased sensitivity for radial superficial currents, whereas MEG senses primarily the tangential current components originating within sulci (Bast *et al.*, 2004). Without difficulties, it is possible to combine MEG with EEG recordings. In a few research centres, it is also possible to combine MEG, EEG and SEEG recordings.

Compared to EEG, MEG benefits from the magnetic transparency of the skull, which facilitates source localization by reducing the risk of errors due to an incorrect head conductivity model, but also by limiting the large-scale mixing of neural sources. This significantly increases the signal-to-noise ratio for MEG in higher frequencies, rendering it a formidable technique for studying high frequency oscillatory activities (Velmurugan *et al.*, 2019). HFO and ictal low voltage fast activities are observed in FCD (Chassoux *et al.*, 2000; Guerrini *et al.*, 2015; Lagarde *et al.*, 2016). Using MEG, gamma events, with or without concomitant interictal spike activity, can be detected and localized independently (Jeong *et al.*, 2013). With MEG, interictal activities as spikes of short duration and steep tilt, needle-like are described (Ueda *et al.*, 2015). Some authors suggest that closed-field effects due to the random orientation of neurons within the FCD, low density of neural cells and small size of especially bottom-of-sulcus FCD as potential reasons for low signal-to-noise ratio spikes (Nakajima *et al.*, 2016; Kasper *et al.*, 2018). Very few studies detailed neurophysiological data according to anatomopathological characteristics. However, one study described more MEG clusters in FCD II than in type I: 52 vs 33%, in a pediatric study comprising 17 FCD II and 10 FCD I patients (Alshafai *et al.*, 2014).

Moreover, in some studies including patients with FCD and particularly with insular epilepsy, HFO sources in the resection zone had a positive predictive value to surgical outcome: when HFO are spatially congruent with the resected cortex, patients have better surgical outcome (Velmurugan *et al.*, 2019; Yin *et al.*, 2019). Encouraged by both the high sensitivity and high accuracy of HFO sources to predict outcome, these authors propose that non-invasive detection of HFO, coupled or not with interictal spikes or related to the pre-ictal period, could be an important asset for the non-invasive presurgical assessment of partial refractory epilepsy.

Nonetheless the most relevant and widespread application of electromagnetic source imagine (EMSI) in clinical practice remains the detection and localization of interictal spikes to help define the EZ. Many studies have demonstrated a very good degree of spatial concordance of the ESI with imaging/metabolic techniques (MRI, PET, SPECT), as well as with SEEG and the resected zone, with a higher number of electrodes increasing the sensitivity of ESI. Comparably to ESI, MEG has a sensitivity and specificity in localizing epileptiform activity of around 70% (up to 95-100% depending on the series) and can add useful information in presurgical evaluation, with a positive predictive value of magnetic source imaging (MSI) for seizure localization of 82–90% (Stefan, 2010). When evaluating the reliability in detecting interictal discharges in MEG compared to EEG, Iwasaki and colleagues (Iwasaki *et al.*, 2006) found no significant difference in terms of both visual identification of spikes and their localisation at a sub-lobar level. Regarding the few ESI studies that focus exclusively on FCD, a good concordance between the sources and the EZ was found. ESI demonstrated high sensitivity and spatial concordance in MRI-negative FCD patients (Russo *et al.*, 2016), as well as magnetic source imaging in three other studies which compared magnetic sources to lesion localization (Kasper *et al.*, 2018, Nakajima *et al.*, 2016) and to the resected zone (Alshafai *et al.*, 2014). Similarly, ESI combined with MSI showed consistent localization of electrical abnormalities in both modalities within the lesional zone (Bast *et al.*, 2004). Furthermore, in all these studies, complete resection of the MEG and/or ESI sources was associated with more favourable surgical outcome, even in MRI-negative patients (Kasper *et al.*, 2018, Nakajima *et al.*, 2016, Bast *et al.*, 2004).

Taking as a whole, these findings indicates that both MSI and ESI are reliable and non-redundant tools for the non-invasive localization of the EZ. They can be complementary in terms of sensitivity for spike detections, since HR-EEG can be negative while MEG is not, and vice-versa (**Figure 2**).

Ictal HR-EEG and MEG

Relationships between irritative and epileptogenic (ictal) zones are variable with good spatial concordance in patients with FCD (Bartolomei *et al.*, 2016). Ictal source localizations have the potential to contribute important clinical information in the presurgical assessment. However, ictal MEG recordings are rare because of logistic difficulties with prolonged MEG recordings. Moreover, movement artifacts interfere with accurate magnetic source localization. Most ictal MEG studies have thus reported only a few cases (Badier *et al.*, 2016). Various types of seizure-onset patterns in FCD including low-voltage fast activity, pre-ictal spiking and rhythmic spikes/spikes-waves have been described (Lagarde *et al.*, 2016). The accuracy of source localization may depend on these ictal patterns and on chosen algorithms. Further research should be done, testing various algorithms according to each ictal pattern and validated by intracerebral data, before encouraging clinical prolonged MEG recordings in order to record seizures (Badier *et al.*, 2016).

With HR-EEG, prolonged recordings are much more easily performed (Rikir *et al.*, 2020). As in MEG, the accuracy of source localization is dependent on the ictal pattern. Indeed, a high level of agreement between source localization and SEEG is obtained for ictal spiking and for low-voltage fast activity. For rhythmic spikes/spikes-waves, source localizations may correspond only to the seizure propagation network (Koessler *et al.*, 2010). Interictal source localization encompasses a risk of false results due to the complex relationships between irritative and epileptogenic (ictal) networks. Inter-ictal analysis has the highest sensitivity while ictal analysis has the highest specificity, especially in FCD patients (Rikir *et al.*, 2020).

MEG in post-operative patients with seizure recurrence

Since magnetic susceptibility is the same for all tissues, including the skull, magnetic signals have negligeable sensitivity to skull defects compared to EEG and are less distorted by anatomic modifications following craniotomy and cortectomy. For this reason, in case of reccurrence of seizures after a first epilepsy surgery, MEG investigation is preferentially proposed: **Figure 3** illustrates a case of MEG recording performed after post-surgical seizure recurrence, which helped to define the complement of cortectomy to be performed, overcoming the relatively limited spatial sampling of SEEG). Indeed, reoperation can be proposed in patients in whom the residual EZ is close relation to the initial region of surgical resection (Vaugier *et al.*, 2018). In that sense, source localization of interictal abnormalities bordering the cortectomy or distant from it, may provide useful arguments for the surgical decision of whether patients have a good chance of seizure control following reoperation.

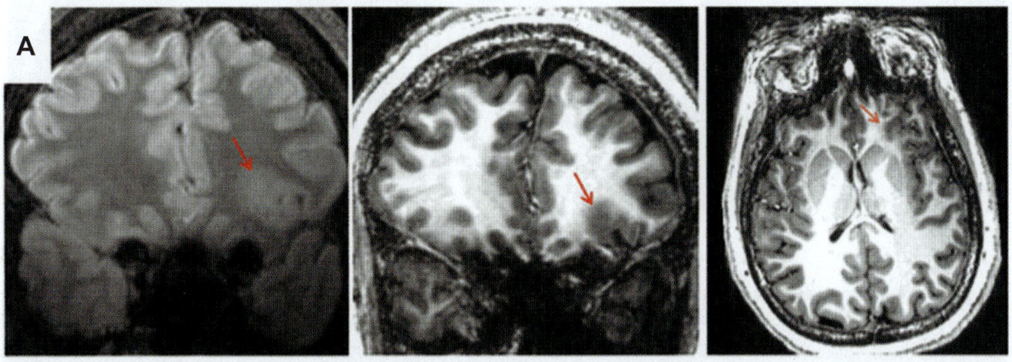

Figure 3

MEG in a post-operative patient with seizure recurrence.

A. MRI. Flair sequence showing a blurring of the gray-white maters interface in the left orbitofrontal cortex. Pathological examination confirmed the presence of FCD IIA in the left orbito-frontal cortex. Left hemisphere is on the right of the reader in all images (usual depiction).

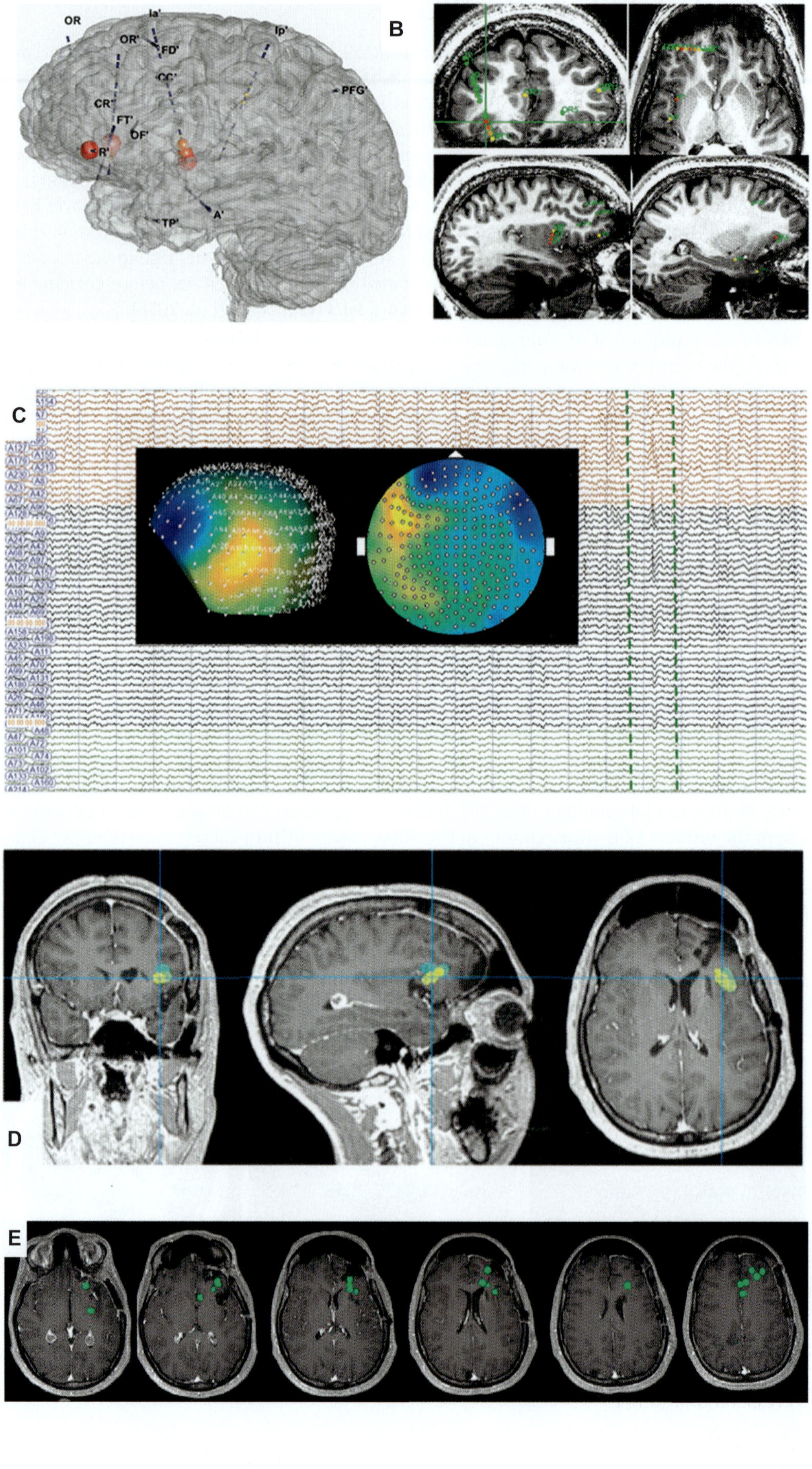

Figure 3

B. Epileptogenicity Index values (Bartolomei *et al.*, 2008) projected into a 3D MESH of the patient's brain with electrodes. Note the involvement of both orbitofrontal cortex and insular cortex. Epileptogenicity Index was maximal on internal contacts of electrode OR' (coronal view), intermediate contacts of R' and internal contacts of Ia' (left anterior insula) which are visible on the sagittal and axial views (note that left hemisphere is on the left of the reader in the coronal and axial images). This case shows an example of FCD II visible in the orbitofrontal cortex but associated with a more extended EZ (orbitofrontal and insular cortices). This case is also illustrated in the chapter: The epileptogenic zone in FCD: SEEG patterns in FCD subtypes. Fabrice Bartolomei (Figure 2) C. MEG signals acquired following post-surgical seizure recurrence (a resection of orbito-frontal cortex, F3 pars orbitalis and anterior insula was performed): several spikes of variable amplitude were recorded, with left dipolar cartography (Marseille MEG 4D device). D. Source localization of a selected spike with an equivalent current dipole in the residual anterior insula. E. Spike dipole sources clustered tightly on and around the cortectomy in the anterior cingulate, anterior insula and ventrolateral prefrontal cortices. In line with these new results and with the revision of SEEG findings, an additional cortectomy has been proposed to resect the residual inferior frontal gyrus with the inferior frontal sulcus, the residual orbito-frontal cortex and the residual anterior insula. Left hemisphere is on the right of the reader in all images (usual depiction) in D and E.

Practical considerations: what relevance for which patients?

• FCD negative-MRI

The relevance of source analysis is maximal in cases with suspected FCD and negative structural MRI. FCD can be difficult to identify with MRI. Some small FCD are not detectable with standard MR sequences. Reinvestigating structural MRI, in some cases with a 7T machine, incorporating the findings from source analysis may prove very important in the presurgical evaluation (Wang *et al.*, 2014; Aydin *et al.*, 2017; Nobile *et al.*, 2021). Interictal source localizations are thus of particular value in localizing epileptogenic cortex in epilepsy surgery patients with FCD, particularly in patients having no visible MRI lesions (Wilenius *et al.*, 2013). Similarly, for HR EEG, Russo and colleagues reported a high concordance (79-100%) between ESI sources and the resected zone especially in temporal epilepsy in a cohort of MRI-negative FCD patients, with favorable outcome when ESI source resection was complete (Russo *et al.*, 2016).

• HR EEG and MEG afford whatever standard EEG characteristics

HR EEG and MEG yield significant additional data during the presurgical evaluation, whatever the patient's standard EEG characteristics. Indeed, in case of sub-continuous interictal activities, HR EEG and MEG do aid in the localization of the sources. In case of negative EEG, HR EEG may highlight some discrete interictal epileptiform activity. Cases of negative HR EEG with positive MEG are also documented, in case of FCD restricted to a bottom of a sulcus (**Figures 2 and 4**) or in case of insular/opercular generators (De Tiege *et al.*, 2012).

Moreover, in case of medial FCD with false lateralizing EEG findings, MEG is particularly useful (Gavaret *et al.*, 2014, Laohathai *et al.*, 2021). Interestingly, higher spatial concordance between MSI and the lesion has been reported for more superficial cortical FCD compared to deep-seated lesions, with a good correlation with surgical outcome for both lesional groups (Nakajima *et al.*, 2016).

Additional value in presurgical work-up: when is it decisive?

• Allowing epilepsy surgery without intracranial recordings

Some studies highlight the importance of the convergence of findings from several functional neuroimaging techniques (FDG-PET, ESI or MSI) to identify the EZ. In selected cases, the multimodal approach may obviate the need for invasive intracranial recordings (Nobile *et al.*, 2021). In a prospective study of 102 patients, interictal source localization provided nonredundant information which contributed to deciding the course of surgery in 33% of the patients, and prevented intracranial recordings in 19% (Tripathi *et al.*, 2021).

HR EEG and MEG are helpful in guiding electrodes implantation

It has been demonstrated that modelling of the spiking volume with MEG is a promising tool to localize non-invasively the SOZ in FCD patients. Combined with brain MRI, MEG modelling of the spiking volume contributes to delineate the spatial extent of the SOZ (Bouet *et al.*, 2017). In many studies, MSI represent a useful tool to guide depth electrode implantation schemes (Wilenius *et al.*, 2013; Abdallah *et al.*, 2017) in conjunction with other non-invasive investigation. As previously explained, MSI and ESI are complementary: for example, scalp EEG has relatively low sensitivity in localising deep-seated structures such as insular cortex, while MEG can detect tangential dipoles arising from insular sulci and help localize the irritative zone in the operculo-insular regions in patients with negative-MRI FCD (Yu *et al.*, 2018). However, we have to keep in mind that the irritative zone, as indicated by the MEG or EEG interictal spikes, may not correspond to the entire epileptogenic network (El Tahry *et al.*, 2016).

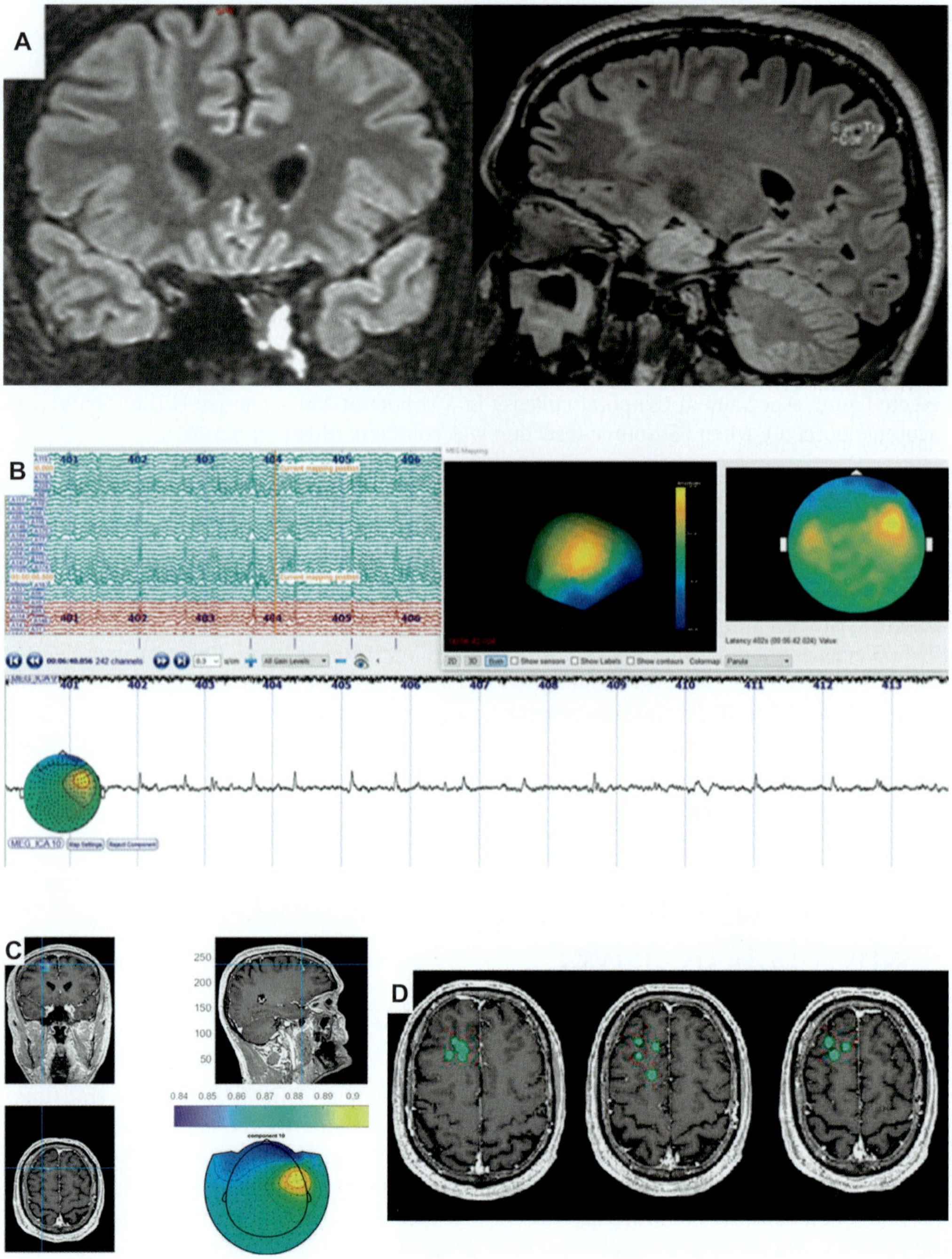

Figure 4

7T MRI and MEG data in a patient with FCD and negative 32-channel EEG.

A. 7T MRI showing increased FLAIR signal of the right superior frontal sulcus with a transmantle sign. B. MEG signals with independent component analysis (ICA) showing spikes with right dipolar cartography (Marseille MEG 4D device). C. Source localization with an equivalent current dipole in the anterior superior frontal sulcus. D. Spike dipole sources clustered tightly in the right prefrontal dysplastic cortex, namely in the superior frontal sulcus and gyrus. This case illustrates a well concordant situation in which surgery could be performed without SEEG.

Conclusions and perspectives

During the presurgical assessment of drug-resistant epilepsies related to FCD, HR EEG and MEG will be used in order to record and localize interictal activity, using traditional equivalent current dipoles or more innovative algorithms. Interictal magnetic and/or electric source imaging are complementary and non-redundant with other non-invasive investigations. HR EEG and MEG will be strikingly interesting in case of suspected FCD despite normal MRI, allowing to re-interpret the cerebral MRI according to source localization. Furthermore, in case of confirmed FCD, EMSI may support the decision of direct surgery without previous intracerebral recordings (Nobile *et al.*, 2021). Moreover, HR EEG and MEG are complementary, being characterized by distinct sensitivity according to the source orientation.

In addition to the well-established localization of interictal spikes using equivalent current dipoles, the reference method for clinical use, further independent biomarkers have been identified as well as methods to allow their identification. Particularly, epileptic ripples or HFO, coupled or not with interictal spikes, have a positive prognostic value, since resection of the area generating these abnormalities is associated with better outcome. Thus, non-invasive mapping with MEG and/or HR-EEG could provide supplementary information for surgical decision and guide electrode implantation. The study of functional connectivity is another promising tool to characterize the epileptic activity and investigate network aspects of different interical and ictal phenomena, and it seems to have potential prognostic correlates. Despite some methodological limitations that should be overcomed and the need of validation studies in large patient cohorts, source connectivity analysis discloses a great potentiality for clinical application.

Finally, the well-established additional value of ESI and MSI to map and define epileptic activity should encourage their widespread use in presurgical evaluation of focal epilepsy and particularly in FCD in which irritative and EZ are often spatially colocalized. As the HR-EEG is relatively inexpensive, its use has already begun to spread, while the main factor limiting the use of MEG remains its cost. Fortunately, engineering research bodes well for the development of more manoeuvrable and less expensive devices.

References

Abdallah C, Maillard LG, Rikir E, *et al.* Localizing value of electrical source imaging: Frontal lobe, malformations of cortical development and negative MRI related epilepsies are the best candidates. *Neuroimage Clinical.* 2017; 16: 319-29.

Ahlfors SP, Han J, Belliveau JW, Hämäläinen MS. Sensitivity of MEG and EEG to source orientation. *Brain Topogr.* 2010; 23 (3): 227-32.

Alshafai L, Ochi A, Go C, *et al.* Clinical, EEG, MRI, MEG, and surgical outcomes of pediatric epilepsy with astrocytic inclusions versus Focal Cortical Dysplasia. *Epilepsia.* 2014; 55 (10): 1568-75.

Aydin Ü, Rampp S, Wollbrink A, *et al.* Zoomed MRI Guided by Combined EEG/MEG Source Analysis: A Multimodal Approach for Optimizing Presurgical Epilepsy Work-up and its Application in a Multi-focal Epilepsy Patient Case Study. Brain Topogr. 2017; 30 (4): 417-433.

Aydin Ü, Pellegrino G, Ali OBK, *et al.* Magnetoencephalography resting state connectivity patterns as indicatives of surgical outcome in epilepsy patients. *Neural Eng.* 2020; 17 (3): 035007.

Badier JM, Bénar CG, Woodman M, *et al.* Ictal magnetic source imaging in presurgical assessment. *Brain Topography* 2016; 29 (1): 182-92.

Baillet S, Mosher JC, Leahy RM. Electromagnetic brain mapping. *IEEE Signal Processing Magazine*, 2001; 18: 14-30.

Bartolomei F, Chauvel P, Wendling F. Epileptogenicity of brain structures in human temporal lobe epilepsy: a quantified study from intracerebral EEG. *Brain* 2008; 131 (Pt 7): 1818-30.

Bartolomei F, Trébuchon A, Bonini F, *et al.* What is the concordance between the epileptogenic zone and the irritative zone? A SEEG quantified study. *Clin Neurophysiol.* 2016; 127 (2): 1157-62.

Bast T, Oezkan O, Rona S, *et al.* EEG and MEG source analysis of single and averaged interictal spikes reveals intrinsic epileptogenicity in Focal Cortical Dysplasia. *Epilepsia* 2004; 45 (6): 621-31.

Boto E, Holmes N, Leggett J, *et al.* Moving magnetoencephalography towards real-world applications with a wearable system. *Nature.* 2018; 555 (7698): 657-661.

Bouet R, Mauguière F, Daligault S, *et al.* The relationship between morphological lesion, magnetic source imaging, and intracranial stereo-electroencephalography in Focal Cortical Dysplasia *Neuroimage Clin.* 2017; 15: 71-79.

Chassoux F, Devaux B, Landré E, *et al.* Stereoelectroencephalography in Focal Cortical Dysplasia: a 3D approach to delineating the dysplastic cortex. *Brain.* 2000; 123 (Pt 8): 1733-51.

De Tiège X, Carrette E, Legros B, *et al.* Clinical added value of magnetic source imaging in the presurgical evaluation of refractory focal epilepsy. *J Neurol Neurosurg Psychiatry.* 2012; 83 (4): 417-23.

El Tahry R, Wang ZI, Kakisaka Y, *et al.* A single tight MEG cluster may only represent a fragment of type I FCD. *Clin Neurophysiol.* 2016; 127 (7): 2570-2.

Englot DJ, Hinkley LB, Kort NS, *et al.* Global and regional functional connectivity maps of neural oscillations in focal epilepsy. *Brain.* 2015; 138 (Pt 8): 2249-62.

Gavaret M, Badier JM, Bartolomei F, Bénar CG, Chauvel P. MEG and EEG sensitivity in a case of medial occipital epilepsy. *Brain Topography* 2014; 27 (1): 192-6.

Guerrini R, Duchowny M, Jayakar P, *et al.* Diagnostic methods and treatment options for Focal Cortical Dysplasia. *Epilepsia* 2015; 56 (11): 1669-86.

Ishii R, Canuet L, Ochi A, *et al.* Spatially filtered magnetoencephalography compared with electrocorticography to identify intrinsically epileptogenic Focal Cortical Dysplasia. *Epilepsy Res.* 2008; 81 (2-3): 228-32.

Jeong W, Kim JS, Chung CK. Localization of MEG pathologic gamma oscillations in adult epilepsy patients with Focal Cortical Dysplasia. *Neuroimage Clin.* 2013 2; 3: 507-14.

Kasper BS, Rössler K, Hamer HM, *et al.* Coregistrating magnetic source and magnetic resonance imaging for epilepsy surgery in Focal Cortical Dysplasia. *Neuroimage Clin.* 2018; 19: 487-496.

Koessler L, Benar C, Maillard L, *et al.* Source localization of ictal epileptic activity investigated by high resolution EEG and validated by SEEG. *Neuroimage* 2010; 51 (2): 642-53.

Lagarde S, Bonini F, McGonigal A, *et al.* Seizure onset patterns in Focal Cortical Dysplasia and neurodevelopmental tumours: relationship with surgical prognosis and neuropathological subtypes. *Epilepsia* 2016; 57 (9): 1426-35.

Lagarde S, Roehri N, Lambert I, *et al.* Interictal stereotactic-EEG functional connectivity in refractory focal epilepsies. *Brain.* 2018; 141 (10): 2966-80.

Laohathai C, Ebersole JS, Mosher JC, *et al.* Practical Fundamentals of Clinical MEG Interpretation in Epilepsy. *Front Neurol.* 2021; 12: 722986.

Mosher JC, Leahy RM. Recursive MUSIC: a framework for EEG and MEG source localization. *IEEE Trans Biomed Eng.* 1998; 45 (11): 1342-54.

Nakajima M, Widjaja E, Baba S, *et al.* Remote MEG dipoles in Focal Cortical Dysplasia at bottom of sulcus. *Epilepsia.* 2016; 57 (7): 1169-78.

Nobile G, Consales A, Tortora D, *et al.* Multimodal approach in the pre-surgical evaluation of focal epilepsy surgery candidates: how far are we from a non-invasive ESI-based "sourcectomy"? *Epileptic Disord* 2021; 23 (4): 661-6.

Rikir E, Koessler L, Gavaret M, *et al.* Electrical Source Imaging in cortical malformation-related epilepsy: a prospective EEG-SEEG concordance study. *Epilepsia* 2014; 55 (6): 918-32.

Rikir E, Maillard LG, Abdallah C, *et al.* Respective Contribution of Ictal and Interictal Electrical Source Imaging to Epileptogenic Zone Localization. *Brain Topography* 2020; 33 (3): 384-402.

Russo A, Lallas M, Jayakar P, *et al.* The diagnostic utility of 3D-ESI rotating and moving dipole methodology in the pre-surgical evaluation of MRI-negative childhood epilepsy due to Focal Cortical Dysplasia. *Epilepsia.* 2016; 57 (9): 1450-7.

Stefan H. Coregistered EEG/MEG for source localization in epilepsy. *Epilepsia.* 2010; 51 Suppl 1: 66-7.

Tripathi M, Kaur K, Ramanujam B, *et al.* Diagnostic added value of interictal magnetic source imaging in presurgical evaluation of persons with epilepsy: A prospective blinded study. *Eur J Neurol.* 2021; 28 (9): 2940-2951.

Ueda Y, Egawa K, Ito T, *et al.* The presence of short and sharp MEG spikes implies Focal Cortical Dysplasia. *Epilepsy Res* 2015; 114: 141-6.

Vaugier L, Lagarde S, McGonigal A, *et al.* The role of stereoelectroencephalography (SEEG) in reevaluation of epilepsy surgery failures. *Epilepsy Behav.* 2018; 81: 86-93.

Velmurugan J, Nagarajan SS, Mariyappa N, *et al.* Magnetoencephalography imaging of high frequency oscillations strengthens presurgical localization and outcome prediction. *Brain.* 2019; 142 (11): 3514-29.

Wang ZI, Alexopoulos AV, Jones SE, *et al.* Linking MRI postprocessing with magnetic source imaging in MRI-negative epilepsy. *Ann Neurol.* 2014; 75 (5): 759-70.

Wilenius J, Medvedovsky M, Gaily E, *et al.* Interictal MEG reveals Focal Cortical Dysplasias: special focus on patients with no visible MRI lesions. *Epilepsy Res.* 2013; 105 (3): 337-48.

Yin C, Zhang X, Chen Z, *et al.* Detection and localization of interictal ripples with magnetoencephalography in the presurgical evaluation of drug-resistant insular epilepsy. *Brain Res.* 2019; 1706: 147-156.

Yu T, Ni D, Zhang X, *et al.* The role of magnetoencephalography in the presurgical evaluation of patients with MRI-negative operculo-insular epilepsy. *Seizure.* 2018; 61: 104-110.

CHAPTER

14. EEG-fMRI in FCD: mapping the epileptogenic networks

Masataka Tanaka, Jean Gotman

Key points

- EEG-fMRI is a noninvasive imaging method to visualize metabolic change during epileptic activities.
- It has been shown that EEG-fMRI is useful to detect the epileptogenic region in patients with FCD lesions, complementing other imaging techniques.

Introduction

Simultaneous recording of scalp EEG and resting-state functional MRI (EEG-fMRI), which measures BOLD signal response related to scalp EEG discharges, is a non-invasive tool to determine the extent of brain tissue involved at the time of an epileptic discharge. The strength of EEG-fMRI is the ability to visualize metabolic changes during epileptic activities with high spatial resolution across the whole brain. In particular, it can "see" the sources of epileptic discharges deep in the brain even if the early electrical epileptic discharge is not visible on the scalp, as long as the discharge propagates sufficiently to eventually become visible on the scalp.

Basic Methodology

In EEG-fMRI analysis, the blood-oxygen-level-dependent (BOLD) signal time-course of each voxel is analyzed as an event-related design. Because MR scanning is used, the recording is inevitably limited in time to approximately one hour and seizures are usually not captured during the recording. The EEG recorded while scanning is heavily contaminated by artefacts but these can largely be removed to recover an EEG of reasonable quality (Allen *et al.*, 1998; Bénar *et al.*, 2003). Timing and duration of each interictal epileptic discharge (IED) are built as a regressor and convolved with a hemodynamic response function (the basic BOLD response to a short neuronal activation), using an event-related type of fMRI analysis. Motion parameters are modelled as confounds, and all regressors are included in the same general linear model to find clusters of voxels having a time course significantly correlated with the model, indicating that the voxels' metabolic activity changes specifically around the time of epileptic discharges; these voxels are called here BOLD clusters. The correlation, which can be positive (increased metabolic activity or activation) or negative (deactivation), is quantified using a statistical value which is usually t-value or F-value. A statistical map of BOLD signal responses correlated to the IEDs, that is referred to as t map or F map, is the result of analyzing an EEG-fMRI study. It is usually superimposed on an anatomical MRI.

Clinical application

BOLD signal responses, despite their interictal origin, have been shown to often co-localize with the SOZ defined with intracranial electrodes (Bénar *et al.*, 2006; Khoo *et al.*, 2017; Thornton *et al.*, 2011). BOLD signal has been demonstrated to usually increase in regions presumably generating IEDs, which are considered to be irritative zones (Bénar *et al.*, 2002); The irritative zone is more extensive than the SOZ in general, and the maximum BOLD responses have been shown to be in good agreement with the SOZ, indicating that the SOZ co-localizes with the location where the metabolic change is highest at the time of IED generation. On the other hand, negative BOLD responses, which are often related to IEDs accompanied by a prominent slow wave, have been proved to be important in localizing the

SOZ as well as positive responses (Kobayashi *et al.*, 2006; Pittau *et al.*, 2013; Rathakrishnan *et al.*, 2010), It is important to note, however, that negative responses are often present in the Default Mode Network and that such responses do not have localizing value (Coan *et al.*, 2014; Fahoum *et al.*, 2012; Fahoum *et al.*, 2013).

EEG-fMRI has demonstrated its ability to provide complementary information to localize epileptic foci in the presurgical evaluation of patients with medically intractable focal epilepsy (Rossi Sebastino *et al.*, 2020; Zijlmans *et al.*, 2007). FCD is a common pathology leading to drug-resistant focal epilepsy for which a surgical treatment is indicated, thus EEG-fMRI for FCD has been explored by several previous studies. The literature is summarized in **Table 1**. Three studies have specifically targeted FCD and the remaining studies have included patients with FCD and others. In most of them, IED-related BOLD clusters were compared to FCD lesions, SOZ or resection areas. Combining these results is difficult because many studies have only a small number of patients and the definition of concordance varies among the studies: some studies evaluated whether any one of the BOLD clusters overlapped with a lesion, SOZ or resection area while others showed whether the primary BOLD cluster (BOLD cluster with the largest absolute *t*-value) was concordant with the lesion. Nevertheless, the literature shows that IED-related BOLD signal responses are generally in good agreement with FCD lesions. Despite the heterogeneity of the published studies, we have combined them and found that BOLD clusters were concordant with lesions in approximately 67% of cases (16 of 24 cases) as well as with SOZ (20 of 31 cases). One can therefore infer that, in patients without an MRI-visible lesion, the BOLD response may provide a reasonable target for a possible FCD.

Table 1

Studies on EEG-fMRI for patients with FCD

Source	Number of patients with FCD included in analysis	What was reported in the study	Percentage of patients with concordant results	FCD type included in the analysis and number of patients for each type
Studies specifically for patients with FCD				
Federico *et al.*, 2005	5 (MRI-visible: 5)	Concordance between BOLD clusters and a lesion	3/5 (60%) (MRI-visible: 3)	FCD with balloon cells: 4
Thornton *et al.*, 2011	12 (MRI-visible: 9, MRI-negative: 3)	Concordance between BOLD clusters and SOZ identified with intracranial EEG	5/12 (41.6%) (MRI-visible: 2, MRI-negative: 3)	Type IIa: 3, Type IIb: 4 (N/A: 5)
Pittau *et al.*, 2017	13 (MRI-visible: 7, MRI-negative: 6)	Concordance between BOLD clusters and a lesion or a resection area	9/13 (69.2%) (MRI-visible: 6, MRI-negative: 3)	Type Ia: 1, Type IIa: 2, Type IIb: 5 (N/A: 5)
Studies partially including patients with FCD				
Diehl *et al.*, 2003	1 (MRI-visible: 1)	Concordance between BOLD clusters and a lesion	1/1 (100%) (MRI-visible: 1)	
Grova *et al.*, 2006	1 (MRI-visible: 1)	Concordance between BOLD clusters and a lesion	1/1 (100%) (MRI-visible: 1)	
Salek-Haddadi., 2006	2 (MRI-visible: 2)	Concordance between BOLD clusters and a lesion	0/2 (0%) (MRI-visible: 0)	
Tyvaert *et al.*, 2008	2 (MRI-visible: 2)	Concordance between the primary BOLD cluster and a lesion	2/2 (100%) (MRI-visible: 2)	
LeVan *et al.*, 2010	2 (MRI-visible: 2)	Concordance between BOLD clusters and a lesion	1/2 (50%) (MRI-visible: 1)	
Thornton *et al.*, 2010	3 (MRI-visible: 3)	A location of BOLD clusters and a surgical outcome	N/A	Type IIa: 3
Grouiller *et al.*, 2011	7 (MRI-visible: 4, MRI-negative: 3)	Concordance between BOLD clusters and a lesion or SOZ identified with intracranial EEG or a resection area	4/7 (57.1%) (MRI-visible: 2, MRI-negative: 2)	

Source	Number of patients with FCD included in analysis	What was reported in the study	Percentage of patients with concordant results	FCD type included in the analysis and number of patients for each type
Pittau *et al.*, 2011	1 (MRI-visible: 1)	Concordance between the primary BOLD cluster and SOZ identified with intracranial EEG	1/1 (100%) (MRI-visible: 1)	
Pittau *et al.*, 2012	2 (MRI-visible: 2)	Concordance between the primary BOLD cluster and spike fields in scalp EEG	2/2 (100%) (MRI-visible: 2)	
van Houdt *et al.*, 2012	1 (MRI-visible: 1)	Locations of BOLD clusters and SOZ identified with intracranial EEG	1/1 (100%) (MRI-visible: 1)	
Hauf *et al.*, 2012	4 (MRI-visible: 3, MRI-negative: 1)	Locations of BOLD clusters, a lesion and a resection area	N/A	
An *et al.*, 2013	11 (MRI-visible: 6, MRI-negative: 5)	Concordance between BOLD clusters and a resection area	6/11 (54.5%) (MRI-visible: 3, MRI-negative: 3)	Possible FCD type I: 1, Type IIa: 4, Type IIb: 5, Type IIIa: 1
Watanabe *et al.*, 2014	14	Difference in t-values of BOLD clusters in spike fields of scalp EEG between FCD and HS	N/A	
Coan *et al.*, 2015	3 (MRI-visible: 2, MRI-negative: 1)	Concordance between BOLD clusters and a resection area	2/3 (66.6%) (MRI-visible: 2)	Type II: 1, HS + FCD type IIa: 1, HS + FCD type IIb: 1
Khoo *et al.*, 2017	9 (MRI-visible: 5, MRI-negative: 4)	Concordance between the primary BOLD cluster and SOZ identified with intracranial EEG	8/9 (88.9%) (MRI-visible: 5, MRI-negative: 3)	
Kowalczyk *et al.*, 2020	3 (MRI-visible: 2, MRI-negative: 1)	Locations of BOLD clusters and a resection area	2/3 (66.6%)	Type IIb: 3
Rossi Sebastiano *et al.*, 2020	5	Concordance between BOLD clusters and SOZ identified with intracranial EEG	4/5 (80%)	Type Ia: 2, Type Ib: 1, Type IIa: 1, Type IIb: 1
Koupparis *et al.*, 2021	8 (MRI-visible: 8)	Concordance between the primary BOLD cluster and a resection area	3/8 (37.5%) (MRI-visible: 3)	
Our latest data				
Tanaka *et al.* (unpublished)	18 (MRI-visible: 18)	Concordance between the primary or secondary BOLD cluster and a lesion	9/18 (50.0%) (MRI-visible: 9) 7/11 (63.6%) in high confident results (MRI-visible: 7)	

BOLD: blood-oxygen-level dependent; FCD: focal cortical dysplasia; HS: hippocampal sclerosis; MRI-negative: patients for whom the MRI finding is normal; MRI-visible: patients for whom focal cortical dysplasia lesions are visible on the MRI; N/A: not available; SOZ: seizure-onset zone.

EEG-fMRI does not always give unambiguous results, for it also frequently reveals a widespread metabolic change involving distant regions. (Kobayashi *et al.*, 2005; Kobayashi *et al.*, 2006). We must determine which of the BOLD clusters are likely to correspond to the SOZ to use EEG-fMRI in clinical practice. Previous studies have shown that the most significant BOLD cluster (the primary BOLD cluster) has a high probability of being the SOZ (An *et al.*, 2013; Kobayashi *et al.*, 2005). Notably, it has been shown that the primary BOLD cluster is likely to be the SOZ when it stands out from the rest of the BOLD clusters, which we call here a high-confidence result (Khoo *et al.*, 2017; Koupparis *et al.*, 2021). Furthermore, it has been shown that surgical outcomes are poor if the primary BOLD cluster is not resected, i.e., EEG-fMRI has a high negative predictive value (An *et al.*, 2013; Coan *et al.*, 2015; Koupparis *et al.*, 2021; Pittau *et al.*, 2017). For FCD, it has also been shown that the primary BOLD cluster must be resected to obtain a good surgical outcome (Pittau *et al.*, 2017; Thornton *et al.*, 2011). EEG-fMRI has so far not had the ability to determine the limits of the resection, i.e. regions that must be resected to obtain seizure freedom (relatively low positive predictive value, Koupparis *et al.*, 2021).

Regarding the FCD pathology, no relationship has been shown between the BOLD signal responses and the histological FCD subtypes. The metabolic demand does not seem to be dependent on the FCD subtype (Pittau *et al.*, 2017).

The ability of EEG-fMRI to detect the SOZ has been similar between lesional and nonlesional epilepsy, which demonstrates the robustness of IED-related EEG-fMRI in localizing the SOZ, independently of the presence of a detectable structural anomaly (Khoo *et al.*, 2017). In MRI-negative FCD, a maximum BOLD signal response is also expected to help in guiding electrode implantation and detecting occult lesions. However, the relationship between MRI-negative FCD and BOLD signal response can only be evaluated in relation to the surgical resection. To analyze precisely the relationship on imaging between FCD lesions and BOLD signal responses, only patients with clearly-defined FCD lesions should be included in the analysis.

Montreal Neurological Institute Cases

We evaluated the concordance between FCD lesions and BOLD clusters in 18 consecutive patients who have FCD lesions clearly defined on MRI and IEDs during EEG-fMRI scans at the Montreal Neurological Institute. A case was considered concordant when the primary BOLD cluster or the secondary BOLD cluster, which is the BOLD cluster with the second largest *t*-value, is located within 10 mm from the edge of FCD lesion. Of 18 patients, 9 cases were concordant (50%). 11 of the 18 scans (61.1%) had high confident results fulfilling the previous study's criteria (Koupparis *et al.*, 2021). Of these 11 scans, 7 cases were concordant (63.6%). Of the 4 discordant cases, there was a large BOLD cluster spreading over 3 lobes or more and including the FCD lesion in 3. An example of concordant case is shown in **Figure 1**. Our results show that if high confident results are obtained, FCD lesions can be identified in about 64% cases by EEG-fMRI alone, and that BOLD signal responses often spread outside of FCD lesions.

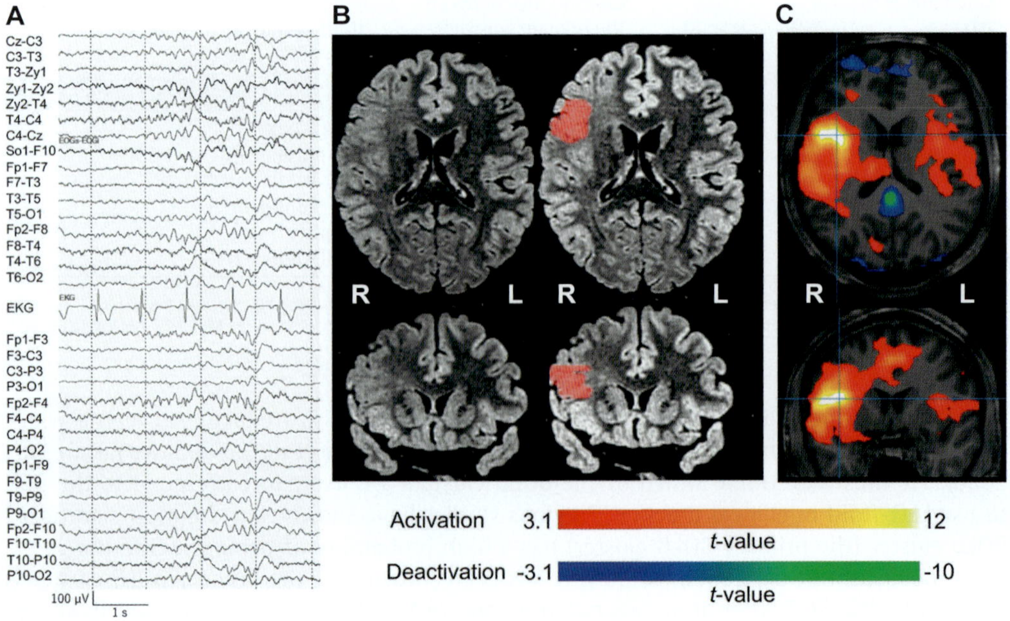

Figure 1

Representative results of EEG-fMRI for focal cortical dysplasia

A. Generalized rhythmic activity (37 events during the EEG-fMRI recording) with a maximum at Fp2, F8, F10, T4 and T10 were marked for analysis. B. MRI shows a dysplasic lesion (marked in red) involving the right inferior and middle frontal gyrus and the right frontal operculum. C. An activation BOLD cluster corresponding to the marked discharges involves the lesion. The voxel with the maximum *t*-value (13.1) of the cluster is inside the lesion.

Conclusion

EEG-fMRI is a useful non-invasive tool to complement other studies including EMSI and nuclear medicine imaging in a presurgical evaluation for FCD. Unlike EMSI, it is sensitive to epileptic discharges initiated deep in the brain and visible on scalp EEG or MEG as a result of propagation (Khoo *et al.*, 2018). If no discharge is visible on scalp EEG, however, then it is generally not possible to find a BOLD response.

References

Allen PJ, Polizzi G, Krakow K, *et al.* Identification of EEG events in the MR scanner: the problem of pulse artifact and a method for its subtraction. *NeuroImage* 1998; 8: 229-39.

An D, Fahoum F, Hall J, Olivier A, *et al.* Electroencephalography/functional magnetic resonance imaging responses help predict surgical outcome in focal epilepsy. *Epilepsia* 2013; 54: 2184-94.

Bénar C-G, Gross DW, Wang Y, *et al.* The BOLD Response to Interictal Epileptiform Discharges. *NeuroImage* 2002; 17: 1182-92.

Bénar C, Aghakhani Y, Wang Y, *et al.* Quality of EEG in simultaneous EEG-fMRI for epilepsy. *Clin Neurophysiol* 2003; 114: 569-80.

Bénar C-G, Grova C, Kobayashi E, *et al.* EEG-fMRI of epileptic spikes: Concordance with EEG source localization and intracranial EEG. *NeuroImage* 2006; 30: 1161-70.

Coan AC, Campos BM, Beltramini GC, *et al.* Distinct functional and structural MRI abnormalities in mesial temporal lobe epilepsy with and without hippocampal sclerosis. *Epilepsia* 2014; 55: 1187-96.

Coan AC, Chaudhary UJ, Frédéric G, *et al.* EEG-fMRI in the presurgical evaluation of temporal lobe epilepsy. *Journal of Neurology, Neurosurgery & Psychiatry* 2016; 87: 642-9.

Diehl B, Salek-haddadi A, Fish DR, Lemieux L. Mapping of spikes, slow waves, and motor tasks in a patient with malformation of cortical development using simultaneous EEG and fMRI. *Magn Reson Imaging* 2003; 21: 1167-73.

Fahoum F, Lopes R, Pittau F, *et al.* Widespread epileptic networks in focal epilepsies: EEG-fMRI study. *Epilepsia* 2012; 53: 1618-27.

Fahoum F, Zelmann R, Tyvaert L, *et al.* Epileptic discharges affect the default mode network--FMRI and intracerebral EEG evidence. *PLoS One* 8 2013: e68038.

Federico P, Archer JS, Abbott DF, Jackson GD. Cortical/subcortical BOLD changes associated with epileptic discharges: an EEG-fMRI study at 3 T. *Neurology* 2005; 64: 1125-30.

Grouiller F, Thornton RC, Groening K, *et al.* With or without spikes: localization of focal epileptic activity by simultaneous electroencephalography and functional magnetic resonance imaging. *Brain* 2011; 134: 2867-86.

Grova C, Daunizeau J, Kobayashi E, *et al.* Concordance between distributed EEG source localization and simultaneous EEG-fMRI studies of epileptic spikes. *NeuroImage* 2008; 39: 755-74.

Hauf M, Jann K, Schindler K, *et al.* Localizing Seizure-Onset Zones in Presurgical Evaluation of Drug-Resistant Epilepsy by Electroencephalography/fMRI: Effectiveness of Alternative Thresholding Strategies. *American Journal of Neuroradiology* 2012; 33: 1818-24.

Khoo HM, Hao Y, von Ellenrieder N, *et al.* The hemodynamic response to interictal epileptic discharges localizes the seizure-onset zone. *Epilepsia* 2017; 58: 811-23.

Khoo HM, von Ellenrieder N, Zazubovits N, *et al.* The spike onset zone: The region where epileptic spikes start and from where they propagate. *Neurology* 2018; 91: e666-74.

Kobayashi E, Bagshaw AP, Jansen A, *et al.* Intrinsic epileptogenicity in polymicrogyric cortex suggested by EEG-fMRI BOLD responses. *Neurology* 2005; 64: 1263-6.

Kobayashi E, Bagshaw AP, Bénar CG, *et al.* Temporal and extratemporal BOLD responses to temporal lobe interictal spikes. *Epilepsia* 2006; 47: 343-54.

Koupparis A, von Ellenrieder N, Khoo HM, *et al.* Association of EEG-fMRI Responses and Outcome After Epilepsy Surgery. *Neurology* 2021; 97: e1523-6.

Kowalczyk MA, Omidvarnia A, Abbott DF, *et al.* Clinical benefit of presurgical EEG-fMRI in difficult-to-localize focal epilepsy: A single-institution retrospective review. *Epilepsia* 2019; 61: 49iaon

LeVan P, Tyvaert L, Moeller F, Gotman J Independent component analysis reveals dynamic ictal BOLD responses in EEG-fMRI data from focal epilepsy patients. *NeuroImage*; 49: 366-78.

Pittau F, LeVan P, Moeller F, *et al.* Changes preceding interictal epileptic EEG abnormalities: Comparison between EEG/fMRI and intracerebral EEG. *Epilepsia* 2011; 52: 1120-9.

Pittau F, Dubeau F, Gotman J Contribution of EEG/fMRI to the definition of the epileptic focus. *Neurology* 2012; 78: 1479-87.

Pittau F, Fahoum F, Zelmann R, *et al.* Negative BOLD response to interictal epileptic discharges in focal epilepsy. *Brain Topogr* 2013; 26: 627-40.

Pittau F, Ferri L, Fahoum F, *et al.* Contributions of EEG-fMRI to Assessing the Epileptogenicity of Focal Cortical Dysplasia. *Frontiers in Computational Neuroscience* 2017; 11.

Rathakrishnan R, Moeller F, Levan P, *et al.* BOLD signal changes preceding negative responses in EEG-fMRI in patients with focal epilepsy. *Epilepsia* 2010; 51: 1837-45.

Rossi Sebastiano D, Tassi L, Duran D, *et al.* Identifying the EZ by four non-invasive imaging techniques versus stereo-EEG in MRI-negative pre-surgery epilepsy patients. *Clinical Neurophysiology* 2020; 131: 1815-23.

Salek-Haddadi A, Diehl B, Hamandi K, *et al.* Hemodynamic correlates of epileptiform discharges: An EEG-fMRI study of 63 patients with focal epilepsy. *Brain Research* 2006; 1088: 148-166.

Thornton R, Laufs H, Rodionov R, *et al.* EEG correlated functional MRI and postoperative outcome in focal epilepsy. *Journal of Neurology, Neurosurgery & Psychiatry* 2010; 81: 922-7.

Thornton R, Vulliemoz S, Rodionov R, *et al.* Epileptic networks in Focal Cortical Dysplasia revealed using electroencephalography-functional magnetic resonance imaging. *Annals of Neurology* 2011; 70: 822-37.

Tyvaert L, Hawco C, Kobayashi E, *et al.* Different structures involved during ictal and interictal epileptic activity in malformations of cortical development: an EEG-fMRI study. *Brain* 2008; 131: 2042-60.

van Houdt PJ, Ossenblok PPW, Colon AJ, *et al.* A framework to integrate EEG-correlated fMRI and intracerebral recordings. *NeuroImage* 2012; 60: 2042-53.

Watanabe S, An D, Safi-Harb M, *et al.* Hemodynamic Response Function (HRF) in Epilepsy Patients with Hippocampal Sclerosis and Focal Cortical Dysplasia. *Brain Topography* 2014; 27: 613-9.

Zijlmans M, Huiskamp G, Hersevoort M, *et al.* EEG-fMRI in the preoperative work-up for epilepsy surgery. *Brain* 2007; 130: 2343-53.

Part IV. IMAGING OF FCD: THE DECISIVE STEP

CHAPTER

15. The role of imaging in FCD: an overview

John S. Duncan

Key points

- MRI provides increasingly sensitive detection and characterization of FCD, with advances in magnet technology and strength, gradients and acquisitions.
- Magnetic resonance spectroscopy reveals abnormalities of neurometabolic profile in FCD but lacks specificity.
- Post-acquisition processing of T1-W, FLAIR and diffusion MRI data provide further sensitivity.
- Electrical and ESI-MSI and EEG-fMRI may be useful for determining the co-location of interictal epileptic discharges with FCD.
- ^{18}F-FDG-PET commonly shows hypometabolism in and around FCD and is particularly helpful in individuals with normal appearing MRI.
- Ligand PET, for example with ^{11}C-flumazenil, methionine and tryptophan, have had some research use but have not had clinical impact.
- Ictal SPECT can be useful for localizing cerebral areas involved in seizure onset and propagation.

Imaging of FCD structure

Some cases of gross FCD could be visualized with X-ray CT, but it was evident from the 1980s that MRI has superior sensitivity for identifying and delineating FCD (Nowell *et al.* 1988, Otsubo *et al.* 1993, Andermann 2000).

The advent of FLAIR in the 1990s (Bergin *et al.* 1995) and 3T MRI in 2000, with a combination of thin slice 2D- and 3D-FLAIR increased the ability to visualise FCD in vivo (Tschampa *et al.* 2015). The cardinal features of FCD are thickening of the grey matter ribbon, blurring of the grey-white interface, increased FLAIR signal in the white matter and abnormal gyral architecture. In FCD IIB, with balloon cells, there is often a striking increase in FLAIR signal extending towards the underlying ventricle, the so called "transmantle sign" reflecting dysmyelination.

FCD I is less easy to discern on MRI (**Table 1**) (Widdess-Walsh *et al.* 2005) and may not be visible in vivo. FCD IIB is the most evident, but may be subtle and discrete and not evident on current MRI, particularly at the bottom of sulci. The optimal sensitivity of MRI detection is contingent

FCD	MRI features	Histology	MRI features
1A	Isolated lesion, radial	Dyslamination	**Blurring of the grey-white junction without increased FLAIR signal**
1B	Isolated lesion, tangential	Dyslamination	**Blurring of the grey-white junction without increased FLAIR signal**
2A	Isolated lesion	Cortical dyslamination and dysmorphic neurons	Abnormal thickening of the cortex with blurring of the grey-white junction and increased signal on FLAIR
2B	Isolated lesion	Cortical dyslamination and dysmorphic neurons Balloon cells	**Focal cortical thickening, often at bottom of a sulcus with blurring of grey-white matter junction** Transmantle sign of increased signal on FLAIR
3A	FCD + hippocampal sclerosis		
3B	FCD + tumour		
3C	FCD + vascular malformation		
3D	FCD + early acquired lesion		

Table 1
Classification of Focal Cortical Dysplasia (Blumcke *et al.*, 2011)

not only on magnet field strength, but also acquisition protocol optimization, with thin slice 2D and 3D FLAIR and T1-volumetric sequences. Critically, images need to be reviewed by a neuroradiologist experienced in epilepsy and a neurologist who knows the nuances of the individual's semiology and EEG, and the likely sites of underlying pathology. Much effort needs to be exerted to identify currently covert FCD, as part of presurgical evaluation.

There is an increased yield of visualizing subtle structural FCD that were not evident on 1.5T and 3T acquisitions, with 7T acquisitions (Opheim *et al.* 2021) (**Figure 1**). A caveat is that not every structural abnormality is causally related to epilepsy (Salehi *et al.* 2021). In a systematic review of 275 patients in 16 studies, the overall extra yield was 31%, with particular yield of FCD, hippocampal sclerosis and gliosis (Van Lanen *et al.* 2021). In general, T2* sequences gave good yield. 3D FLAIR was best for detecting FCD and 3D T2* clarified the internal structure and extent of dysplasia.

Morphometric analysis can help to detect subtle FCD. The Morphometric Analysis Program highlights FCD on the junction image (blurred grey/white matter junction) and extension image (grey matter extending into white matter (Huppertz *et al.* 2005). Using an MP2RAGE2 sequence that improves homogeneity of T1-contrast, and corrects B_1 inhomogeneities, junction images from morphometric analysis shows abnormalities with greater sensitivity and precision, than on standard MPRAGE junction images (Demerath *et al.* 2020, Urbach *et al.* 2021) (**Figure 2**).

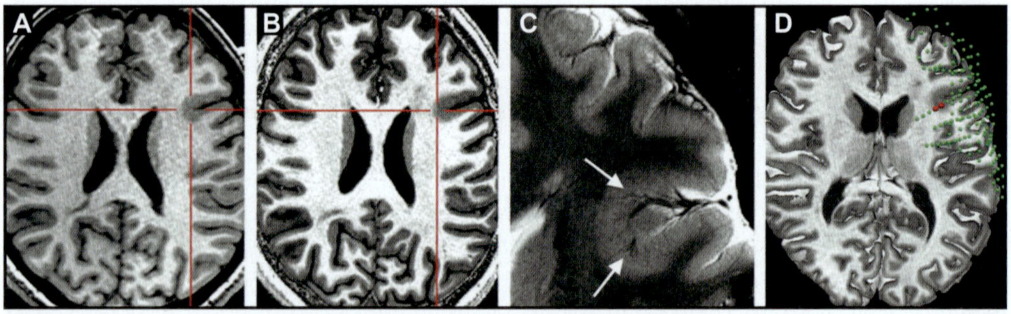

Figure 1

Increased sensitivity to detect Focal Cortical Dysplasia at 7T.

A. Axial 3T T_1-weighted MPRAGE (read as normal).

B. Axial 7T T_1-weighted MP2RAGE.

C. Axial 7T T_2*-weighted GRE. Vascular changes associated with FCD évident.

D. Seizure onset with intracranial-EEG (reproduced from Opheim *et al.* 2021).

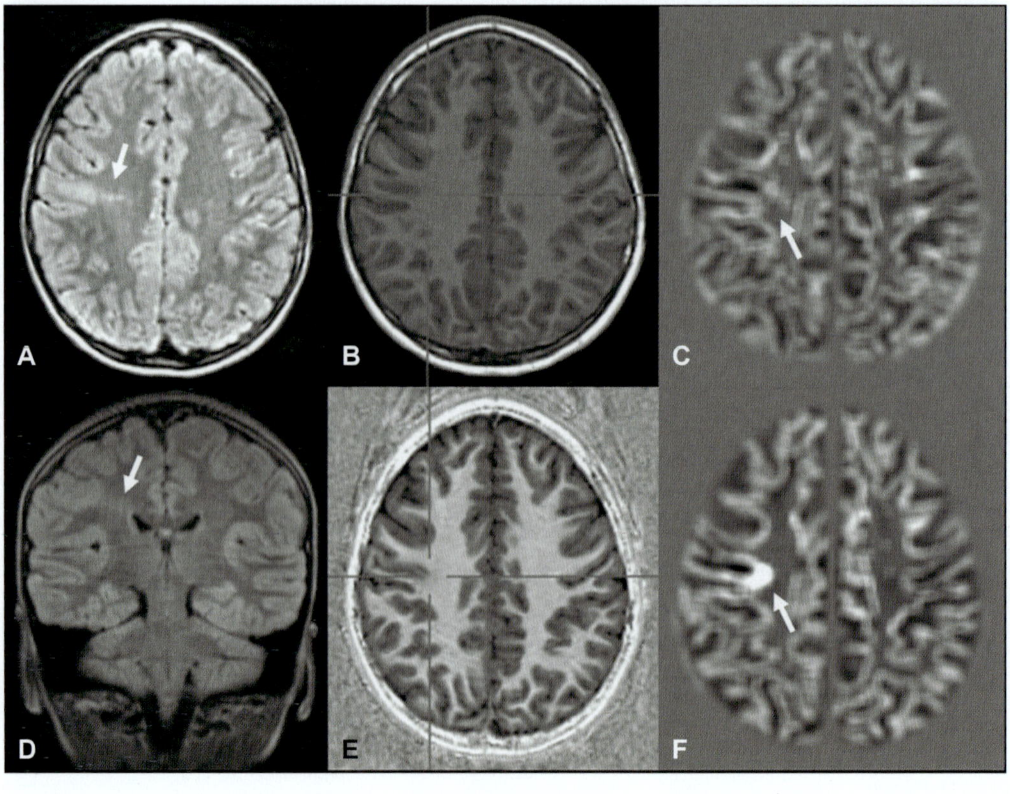

Figure 2

Junction images improved with refined MPRAGE2.

FCD with the transmantle sign of the right precentral gyrus. The lesion is visible on FLAIR (A and D) and MP2RAGE-based junction images (F). In an MPRAGE-based junction image (C) for comparison, the lesion is not clearly seen. Strong T1WI contrast is seen in a uniform MP2RAGE image (E) compared with MPRAGE (B). (reproduced from Demerath *et al.* 2020)

The Multicentre Epilepsy Lesion Detection Project (MELD) is an automated analysis program that uses a trained neural network classifier based on cortical surface data, with increased detection of FCD (Adler *et al.* 2016) and a high degree of co-localization with seizure onset identified on SEEG (Wagstyl *et al.* 2020). Ongoing work in a multicentre study has shown that FCD have a predilection for localization in superior frontal sulcus, pole and temporal pole.

Multicentre assessment of a Deep Learning Detection Algorithm has shown a 93% sensitivity to detect FCD, with an average of 6 false positives per patient, and a sensitivity to detect FCD in visually normal MRI of 85% (Gill *et al.* 2021). In all analysis programmes applied to individual patient care, there is a balance of sensitivity and specificity to be struck. Methods with high sensitivity and low specificity are useful to apply as a screening tool. High specificity, with low sensitivity is helpful to confirm relevance of a putative abnormality. It is always crucial to critically appraise the concordance of findings with electroclinical data.

Further analysis of MRI data promises more detailed classification of FCD in vivo, that may facilitate individualized treatment planning. Unsupervised machine learning analysis of MRI of 46 patients with histologically-verified FCD IIB and IIA, based on cortical thickness, FLAIR intensity, T1W/FLAIR ratio and T1W and FLAIR gradients has shown lesional variability on a millimetric scale, reflecting cellular variability across and within FCD and identified four classes with distinct profiles within a given FCD (Lee *et al.* 2020).

Diffusion MR imaging

Diffusion tensor imaging (DTI) in FCD has shown reduced fractional anisotropy (FA) in the vicinity of FCD, reduction of tract volume (Lee *et al.* 2004), and FA between FCD and subcortical white matter (Diehl *et al.* 2010), also in thalamocortical pathways ipsilateral to FCD (Rezayev 2018). Further, the local efficiency of structural connectivity was reduced in those with FCD (Lee *et al.* 2021), indicating the network-effects of apparently localized FCD.

Diffusion tensor imaging based measures and T2-weighted MRI, showed similar ability to detect FCD, but when these were combined in a multimodal Gaussian processes for machine learning (GPML) classifier, there was improved performance (Wang *et al.* 2018). Recently developed models of diffusion MRI such as the spherical mean technique (SMT) and neurite orientation dispersion and density imaging (NODDI) provide measurements and maps of abnormality that are more specific for abnormal microstructure, than are measures of FA and mean diffusivity (MD). Intracellular volume fraction (ICVF), now often referred to as neurite density index (NDI), was reduced in FCD and abnormalities were more visually evident than on T1-weighted, FLAIR, FA or MD images (Winston *et al.* 2014). Further, the visibility of FCD on NODDI ICVF maps was better than in FLAIR and T1-weighted imaging in 15% patients, and SMT intra-neurite volume fraction (INVF) in 9%. Lesion detection on ICVF was better than FA or MD in 82%, and INVF was better than MD and FA in 61%. FCD was associated with reduced ICVF and INVF, and increased radial, and axial diffusivities with greater changes in FCD IIB than IIA (Lorio *et al.* 2020).

Magnetic resonance spectroscopy

The in vivo biochemistry of FCD can be probed with magnetic resonance spectroscopy (MRS). Limitations of in vivo MRS are the size of the voxels needed to give sufficient signal to noise, and the inability to distinguish between metabolic and neurotransmitter pools of neuroactive metabolites. Increased choline and decreased N-acetyl-aspartate concentration has been reported in FCD (Tschampa *et al.* 2015). This metabolic signature is not unique to FCD and has been reported in a range of other aetiologies of epilepsy. Raised γ-aminobutyric acid (GABA) levels, which also contained signals from macromolecules and homocarnosine, with no change in glutathione, and the combination of glutamate and glutamine (Gong *et al.* 2021). It remains unclear therefore whether the reported increase was due to GABA or macromolecules, and the compartment in which the GABA was located.

Imaging epileptogenicity in FCD

Simultaneous scalp EEG-fMRI can assist identification of the epileptogenic focus in pharmacoresistant focal epilepsy by mapping haemodynamic changes associated with IED (Van Eyndhoven *et al.* 2021). In 23 patients with FCD having presurgical evaluation, 11 had IED during EEG-fMRI with significant associated haemodynamic changes. The EEG-fMRI results were compatible with a single SOZ on intracranial EEG in 5 of 11, and four of these had greater than 50% reduction in seizures after resection. The remaining six had widespread or discordant regions of IED-related changes in fMRI signal. Five of these 6 had either a poor surgical outcome or a widespread SOZ that ruled out surgery. The implication is that EEG-fMRI may provide useful data about the SOZ in FCD and that discordant regions of IED-related haemodynamic changes implicated a widespread SOZ in association with FCD and are predictive of poor seizure outcome from resection (Thornton *et al.* 2011). In 20 patients with FCD and focal epilepsy, BOLD responses on EEG-fMRI that were concordant with the spike field were recorded in 13 and in nine of these at least one BOLD response was concordant with the FCD. This suggests a potential role of EEG-fMRI for confirming the epileptogenicity of FCD and to aid localization of the irritative zone in those with normal MRI. Further, the finding of distant BOLD changes indicates the widespread nature of the epileptic network associated with FCD (Pittau *et al.* 2017).

Electrical source imaging (ESI) based on scalp EEG combined with MRI data has been demonstrated to localize IED (Tamilia 2020). ESI derived from scalp EEG was thought to be helpful in delineating the irritative zone in 41 individuals with MCD, with highest rate of concordance being found in FCD (Abdallah *et al.* 2017). ESI applied to intracranial IED and ictal epileptic activity may assist the localization of the EZ in relation to FCD (Alhilani *et al.* 2020).

MSI of interictal epileptic activity in individuals with FCD has shown a localization within 12+/-8mm of MRI lesion, with seizure-free outcome related to complete excision of the magnetic source (Kasper *et al.* 2018).

In summary, it appears that ESI of scalp and intracranial EEG data, and MSI data may be a valuable addition to localization of epileptic activity in individuals with drug-resistant focal epilepsy and FCD who are being considered for epilepsy surgery. ESI can be recording for a longer duration and at a fraction of the cost of MEG data for MSI. The advent of optically pumped magnetoencephalography (OP-MEG), however, offers the opportunity for prolonged MEG recordings (Seymour *et al.* 2021).

Isotope imaging of FCD

Interictal hypometabolism visualized with ^{18}F-fluoro-deoxyglucose PET has a long established role in lateralizing and broadly localizing the likely source of refractory focal epilepsy, particularly in individuals with normal-appearing MRI. An important clinical point is that if there is an area of focal hypometabolism, review of MRI may lead to identification of a subtle FCD, commonly at the bottom of a sulcus (Berlangieri *et al.* 2020) (**Figure 3**). As would be expected, co-registration of MRI and PET data and integration with clinical and EEG data improves the ability to localize FCD (Desarnaud *et al.* 2018).

Both decreased and increased binding of ^{11}C-flumazenil to $GABA_A$ receptors has been shown in FCD (Richardson *et al.* 1996, Arnold *et al.* 2000). ^{11}C-methionine PET has been suggested to aid the differentiation of FCD from mixed glial-neuronal tumours (Phi *et al.* 2010). This is not widely available however, and the clinical impact of this method is not established. ^{11}C-alpha-methyl-L-tryptophan PET has been suggested to be helpful in determining which tuber, in individuals with tuberous sclerosis, is giving rise to seizures (Chugani *et al.* 2013), and was suggested 20 years ago to be potentially useful for identifying occult FCD (Fedi *et al.* 2001). These results however have not been widely replicated and reliance on an on-site cyclotron to produce ^{11}C-labelled isotopes precludes clinical application.

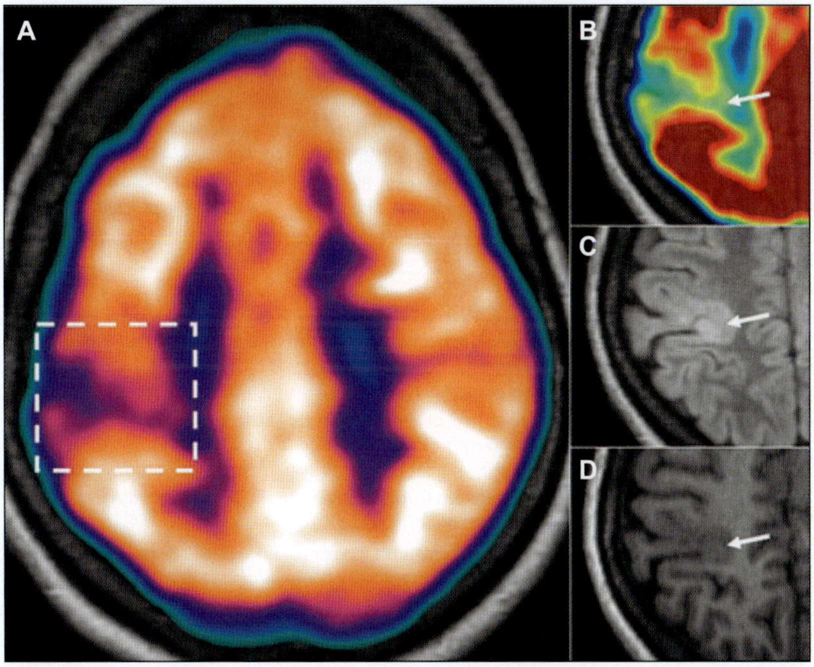

Figure 3

Bottom of sulcus Focal Cortical Dysplasia on ^{18}F-FDG PET and MRI.

A. Coregistered ^{18}F-FDG-PET and MRI data. Focal hypometabolism is shown in the dashed box

B. Area of PET hypometabolism

C. FLAIR image shows T2 hyperintensity

D. Hypointensity on T1-weightedMRI (reproduced from Berlangieri *et al.* 2020)

Ictal single-photon emission computerized tomography (SPECT) has been used for decades to assist the localization of the SOZ and is useful to assist the identification of FCD and localization of the site of seizure onset (Gupta *et al.* 2004). Successful ictal SPECT requires a high degree of multidisciplinary organization on the EEG monitoring unit and Nuclear Medicine Department. A limitation is that with short seizures, lasting less than 30 seconds, it is inevitable that even with an injection made within 5 seconds of clinical and/or scalp EEG seizure onset, the perfusion pattern demonstrated will be of areas that represent seizure spread or are post-ictal. It is also noteworthy that ictal hyperperfusion shown with SISCOM frequently overlays FCD and that complete resection of the area of hyperperfusion is not essential to get a seizure free outcome (Dupont *et al.* 2006).

Conclusion

The structure and function of FCD may be visualized with a range of techniques that are based on MRI, nuclear medicine, electrical and magnetic abnormalities. Together these methods can produce multimodal 3D maps of FCD, that may be integrated to better understand the underlying neurobiology and to guide clinical practice.

Other chapters address the details of the individual structural and functional imaging techniques described.

References

Abdallah C, Maillard LG, Rikir E, *et al.* Localizing value of electrical source imaging: Frontal lobe, malformations of cortical development and negative MRI related epilepsies are the best candidates. *Neuroimage Clin.* 2017; 16: 319-29.

Adler S, Wagstyl K, Gunny R, *et al.* Novel surface features for automated detection of Focal Cortical Dysplasias in paediatric epilepsy. *Neuroimage Clin.* 2016; 14: 18-27.

Alhilani M, Tamilia E, Ricci L, *et al.* Ictal and interictal source imaging on intracranial EEG predicts epilepsy surgery outcome in children with Focal Cortical Dysplasia. *Clin Neurophysiol.* 2020; 131: 734-43.

Andermann F. Cortical dysplasias and epilepsy: a review of the architectonic, clinical, and seizure patterns. *Adv Neurol.* 2000; 84: 479-96.

Arnold S, Berthele A, Drzezga A, *et al.* Reduction of benzodiazepine receptor binding is related to the seizure-onset zone in extratemporal Focal Cortical Dysplasia. *Epilepsia.* 2000; 41: 818-24.

Bergin PS, Fish DR, Shorvon SD, Oatridge A, deSouza NM, Bydder GM. Magnetic resonance imaging in partial epilepsy: additional abnormalities shown with the fluid attenuated inversion recovery (FLAIR) pulse sequence. *J Neurol Neurosurg Psychiatry.* 1995; 58: 439-43.

Berlangieri SU, Mito R, Semmelroch M, Pedersen M, Jackson G. Bottom-of-sulcus dysplasia: the role of ^{18}F-FDG PET in identifying a focal surgically remedial epileptic lesion. *Eur J Hybrid Imaging.* 2020; 4: 23.

Bernasconi N, Bernasconi A. Multicenter validation of a deep learning detection algorithm for Focal Cortical Dysplasia. *Neurology.* 2021; 97: e1571-82.

Blümcke I, Thom M, Aronica E, *et al.* The clinicopathologic spectrum of Focal Cortical Dysplasias: a consensus classification proposed by an ad hoc Task Force of the ILAE Diagnostic Methods Commission. *Epilepsia.* 2011; 52: 158-74.

Chugani HT, Luat AF, Kumar A, Govindan R, Pawlik K, Asano E. α-[11C]-Methyl-L-tryptophan--PET in 191 patients with tuberous sclerosis complex. *Neurology.* 2013; 81: 674-80.

Demerath T, Rubensdörfer L, Schwarzwald R, *et al.* Morphometric MRI analysis: improved detection of Focal Cortical Dysplasia using the MP2RAGE sequence. *AJNR Am J Neuroradiol* 2020; 41: 1009-14.

Desarnaud S, Mellerio C, Semah F, *et al.* ^{18}F-FDG PET in drug-resistant epilepsy due to Focal Cortical Dysplasia type 2: additional value of electroclinical data and coregistration with MRI. *Eur J Nucl Med Mol Imaging.* 2018; 45: 1449-60.

Diehl B, Tkach J, Piao Z, *et al.* Diffusion tensor imaging in patients with focal epilepsy due to cortical dysplasia in the temporo-occipital region: electro-clinico-pathological correlations. *Epilepsy Res.* 2010; 90: 178-87.

Dupont P, Van Paesschen W, Palmini A, *et al.* Ictal perfusion patterns associated with single MRI-visible focal dysplastic lesions: implications for the noninvasive delineation of the epileptogenic zone. *Epilepsia.* 2006; 47: 1550-7.

Fedi M, Reutens D, Okazawa H, *et al.* Localizing value of alpha-methyl-L-tryptophan PET in intractable epilepsy of neocortical origin. *Neurology.* 2001; 57: 1629-36.

Gill RS, Lee HM, Caldairou B, *et al.* Multicenter validation of a deep learning detection algorithm for Focal Cortical Dysplasia. *Neurology.* 2021; 97: e1571-82.

Gong T, Liu Y, Chen Y, Lin L, Lin Y, Wang G. Focal Cortical Dysplasia in epilepsy is associated with GABA increase. *Neuroimage Clin.* 2021; 31: 102763.

Gupta A, Raja S, Kotagal P, Lachhwani D, Wyllie E, Bingaman WB. Ictal SPECT in children with partial epilepsy due to Focal Cortical Dysplasia. *Pediatr Neurol.* 2004; 31: 89-95.

Huppertz HJ, Grimm C, Fauser S, *et al.* Enhanced visualization of blurred gray-white matter junctions in Focal Cortical Dysplasia by voxel-based 3D MRI analysis. *Epilepsy Res.* 2005; 67: 35-50.

Kasper BS, Rössler K, Hamer HM, *et al.* Coregistrating magnetic source and magnetic resonance imaging for epilepsy surgery in Focal Cortical Dysplasia. *Neuroimage Clin.* 2018; 19: 487-96.

Lee DA, Lee HJ, Kim HC, Park KM. Alterations of structural connectivity and structural co-variance network in Focal Cortical Dysplasia. *BMC Neurol.* 2021; 21: 330.

Lee HM, Gill RS, Fadaie F, *et al.* Unsupervised machine learning reveals lesional variability in Focal Cortical Dysplasia at mesoscopic scale. *Neuroimage Clin.* 2020; 28: 102438.

Lee SK, Kim DI, Mori S, *et al.* Diffusion tensor MRI visualizes decreased subcortical fiber connectivity in Focal Cortical Dysplasia. *Neuroimage.* 2004; 22: 1826-9.

Lorio S, Adler S, Gunny R, *et al.* MRI profiling of Focal Cortical Dysplasia using multi-compartment diffusion models. *Epilepsia.* 2020; 61: 433-44.

Nowell MA, Grossman RI, Packer R, *et al.* Focal Cortical Dysplasia on magnetic resonance imaging: a case report. *J Comput Tomogr.* 1988; 12: 61-3.

Opheim G, van der Kolk A, Markenroth Bloch K, *et al.* 7T Epilepsy Task. Force consensus recommendations on the use of 7T MRI in clinical practice. *Neurology* 2021; 96: 327-41.

Otsubo H, Hwang PA, Jay V, *et al.* Focal Cortical Dysplasia in children with localization-related epilepsy: EEG, MRI, and SPECT findings. *Pediatr Neurol.* 1993; 9: 101-7.

Phi JH, Paeng JC, Lee HS, *et al.* Evaluation of Focal Cortical Dysplasia and mixed neuronal and glial tumors in pediatric epilepsy patients using 18F-FDG and 11C-methionine PET. *J Nucl Med.* 2010; 51: 728-34.

Pittau F, Ferri L, Fahoum F, Dubeau F, Gotman J. Contributions of EEG-fMRI to assessing the epileptogenicity of Focal Cortical Dysplasia. *Front Comput Neurosci.* 2017 20; 11: 8.

Rezayev A, Feldman HA, Levman J, Takahashi E. Bilateral thalamocortical abnormalities in Focal Cortical Dysplasia. *Brain Res.* 2018; 1694: 38-45.

Richardson MP, Koepp MJ, Brooks DJ, Fish DR, Duncan JS. Benzodiazepine receptors in focal epilepsy with cortical dysgenesis: an 11C-flumazenil PET study. *Ann Neurol.* 1996; 40: 188-98.

Salehi F, Nadeem IM, Kwan BYM, *et al.* Ultra-high field 7-Tesla magnetic resonance imaging and electroencephalography findings in epilepsy. *Can Assoc Radiol J* 2021; 30: 8465371211031802.

Seymour RA, Alexander N, Mellor S, *et al.* Using OPMs to measure neural activity in standing, mobile participants. *Neuroimage* 2021; 244: 118604.

Tamilia E, Dirodi M, Alhilani M *et al.* Scalp ripples as prognostic biomarkers of epileptogenicity in pediatric surgery. *Ann Clin Transl Neurol* 2020; 7: 329–42.

Thornton R, Vulliemoz S, Rodionov R, *et al.* Epileptic networks in Focal Cortical Dysplasia revealed using electroencephalography-functional magnetic resonance imaging. *Ann Neurol.* 2011; 70: 822-37.

Tschampa HJ, Urbach H, Malter M, Surges R, Greschus S, Gieseke J. Magnetic resonance imaging of Focal Cortical Dysplasia: Comparison of 3D and 2D fluid attenuated inversion recovery sequences at 3T. *Epilepsy Res.* 2015; 116: 8-14.

Tschampa HJ, Urbach H, Träber F, *et al.* Proton magnetic resonance spectroscopy in Focal Cortical Dysplasia at 3T. *Seizure.* 2015; 32: 23-9.

Urbach H, Heers M, Altenmueller DM, *et al.* "Within a minute" detection of Focal Cortical Dysplasia. *Neuroradiology.* 2021.

Van Eyndhoven S, Dupont P, Tousseyn S, *et al.* Augmenting interictal mapping with neurovascular coupling biomarkers by structured factorization of epileptic EEG and fMRI data. *NeuroImage* 2021; 228: 117652.

Van Lanen RHGJ, Colon AJ, Wiggins CJ, *et al.* Ultra-high field magnetic resonance imaging in human epilepsy: A systematic review. *Neuroimage Clin* 2021; 30: 102602.

Wagstyl K, Adler S, Pimpel B, *et al.* Planning stereoelectroencephalography using automated lesion detection: Retrospective feasibility study. *Epilepsia.* 2020; 61: 1406-16.

Wang Y, Zhou Y, Wang H, *et al.* Voxel-based automated detection of Focal Cortical Dysplasia lesions using diffusion tensor imaging and T2-weighted MRI data. *Epilepsy Behav.* 2018; 84: 127-134.

Widdess-Walsh P, Kellinghaus C, Jeha L, *et al.* Electro-clinical and imaging characteristics of Focal Cortical Dysplasia: correlation with pathological subtypes. *Epilepsy Res.* 2005; 67: 25-33.

Winston GP, Micallef C, Symms MR, Alexander DC, Duncan JS, Zhang H. Advanced diffusion imaging sequences could aid assessing patients with Focal Cortical Dysplasia and epilepsy. *Epilepsy Res.* 2014; 108: 336-9.

CHAPTER

16. Morphological and functional MRI for FCD in clinical practice

Charles Mellerio

Key points

- An optimized protocol is essential for FCD visualization. Three high-resolution sequences are mandatory: 3D gradient echo T1-weigted, 3D FLAIR and 2D coronal spin echo T2-weighted.
- Additional sequences and optional advanced images can be added to improve lesion detection.
- MR signature of FCD includes thickened and blurred gray-white matter interface, cortical and subcortical signal change that occasionally linearly tapper to the ventricle surface leading to a transmantle sign and sulco-gyral abnormalities. Even though highly characteristic, these MR signs are often very subtle or absent.
- Functional reorganization may be observed in dysplastic regions. Functional MRI is helpful to identify eloquent areas in the vicinity of the dysplastic cortex and prevent postoperative deficits.

Introduction

In the past years, MRI has led to dramatic advances in the ability to study brain structures, owing to higher magnetic field strength, multiplication of phased array head coil elements, new advanced sequences, dedicated protocols and better post-processing solutions. These rapid technical advances in MRI have allowed identification of the underlying etiology in a growing percentage of patients with epilepsy, thus contributing to a steady increase of surgical candidates. Importantly, in addition to detection and characterization of lesions by morphological MRI, imaging also plays a crucial role in the localization of eloquent cortical areas through functional MRI to reduce the risk of postoperative deficits.

Although MRI has been of enormous importance to identify dysplastic lesions, FCD is still one of the most difficult lesions to detect with imaging techniques, because of their often small size and contrast similarity to normal contiguous cortex. Optimization of MR protocols and careful review of images - often incorporating clinical and neurophysiological data - are thus essential to the best management of patients.

In this chapter, I will detail the "ideal" protocol for FCD imaging, highlighting the mandatory sequences. The typical MR semiology of FCD will then be analyzed, emphasizing the features of FCD II, the most recognizable and characteristic subtype. Following this, I will insist on the main pitfalls that may lead the clinician to overlook or mischaracterize a FCD lesion and, finally, the role of functional MRI in the preoperative workup will be discussed.

MRI technique for FCD detection: what is mandatory?

A "standard" MR protocol is ineffective for detecting FCD (Oertzen *et al.*, 2002) and the detection of FCD is improved when reviewed by experts who have been provided with clinical information and results from other investigations (Gaillard *et al.*, 2009; Bernasconi *et al.*, 2019). Moreover, an optimized protocol combining volumetric acquisition is required, with high spatial and contrast resolution allowing multiplanar reformatting, delineation of gyral structures and identification of subtle cortical lesions (Wellmer *et al.*, 2013).

• Which sequences?

A recent taskforce of the international league against epilepsy (ILAE) defined an harmonized imaging protocol that can be considered as the minimal standards for FCD MR imaging (Bernasconi *et al.*, 2019; Wang *et al.*, 2020). The basic "essential" and advanced optional sequences are listed in table 1. Injection of a contrast medium (Gadolinium) is not required in most cases.

Table 1

Imaging protocol for patients referred for Focal Cortical Dysplasia: Mandatory and optional sequences

Mandatory sequences (according to ILAE)	Requirement	Benefits
High-resolution 3D T1	Gradient Echo (SPGR, MPRAGE, TFE...) Isotropic millimetric voxel resolution (< 1 × 1 × 1 mm^3, no interslice gap)	Excellent spatial resolution Optimal evaluation of brain anatomy and morphology Multiplanar/curvilinear/volumetric reformat May detect subtle sulco-gyral and cortical abnormalities
High-resolution 3D fluid-attenuated inversion recovery (FLAIR)	Isotropic millimetric voxel resolution (< 1 × 1 × 1 mm^3, no interslice gap)	Excellent contrast resolution of subcortical abnomalies Multiplanar reformat Nulling of CSF signal enhances visibility of cortical pathologies such as abnormal cells Caution: Not sensitive in neonates and infants<2 years, as the myelination process is not yet complete
High in-plane resolution coronal spin echo T2	Submillimetric voxel resolution (eg, 0.4 × 0.4 × 2 mm, no interslice, oriented in the axis perpendicular to hippocampus	Excellent in plane contrast resolution Delination of the cortex and especially of hippocampus (digitations loss, dedifferentiation)
Axial T2 Gradient echo (or susceptibility weighted imaging)		Calcification sensitive sequences for differential diagnosis (trauma/scar, vascular malformations/cavernomas, tuber with calcifications)
Additional/optional sequences		
Volumetric T2 with double inversion recovery	Slice thickness < 2mm	Suppression of the signal from both white matter and CSF May provide better contrast for cortical lesion detection
Arterial spin labeling (ASL)	Post labelling delay depending on the age of the patient (1 to 1.5s in children/>1.5 s in adults)	Quantitative maps of cortical perfusion Post ictal hyperperfusion of the EZ Interictal hypoperfusion of the FCD
Volumetric T1-weighted sequence with contrast media injection		Not necessary/ not systematic Helps characterization of differential diagnosis in epilepsy (tumors, vascular malformations)
Functional MRI and diffusion tensor imaging	Paradigms depending on the location of the lesion	Surgical planning and prediction of the functional outcome after corticectomy

Moreover, advanced sequences developed in recent years can be added. Their selection is, however, subject to duration of acquisition and patient tolerance. For example, 3D T2 Double Inversion Recovery weighted sequences (Rugg-Gunn *et al.*, 2006; Li *et al.*, 2011) with a reduction of both CSF (as in FLAIR sequence) and white matter signal, may help enhancing cortical contrast/noise ratio, and thus better delineate FCD borders. In addition, arterial spin labelling (ASL) provides a cartography of the cerebral blood flow and can be easily added to the routine MRI evaluation. To provide efficient data on cortical perfusion, this cartography needs to overlap with anatomical 3DT1 or 3DFLAIR, in order to reveal a focal zone of cortex that is hypo-perfused compared to the adjacent cortex. This hypoperfusion has been shown to be co-localized with FCD, and therefore can give an additional clue for the detection of the lesion (Pendse *et al.*, 2010). When located in the temporal lobe, FCD can be associated with hippocampal sclerosis (double pathology). Therefore, a particular attention should be given to mesial temporal structures, using thin (< 2mm) coronal T2-weighted slices, perpendicular to the long axis of the hippocampus.

• Which magnetic field? MR field 1.5 vs 3T vs 7T

MR-scanners with higher field magnet are associated with higher signal-to-noise ratio and spatial resolution, and therefore clearly benefit FCD imaging. Studies comparing 3T with 1.5T MRI in patients with epilepsy demonstrate that increasing field is associated with an improvement in lesion characterization and delineation (Phal *et al.*, 2008; Zijlmans *et al.*, 2009; Mellerio *et al.*, 2014; Rubinger *et al.*, 2016). This advance of 3T over 1.5T implies that it is currently inadvisable to conclude MR exams as "negative" if performed only at 1.5T MRI. In these cases, it is recommended to redo the exam with a 3T magnet.

The recent advent of 7T MRI follows this field tendency in epilepsy imaging (Opheim *et al.*, 2021), with further improvements in signal and resolution, yet increased susceptibility sensitivity, which makes it technically challenging for clinical routine (see also previous chapter).

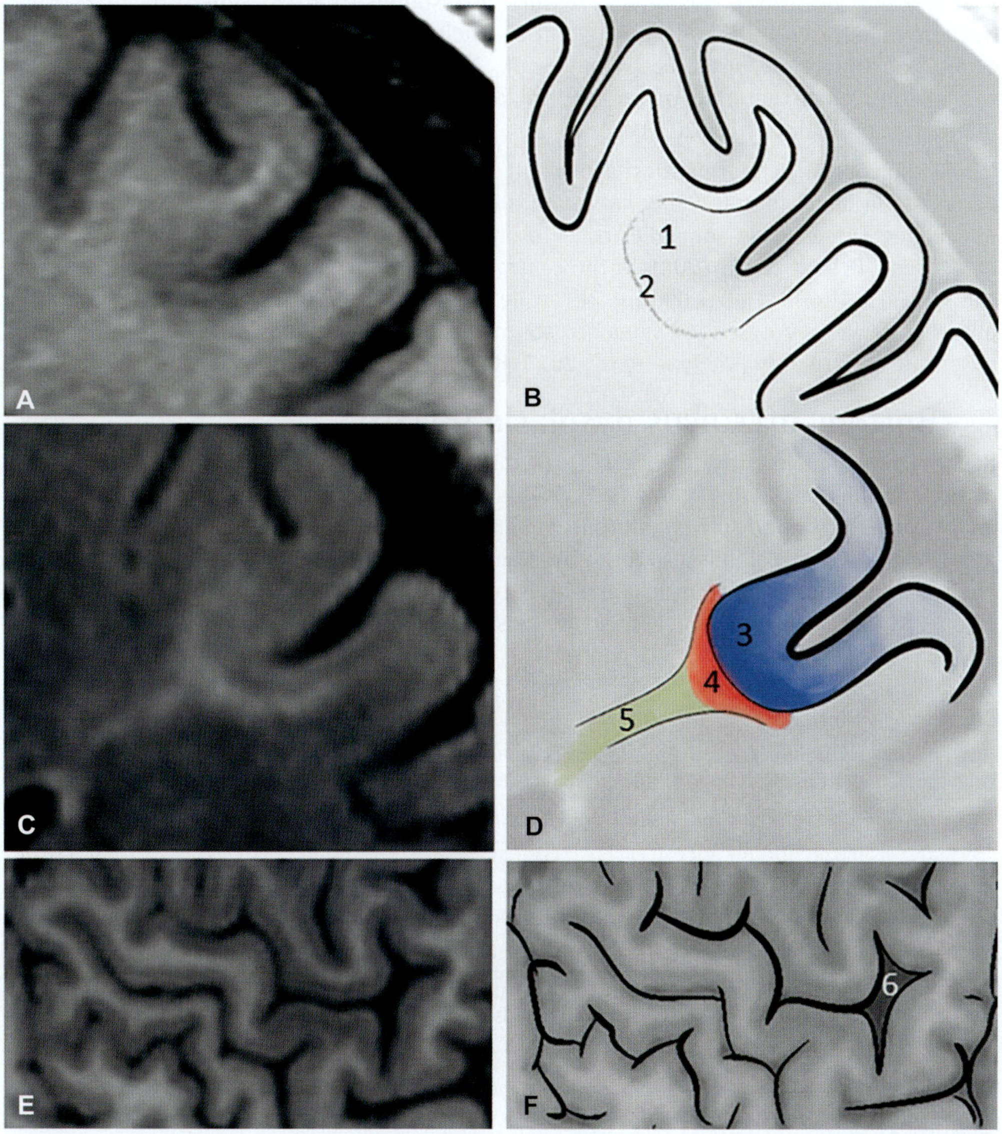

Figure 1

Coronal view, 3DT1 (A) and FLAIR (C) weighted MRI with a superimposed drawing of grey-matter limits (B, D) and signal changes on FLAIR (C). Curvilinear reformat (E) of the cortical surface on 3DT1 acquisition, with a superimposed drawing of the sulci (F). FCD is characterized by one or more of the following signs: 1- blurring of the grey-white matter interface; 2- cortical thickening; 3- increased cortical FLAIR signal, maximal at the deep part of the sulcus (in blue); 4- increased subcortical white matter FLAIR signal (in red); 5- funnel shape signal from this cortical lesion to the ventricle wall (transmantle sign in yellow); 6- atypical sulcal morphology with enlargement of the sulcus at the base of the lesion.

MRI characteristics of FCD: nonspecific features and unique signature

Among the different subtypes, FCD II (A and B) refer to a more homogeneous pathological entity than types I and III, and thus have a more typical and reproducible "signature" in MR imaging, In the next paragraph, the MR features of FCD II are described, followed by a consideration of the characteristic features of subtypes I and III.

Typical MR features include abnormalities of the cortex and of the underlying white matter (**Figure 1** and **Table 2**). Some are better visualized on 3DT1 sequences, such as cortical thickening and blurring of the gray-white matter (GWM) interface, corresponding to the presence of dysmorphic neurons and balloon cells in the cortex and the sub-cortical junction. GWM blurring can be very subtle and needs to be observed in at least two different axes to avoid being confounded with partial volume effect. Some other features, such as increased signal of the cortex and subcortical white matter, are better detected on 3D FLAIR and T2 weighted images (Mellerio *et al.*, 2012). They have been related to a high density of balloon cells in the cortex (Widdess-Walsh, Kellinghaus and Jeha, 2005) and to the presence of ectopic neurons or axonal loss in underlying white matter. This subcortical hyperintensity can linearly extend to the ventricle surface, reproducing the path of migrating neuroblasts during the fetal period, currently described as a "transmantle sign" (Barkovich *et al.*, 1997). This typical feature corresponds to a MR "signature" of FCD, has been demonstrated to be better visible at 3T (Mellerio *et al.*, 2014) and is associated with a good postoperative outcome (Wang *et al.*, 2013). As this sign does not systematically taper along an orthogonal plane, multiplanar reformatting may be needed to correct identification (Saini *et al.*, 2010).

Finally, sulco-gyral abnormalities, a difficult feature to assess because of inter-individual variability in sulcal anatomy, should be carefully searched on curvilinear or volume-rendering 3D images. These subtle anomalies refer to unusual depth, uncommon angulation or shape of a sulcus (Besson *et al.*, 2008). In the central region, a specific sulcal pattern reproducing the "power button" symbol (**Figure 2**) can be identified in half of the patients, even when all other previously described signs are absent and is strongly indicative of an underlying dysplastic abnormality (Mellerio *et al.*, 2015; Roca *et al.*, 2015).

• Bottom-of-sulcus dysplasia (BOSD)

BOSD is a distinctive entity among FCD II with a typical imaging feature on MRI (**Figure 3**), distinguishable from other forms of FCD. It is defined as a small lesion limited to depth of an unusually profound sulcus with cortical and/or subcortical abnormalities (Harvey *et al.*, 2015). A transmantle sign is also often observed and the other cortical and subcortical signal changes are arranged symmetrically, relative to an axis perpendicular to the cortex (Mellerio *et al.*, 2012). Moreover, in sulcal FCD, the axis of symmetry often overlaps the trajectory of

Table 2

Main signs of Focal Cortical Dysplasia in MRI

A. Better visible on 3DT1
1. Abnormal cortical thickness, defined as a thickening (or thinning) of at least 50% of the normal cortex, on at least two orthogonal plans, to rule out partial volume effects
2. Blurring of the GWM junction, visible on at least one sequence and in 2 orthogonal plans
B. Better visible on 3DFLAIR – T2
1. Abnormal cortical signal intensity, defined as signal changes involving the entire thickness of the cortex. The maximum of the hyperintensity is located at the bottom of the sulcus.
2. Abnormal signal intensity of subcortical white matter, relative to normal cortex.
3. Abnormal signal intensity of deep white matter, the so-called transmantle sign, defined as a subcortical white matter signal intensity change, tapering towards the ventricle
C. Better visible on Volume rendering or curvilinear reformat
1. Sulcal morphology, defined as an abnormality of the depth, angulation or shape of a sulcus, as compared to the contralateral side, on reformatted sequences.

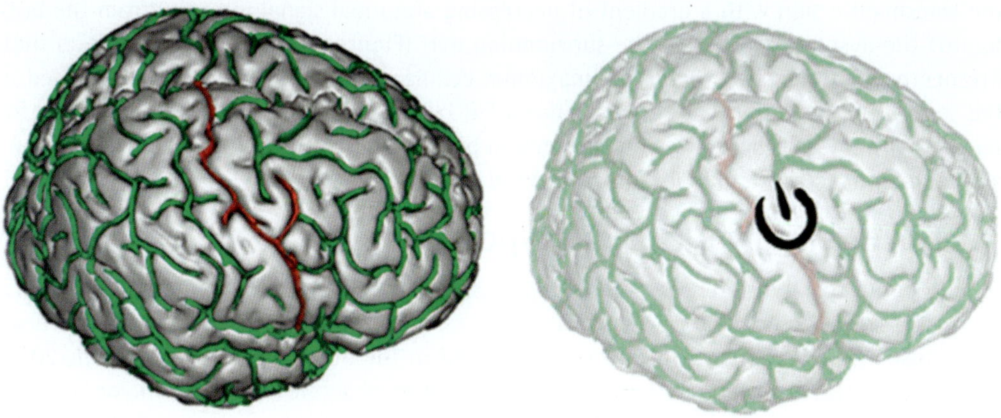

Figure 2

Abnormal sulcal pattern in a patient with precentral FCD on a 3D reformat of the lateral surface of the brain: This interposition of a pre-central sulcal segment between the central sulcus and one of its hook-shaped anterior ascending branches, termed "power button sign" (PBS) is typical of FCD in the central region.

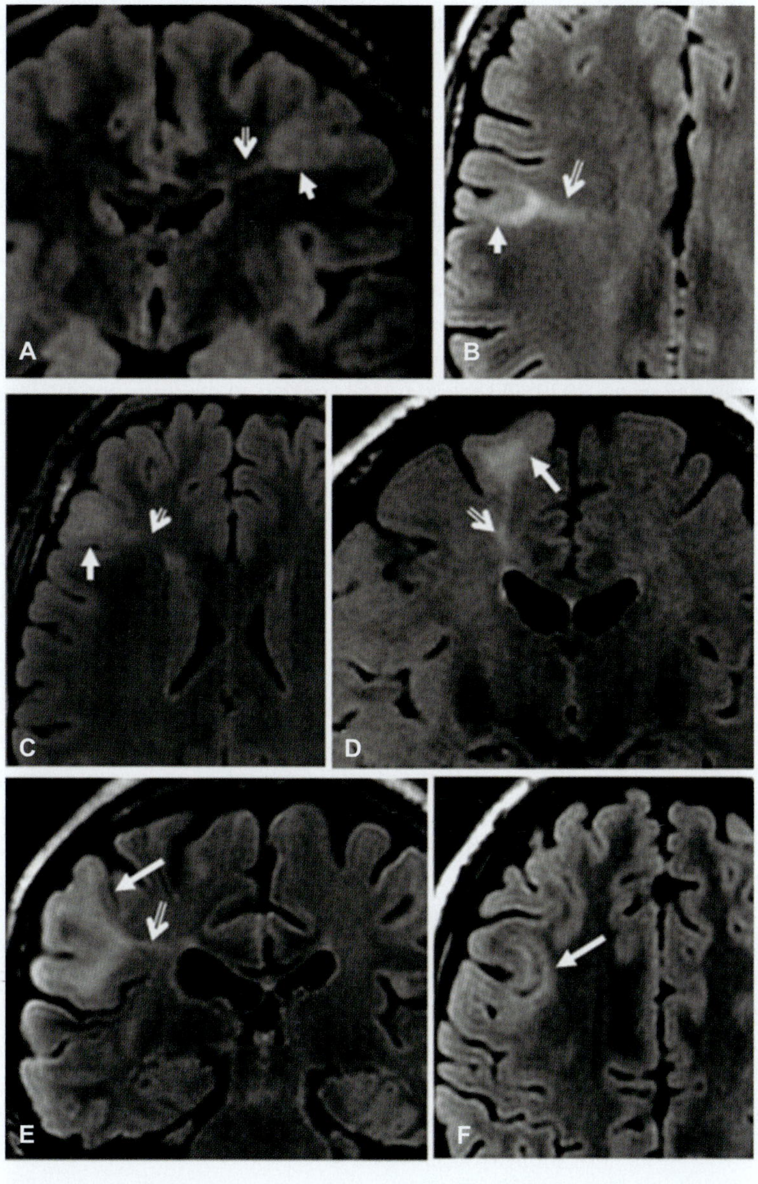

Figure 3

Different types of FCD (arrow - when present, the transmantle sign is pointed out with a double arrow). A and B. Bottom of the sulcus FCD in two different patients on a coronal (A) and axial (B) 3D FLAIR reformat. Note that the maximum signal change is located at the deep part of the dysplastic sulcus. C and D. Gyral FCD in 2 different patients on axial (C) and coronal (D) 3D FLAIR reformat. The maximal signal change is centered on the superficial part of the cortex. E. Broad FCD in a patient on coronal 3D FLAIR reformat where more than one dysplastic gyrus is involved. F. Subtle FCD in a patient on axial 3D FLAIR reformat, where a very slight signal change is limited to the cortex, without transmantle sign. Note that the atypical curved sulco-gyral conformation pointing to the lesion.

the transmantle sign with a gradient of decreasing abnormal signal intensity from the bottom of the dysplastic sulcus to the surrounding gyri (**Figures 1 and 3**). This suggests that, irrespective of the size of the lesion, maximum cellular abnormalities are deeply located in the sulcus. The detection and identification of BOSD is valuable because the prognosis for seizure control is excellent after focal resection both in adults (Harvey *et al.*, 2015; Macdonald-Laurs *et al.*, 2021) and in infants (Jain *et al.*, 2021).

• Differentiating FCD subtypes

Despite pathological differences, FCD subtypes cannot be reliably discriminated on MRI. Most of the MR signs, such as abnormal cortical thickness, gray-white matter blurring, and cortical/subcortical T2 signal abnormalities can be observed in the other subtypes (Kim *et al.*, 2012; Hong *et al.*, 2017) even though there is a tendency for more subtle anomalies in types I and III (Jayalakshmi *et al.*, 2021). The only MR sign that provides a reliable distinction between subtypes is the transmantle sign, which is very rare in type I (Kim *et al.*, 2012), much more frequent in type II and especially in type IIB (Colombo *et al.*, 2012; Kim *et al.*, 2012; Mühlebner *et al.*, 2012).

Regardless of MR signs, the FCD subtype can be hypothesized from the localization of the lesion, as the distribution of FCD differs according to the histopathological subtype (Wagstyl *et al.*, 2022). In this large multicentric study of 580 patients, it has been shown that a greater proportion of FCD I and III were located in the temporal lobe and especially in the temporal pole, while FCD II were mainly located in the frontal lobes.

Limits and pitfalls of visual analysis

The possibility of under- or over- diagnosis of an FCD lesion must always be kept in mind. The most common mistake is to overlook a visible lesion and to incorrectly interpret the imaging as normal or "negative" MRI. This frequent mistake on initial imaging (up to 40% of the cases in surgical series) leads to delayed referral for surgery (Chang *et al.*, 2011; Jayalakshmi *et al.*, 2021), thereby depriving patients of effective treatment for years and compromising outcome (Lamberink *et al.*, 2020). A second pitfall consists in overinterpreting images that do not correspond to a FCD and leads to a wrong positive diagnosis or to the incorrect localization of a FCD located elsewhere.

• False negative MRI

The ILAE neuroimaging task force insists on the importance of repeating MRI using the optimal protocol, the best image resolution, magnetic field strength, number of phased-array head coils, and neuroimaging expertise of the reader. Even more importantly, these images should be evaluated considering all the clinical and electrical data to focus on the most plausible epileptogenic area. It is therefore important to repeat the MRI if it has not been performed under optimal conditions.

One of the main issues lies in the fact that the characterization of a mild cortical thickening may be difficult due to the curve of the cortical surface. Thus, a subtle thickening of the cortex can be mistaken for a partial volume effect or missed because the cortex is not seen in the same plane that the sulcus. One way to solve this problem of the cortical curvature is to "unroll" the cortical surface on a 2D plane through a curvilinear reformatting (**Figure 4**). In this type of reformatting, the cortex is unrolled concentrically and thus can be analyzed in the axis of the folding. Subtle cortical thickening and/or cortical blurring can thus be unmasked. In the same way, volume reformatting of the cortical surface allows better appreciation of the layout and interconnections of the sulci, and thus to detect an abnormal configuration of the sulcal anatomy (a power button sign in the central region, for example). However, despite all the major advances in MR imaging techniques, true MRI-negative FCD do exist and require other investigations as described in the following chapters.

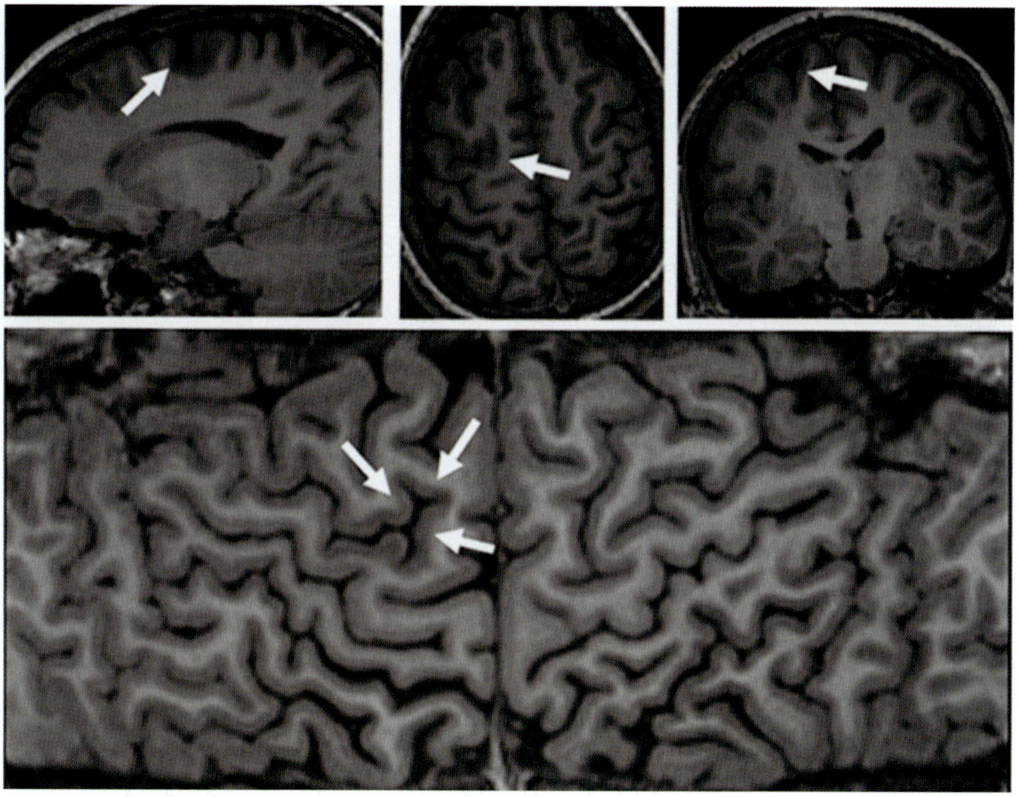

Figure 4

Example illustrating the importance of curvilinear reformat of the cortical surface. A focal area of grey matter in the right frontal region (arrow) appears to have a mild thickened appearance on the axial plane, less obvious on coronal and sagittal views, possibly resulting from a partial volume effect. The curvilinear view helps to compare the cortical thickness of this sulcus to the whole cortical surface, confirming this abnormal thickness.

False positive MRI

When MRI features are typical, combining all FCD signs (including the presence of a transmantle sign) and are associated with a typical electroclinical presentation, there is almost no differential diagnosis. On the other hand, some atypical appearances can be misinterpreted and confounded with other diagnosis. Of note, excessive diagnosis of FCD could be as unfavorable to the patient as an overlooked lesion. In addition, due to the strong intrinsic electrical activity of this lesion and the absence of asymptomatic forms described so far in the literature, a fortuitous discovery of FCD is unlikely. This condition must impose caution and evoke other diagnostic hypotheses.

Among the cortical lesions that can be confused with FCD and illustrated in **Figure 5**, the following deserve particular attention:

Tuberous sclerosis

There is a continuum in MRI between cortical tubers and FCD. Thus, their imaging appearance can be similar, including the presence of radial subcortical bands similar to the transmantle sign. The presence of a pronounced subcortical hyperintensity (due to a high concentration of balloon cells), of more than one cortical lesion (even if multiple FCD are possible) and of cortical calcifications suggest tuberous sclerosis and should prompt genetic investigation.

Low grade glial tumors

Focal thickening of the cortex can occur in infiltrated tumors of the cortex such as oligodendrogliomas, as well as in some FCD (Widdess-Walsh, Diehl and Najm, 2006). It should be noted that MRI spectrometry in FCD lesions is often non-specific, sometimes resembling tumor lesions (Leite *et al.*, 2007) and therefore does not allow reliable discrimination. However, the cortical thickening of the low-grade gliomas is often associated with loss of delimitation of the subcortical-cortical junction which is more pronounced than

CHAPTER

17. Critical perspective of automatic detection of FCD: what should the clinician use?

Fernando Cendes

Key points

- MRI visual analysis of the signal characteristics of a suspect lesion, with or without postprocessing, is fundamental to the surgical approach in patients with FCD.
- Visual inspection of digitally stored 3D MRIs should be done in an imaging platform that allows multiplanar reformatting to best evaluate suspect FCD lesions, in the context of seizure semiology, EEG data and other imaging modalities
- An MRI *reported as normal* might show mild structural abnormalities that were not initially detected, and thus a negative MRI may become positive with further visual or postprocessing analyses.
- MRI findings in FCD are often subtle and sometimes not seen, even with ideal imaging, pointing to the additional role of automatic detection of subtle changes
- There are several methods for computer-assisted analysis of images for detecting FCD and some have already been used in the clinical setting.
- Although not yet readily available for clinical practice, artificial intelligence approaches such as machine-learning and deep learning have shown great potential for automatic detection of FCD lesions in MRI-negative focal epilepsies

Imaging as the crucial tool in the diagnosis of FCD

High-resolution structural MRI plays a vital role in defining the etiology and prognosis of medical and surgical treatment in patients with epilepsies. Therefore, structural MRI must be optimally acquired, including 3D T1-weighted and FLAIR sequences, and carefully reviewed by trained experts within the context of all available clinical and EEG data (Bernasconi *et al.*, 2019; Wang *et al.*, 2020a). Multiplanar reformatting of high-resolution MRI and correlation with functional multimodal imaging improves the detection of subtle lesions (Cendes *et al.*, 2016). Detection of a lesion on a previous negative MRI has a substantial impact on determining the etiology of epilepsy, reducing the need for invasive investigations, and planning surgical treatment and postoperative outcomes in patients with pharmacoresistant seizures (Widjaja *et al.*, 2020). The high diagnostic yield of MRI to identify the common pathological findings in individuals with focal seizures, including hippocampal sclerosis, vascular anomalies, low-grade glial neoplasms, and MCD along with other lesions, has been well established, and quantitative postprocessing may help to complement the evaluation of subtle MCD, in particular, FCD (Blumcke *et al.*, 2021).

The results from an MRI visual analysis of signal characteristics of a suspect lesion, its location and extent, with or without postprocessing, are fundamental to the surgical approach in patients with FCD. The visual inspection of digitally stored 3D MRI (usually in DICOM format), acquired with the smaller isotropic voxel size as possible, should be done in an imaging platform that allows multiplanar reformatting. Fortunately, there are numerous options of user-friendly DICOM viewers that run on most desktop computers, so it does not need to be exclusive to neuroradiologists and can be incorporated into every epileptologist's routine. Such an approach allows changing the angulations of planes *dynamically* to avoid false abnormalities due to the partial volume effect of cutting parallel of deep sulci, with the original native thin high-resolution format (not with reconstructed thicker cuts) by simultaneous inspection of images in all three orthogonal planes (coronal, axial, and sagittal) (Bernasconi *et al.*, 2019; Cendes *et al.*, 2016). These DICOM viewers also allow the inspection of different MRI acquisitions (e.g., T1-weighted and FLAIR) side-by-side and evaluate morphology and signal changes simultaneously, increasing diagnostic accuracy (**Figure 1**).

MRI findings in many patients with FCD are often subtle, and sometimes not seen, even with ideal imaging. The MRI features range from abnormal signal changes to subtle, almost invisible, abnormalities.

MRI is normal in most patients with FCD I, or it may show mild hyperintensity of the white matter in T2/FLAIR images with loss of gray-white matter differentiation or focal volume loss and thin cortex (Blümcke *et al.*, 2021).

MRI findings in FCD IIA include abnormal focal patterns of sulci and gyri, cortical dimple, mild cortical thickness changes, gray-white matter blurring, and at times a subtle hyperintense T2/FLAIR signal in the subcortical and deep white matter (**Figure 1**) (Cendes *et al.*, 2016).

FCD IIB, or FCD with balloon cells, presents with a gradient of morphologic changes, from dysplastic lesions that can be easily identified by conventional MRI techniques to minor structural abnormalities, including small areas of discrete cortical thickening or blurring of the gray-white matter interface that often go unrecognized. It often shows deep sulci, abnormal cortical gyration, and hyperintense T2/FLAIR signal in the subcortical white matter, sometimes with a wedge shape that extends to the ventricle ependymal surface (transmantle sign). FCD IIB may be localized only in the bottom of the sulcus (**Figure 2**). Although most patients with FCD II show MRI abnormalities, almost one-third remain MRI negative. FCD III lesions share the typical features of the associated lesions (Cendes *et al.*, 2016).

MOGHE has been described as a new entity within the spectrum of FCD (Blümcke *et al.*, 2021; Mendes Coelho *et al.*, 2021; Schurr *et al.*, 2017).

The MRI characteristics in patients with MOGHE appear to be age-related. They seem to change with brain maturation, including changes in gyral and sulcal morphology, mild cortical thickening, a slight increase in signal intensity in the subcortical white matter, and a mild cortical-subcortical blurring, which are similar to those of FCD IIA (Mendes Coelho *et al.*, 2021; Schurr *et al.*, 2017). In addition, young children may present with an extensive and pronounced cortical-subcortical blurring that gives a false impression of cortical thickening (Hartlieb *et al.*, 2019).

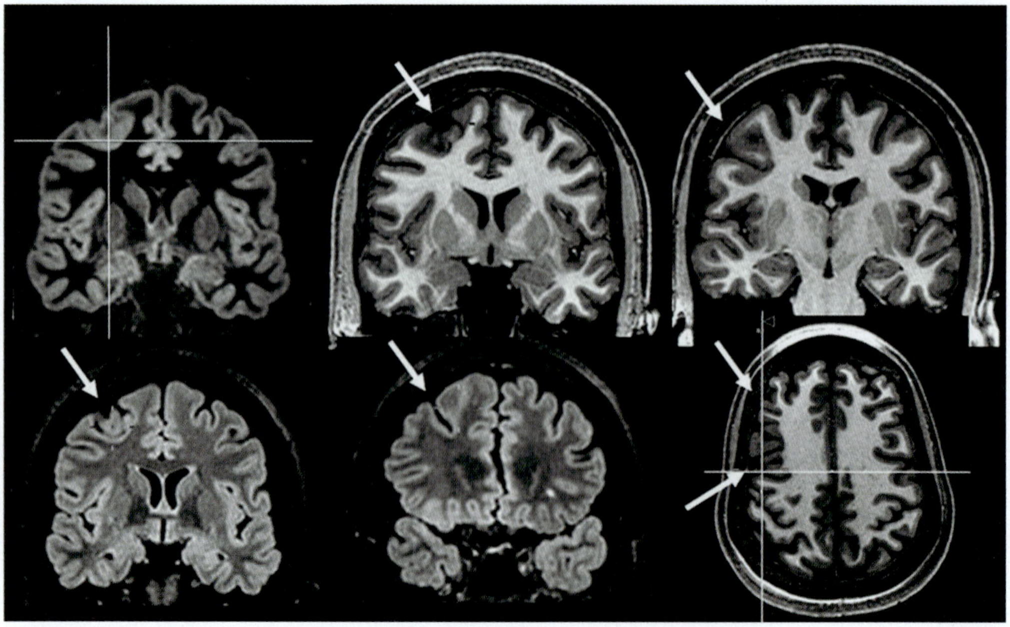

Figure 1

MRI multiplanar reconstructions in a patient with frontal-lobe seizures whose previous MRI were considered negative.
Reconstructions from 3D double inversion recovery (DIR), 3D T1-weighted, and 3D fluid-attenuated inversion recovery (FLAIR) images (all with 1-mm thickness). The area with FCD in the left frontal lobe presents with a slightly thickened cortex associated with abnormal gyri and cortical dimple (arrows). The FLAIR and DIR images did not show a clear abnormal signal, except for a slightly blurred cortical-subcortical transition. The postoperative histopathology showed classic signs of FCD II-A. The patient became seizure free after complete removal of the lesion.

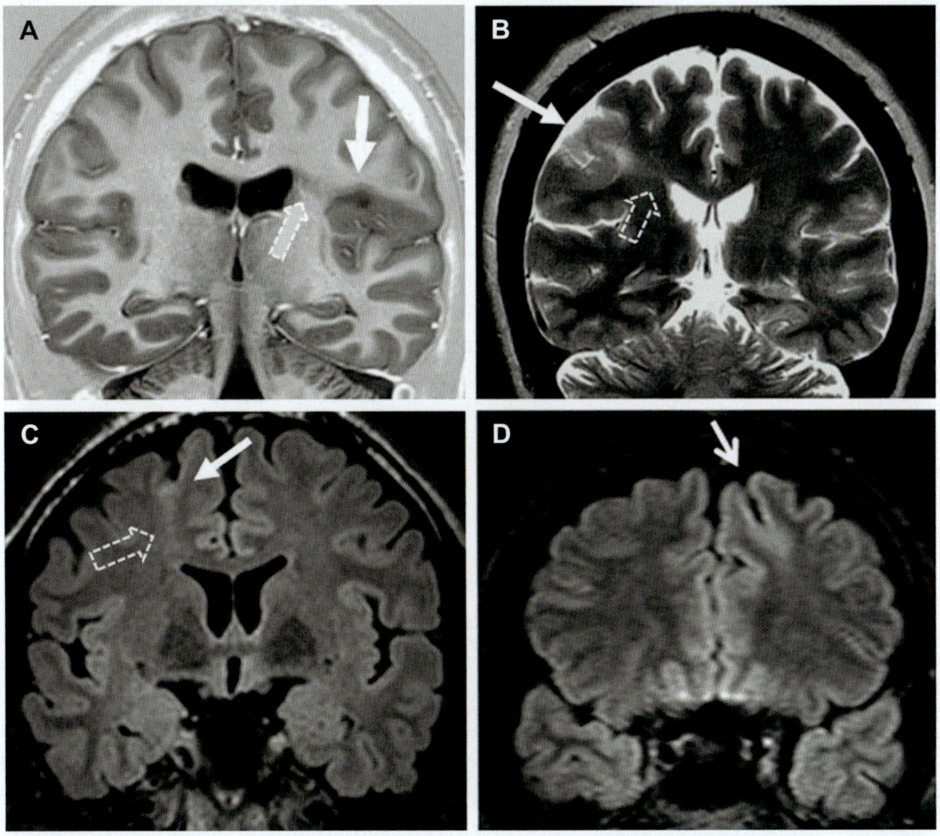

Figure 2

Coronal MRI from 4 patients with Focal Cortical Dysplasia (FCD) type II-B.

A. Coronal T1-weighted inversion recovery (IR) image in a patient with FCD II-B in the left insula. Note the cortical thickening and blurring of the cortical-subcortical interface (arrow) and a transmantle sign (open arrow). B. Coronal T2-weighted image in a patient with frontal lobe seizures showing focal cortical thickening, blurring of the cortical-subcortical transition with subcortical hyperintense T2-weighed signal, abnormal gyri, cortical dimple (arrow), and a transmantle sign (open arrow). C. Coronal FLAIR image showing typical changes of the bottom of the sulcus dysplasia (arrow) with a transmantle sign (open arrow) in a patient with right frontal lobe epilepsy. D. Coronal FLAIR image showing a thickened cortex localized in a deep sulcus with a hyperintense FLAIR signal (bottom of the sulcus dysplasia) in a patient with left frontal epilepsy. Histopathology showed FCD II-B in all four patients, and all became seizure-free after surgery, except for the patient in (B), who improved but remained with focal seizures because the lesion could not be removed completely due to the proximity of the motor area.

The quest for the Holy Grail: what to do when the visual analysis is negative in focal refractory epilepsies in clinical practice

It is important to emphasize that an MRI reported as normal might still show mild structural abnormalities that were not initially detected and thus, a negative MRI may become positive with further visual or postprocessing analyses (Bernasconi *et al.*, 2019). The most practical approach is the multiplanar reconstructions of 3D T1-weighted and FLAIR images in the context of seizure semiology, EEG data and other imaging modalities (Federico *et al.*, 2020).

A negative study on a low field MRI without an epilepsy-dedicated protocol suggests a non-adequate imaging acquisition. The frequency of false negative MRI depends on the expertise of the examiners and the quality of the scans. Using sequences considered optimal for the investigation of epilepsies (Bernasconi *et al.*, 2019), structural MRI will show a lesion in up to 91% of patients with pharmacoresistant focal epilepsy when evaluated by experts in epilepsy imaging, as opposed to 39% with a suboptimal protocol read by non-experts (Von Oertzen *et al.*, 2002).

Additional functional imaging modalities, such as interictal fluorodeoxyglucose positron emission tomography (FDG-PET) and subtraction of ictal/interictal SPECT, and its co-registration with structural MRI may add important information in patients with subtle lesions, that help to increase the confidence of the structural MRI diagnosis (Cendes *et al.*, 2016). Also, statistical parametric mapping (SPM) postprocessing of ictal-interictal SPECT subtraction images can improve the detection of subtle lesions (Sulc *et al.*, 2014).

Positron emission tomography (PET) is the most performed interictal functional neuroimaging technique that may reveal a focal hypometabolic region concordant with seizure onset. FDG-PET demonstrates focal hypometabolism in 71-89% of patients undergoing presurgical evaluation, with a 56-90% agreement with the SOZ as determined by intracranial EEG (Tomás *et al.*, 2019). When appropriately coregistered with MRI, FDG-PET has a sensitivity of up to 95% for detecting MRI-occult FCD lesions (Chassoux *et al.*, 2010), particularly in young children, because incomplete myelination hinders the MRI detection of small FCD (Salamon *et al.*, 2008). Quantitative FDG-PET studies for determining focal hypometabolism may be more accurate than visual analysis and may increase the yield for detecting subtle lesions (Mendes Coelho *et al.*, 2017).

Emerging advanced postprocessing methods and artificial intelligence for automatic detection of FCD

Advanced postprocessing of functional imaging modalities, such as resting-state functional MRI (fMRI), and EEG-fMRI, may help to reduce the need for invasive investigations and predict prognosis (Duncan & Trimmel, 2022). For example, EEG-fMRI studies have shown that the maximum signal change in the fMRI often corresponds to the presumed epileptogenic zone and may help reevaluate previously normal MRI (Khoo *et al.*, 2017). Clinical applications of EEG-fMRI are already becoming a reality in a few centers (Kowalczyk *et al.*, 2020; Van Eyndhoven *et al.*, 2021), including for surgical outcome prediction (Koupparis *et al.*, 2021).

There are several methods for computer-assisted analysis of images for detecting FCD (Adler *et al.*, 2017; Ahmed *et al.*, 2015; Demerath *et al.*, 2020; Urbach *et al.*, 2022). Methods such as voxel-based morphometry (VBM), voxel-based relaxometry (VBR), voxel-based diffusivity (VBD), automatic morphometry using FreeSurfer for measuring volumes and cortical thickness, among others, can use statistical methods to demonstrate the areas of the brain that differ from normal control values (Duncan & Trimmel, 2022; Martin *et al.*, 2017; Whelan *et al.*, 2018).

Some MRI postprocessing using different approaches have already been used in the clinical setting. For example, maps generated by morphometric analysis program (MAP), used as input for a trained automated artificial neural network (ANN), has identified structurally abnormal subtle FCD lesions, particularly with 3T MRI, although there are false-positives (Urbach *et al.*, 2022).

Also, higher field MRI (7T) with postprocessing reported the detection of subtle FCD lesions in 22% or more patients with focal epilepsies and negative 3T MRI (De Ciantis *et al.*, 2016; Wang *et al.*, 2020b).

Big data and artificial intelligence approach: How may these methods help detect FCD and understand surgical failures?

Advances in computer hardware and software now allow analyses of big data of structural and multimodal imaging. The use of artificial intelligence (AI) approaches, including machine learning (ML) and deep learning (DL), can segment and calculate the volume or shape of brain structures on MRI, among other MRI features, with little or no human intervention (Cendes &

McDonald, 2022). Although not yet readily available for clinical practice, ML and DL have shown great potential for automatic detection of FCD lesions in MRI-negative focal epilepsies (Adler *et al.*, 2017; Beheshti *et al.*, 2021; Demerath *et al.*, 2020; El Tahry *et al.*, 2020; Gill *et al.*, 2021; Kini *et al.*, 2016; Wagstyl *et al.*, 2022). One successful example of big data AI applications is the *Enhancing Neuroimaging Genetics through Meta-analysis* (ENIGMA) brain-imaging consortium that showed associations between MRI changes not visible by the naked eye with several clinical characteristics in thousands of patients with epilepsy (Sisodiya *et al.*, 2020).

A recent automated ML algorithm using a deep convolutional neural network (CNN) classifier, summarized in **Figure 3**, was trained and validated on a multicenter MRI dataset of patients with histologically confirmed FCD from 9 epilepsy centers worldwide (Gill *et al.*, 2021). The algorithm used both 3D T1-weighted and 3D FLAIR MRI acquired as part of the presurgical investigation. Manually segmented lesions by two experts were used to train the model. This algorithm had a sensitivity of 93% using a leave-one-site-out cross-validation and 83% when tested on an independent cohort and retaining a high specificity of 89% in healthy and disease controls. Furthermore, it detected MRI-negative FCD, as illustrated in **Figure 4**, with 85% sensitivity (Gill *et al.*, 2021). More important, their results were generalizable across cohorts, independent of age, MRI scanner, and acquisition parameters (Gill *et al.*, 2021).

Of course, such automated AI procedures are not enough to be used as a "stand-alone" method of MRI analyses and will not substitute the imaging experts. However, the visual analysis of subtle FCD is time consuming, and the level of expertise varies considerably among centers, explaining the variable, and sometimes high, percentage of negative MRI in patients with pharmacoresistant focal seizures (Von Oertzen *et al.*, 2002). Therefore, automated computer algorithms such as the one presented by Gill *et al.* (2021) in parallel to the visual analyses may enhance the confidence of experts and non-experts in evaluating subtle FCD and have promise for clinical translation.

Another approach was taken by the MELD project that included a retrospective cohort of 580 patients with FCD (Wagstyl *et al.*, 2022). Here, the AI was not used to detect the lesion. Instead, they trained logistic regression models to test for associations between clinical data and the location of FCD lesions that were delineated on T1-weighted MRI scans by imaging

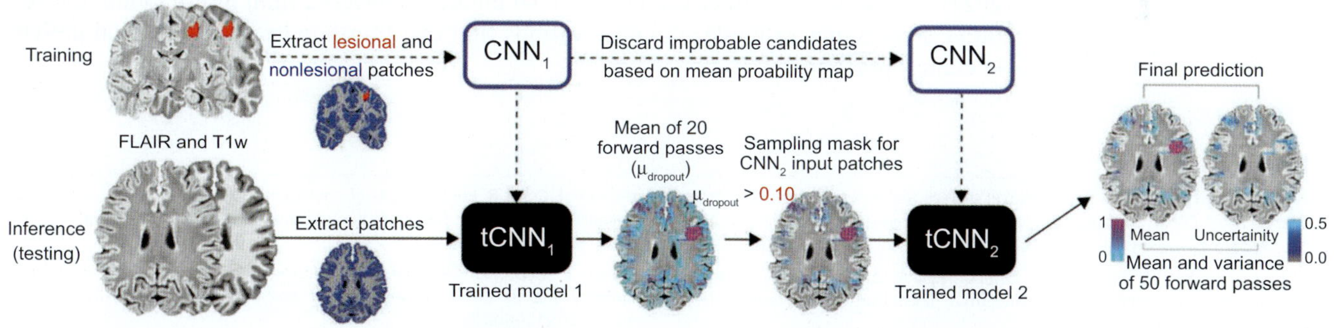

Figure 3

Classifier Design of a Deep Learning Detection Algorithm for Focal Cortical Dysplasia.

Training and inference (or testing) workflow. In the cascaded system, the output of convolutional neural network (CNN) -1 serves as an input for CNN-2. CNN-1 maximizes the detection of lesional voxels; CNN-2 reduces the number of misclassified voxels, removing false positives (FPs) while maintaining optimal sensitivity. The training procedure (indicated by dashed arrows) operating on T1-weighted (T1w) and fluid-attenuated inversion recovery (FLAIR) MRI extracts 3-dimensional patches from lesional and nonlesional tissue to yield tCNN-1 (trained model 1) and tCNN-2 (trained model 2) models with optimized weights (indicated by vertical dashed-dotted arrows). These models are then used for participant-level inference. For each unseen participant, the inference pipeline (solid arrows) uses tCNN-1 and generates a mean (μdroupout) of 20 predictions (forward passes); the mean map is then thresholded voxel-wise to discard improbable lesion candidates (μdroupout > 0.1). The resulting binary mask serves to sample the input patches for the tCNN-2. Mean probability and uncertainty maps are obtained by collating 50 predictions; uncertainty is transformed into confidence. The sampling strategy (identical for training and inference) is illustrated only for testing. Reproduced with permission from Gill RS, *et al.* 2021.

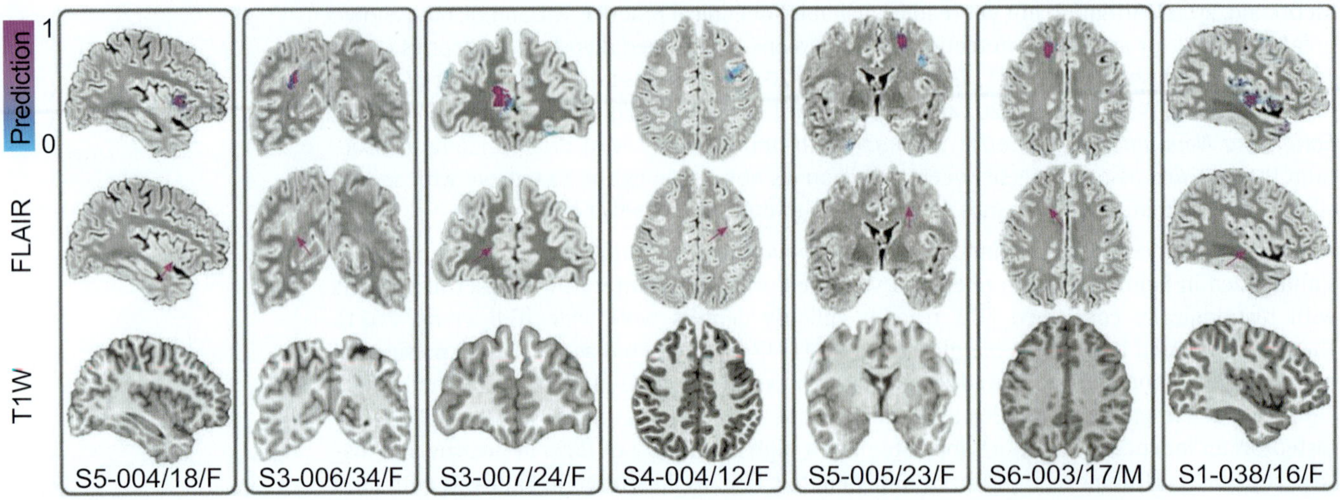

Figure 4

Examples of Representative FCD Detected by a Deep Learning Algorithm for Focal Cortical Dysplasia.

Seven representative MRI-negative Focal Cortical Dysplasia (FCD) lesions across sites (Ss) are shown (top row: prediction overlaid on the fluid-attenuated inversion recovery [FLAIR]; flame scale indicates the probability strength). Bottom labels are interpreted as site-patient-identification/age/sex. Arrows indicate the ground-truth lesion location. T1w = T1 weighted. Reproduced with permission from Gill RS, *et al.* 2021.

experts. As inferred by smaller independent studies, their data-driven atlases demonstrated a non-uniform distribution of FCD with higher concentrations in the superior frontal sulcus, frontal pole, temporal pole, and superior temporal gyrus. Lesions in primary sensory areas associated with earlier epilepsy onset and lesions in association cortices with later epilepsy onset. Postoperative seizure freedom varied according to the FCD location, from around 30% in the vicinity of very eloquent cortices to 75% in temporal and frontal gyri. Also, the likelihood of seizure freedom decreased with a longer duration of epilepsy (Wagstyl *et al.*, 2022). This study is another example of how big data collected from international collaborative studies generate essential observations that can translate back to individual patients in clinical practice.

References

Adler S, Wagstyl K, Gunny R, *et al.* Novel surface features for automated detection of Focal Cortical Dysplasias in paediatric epilepsy. *Neuroimage Clin* 2017; 14: 18-27.

Ahmed B, Brodley CE, Blackmon KE, *et al.* Cortical feature analysis and machine learning improves detection of "MRI-negative" Focal Cortical Dysplasia. *Epilepsy Behav* 2015; 48: 21-8.

Beheshti I, Sone D, Maikusa N, *et al.* Accurate lateralization and classification of MRI-negative 18F-FDG-PET-positive temporal lobe epilepsy using double inversion recovery and machine-learning. *Comput Biol Med* 2021; 137: 104805.

Bernasconi A, Cendes F, Theodore WH, *et al.* Recommendations for the use of structural magnetic resonance imaging in the care of patients with epilepsy: A consensus report from the International League Against Epilepsy Neuroimaging Task Force. *Epilepsia* 2019; 60: 1054-68.

Blumcke I, Cendes F, Miyata H, *et al.* Toward a refined genotype-phenotype classification scheme for the international consensus classification of Focal Cortical Dysplasia. *Brain Pathol* 2021; 31: e12956.

Blümcke I, Coras R, Busch RM, *et al.* Toward a better definition of Focal Cortical Dysplasia: An iterative histopathological and genetic agreement trial. *Epilepsia* 2021; 62: 1416-28.

Cendes F, McDonald CR. Artificial Intelligence Applications in the Imaging of Epilepsy and Its Comorbidities: Present and Future. *Epilepsy Currents* 2022: 15357597211068600.

Cendes F, Theodore WH, Brinkmann BH, *et al.* Neuroimaging of epilepsy. *Handb Clin Neurol* 2016; 136: 985-1014.

Chassoux F, Rodrigo S, Semah F, *et al.* FDG-PET improves surgical outcome in negative MRI Taylor-type Focal Cortical Dysplasias. *Neurology* 2010; 75: 2168-75.

De Ciantis A, Barba C, Tassi L, *et al.* 7T MRI in focal epilepsy with unrevealing conventional field strength imaging. *Epilepsia* 2016; 57: 445-54.

Demerath T, Rubensdörfer L, Schwarzwald R, *et al.* Morphometric MRI Analysis: Improved Detection of Focal Cortical Dysplasia Using the MP2RAGE Sequence. *AJNR Am J Neuroradiol* 2020; 41: 1009-14.

Duncan JS, Trimmel K. Advanced neuroimaging techniques in epilepsy. *Curr Opin Neurol* 2022; 35: 189-95.

El Tahry R, Santos SF, Vrielynck P, *et al.* Additional clinical value of voxel-based morphometric MRI post-processing for MRI-negative epilepsies: a prospective study. *Epileptic Disord* 2020; 22: 156-64.

Federico P, Ng DW, Bernasconi A, *et al.* ILAE Neuroimaging Task Force highlight: Review MRI scans with semiology in mind. *Epileptic Disord* 2020; 22: 683-7.

Gill RS, Lee HM, Caldairou B, *et al.* Multicenter Validation of a Deep Learning Detection Algorithm for Focal Cortical Dysplasia. *Neurology* 2021; 97: e1571-82.

Hartlieb T, Winkler P, Coras R, *et al.* Age-related MR characteristics in mild malformation of cortical development with oligodendroglial hyperplasia and epilepsy (MOGHE). *Epilepsy Behav* 2019; 91: 68-74.

Khoo HM, Hao Y, von Ellenrieder N, *et al.* The hemodynamic response to interictal epileptic discharges localizes the seizure-onset zone. *Epilepsia* 2017; 58: 811-23.

Kini LG, Gee JC, Litt B. Computational analysis in epilepsy neuroimaging: A survey of features and methods. *Neuroimage Clin* 2016; 11: 515-29.

Koupparis A, von Ellenrieder N, Khoo HM, *et al.* Association of EEG-fMRI Responses and Outcome After Epilepsy Surgery. *Neurology* 2021; 97: e1523-36.

Kowalczyk MA, Omidvarnia A, Abbott DF, *et al.* Clinical benefit of presurgical EEG-fMRI in difficult-to-localize focal epilepsy: A single-institution retrospective review. *Epilepsia* 2020; 61: 49-60.

Martin P, Winston GP, Bartlett P, *et al.* Voxel-based magnetic resonance image postprocessing in epilepsy. *Epilepsia* 2017; 58: 1653-64.

Mendes Coelho VC, Morita-Sherman M, Yasuda CL, *et al.* Magnetic resonance imaging findings and clinical characteristics in mild malformation of cortical development with oligodendroglial hyperplasia and epilepsy in a predominantly adult cohort. *Epilepsia* 2021; 62: 1429-41.

Mendes Coelho VC, Morita ME, Amorim BJ, *et al.* Automated Online Quantification Method for (18) F-FDG Positron Emission Tomography/CT Improves Detection of the Epileptogenic Zone in Patients with Pharmacoresistant Epilepsy. *Front Neurol* 2017; 8: 453.

Schurr J, Coras R, Rössler K, *et al.* Mild Malformation of Cortical Development with Oligodendroglial Hyperplasia in Frontal Lobe Epilepsy: A New Clinico-Pathological Entity. *Brain Pathol* 2017; 27: 26-35.

Sisodiya SM, Whelan CD, Hatton SN, *et al.* The ENIGMA-Epilepsy working group: Mapping disease from large data sets. *Hum Brain Mapp* 2020. 29; 43 (1): 113-28.

Sulc V, Stykel S, Hanson DP, *et al.* Statistical SPECT processing in MRI-negative epilepsy surgery. *Neurology* 2014; 82: 932-9.

Tomás J, Pittau F, Hammers A, *et al.* The predictive value of hypometabolism in focal epilepsy: a prospective study in surgical candidates. *Eur J Nucl Med Mol Imaging* 2019; 46: 1806-16.

Urbach H, Heers M, Altenmueller DM, *et al.* "Within a minute" detection of Focal Cortical Dysplasia. *Neuroradiology* 2022; 64: 715-26.

Van Eyndhoven S, Dupont P, Tousseyn S, *et al.* Augmenting interictal mapping with neurovascular coupling biomarkers by structured factorization of epileptic EEG and fMRI data. *Neuroimage* 2021; 228: 117652.

Von Oertzen J, Urbach H, Jungbluth S, *et al.* Standard magnetic resonance imaging is inadequate for patients with refractory focal epilepsy. *J Neurol Neurosurg Psychiatry* 2002; 73: 643-7.

Wagstyl K, Whitaker K, Raznahan A, *et al.* Atlas of lesion locations and postsurgical seizure freedom in Focal Cortical Dysplasia: A MELD study. *Epilepsia* 2022; 63: 61-74.

Wang I, Bernasconi A, Bernhardt B, *et al.* MRI essentials in epileptology: a review from the ILAE Imaging Taskforce. *Epileptic Disord* 2020a; 22: 421-37.

Wang I, Oh S, Blümcke I, *et al.* Value of 7T MRI and post-processing in patients with nonlesional 3T MRI undergoing epilepsy presurgical evaluation. *Epilepsia* 2020b; 61: 2509-20.

Whelan CD, Altmann A, Botía JA, *et al.* Structural brain abnormalities in the common epilepsies assessed in a worldwide ENIGMA study. *Brain* 2018; 141: 391-408.

Widjaja E, Jain P, Demoe L, *et al.* Seizure outcome of pediatric epilepsy surgery: Systematic review and meta-analyses. *Neurology* 2020; 94: 311-21.

CHAPTER

18. PET and SPECT: searching for FCD and identifying the epileptogenic zone

Part 1. PET in FCD

Francine Chassoux

Key points

- ^{18}F-FDG-PET is highly sensitive for the detection of FCD, especially FCD II, in negative MRI cases.
- It can be used both in adults and children, although sedation may be necessary in youngest and agitated children
- Visual analysis is used in clinical routine. Statistical analysis may be helpful, but a control population is needed.
- Coregistration with MRI greatly improves PET sensitivity.
- Hypometabolism is usually observed in the interictal state and the site of maximal hypometabolism has proven to be concordant with the dysplastic cortex and the EZ.
- Hypermetabolism is rarely observed in adults. It is more frequent in children with high seizure frequency and is usually related to ictal PET.
- Hybrid PET/MR provides a better quality of images and improves FCD detection in previously negative examination.
- In well localized PET abnormalities, and concordant electroclinical data, PET/MR guided surgery may be performed with successful outcome.
- In large or multilobar hypometabolism, where SEEG remains indicated, PET findings are helpful for the planning of depth electrodes implantation and the accurate EZ determination.
- New radiotracers investigating $GABA_A$ central benzodiazepine receptors (FMZ), serotonin receptor binding (AMP), or inflammation markers (TSPO) are mainly used in research protocols.

Introduction

^{18}F-Fluoro-Desoxy-Glucose Positron Emission Tomography (^{18}F-FDG-PET) has gradually become an important part of the presurgical workup for epilepsy surgery for more than 40 years, especially in mesial temporal lobe epilepsy (MTLE). In extratemporal epilepsy, a low sensitivity was initially reported, until further studies demonstrated its value especially for the detection of FCD when MRI was negative (Salamon *et al.*, 2008, Chassoux *et al.*, 2010).

In this chapter, we will discuss the role of ^{18}F-FDG-PET and the metabolic changes as biomarkers of the epileptogenic zone (EZ) and the dysplastic tissue. We will emphasize some methodological and technical issues to improve ^{18}F-FDG-PET usefulness in clinical routine and for surgical planning. Finally, we also will assess the place of other radiotracers and new hybrid PET-MR machines in the diagnosis of FCD.

^{18}F-FDG-PET in Epilepsy: Metabolic biomarker of the epileptogenic zone

In MTLE, the first recognized indication of ^{18}F-FDG-PET, it has been well established that interictal hypometabolism is helpful for the localization and lateralization of the epileptic focus (Engel *et al.*, 1982), being found in up to 90% of the cases. However this hypometabolism was more extensive than the structural lesions found on MRI (most commonly hippocampal sclerosis) and involved other areas in the temporal lobe, such the temporal pole, the lateral and basal temporal cortex, as well as extratemporal cortical and subcortical regions, especially the frontal lobe, the insula and the basal ganglia (Theodore *et al.*, 1988; Semah *et al.*, 1995; Arnold *et al.*, 1996; Ryvlin *et al.*, 1998). Although hypometabolism includes the EZ and remote areas, its extent and topography vary greatly at the individual level. Mechanisms of hypometabolism are incompletely understood and assumed to be multifactorial, including the effect of structural lesions and neuronal loss, the decrease of synaptic activity or density, and postictal depression of electrical activity. It may be influenced by subclinical seizures and other factors related to the epilepsy, such as duration of the disease, seizure frequency, delay between the last seizure and PET examination, type of the last seizure (especially if generalized or an unusual seizure type) and anti-seizure drugs (Theodore *et al.*, 1988; Engel *et al.*, 1990; Henry *et al.*, 1994; Gaillard *et al.*, 1995; Savic *et al.*, 1997). It has been also related to the extent of the EZ, including the SOZ and the areas of propagation of ictal discharges (Chassoux *et al.*, 2004, 2016; Wong *et al.*, 2010; Guedj *et al.*, 2015). Finally, PET findings correlated with the surgical prognosis (Radtke *et al.*, 1993; Dupont *et al.*, 2000; Vinton *et al.*, 2007; Chassoux *et al.*, 2017; Cahill *et al.*, 2019). All this knowledge has been widely disseminated and the use of ^{18}F-FDG-PET has been assessed in large cohorts, proving its usefulness in clinical routine in adults as in children (Rathore *et al.*, 2014; Rubinger *et al.*, 2015; Steinbrenner *et al.*, 2022).

FDG-PET in FCD: Metabolic biomarkers of the dysplastic tissue

Despite the low sensitivity previously reported in extratemporal epilepsies (Knowlton *et al.*, 2008), ^{18}F-FDG-PET proved early to be highly sensitive for the detection of FCD (Chugani *et al.*, 1990; Lee *et al.*, 2001; Kim *et al.*, 2002). Advances of MR techniques over the next decade have blurred the role of ^{18}F-FDG-PET, however subsequent studies have highlighted its value, especially in negative MRI cases, whatever the FCD localization (Salamon *et al.*, 2008; Chassoux *et al.*, 2010). As FCD II are predominantly located in extra-temporal areas, often involving eloquent areas, and are often of small size and difficult to detect even with optimal MRI (Chassoux *et al.*, 2012; Colombo *et al.*, 2012; Mellerio *et al.*, 2012; Bernasconi *et al.*, 2019), improving their identification and localization is crucial for referring patients to surgery and guide the cortical resection. In a previous study, we demonstrated that ^{18}F-FDG-PET was able to detect the FCD II in 22/23 patients operated in extratemporal areas, despite a negative/doubtful MRI, allowing an excellent seizure outcome (87% of seizure-free) for these difficult-to-treat patients (Chassoux *et al.*, 2010). Although MRI was not optimal at that time, comparison with ^{18}F-FDG-PET unequivocally demonstrated the PET superiority (**Figures 1-2**). In addition, finding a strong focal hypometabolism may help to detect a subtle lesion previously missed on MRI.

A major issue remains the relatively low sensitivity of ^{18}F-FDG-PET alone, which increases dramatically after the integration of electroclinical features and the coregistration of PET and MRI (Salamon *et al.*, 2008; Chassoux *et al.*, 2010; Rubi *et al.*, 2011; Desarnaud *et al.*, 2018; Ding *et al.*, 2018; Tan *et al.*, 2018). In a large series of 103 FCD II histologically proven, we showed that visual analysis of ^{18}F-FDG-PET alone allowed to detect 44% of the lesions, increasing to 71% after considering the electroclinical data and 83% after superimposition of PET on MRI (Desarnaud *et al.*, 2018). The additional value of the coregistration was particularly obvious for small, deeply located FCD II, for which the spatial resolution of PET was too low for the detection of the lesion but "compensated" by the fusion with MRI. These data should be considered when searching for FCD in MRI-negative cases and support the coregistration of PET and MRI as a standard protocol.

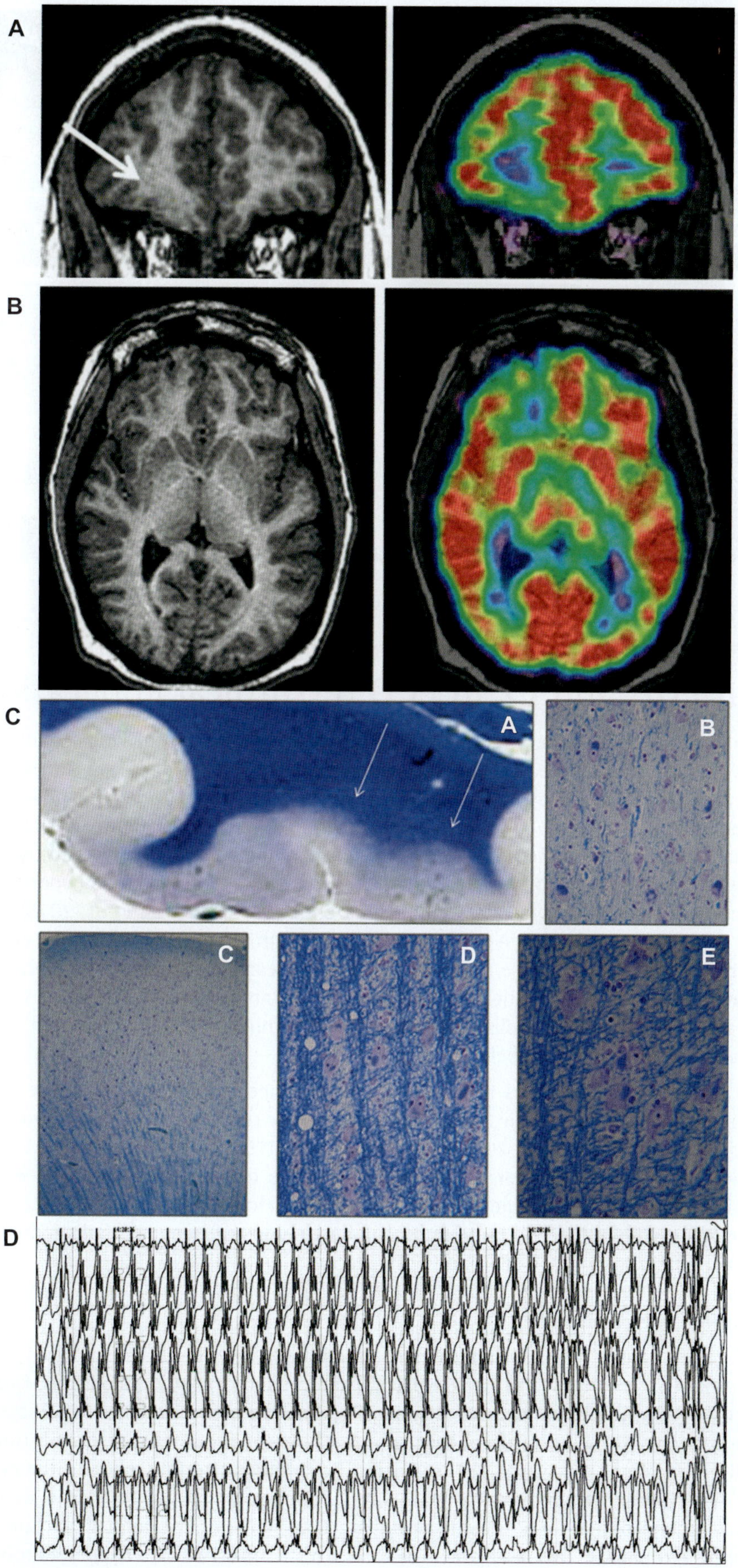

Figure 1

MRI, ^{18}F-FDG-PET, neuropathology and SEEG correlations in a right fronto-orbitar FCD IIB. 18 year-old female, sleep-related right frontal lobe epilepsy, daily seizures, onset at 3.

A. 1.5T T1-MRI, coronal view, superimposition of ^{18}F-FDG-PET on MRI; B. Axial view, same sequences. MRI was initially considered negative, but revised positive after PET showing a strong hypometabolism involving the right frontobasal region and allowing to detect a mild blurring of the gray-white matter junction on MRI (arrow); C. Cortical specimen, "en bloc" resection showing a localized blurring of the gray and white matter junction (Klüver Barrera, magnification AX4, arrows), cortical dyslamination and typical cytomegalic neurons and balloon cells (B-C-D-E X10-40) – *Courtesy of Prof. Catherine Daumas-Duport*; D. SEEG, interictal activity recorded within the hypometabolic area, typical interictal FCD II pattern with continuous rhythmic spiking. The patient has been seizure-free for 20 years without anti-seizure treatment after the cortical resection corresponding to the hypometabolic area.

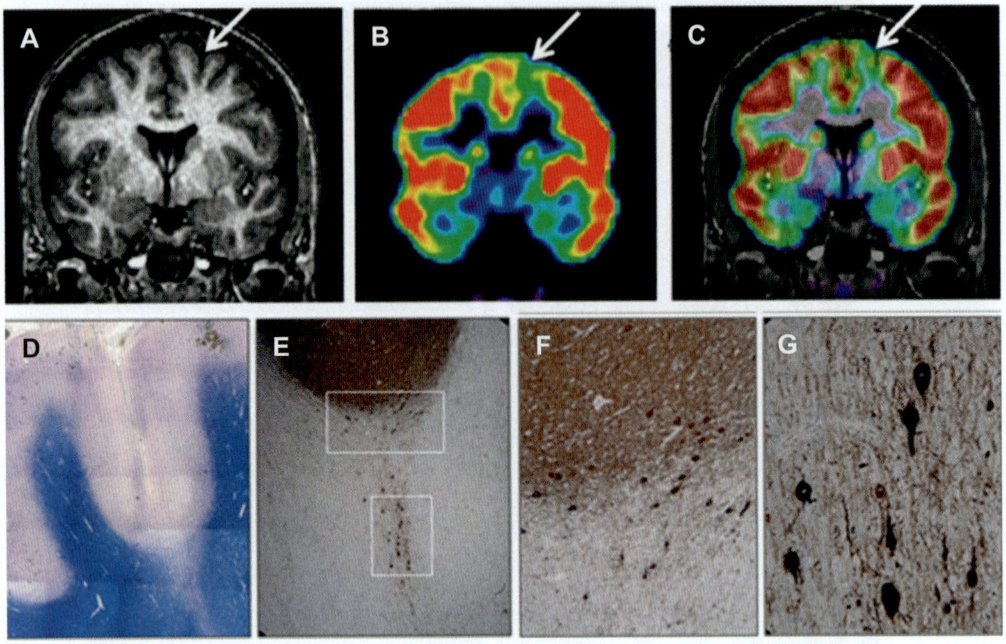

Figure 2
MRI, ^{18}F-FDG-PET and neuropathologic correlations in a left frontal FCD IIA.
17 year-old female, sleep-related frontal lobe epilepsy, left SMA semiology, daily seizures, onset at 3. A. 1.5T T1-MRI, coronal view, considered negative; B. ^{18}F-FDG PET showing a clearcut focal hypometabolism involving the left posterior frontal convexity, near the midline; C. Superimposition of PET on MRI, hypometabolism involving a single gyrus in the posterior part of the left superior frontal sulcus with a transmantle sign (Bottom of the sulcus dysplasia: BOSD); D. Cortical specimen, "en bloc" resection showing the histologic hallmark of the transmantle sign with a deep extension within the white matter from the bottom of the sulcus (Klüver Barrera, magnification X4), E. (NeuN, magnification X10), cytomegalic neurons predominant at the bottom of the sulcus (FX20), linear extension within the white matter (GX40), no balloon cells identified in the surgical specimen (FCD IIA) – *Courtesy of Prof. Catherine Daumas-Duport.* The patient is seizure-free for 20 years without anti-seizure treatment after the resection of the hypometabolic gyrus.

Relationship between interictal metabolic patterns and EZ in FCD II: surgical implications

The high intrinsic epileptogenicity of FCD II sustained by a continuous spiking activity could, in theory, lead to increased focal metabolic activity (hypermetabolism). However, the interictal metabolic pattern usually observed in FCD II consists in a focal or regional hypometabolism, corresponding to a decrease of cerebral metabolic rate of glucose (CMRglu). Comparison with SEEG data have demonstrated that the site of maximal hypometabolism was always concordant with the dysplastic cortex and the SOZ (**Figures 3-4**), while relative hypometabolism corresponded to areas of ictal spread (Chassoux *et al.*, 2010; Guerrini *et al.*, 2015). The reasons of such hypometabolism in cortical lesions with high spiking activity are not elucidated. It can be assumed that glucose uptake is strongly decreased in the dysplastic cortex due to abnormal neuronal and synaptic activity. This notwithstanding, in a few cases - especially in young children – hypermetabolism can be observed within the FCD, likely related to continuous subclinical seizures (see below).

Importantly, in selected cases topographic concordance between the FCD, the extent of the EZ and the hypometabolic areas may allow direct resective surgery without invasive monitoring (Chassoux *et al.*, 2010, Guerrini *et al.*, 2015, Flaus *et al.*, 2021). When focal hypometabolism is found, corresponding to a single gyrus and concordant with electroclinical data, a PET/MR guided surgery may be performed, with a favorable outcome (**Figure 2**). In contrast, when large or multilobar regions of hypometabolism are seen, or when hypometabolism is discordant with electroclinical data, SEEG remains necessary. In these cases, the planning of depth electrode implantation will benefit from the PET findings (**Figures 3-5**).

There was no specific SEEG signature in hypometabolic zones, that at times extended beyond the FCD lesion, but rather electrical patterns indicating propagation of interictal and ictal discharges, and the spatiotemporal spread from the SEEG patterns seen at the ictal onset zone. These patterns, in turn, pointed to the main pathways of evolution of the ictal discharge from the site of seizure onset. The findings strongly relate to the proximity of the FCD from large white matter pathways: if the lesion is close to a large, dense fiber pathway (occipito-temporal, arcuate or uncinate fasciculi, or the corpus callosum fibers), discharges propagate fast and reach distant sites – and the PET hypometabolic zones

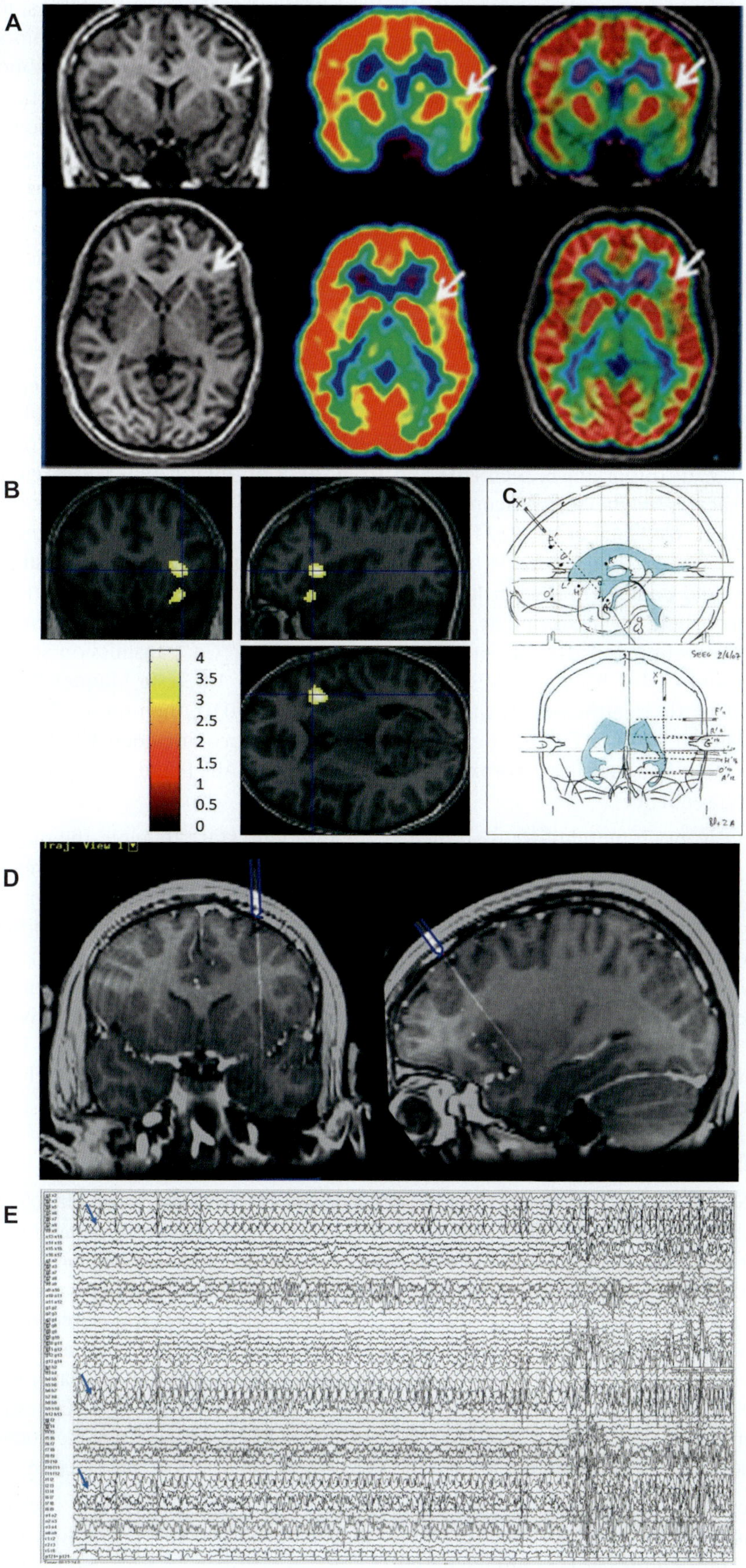

Figure 3

^{18}F-FDG-PET and SEEG correlations in a left insular FCD IIA.

16 year-old female, sleep-related epilepsy, hypermotor seizures, several seizures per night, onset at 1.5.

A. 1.5T T1-MRI, ^{18}F-FDG-PET, superimposition of PET on MRI, coronal and axial views. Left anterior insular and temporopolar hypometabolism.
B. Statistical parametric analysis (SPM5), comparison with 30 healthy controls (p=0.005): hypometabolism maximal in the insula (left side on the right); C. SEEG, depth electrode implantation scheme, sampling the left frontal (F', G', O', R'), insular (X', H', L') and temporal areas (A'); D. Trajectory of the oblique electrode X' on MRI (by convention, the electrode contacts are numbered from the depth to the surface, contacts 5 to 9 are located in the insula, whereas contacts 1-4 are located in the fronto-orbitar area and 10-18 in the white matter then in the middle frontal gyrus;
E. SEEG recordings, interictal activity showing subcontinuous rhythmic spikes and slow waves without background activity, well localized within the anterior insula (middle contacts of the electrode X', deep contacts of the electrodes H' and L' (arrows), ictal onset zone in the same areas. After a focal resection of the anterior insula (FCD IIA found in the cortical specimen), the patient was seizure free for 6 months then relapsed; after stereotaxic thermocoagulations of the adjacent part of the resection, she has been almost seizure free for 12 years (Engel class II).

reflect their trajectory. However, if the lesion is distant from these pathways, discharges as well as the PET hypometabolism remain local. The rate of glucose consumption is the key aspect to understand the relations between propagation of epileptic abnormalities and metabolism, including the post-ictal depression of activity which reflects the intensity of the discharges over each territory. Therefore, there is a gradient of hypometabolism away from the lesion – from most to least severe –pointing to the direction and intensity (speed) of the propagation of epileptic discharges to adjacent and distant cortical regions (Figures 4-5).

Technical and practical considerations

• Principles and methods of PET examination

Our experience with FDG-PET in patients investigated for drug-resistant epilepsy is based on more than 1200 exams between 2000 and 2020 at SHFJ (CEA, Orsay, France), using high resolution 3D PET camera (HR+ CTI Exact Siemens, Knoxville, TN, USA), then from 2009 on a PET-CT with (Biograph 6, Siemens) and from 2018 an hybrid PET-MR machine (SIGNA GE Healthcare, Milwaukee, Wisconsin, USA) based on a 3T MR scanner (for more technical information, see Flaus *et al.*, 2021). ^{18}F-FDG was injected intravenously at a mean dose of 3MBq/kg of body-weight after 4 hours fasting. Image acquisition started 30 min after the injection and ended 15-20 min later. Patients were studied in awake and resting state, in a quiet, dimly lit environment and carefully monitored for head movements and ictal events. Correction for attenuation was done using ^{68}Ga–^{68}Ge transmission scans for HR+ cameras and CT for Biograph. MRI were performed on a 1.5 Tesla Magnet (Signa Excite, General Electric Healthcare, Milwauke, WI, USA) before 2010, then on a 3 Tesla MRI (Discovery MR750; General Electric Healthcare). The MRI protocol included 3D T1-weighted 1.2 mm thick contiguous slices, coronal T2-weighted and FLAIR (Fluid Attenuation Inversion Recovery) sequences.

Importantly, brain metabolism is studied at the interictal state to avoid the major changes due to ictal (CMRglu strongly increased) and postictal (CMRglu strongly decreased) states during glucose uptake time (30 min). In addition, head and body movements during a seizure would compromise PET acquisition and the localization of abnormalities. Ideally, the interictal metabolic state should be evaluated at least 6 hours after the last seizure, a delay which is not always possible in patients with FCD, who have several seizures per day. Then peri-ictal examinations are not rare and may contribute to false negative or wrong results. In case of doubt, repeated examination must be discussed. Overall, it is recommended to avoid periods with unusually high seizure frequency or seizure clusters when performing ^{18}F-FDG-PET.

• Ictal PET

Unlike SPECT, for which ictal scans can be planned, ictal PET scans are rarely feasible because of the relatively short half-life of ^{18}F-FDG (110 min). However, patients with frequent seizures may experience a seizure during the 30-min ^{18}F-FDG uptake period. It has been reported that if a seizure occurs early (the first 10 min) during tracer uptake and lasts for more than a few minutes, hypermetabolism may be observed, while brief seizures or seizures occurring later will usually not show hypermetabolism (Chugani, 2021). In our experience, hypermetabolism is rarely observed and never in FCD cases, despite seizures occurring during PET acquisition, probably due to usual short seizure duration. In contrast, a large hypometabolism may be observed, suggesting a postictal pattern. In other cases, a composite pattern combining hyper and hypometabolism can be seen. These data are difficult to interpret and as peri-ictal PET, ictal PET may need to be repeated.

EEG recordings during the PET examinations are not performed in clinical routine but the patients should be carefully monitored for ictal events and asked for any subclinical manifestation during the ^{18}F-FDG uptake period.

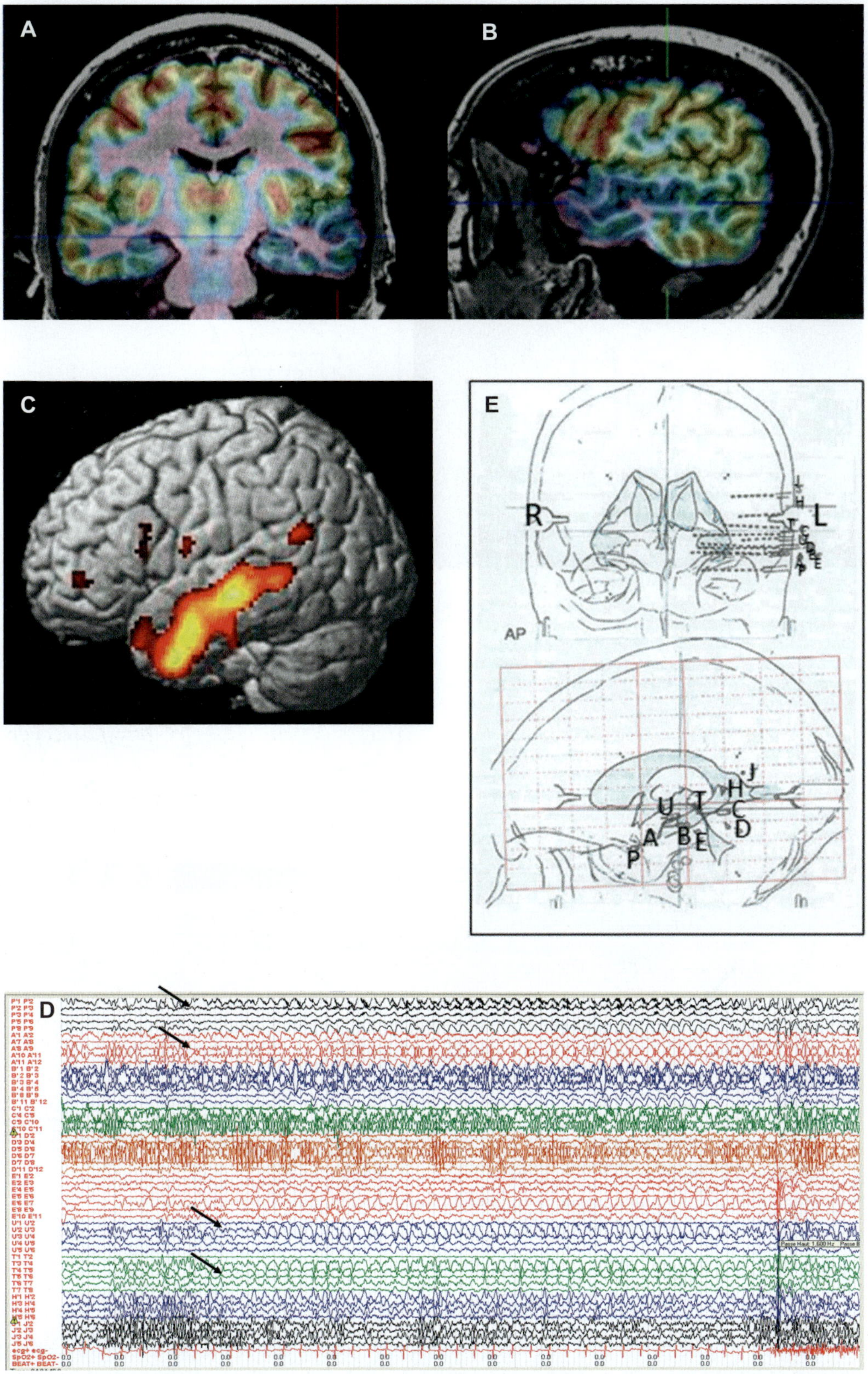

Figure 4

^{18}F-FDG-PET and SEEG correlations in a left temporal FCD IIB.

42 year-old female, sleep-related epilepsy, left temporal semiology, several seizures per month, onset at 5. 3T MRI negative.
A. Superimposition of PET on MRI, coronal view showing a regional hypometabolism involving the left temporal lobe (predominant in the lateral and anterior part); B. Sagittal view; C. Hypometabolic areas on a 3D brain render of SPM images (SPM5, p=0.005), maximal in the temporal pole, superior and middle temporal gyri (STG-MTG); D, E. SEEG recordings and scheme of depth electrode implantation; subclinical discharge involving the temporal pole (P'), the anterior part of the MTG (A') and STG (T'), with a slower activity on other adjacent electrodes (U', B'lateral, E'), less visible on H', without involvement of posterior areas (D', J') and hippocampus (B'-C', mesial contacts). Note the correspondence between the gradient of hypometabolism (from more to less severe) and the speed of the ictal discharge (from faster to slower). FCD IIB was located in the anterior part of the superior temporal sulcus up to T', the posterior limit of the resection was between T'and H'. The patient has been seizure free for 8 years and anti-seizure drugs stopped.

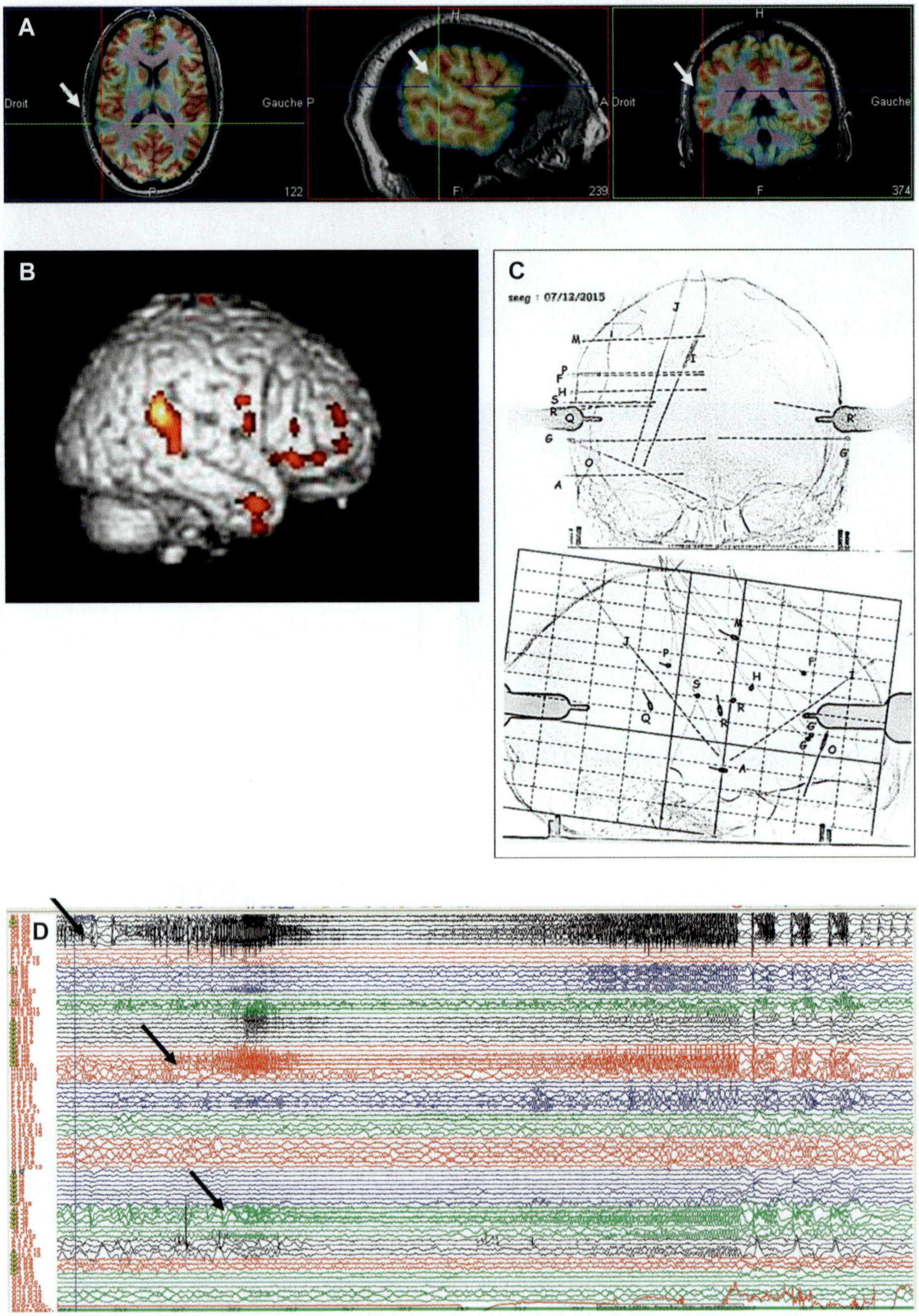

Figure 5

^{18}F-FDG-PET and SEEG correlations in a right posterior temporal FCD IIB. 30 year-old male, sleep-related epilepsy, frontal (hypermotor) semiology, several seizures per night, onset at 10. 3T MRI negative. A. Superimposition of PET on MRI, axial, sagittal and coronal views, showing a focal hypometabolism involving the right posterior superior temporal gyrus (STG, arrow); B. Hypometabolic areas on a 3D brain render of SPM images (SPM5, p=0.005), maximal in the STG corresponding to the visually detected hypometabolism, mild other hypometabolis areas in the frontal and temporal areas; C. Scheme of depth electrode implantation, large sampling of the right frontal (H, M, R, F, G, O), insular (J, I), parietal (P, S) and temporal areas (Q': STG, corresponding to the hypometabolic gyrus, A: amygdala and middle temporal gyrus), with 2 electrodes on the left side (G', R'); D. SEEG, typical interictal and ictal FCD pattern on Q', continuous rhythmic spiking and ictal onset with transitional high amplitude fast activity before the low voltage fast activity, early spread to remote frontal areas (especially H), and insular electrode (J), less rapid on other electrodes (S, R, G, A). Note the concordance between the main hypometabolism and the ictal onset zone on the one hand, the gradient of hypometabolism and the propagation of the ictal discharge on the other hand, the remote hypometabolic areas corresponding to the main ictal spread pathways. The patient has been seizure free for 5 years after a resection limited to the hypometabolic gyrus (FCD IIB).

Specificities in children

^{18}F-FDG-PET may be performed in children including infants, under the same general conditions as in adults. EEG can be performed during the PET scan in young children to assess the occurrence of subclinical seizures. In children <6 years or agitated, sedation using Pentobarbital (5mg/kg IR) is usually necessary, under the supervision of pediatrists. Sevoflurane or propofol may also be used. It has been shown that such drugs did not impact the CMRGlu. The absorbed dose has been calculated at 5mSv for PET alone and 25mSv for PET-CT. To reduce the radiation exposure, PET/MR if available is a good option (see below). Variation in brain size during childhood (< 6y) demands a specific pediatric FDG template for SPM. In addition, non-linear regional changes of brain metabolism occur during childhood, implying the need for a pediatric control population for statistical comparisons (Archambaud *et al.*, 2013).

Analysis of images

In clinical routine, images are visually analyzed using a semi-quantitative grading of the metabolic changes. The look-up table (LUT) roughly equally divided the colour scale with upper scale normalization of 80% and background noise of 20%, followed by a new upper scale normalization if necessary. Hypometabolism is classified as mild, moderate or severe according to the percentage of standard uptake variation (SUV) reduction (10-15, 15-20, >20), and subtle/doubtful if <10%. The "rainbow scale" offers a large spectrum of colours easy to differentiate by the human eye, each colour indicating approximatively 15% of SUV. After having previously used a homemade software (Anatomist, available on <http://brainvisa.info>), PET and MRI images superimposition are now performed on the PET working stations using the tools provided by the manufacturers.

Statistical analyses may provide additional information but needs a control population according to age, using the same protocol and the same PET camera. For ethical reasons, it is difficult to build a database of ^{18}F-FDG-PET scans of normal children, hence comparison may be achieved with pediatric pseudo-controls (epileptic children with normal MRI and normal PET) as described by Archambaud *et al.* (2013). Our previous study in MRI-negative FCD using SPM5 demonstrated a concordance with visual analysis in most cases, despite some limitations, especially for small lesions deeply located in the medial aspect of the brain or at the bottom of the sulci, where metabolism does not clearly differ from that of the white matter. In addition, SPM analysis allowed to objectively determine the site of maximal hypometabolism and provided additional elements to delineate the dysplastic lesion (**Figures 3-5**). Overall, while not improving visual assessment, SPM analysis provided objective data and supported the localization of the visually detected hypometabolism. Therefore, combination of visual PET/MRI coregistration and SPM analysis may be helpful, provided an adequate control population is available. Of note, some Centers currently include the statistical analysis in their clinical work-up, especially in negative MRI and extratemporal cases (Mayoral et al 2016, Mendes-Coelho *et al.*, 2017).

PET/MR hybrid imaging: a new step for FCD detection

More recently, new hybrid PET/MR imaging has been developed, allowing simultaneous acquisition of brain metabolism images provided by ^{18}F-FDG PET and morphological or functional images by MRI under the same clinical conditions. This new technique aimed to improve the suboptimal co-registration when PET and MRI images were obtained separately on different machines. In addition, PET/MR decreased the radiation exposure compared with PET-CT, a notable advantage especially in children. The reliability of PET/MR has been assessed in focal epilepsy and an increased accuracy for the localization of the EZ and the detection of structural lesions has been shown compared with PET-CT and MRI performed separately (Ding *et al.*, 2014; Shin *et al.*, 2015; Paldino *et al.*, 2017; Oldan *et al.*, 2018; Poirier *et al.*, 2021; Kikuchi *et al.*, 2021).

In a recent study based on 25 patients, we found that the PET/MR had a 13% increase of sensitivity compared to PET coregistered with MRI, both being previously obtained separately. In this series, PET/MR allowed the detection of structural lesions (including 5 FCD II) in 6 patients in whom the MRI was initially considered negative (Flaus *et al.*, 2021). In addition, changes in surgical decision-making was substantial for 10 patients (40%), consisting in avoiding invasive monitoring in 6 and modifying the planning in 4 others. In the 14 patients who underwent corticectomy, a seizure-free outcome was obtained in 12 (follow-up>1 year). PET/MR appears to reach a new, higher level of resolution for detection of FCD compared to the reference imaging. Reasons for this improvement may relate to better coregistration of PET and MRI provided by PET/MR, a better detection of small lesions due to the simultaneous acquisition of high-resolution 3D-T1 MRI sequences (especially when located at the bottom of the sulcus) and a better analysis of FLAIR images guided by PET (**Figure 6**). Indeed, despite advances in fusion software, it may be difficult to obtain optimal co-registration of PET and MR images acquired separately on different machines, at different times and under different conditions, including the postictal state. In addition, visual analysis of 3D-T1 and FLAIR images is greatly facilitated by the simultaneous acquisition of PET. This argues for the simultaneous acquisition of PET and MRI especially when searching for small FCD in MRI-negative cases.

Place of other radiotracers

Beside ^{18}F-FDG, several radiotracers have been developed to improve the sensitivity and specificity of PET for delineation of the EZ and identification of epileptogenic lesions. ^{11}C-Flumazenil (FMZ), a reliable in vivo marker of $GABA_A$-central benzodiazepine receptor (cBZR) binding, has been assessed in MTLE and in MCD, including FCD. In patients with MTLE, ^{11}C-FMZ-PET allowed a similar rate of localization of the EZ compared to ^{18}F-FDG, but showing more restricted, localized abnormalities - and therefore providing additional information on the EZ delineation (Ryvlin *et al.*, 1998). In addition, ^{11}C-FMZ-PET was more informative than ^{18}F-FDG-PET in frontal lobe epilepsies without a lesion visible on MRI, although it did not help to localize the EZ in FCD cases. Another study showed a significant decrease of cBZR binding within the FCD but increased binding in the vicinity, suggesting the FCD extent to be larger than MRI findings (Hammers *et al.*, 2001). Although promising, ^{11}C-FMZ-PET was difficult to use in clinical routine due to short ^{11}C half-life (20 min) and has been limited to research protocols. In addition, benzodiazepine drugs could not be administered during a month before the PET, a difficult requirement in patients with high seizure frequency and seizure clusters.

In Tuberous Sclerosis, α-^{11}C-methyl-L-tryptophan (AMT) was used to identify the epileptogenic tubers, showing a high specificity despite a low sensitivity (Chugani *et al.*, 2011). These results were partially reproduced in other Centers and remain to be confirmed (Rubi *et al.*, 2013). ^{11}C-AMT-PET was also proposed in FCD, in which abnormalities were typically smaller

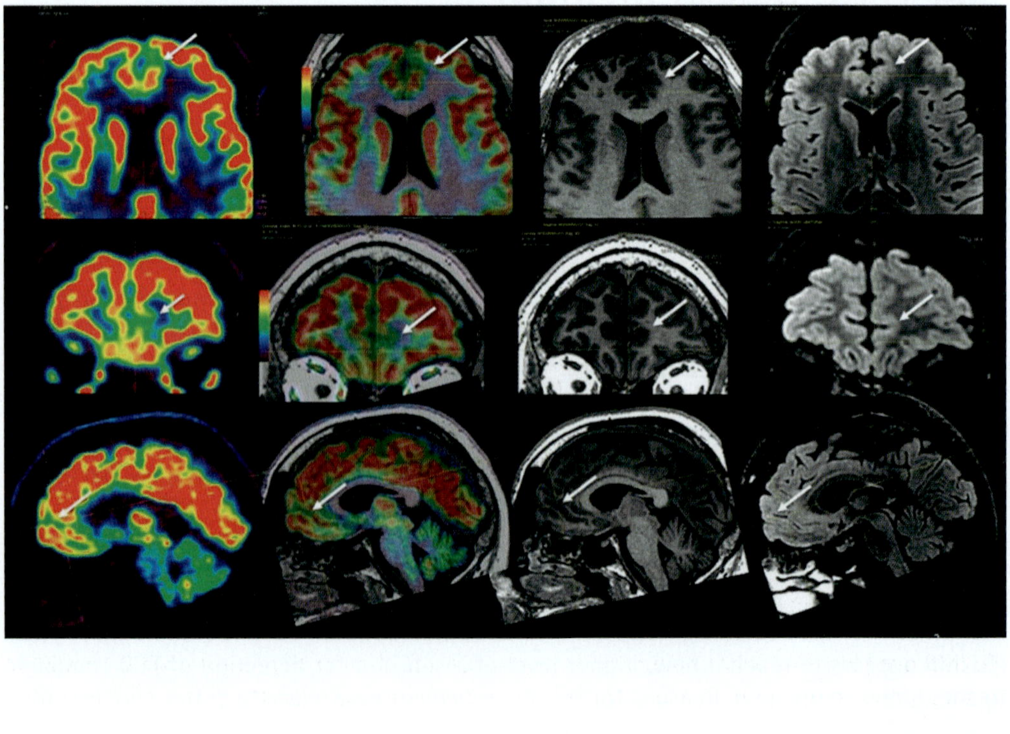

Figure 6

^{18}F-FDG-PET/MR in a right anterior mesial FCD IIB.
55 year-old male, frontal lobe epilepsy, difficult to lateralize, daily seizures, onset at 5. Negative 3T-MRI. Simultaneous acquisition of PET, 3DT1 and 3D-FLAIR MRI, axial, coronal and sagittal coregistration of PET on MRI; focal hypometabolism involving the left anterior mesial frontal lobe (arrows), corresponding to a single gyrus. Careful analysis of MRI, guided by the hypometabolism, allows the detection of a mild blurring of the gray-white matter junction, with a sharp hypersignal into the white matter on FLAIR sequences. The patient was seizure free for 3 years after a resection limited to the hypometabolic gyrus (FCD IIB), performed without SEEG (PET/MR guided surgery).

than the hypometabolism shown by ^{18}F-FDG-PET. ^{11}C-AMT-PET was also reported able to detect epileptogenic regions missed by both MRI and ^{18}F-FDG-PET (Chugani *et al.*, 2011). For these authors, the neuropathological similarities between tubers and FCD II suggested a common mechanism of epileptogenesis, for which ^{11}C-AMT-PET could be a biomarker. However, as for ^{11}C-FMZ, AMT labeled with ^{11}C must be synthesized on site using a cyclotron due to the short half-life of only 20 min, limiting access to ^{11}C-AMT-PET until AMT can be labeled with ^{18}F, a PET radionuclide widely available with a longer half-life (110 min).

The last class of radioligands that may be used in focal epilepsies due to FCD are based on the neuroinflammatory processes identified in epileptogenic foci, such as hippocampal sclerosis but also in dysplastic lesions. Several markers have been developed for the "peripheral benzodiazepine receptor" (PBR) or translocator protein 18kDa (TSPO), located on brain glial and ependymal cell mitochondrial membranes and expressed at high levels on activated astrocytes and microglia. Preliminary studies have suggested that ^{11}C-PK11195 can identify brain inflammation in a case report of frontal lobe epilepsy due to FCD (Butler *et al.*, 2013). A recent study has confirmed increased TSPO binding in ictal-onset regions with other markers of neuroinflammation (^{11}C-PBR or DPA-713), suggesting the presence of inflammation both ipsilateral and contralateral to the seizure focus. FCD II was found in five of six patients who had surgery, consistent with previous reports of increased inflammatory markers in pathological specimens. However, according to the authors' view, the complexity of the method, inherent variability, and presence of increased binding in regions outside seizure foci will limit the applicability of the technique (Dieckstein *et al.*, 2019). The high affinity of another TSPO ligand ^{18}F-DPA-714 has been evaluated in animal models and is currently under investigation in epileptic patients (Bouilleret et Deuderweadere, 2021). Because of its high bioavailability in brain tissue and its reduced nonspecific binding, ^{18}F-DPA-714 appears a ligand of choice for developing a novel imaging approach in epilepsy.

Limitations and pitfalls

As the technique is mainly used at the interictal state, ^{18}F-FDG-PET does not provide direct information about the EZ and the temporospatial dynamic of seizure spread. However, it provides valuable information on the location of FCD, a specific kind of lesion in which the dysplastic tissue and SOZ are most often colocalized. In addition, large hypometabolic areas usually encompass the SOZ and ictal discharge spread, and the topography of the hypometabolism may be helpful for SEEG planning if indicated. On the other hand, ictal PET may provide precise localization findings but is difficult to obtain and to interpret.

A second limitation is the lack of information about other FCD subtypes, especially for FCD I in which no reliable data are available. Further investigations will be facilitated by the clarification of their definition and electroclinical features, as the use of more specific radiotracers in the future.

One of the main pitfalls consists in the temporal lobe involvement, that can appear predominant even in cases of extratemporal SOZ, reflecting secondary spread of ictal discharges to the temporal lobe (Chassoux *et al.*, 2010). This mainly occurs in fronto-basal or anterior mesial frontal FCD, in which early temporal involvement may be observed. This finding can also be made in FCD located in the anterior part of the insula, or in posterior cortex with temporal spread. In such cases, a careful analysis of electroclinical data may allow identification of a focal hypometabolism corresponding to the SOZ, that will be confirmed by intracranial recordings if the depth electrodes are adequately placed.

Conclusion

^{18}F-FDG-PET has proved its high sensitivity for the detection of FCD in adults and children, and its reliability in MRI-negative FCD II, a crucial issue when searching for these epileptogenic lesions as an important step before referring these patients to an epilepsy surgery program. To improve PET sensitivity, integration of electroclinical data and coregistration with MRI are mandatory. The site of maximal visually-detected hypometabolism has proven to be concor-

Part 2. SPECT in FCD

Martin Kudr

Key points

- Although ictal SPECT (SISCOM) is not part of standard presurgical workup, it could be useful in the localization of the EZ, especially in MRI negative or other difficult cases.
- Injection time, seizure type, seizure duration, hyperperfusion pattern and other technical aspects must be considered for correct SPECT performance and interpretation.
- Ictal SPECT is a useful and safe diagnostic method for children, including infants.

Introduction

Ictal SPECT is a functional neuroimaging method that uses visualization of regional cerebral perfusion (rCP) for localising the EZ in focal epileptic seizures. Although the examination is logistically demanding, it could be useful in FCD cases with normal or doubtful MRI findings by guiding the extent and location of resective epilepsy surgery or electrode implantation.

Technical considerations of ictal SPECT examination

• Methodological background

The localizing value of the method is based on cerebral metabolic and perfusion coupling - the increase in neuronal metabolic activity during seizures is associated with increase in rCP and conversely, the decrease in metabolic activity during the interictal period is associated with a decrease in rCP (Van Paesschen, 2004). Tracers used for perfusion SPECT studies are lipophilic substances 99m Tc-hexamethylene propylene amine (99m Tc-HMPAO) and 99m Tc-ethyl cysteinate dimer (99m Tc-ECD) (Kapucu *et al.*, 2009). Most of the tracers cross the blood-brain barrier a few seconds after the injection (with first pass brain uptake about 60% in 99m Tc-ECD and 85% in 99m Tc-HMPAO). Within the cells the tracer forms a non-diffusible compound with long retention time and low subsequent redistribution, hence creating an image of brain perfusion at the time of tracer injection (Van Paesschen, 2004). With a long half-life of both tracers, the SPECT scans can be acquired up to 4 hours after the injection (99mTc-ECD is stable 6 to 8 hours, and the stabilized form of 99m Tc-HMPAO for 4 h).

• The SISCOM era

The yield of ictal SPECT can be increased by co-registration of subtracted ictal and interictal SPECT images with MRI (SISCOM). Concordance of SISCOM focus with the site of surgery was shown to predict favourable postsurgical outcome (Kudr *et al.*, 2013a; O'Brien *et al.*, 2004) and has been demonstrated in a prospective study to alter the consensus decision-making process in epilepsy surgery (Tan *et al.*, 2008). Methods such as ictal-interictal SPECT analysis by SPM (ISAS) and statistical ictal SPECT co-registered to MRI (STATISCOM) further improve the localisation of the EZ by compensating the physiologic variance in cerebral blood flow that shows significant asymmetries in multiple areas (Kazemi *et al.*, 2009; McNally *et al.*, 2005; Sulc *et al.*, 2014). A summary of data processing comparing all three methods is presented in **figure 1** (Sulc *et al.*, 2014).

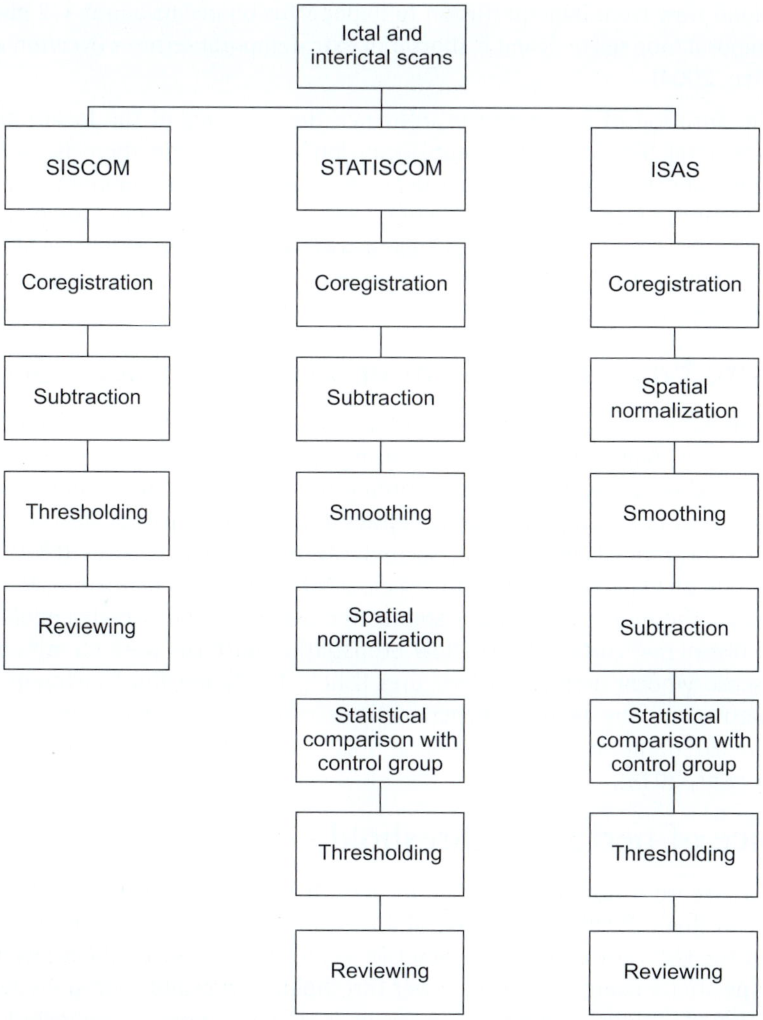

Figure 1
Summary of image processing (Sulc *et al.*, 2014).

• Injection time and seizure duration

One of the most important factors for correct ictal SPECT localisation is the shortest possible delay between the time of seizure onset and the time of injection – early injections of the tracer are associated with the best sensitivity and specificity. Lee and colleagues proved that injection delays of less than 20 seconds were significantly correlated with a correct localisation (Lee *et al.*, 2006). Other authors also recognised early injection time as crucial for success and accurate interpretation of ictal SPECT data. For instance, O'Brien and colleagues reported late injections (>45 seconds after seizure onset) significantly more frequently in patients with non-localising or falsely localising SPECT data. The same study demonstrated that late injections reduced the clarity of SISCOM localisation, as shown by the inability of reviewers to agree on localisation or to label the study as non-localising (O'Brien *et al.*, 1998). Kudr and colleagues showed that well-localized SPECT findings were significantly associated with early radiotracer injections (<30 seconds) (Kudr *et al.*, 2013b).

The explanation for the association between correctly localising SPECT findings and early radiotracer injections is the fact that regions of ictal hyperperfusion primarily reflect the site of predominant seizure activity at the time of radioisotope injection (Stefan *et al.*, 2000; Van Paesschen *et al.*, 2007) and thus, for early injections, there is a greater probability that the predominant seizure activity will be centred focally around the EZ. In contrast, when the injection is late, there is more time for spread of seizure activity and correspondent perfusion changes in secondary areas. Another important factor is the "postictal switch phenomenon". After injection in an arm vein, it takes about 30 seconds until the tracer reaches the brain.

Switch of blood flow from hyperperfusion to hypoperfusion occurs about 1-2 minutes post-ictally in temporal lobe seizures and is shorter in extratemporal seizures (Newton *et al.*, 1992; Van Paesschen, 2004).

Similarly, the duration of a seizure can influence the accuracy of the localization. In very short seizures, ictal SPECT could be non-localizing and although there is no observation based on large cohorts of patients, it has been estimated that extratemporal seizures should last ≥10–15 seconds after ictal SPECT injection to give localizing information (Van Paesschen, 2004). In contrast, longer seizure duration was associated with more extensive SPECT findings (Kudr *et al.*, 2013b), although the study evaluated more the extent of SPECT hyperperfusion focus than the accuracy of the localization.

Seizure type and localization accuracy of ictal SPECT

Despite scarce data, the type of injected seizure is also likely relevant for SPECT accuracy. Van Paesschen and colleagues described localizing information in around 40% of simple partial seizures (focal onset aware seizures according to new classification). Shin and colleagues described best results in temporal lobe epilepsies with complex partial seizures (focal onset with impaired awareness). In contrast, secondarily generalized seizures (FBTCS) may give multiple regions of hyperperfusion (Shin *et al.*, 2002; Van Paesschen, 2004; Van Paesschen *et al.*, 2000). Furthermore, some SPECT studies focused on specific ictal semiology or brain region. Two distinctive cortical blood-flow propagation patterns were identified in supplementarary sensorymotor area (SSMA) seizures (Laich, 1997) and three different patterns of ictal hyperperfusion were seen for hyperkinetic seizures, varying according to the subtype (Kheder *et al.*, 2020). In insular seizures, ictal SPECT can be localising but falsely lateralising (Sala-Padro *et al.*, 2019).

Choice of perfusion threshold

In SISCOM, a z-score threshold 2 is generally accepted and routinely used. Different z-score thresholds may hyperfocus or overextend the distribution of ictal hyperperfusion, thus impacting in the clinical evaluation of SISCOM. A higher z-score results in lower sensitivity and higher specificity compared with a lower threshold. Newey and colleagues evaluated the localizing value of various z-scores (1, 1.5, 2, and 2.5) in a seizure-free cohort of 26 patients following resective epilepsy surgery and examined the localising information of perfusion patterns observed at each z-score. The study showed that a z score of 1.5 represents a highly sensitive and specific SISCOM threshold that should be examined in conjunction with the traditionally used z score of 2 to enhance the chances of correct localization (Newey *et al.*, 2013). A more recent study of De Coster and colleagues on a larger cohort of 80 cases found no significant differences in the localizing value of the ictal onset zone using a threshold of 1.5 or 2, but interrater agreement and reader confidence were higher using a z-score threshold of 2. The authors, thus, advocate using a z-score 2 in routine clinical practice (De Coster *et al.*, 2018).

Clinical implications

Granting all the aspects considered to this point, it is hardly surprising that correct acquisition and interpretation of the ictal SPECT demands a stepwise process combining epileptology and logistics. In the first place, the rationale to perform an ictal SPECT for a particular patient should be considered. That consideration should follow a full presurgical work up, including patient and seizure history, video-EEG examination and MRI acquired with epilepsy surgery protocol, often complemented by FDG-PET. Furthermore, information on the type, duration, frequency and usual time of day of the seizures is important for the decision to proceed with an ictal SPECT examination. Ideal candidates are patients with frequent focal seizures longer than ≥10–15 seconds that are not evolving to FBTCS. On the other hand, ictal SPECT often fails to localize the ictal onset zone in cases with very short seizures or seizures with very fast propagations such as frontal lobe seizures with sudden motor phenomena (tonic, hyperkinetic and SSMA-type seizures) or opercular-insular seizures.

Injection of the tracer should be performed concomitant with video-EEG monitoring by a doctor or technician who is able to recognize the very initial manifestations of the seizure and, if possible, also the initial ictal EEG changes. In children, the presence of parents is mandatory, also because they are often able to recognize the very early phases of habitual seizures - and sometimes even the seizure prodromes. The tracer should be available in the patient's room at the time when the seizure is expected, and the patient must have a functional intravenous cannula that allows fast injection. In some centres including ours, anti-seizure therapy is reduced or withdrawn in patients with low seizure frequency to increase the likelihood of seizure occurrence. For the same reason, sleep deprivation can be useful, especially in children with seizures that occur during sleep (the patient has partial sleep deprivation during night and is allowed to sleep during the day when the tracer is ready). In such cases, the availability of medical staff able to treat generalized seizures and status epilepticus is necessary. As two final points, Barba *et al.* (2012) described the efficacy and safety of ictal SPECT performed during seizures provoked by pentylentetrazol in a large cohort of 52 patients, and Setoain and colleagues studied an automated injection system that could have some advantage compared to the traditional manual injection such as better adjustment of the injection dose and reduced rate of radiation exposure for patients and nurses, with mean average injection time similar in both methods (Setoain *et al.*, 2021). These latter approaches are not in routine clinical use.

In contrast to ictal SPECT, for interictal injections the tracer must be administered when the patient does not have seizure(s); hence, the anti-seizure medication must be returned, or even increased. Similarly, video-EEG monitoring during interictal SPECT injection may be useful to rule out subclinical seizures.

SPECT scans can be acquired up to four hours after the injection. In small children (up to six years) general anaesthesia is necessary during SPECT acquisition. Cooperation between neurologist, nuclear medicine expert, anaesthesiologist and the patient or his family is mandatory for a successful ictal SPECT examination.

Ictal SPECT perfusion patterns related to FCD

Dupont and colleagues described four different SISCOM hyperperfusion patterns in focal seizures due to dysplastic lesions visible on MRI (Dupont *et al.*, 2006; Van Paesschen *et al.*, 2007). In the first pattern, the highest z score and largest SISCOM cluster was observed within or near the dysplastic lesion and was most often seen in cases with very short injection time. The second pattern was characterized by bilobulated, "hourglass" appearance with the two lobules connected by a trail of hyperperfusion. The lobule with the lower z score represented the ictal onset zone and the lobule with maximum z score propagated ictal activity. Perfusion pattern 3 was similar to pattern 2, except that the cluster with the maximum z score was a separate cluster. However, when the SISCOM was thresholded at $z = 1$ instead of 2, the two clusters were connected in a multilobulated structure by narrow trails of hyperperfusion. This pattern was observed mostly in frontal lobe seizure with late ictal injection or when short seizures were injected. In the fourth perfusion pattern there was no hyperperfusion within or near the dysplastic lesion in the only patient with injection during a FBTCS. The mentioned patterns are in accordance with our clinical experience and should be considered when evaluating a SISCOM. **Figure 2** shows a pattern with maximum Z score in left opercular-insular cortex, **Figure 3** shows a bilobulated, "hourglass" pattern in right orbitofrontal and insular cortex and **Figure 4** shows typical non-localizing pattern with multiple foci of hyperperfusion.

In some disputable or non-localizing SPECT results the subcortical activations can provide indirect information about lateralisation of EZ. Contralateral cerebellar activation and ipsilateral basal ganglia/thalamic activation was described in examinations where cortical hyperperfusion was present (Krsek *et al.*, 2013; Sojkova *et al.*, 2003; Won *et al.*, 1999). However, in the study of Krsek and colleagues subcortical activation did not lateralised the EZ in SPECT studies lacking cortical hyperperfusion.

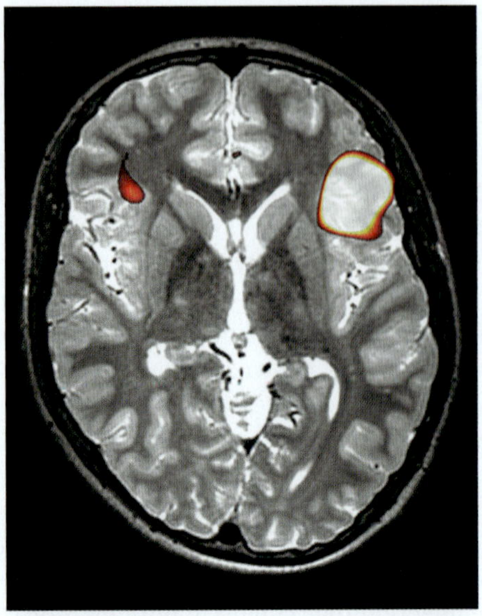

Figure 2

Pattern with maximum Z score in left opercular-insular and frontal cortex. 16 years old boy. Initially subclinical seizure during sleep with clear ictal pattern in left frontopolar (Fp) and frontal (F) electrodes (33 seconds), after waking up short behavioral arrest (25 seconds). Injection time 40 seconds. SISCOM finding partially congruent with PET and SEEG findings. Successful surgery of left anterior insula and frontal operculum, FCD IIB confirmed.

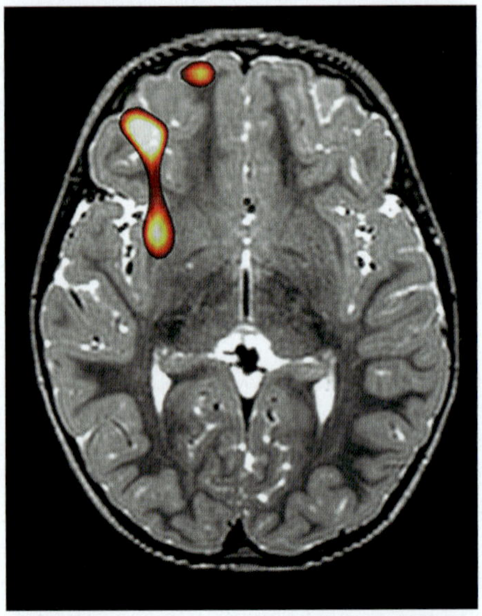

Figure 3

Bilobulated, "hourglass" pattern in right orbitofrontal and insular cortex. 4 years and 3 months old girl. Injected seizure - suspect epigastric aura followed by focal tonic signs (left sided extremities) and later automatic and hyperkinetic movements (mostly right sided extremities). Seizure duration 56 seconds. Injection time 30 seconds. Insular part of the SISCOM focus congruent with MRI, PET and SEEG findings. Successful surgery of right anterior insula and frontal operculum. Histology from operculum negative, from insula not available due to the use of cavitron ultrasonic surgical aspirator during surgery.

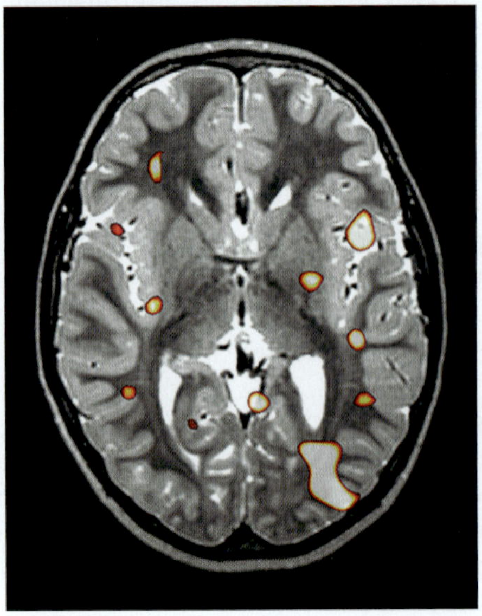

Figure 4

Non-localizing pattern with multiple and less extensive hyperperfusion focuses. 7 years and 11 months old boy. Focal tonic seizure quickly evolving to BTCS (3 minutes) followed by prolonged phase with spasms ended by application of rectal DZP (5 minutes). Injection time 49 seconds. Successful surgery of posterior insula based on SEEG implantation. FCD IA confirmed.

Role of ictal SPECT in MRI-negative cases

Patients with intractable focal epilepsy and normal MRI represent the most difficult-to-manage group of epilepsy surgery candidates. There is no exclusive diagnostic test to localize the EZ, however the ability to define and fully remove MRI-invisible dysplastic cortex is the most powerful variable that influences outcome in FCD patients (Cascino, 2004; Jayakar *et al.*, 2008; Paolicchi *et al.*, 2000). Multimodal diagnostic approach is necessary in MRI-negative cases and ictal SPECT (SISCOM) can be one of the tests that can help in the presurgical workup, mostly by guiding the localization and extent of invasive EEG monitoring. In some selected cases with concordant results of SPECT with other methods the one-stage surgical procedure can be performed.

Studies on this topic have used different approaches to determine the localization value of ictal SPECT as well as different postprocessing methods and thus the data are poorly comparable. Some studies show a very good diagnostic yield of the method in MRI negative cases, however the proper evaluation of the details regarding seizure type and injection time should be considered when considering the specificity and sensitivity of ictal SPECT in these studies. A brief comparison of published studies is shown in table 1.

Table 1

Comparison of SISCOM sensitivity in MRI negative cases and FCD in different studies.

	Seo *et al.* 2011	Krsek *et al.* 2013	Kudr *et al.* 2013	Perissinotti *et al.* 2014	Fernández *et al.* 2015
Cases (all pathologies)	14	106	14	54	25
MRI negative or non-informative	14	34	14	33	12
Histologically proved FCD/MCD	14	34	14	3	3
SPECT/SISCOM concordant with EEG/iEEG	11	NA	11	2	2
Favourable outcome when:					
completely resected	NA	6/6	3/3	NA	NA
partially resected	NA	7/14	4/8	NA	NA
non resected	NA	0/2	1/2	NA	NA
non-localizing	NA	6/12	1/1	NA	NA

In a large paediatric cohort evaluating the relationship of completeness of the SPECT hyperperfusion zone removal to surgical outcome, Krsek and colleagues described a subgroup of 34 children with non-lesional MRI in whom the authors used visual evaluation of ictal SPECT (not SISCOM or other postprocessing method). The six patients with completely resected zones of hyperperfusion had favourable postsurgical outcomes. In contrast, patients with non-resected hyperperfusion zones had unfavourable outcomes. Seven of 14 patients with partially resected hyperperfusion zones and six of 12 patients with non-localizing SPECT had favourable postsurgical outcomes (Krsek *et al.*, 2013). Kudr and colleagues studied SISCOM results in a group of 14 MRI-negative patients with histologically proven FCD. SISCOM findings were localized for all but one patient. Complete resection of the SISCOM focus (three cases) was predictive of favourable postsurgical outcome. Favourable outcome was also encountered in half (four of eight) cases with incomplete resection and one of two cases with no resection of the SISCOM focus (Kudr *et al.*, 2013a). Although based on a small cohort this study showed that SISCOM can very well localize the EZ in MRI negative FCD cases and that favourable outcome can be achieved also in cases with non-complete SISCOM focus resection. This might be explained by the fact that hyperperfusion areas represent different modes of seizure propagation as described above. In the study of Fernandez and colleagues, SISCOM was obtained in 25 patients with different pathologies and showed an area of hyperperfusion concordant with the presumed SOZ on EEG in two of three patients with normal MRI and FCD and five of ten patients with other or unknown pathology. Interestingly, SISCOM hyperperfusion was less extensive than PET hypometabolism (Fernández *et al.*, 2015). Similar results were found by Perissinotti and colleagues: SISCOM was able to localize the presumed EZ in 19 of 33 (57.6%) paediatric patients with noninformative MRI including two of three cases with proven FCD (Perissinotti *et al.*, 2014). In the study of Seo and colleagues SISCOM showed lobar concordance with intracranial EEG in 11 of 14 patients with FCD (79%) (Seo *et al.*, 2011).

The sensitivity of MRI is increasing in recent years due to special protocols for epilepsy, widespread use of higher magnetic-field and increasing skills of radiologists. This factor can influence the role of ictal SPECT examinations. On the other hand, some of the MRI-negative cases can became "subtle-lesion" cases during the presurgical workup exactly because ictal SPECT or other multimodal diagnostic tests provided valuable information.

Comparing the usefulness, availability and logistic difficulties, it is clear that FDG-PET is slowly becoming an essential part of epilepsy presurgical workup in FCD, whereas ictal SPECT should be reserved for special cases, when the integration of other sets of evaluation cannot localize the EZ. However, ictal SPECT could be useful to guide SEEG electrode implantation.

Ictal SPECT in children

Although feasibility of ictal SPECT in a real-life clinical setting in children was not systematically studied, application of radionuclide during ictal SPECT examination in children (especially in the infants and smaller children) raises some important methodological questions. As mentioned, the tight cooperation with family and the presence of the parents is mandatory. The general experience is that children up to six years require general anaesthesia during SPECT acquisition, up to four hours after the injection. Global cerebral blood flow changes rapidly in normal infants and young children, increasing after birth and peaking by age five or six years; it then diminishes slowly until it reaches adult levels between ages 15-19 years (Chiron *et al.*, 1992). Furthermore, over the first year of life, rCBF increases more rapidly in occipital rather than frontal cortex, causing an increased postero-anterior gradient (Chiron *et al.*, 1996). In infants, seizure semiology differs markedly from that in older children. Seizures in early life are more frequent and have a more limited repertoire of ictal manifestations, often lacking features indicative of localized onset such as auras (Acharya *et al.*, 1997).

Despite these age-related differences, the findings in purely paediatric as well as mixed-aged cohort studies on ictal SPECT revealed good sensitivity and specificity and ictal SPECT is thus considered to be an effective localizing tool for planning epilepsy surgery in paediatric patients with FCD (Buchhalter and So, 2004; Foiadelli *et al.*, 2020; Gupta *et al.*, 2004; Kaminska, 2003; Krsek *et al.*, 2013; O'Brien *et al.*, 2004; Perissinotti *et al.*, 2014; Seo *et al.*, 2011). Kudr and colleagues studied the localizing value of ictal SPECT (without any postprocessing) in 13 infants with intractable focal epilepsy caused by FCD. All ictal SPECT findings revealed localised hyperperfusion. All five patients with complete resection of the hyperperfusion zone were seizure-free compared to only one of eight patients with incomplete or no excision of hyperperfusion zones (Kudr *et al.*, 2016). These results argue strongly in favour of the utilization of ictal SPECT in this demanding subgroup of epilepsy surgery candidates.

References

Acharya J.N, Wyllie E, Luders H.O, Kotagal P, Lancman M, Coelho M. Seizure symptomatology in infants with localization-related epilepsy. *Neurology* 1997; 48, 189-96.

Barba C, Barbati G, Di Giuda D, *et al.* Diagnostic yield and predictive value of provoked ictal SPECT in drug-resistant epilepsies. *J. Neurol* 2012; 259, 1613-22.

Buchhalter J.R, So E.L. Advances in computer-assisted single-photon emission computed tomography (SPECT) for epilepsy surgery in children. *Acta Paediatr.* 2004; 93, 32-5.

Cascino G.D. Surgical treatment for extratemporal epilepsy. *Curr. Treat. Options Neurol.* 2004; 6, 257-62.

Chiron, C, Nabbout, R, Pinton, F, Nuttin, C, Dulac, O, Syrota, A. Brain functional imaging SPECT in agyria-pachygyria. *Epilepsy Res.* 1996; 24, 109-117.

Chiron, C, Raynaud, C, Mazière, B, *et al.* Changes in regional cerebral blood flow during brain maturation in children and adolescents. *J. Nucl. Med. Off. Publ. Soc. Nucl. Med.* 1992; 33, 696-703.

De Coster, L, Van Laere, K, Cleeren, E, *et al.* On the optimal z-score threshold for SISCOM analysis to localize the ictal onset zone. *EJNMMI Res.* 2018; 8, 34.

Dupont, P, Van Paesschen, W, Palmini, A. *et al.* Ictal Perfusion Patterns Associated with Single MRI-Visible Focal Dysplastic Lesions: Implications for the Noninvasive Delineation of the Epileptogenic Zone. *Epilepsia* 2006; 47, 1550-7.

Fernández, S, Donaire, A, Serès, E, *et al.* PET/MRI and PET/MRI/SISCOM coregistration in the presurgical evaluation of refractory focal epilepsy. *Epilepsy Res.* 2015; 111, 1-9.

Gupta, A, Raja, S, Kotagal, P, Lachhwani, D, Wyllie, E, Bingaman, W.B. Ictal SPECT in children with partial epilepsy due to Focal Cortical Dysplasia. *Pediatr. Neurol.* 2004; 31, 89-95.

Jayakar, P, Dunoyer, C, Dean, P, *et al.* Epilepsy surgery in patients with normal or nonfocal MRI scans: Integrative strategies offer long-term seizure relief. *Epilepsia* 2008; 49, 758-64.

Kaminska, A. Chiron C, Ville D *et al.* Ictal SPECT in children with epilepsy: comparison with intracranial EEG and relation to postsurgical outcome. *Brain* 2003; 126, 248-60.

Kapucu, Ö.L, Nobili, F, Varrone, A, *et al.* EANM procedure guideline for brain perfusion SPECT using 99mTc-labelled radiopharmaceuticals, version 2. *Eur. J. Nucl. Med. Mol. Imaging* 2009; 36, 2093-102.

Kazemi, N.J, Worrell, G.A, Stead, S.M, *et al.* Ictal SPECT statistical parametric mapping in temporal lobe epilepsy surgery. *Neurology* 2009; 74, 70-6.

Kheder, A, Thome, U, Aung, T, *et al.* Investigation of networks underlying hyperkinetic seizures utilizing ictal SPECT. *Neurology* 2020; 95, e637-42.

Krsek, P, Kudr, M, Jahodova, A, *et al.* Localizing value of ictal SPECT is comparable to MRI and EEG in children with Focal Cortical Dysplasia. *Epilepsia* 2013; 54, 351-358.

Kudr, M, Krsek, P, Marusic, P, *et al.* SISCOM and FDG-PET in patients with non-lesional extratemporal epilepsy: correlation with intracranial EEG, histology, and seizure outcome. *Epileptic Disord. Int. Epilepsy J. Videotape* 2013a; 15, 3-13.

Kudr, M, Krsek, P, Maton, B, *et al.* Predictive factors of ictal SPECT findings in paediatric patients with Focal Cortical Dysplasia. *Epileptic Disord. Int. Epilepsy J. Videotape* 2013b; 15, 383-91.

Kudr, M, Krsek, P, Maton, B, *et al.* Ictal SPECT is useful in localizing the epileptogenic zone in infants with cortical dysplasia. *Epileptic Disord. Int. Epilepsy J. Videotape* 2016; 18, 384-390.

Laich, E,. Supplementary sensorimotor area epilepsy. Seizure localization, cortical propagation and subcortical activation pathways using ictal SPECT. *Brain* 1997; 120, 855-864.

Lee, S.K, Lee, S.-Y, Yun, *et al.* Ictal SPECT in neocortical epilepsies: clinical usefulness and factors affecting the pattern of hyperperfusion. *Neuroradiology* 2006; 48, 678-684.

McNally, K.A, Paige, A.L, Varghese, G, *et al.* Localizing value of ictal-interictal SPECT analyzed by SPM (ISAS). *Epilepsia* 2005; 46, 1450-64.

Newey, C.R, Wong, C, Irene Wang, Z, Chen, X, Wu, G, Alexopoulos, A.V. Optimizing SPECT SISCOM analysis to localize seizure-onset zone by using varying z scores. *Epilepsia* 2013; 54, 793-800.

Newton, M.R, Berkovic, S.F, Austin, M.C, Rowe, C.C, McKay, W.J, Bladin, P.F,. Postictal switch in blood flow distribution and temporal lobe seizures. *J. Neurol. Neurosurg. Psychiatry* 1992; 55, 891-894.

O'Brien, T.J, So, E.L, Cascino, G.D, *et al.* Subtraction SPECT coregistered to MRI in focal malformations of cortical development: localization of the EZ in epilepsy surgery candidates. *Epilepsia* 2004; 45, 367-376.

O'Brien, T.J, Zupanc, M.L, Mullan, B.P, *et al.* The practical utility of performing peri-ictal SPECT in the evaluation of children with partial epilepsy. *Pediatr. Neurol.*1998; 19, 15-22.

Paolicchi, J.M, Jayakar, P, Dean, P, *et al.* Predictors of outcome in pediatric epilepsy surgery. *Neurology* 2000; 54, 642-7.

Perissinotti, A, Setoain, X, Aparicio, J, *et al.* Clinical Role of Subtraction Ictal SPECT Coregistered to MR Imaging and ^{18}F-FDG PET in Pediatric Epilepsy. *J. Nucl. Med.* 2014; 55, 1099-105.

Sala-Padro, J, Fong, M, Rahman, Z, *et al.* A study of perfusion changes with Insula Epilepsy using SPECT. *Seizure* 2019; 69, 44-50.

Seo, J.H, Holland, K, Rose, D, *et al.* Multimodality imaging in the surgical treatment of children with nonlesional epilepsy. *Neurology* 2011; 76, 41-8.

Setoain, X, Campos, F, Donaire, A, *et al.* How to inject ictal SPECT? From manual to automated injection. *Epilepsy Res.* 2021; 175.

Shin, W.C, Hong, S.B, Tae, W.S, Kim, S.E,. Ictal hyperperfusion patterns according to the progression of temporal lobe seizures. *Neurology* 2002; 58, 373-80.

Sojkova, J, Lewis, P.J, *et al.* Does asymmetric basal ganglia or thalamic activation aid in seizure foci lateralization on ictal SPECT studies? *J. Nucl. Med.* 2003; 44, 1379-86.

Stefan, H, Hopp, P, Platsch, G, Kuwert, T. SPECT: ictal perfusion in localization-related epilepsies. *Adv. Neurol.* 2000; 83, 41-50.

Sulc, V, Stykel, S, Hanson, D.P. *et al.* Statistical SPECT processing in MRI-negative epilepsy surgery. *Neurology* 2014; 82, 932-9.

Tan, K.M, Britton, J.W, Buchhalter, J.R, *et al.* Influence of subtraction ictal SPECT on surgical management in focal epilepsy of indeterminate localization: A prospective study. *Epilepsy Res.* 2008; 82, 190-3.

Van Paesschen, W. Ictal SPECT. *Epilepsia* 2004; 45, 35-40.

Van Paesschen, W, Dupont, P, Sunaert, S, Goffin, K, Van Laere, K,. The use of SPECT and PET in routine clinical practice in epilepsy. *Curr. Opin. Neurol.* 2007; 20, 194-202.

Van Paesschen, W, Dupont, P, Van Heerden, B, *et al.* Self-injection ictal SPECT during partial seizures. *Neurology* 2000; 54, 1994-7.

Won, H.J, Chang, K.H, Cheon, J.E, *et al.* Comparison of MR imaging with PET and Ictal SPECT in 118 patients with intractable epilepsy. *Am. J. Neuroradiol.* 1999; 20, 593-9.

PART V. SURGICAL THERAPY FOR FCD: A CURATIVE PERSPECTIVE

CHAPTER

19. Surgery for FCD: principles and outcome

Francesco Cardinale, Martina Revay, Piergiorgio d'Orio, Flavia Maria Zauli, Belén Abarrategui, Giorgio Lo Russo, Ivana Sartori

Key points

- The diagnostic/therapeutic pathway must always be guided by the fundamental principle of consistent anatomic/electro/clinical correlations, in FCD as in other underlying causes of epilepsy.
- The EZ in FCD can be variable: sometimes it corresponds perfectly to the lesion, but other times it may be larger than or include only part of the dysplasia.
- During the last decades, the proportion of resections without invasive investigations significantly increased, particularly when the lesion can be clearly outlined on MRI and is concordant with electrical-clinical signs.
- Overall, surgical treatment is effective, although not all patients are seizure-free after surgery. Predictors of seizure outcome should be well considered for indication for treatment and for pre-surgical counselling.
- We report a retrospective multivariate analysis of a surgical series of 641 histologically proven FCDs and describe the planning and surgical methods adopted at the "Claudio Munari" Center for Epilepsy Surgery, Milano, Italy.
- Histopathology is a crucial determinant of surgical outcome: All other variables aside, patients with FCD IIA have twice the risk of seizure recurrence and those with FCD I four times the risk of post-operative recurrence than patients with FCD IIB.
- In addition to FCD subtypes, complete resection of the lesion, positive MRI, shorter disease duration, absence of neurological deficits or cognitive impairment and smaller EZ are the best predictors of surgical success.
- Completeness of FCD resection can be achieved when pre-surgical planning is multimodal and includes 3D reconstructions of the brain surface and vasculature.

Prologue

• Illustrative case 1

Weruska, left-handed: first seizures at age 5, characterized by tingling in the left mandibular region, jerks of the chin, repeated singultus, salivation, uncoordinated movements with the upper limbs and widespread stiffness, without loss of consciousness. Immediate ictal aphasia, lasting a few seconds (sometimes longer) after the end of the episode. Interictal neurological examination was normal. Long-term non-invasive video-EEG monitoring confirmed ictal semiology in four sleep-related episodes, characterized electrographically by theta activity with super-imposed fast rhythms on the right fronto-parietal region. Magnetic resonance (MRI) showed a lesion in the inferior third of the right fronto-central region with the typical features of a FCD. Now a professional typewriter, she was seen by us at age 38 because of daily seizures, refractory to medication. Considering the strong coherence between ictal clinical-electrical signs and the anatomical location, the eloquent cortex region and the MRI typical appearance of a FCD II (highly intrinsically epileptogenic), a simple lesion-oriented surgical resection with intraoperative mapping and monitoring was indicated. Accurate presurgical planning was considered mandatory (**Figure 1**): multiplanar reconstructions, 3D-estimation of brain surface and cortical thickness mapping clarified that the lesion was seated in the depth of the central sulcus, and functional MRI (f-MRI) indicated right-hemisphere dominance for language. Fiber tracking reconstructed the arcuate fasciculus and the cortico-spinal tract (CST) running immediately lower and mesial to the lesion, respectively. The patient underwent surgical resection with immediate and permanent seizure freedom. Temporary speech impairment and left upper limb motor deficit, started the

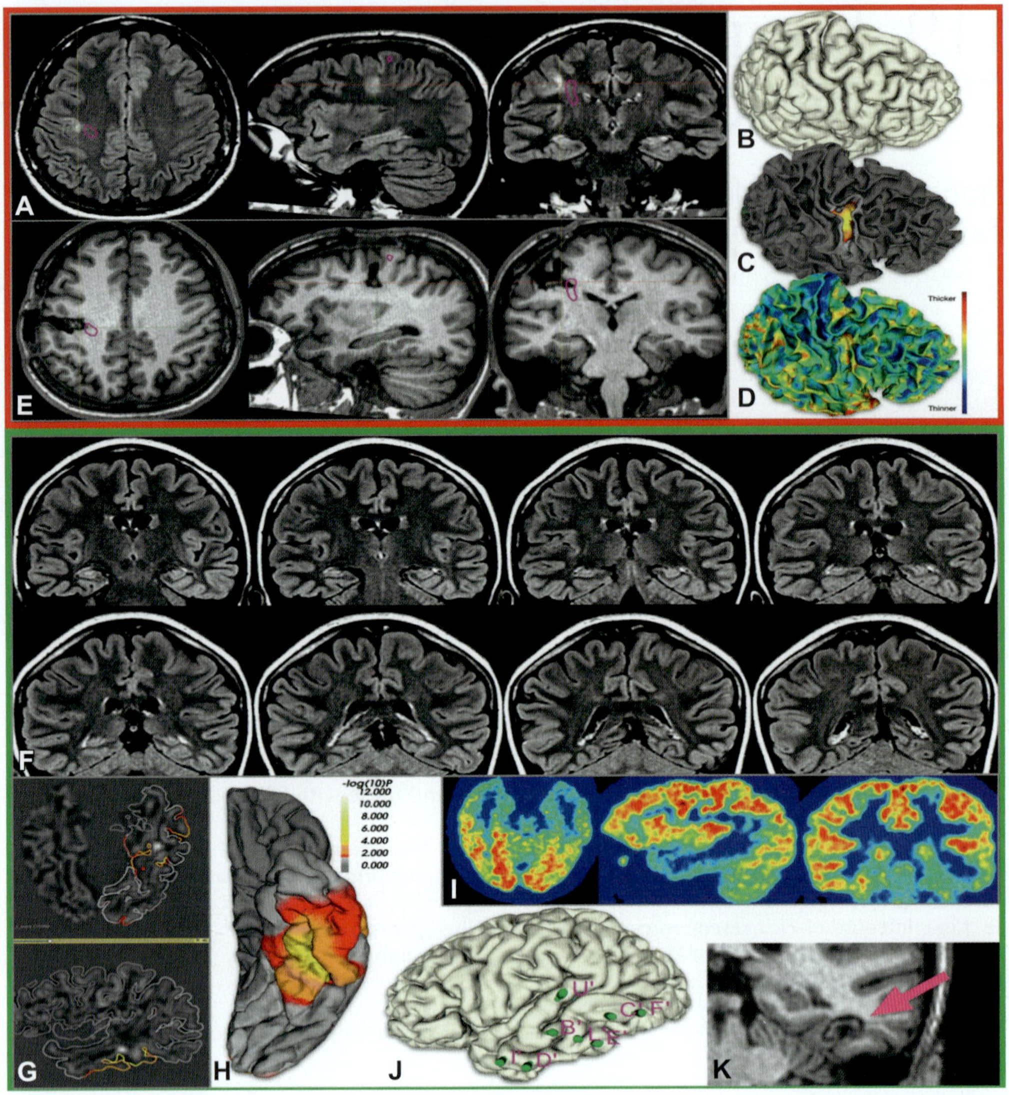

Figure 1

Illustrative case 1 (red frame). A. Multiplanar FLAIR views showing a FCD II in the right precentral-central region. Based only on these 2D slices, it is not easy to assess the exact location of the lesion. The purple contour represents the intersection between the slides and the reconstruction of the CST probabilistically estimated with FSL software package. B. Pial surface, estimated by Freesurfer software package. The lesion, hidden in the depth of a sulcus, is not visible. C. White "surface": it is possible to see the lesion in the depth of the central sulcus, enhanced by P-value mapping computed with the method of SUPR-FLAIR statistical analysis performed retrospectively because it was not available when the patient was studied and treated (Cardinale *et al.*, 2017). D. Cortical thickness mapping confirms that the lesion is seated in the central sulcus. In fact, the posterior bank of the sulcus is thinner (darker blue), thus it corresponds to the posterior wall of the central sulcus (primary somato-sensory cortex). E. Postoperative MRI shows the complete resection of the FCD. The deepest part of the "cavity", triangular in the coronal view, is likely due to an ischemic damage. It intersects the CST and thus justifies the postoperative temporary motor deficits.

Illustrative case 2 (green frame). F. Coronal FLAIR slices: a small tapering is visible between the bottom of the occipital-temporal sulcus and the temporal horn (first row, columns 3 and 4). G. MAP18 software computation reveals a small area of significant grey/white matter interface blurring, visible as a white spot (higher z-scores) in the axial and sagittal views. H. SUPR-FLAIR statistical analysis reveals an area of cortical hyper-intensity, particularly significant at the lesion level as indicated by the yellow area in the 3D view and in the slice intersections of the 3D surface model with 2D planes. Of note, this hyper-intensity is visible only with statistical analysis and not at visual inspection. I. Multiplanar reconstructions of fdg-PET shows a global hypo-metabolism of the left temporal lobe. J. The 3D view depicts the SEEG implantation. The occipital-temporal sulcus is explored by some leads of electrodes L' and E'. K. The effect of radio-frequency thermal ablation (arrow) performed by means of SEEG electrodes just before their removal.

day after operation, completely recovered in a few days or weeks, respectively. The patient is seizure free for nine years, without any drug-treatment, able to practice her activity of type-writer with full efficiency with both hands.

• Illustrative case 2

Giada, also left-handed, had first seizures when she was 5, characterized by eye blinking, oral and left superior limb automatisms and disconnection. Drug-resistant seizures, mostly sleep related, occurred almost daily. She came to see us at age 30 and long-term scalp EEG monitoring suggested left temporal origin of seizures. MRI was reported as non-informative at first visual inspection. Interictal 18F-fluorodeoxyglucose-positron emission tomography (FDG-PET) scan showed a coherent hypometabolism affecting the mesial and lateral aspects of the left temporal lobe (**Figure 1**). Due to age at seizure onset, high seizure frequency, sleep-related occurrence (Nobili *et al.*, 2009) and left temporal localization of both PET hypometabolism and EEG ictal onset (compatible with the ictal signs), a predominantly temporal lobe stereo-electroencephalography (SEEG) was indicated. Image processing suggests a basal temporal FCD, highlighted by a small area of white/grey matter blurring unveiled by MAP18 software package (Wagner *et al.*, 2011) and subtle cortical hyper-intensity of Fluid Attenuation Inversion Recovery (FLAIR) unveiled by SUPR-FLAIR statistical analysis (Cardinale F *et al.*, 2017a). A second look at the MRI reinforced the suspicion of a FCD; however, the indication for SEEG was maintained. SEEG monitoring confirmed the suspected FCD site as the ictal onset zone, with electrical stimulation eliciting a seizure which the patient recognized as habitual. Radiofrequency thermal ablation was carried out by means of SEEG electrodes and the patient is still seizure free more than three years later, tapering anti-seizure medication.

• Illustrative case 3

Giorgio, right-handed, suffered from his first seizures at 6 years of age. The episodes occurred pluri-daily, both in wakefulness and during sleep, and were characterized by stiffness of the right upper limb (flexed at the elbow), right-flexion of the head and tonic right deviation of the mouth rhyme. Drug treatment stopped seizures for a long period but, ten years later, pluri-daily ictal episodes recurred, mostly sleep-related. At outpatient visit, the patient told that seizures now start with a general strange feeling followed by a sort of "nausea localized at the throat". The subsequent objective signs are the same described at ictal onset. The patient would remain conscious all along the episode, lasting about 20 seconds, even if he is not able to speak. The findings of a recent video-EEG monitoring showed a possible origin of the seizure in the left fronto/central region. MRI was negative, f-MRI demonstrated left-hemisphere dominance for language (**Figure 2**). FDG-PET showed a wide hypo-metabolism in the mesial aspect of the left frontal region. SEEG delineated a left fronto/mesial EZ, including the posterior part of the superior and mesial frontal gyri and of the corresponding segment of the cingulate gyrus. The cortical resection was performed and FCD IIA was histologically diagnosed. No ictal episodes occurred after the surgery and the patient is still seizure-free nine years after the resection, without any drug treatment.

• Illustrative case 4

Cinzia suffered from simple febrile seizures at 2 years of age. Weekly recurrent unprovoked seizures, mainly during wakefulness, started when she was 10, characterized by rising epigastric sensation, preserved initial ability to speak, then staring and psychomotor arrest. Interictal sleep EEG showed spikes on the right temporal region and less frequently on the left. MRI showed right hippocampal sclerosis with atrophy and blurring of the grey/white matter junction of the temporal pole (**Figure 2**). Moreover, and surprisingly, there was also a lesion at the triangular part of the right inferior frontal gyrus, with MRI features suggestive of FCD or low-grade tumor. This notwithstanding, the clinical history and seizure semiology strongly suggested a right temporal lobe origin. The "innocence" of the cortical frontal lesion was demonstrated through SEEG investigation, and the patient underwent right antero-mesial temporal lobectomy at 46 years of age. Eight years after surgery the patient is seizure-free (only one seizure occurred in the first postoperative year), with minimal drug treatment.

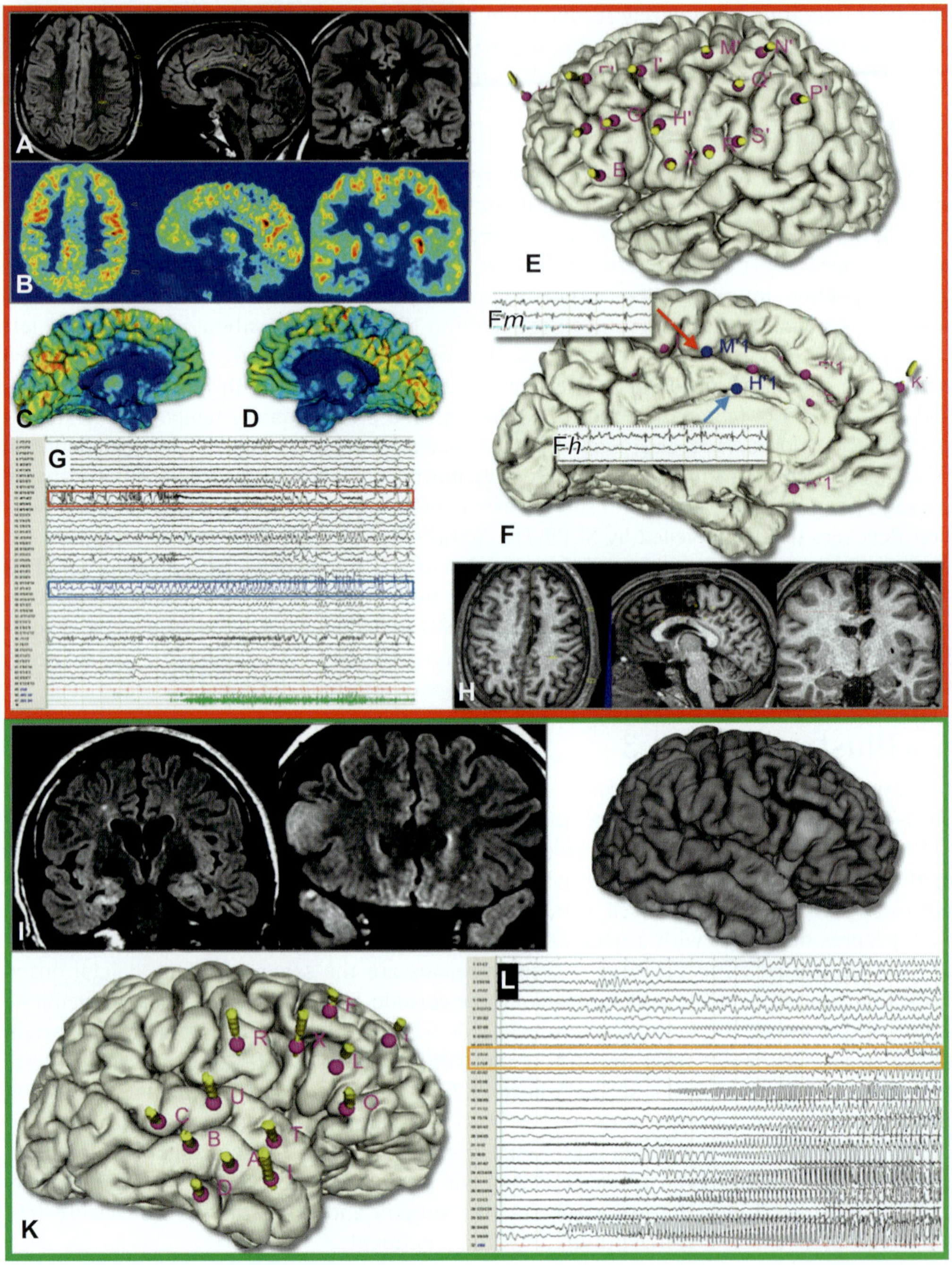

Figure 2

Illustrative patient 3 (red frame). A. FLAIR multiplanar views cut at the level of the histologically-proven FCD IIA: MRI is not informative. B. FDG-PET shows left cingulate hypo-metabolism, visible also in C and D, where metabolic data is mapped on the two hemispheres. E and F show the 3D rendering of SEEG implantation. Fm shows interictal spikes recorded from the lowest portion of the mesial frontal gyrus sampled by the inner contacts of the electrode M'. Fh shows recurrent interictal spikes recorded from the portion of the cingulate gyrus sampled by the inner contacts of the electrode H'. G. SEEG traces demonstrate the ictal onset at the level of inner contacts of the electrodes M' (red frame) and H' (blue frame). H. Multiplanar reconstruction of post-operative MRI.

Illustrative patient 4 (green frame). I. MRI shows both the right hippocampal sclerosis and an area of FLAIR hyper-intensity at the level of the frontal convexity. J. SUPR-FLAIR technique renders the lesion as a brighter area at the level of the triangular part. K. 3D rendering shows the SEEG implantation covering the temporal lobe, the lesional area and the possible pathways of supra-sylvian spreading. L. SEEG shows ictal activity starting and recruiting at the level of extra-lesional traces (especially the inferior ones, recording from the temporal lobe), while the contacts recording from within the frontal lesion are not involved (orange frame).

Preliminary comments

What can we learn from these cases? An FCD can be obvious at visual inspection of MRI, or difficult or even impossible to see and advanced imaging processing aimed at detecting occult FCD can be helpful. FDG-PET scans also are often useful, but the hypometabolic area is sometimes larger than the epileptogenic lesion. Multimodal integration, merging data from different imaging modalities and 3D reconstruction of brain surface is helpful for achieving an accurate topographic diagnosis that helps planning SEEG implantation and/or resection of the epileptogenic zone. However, the most important principle is that presurgical work-up must establish the degree of convergence of anatomical, electrical and clinical findings.

Introduction

Lesionectomy versus corticectomy: is it still a matter of debate? How to plan the resection in the different histopathological types of FCD? Why apparently complete resections do not always lead to complete seizure control?

From a surgical perspective, these questions can be a bit surprising for surgeons new to the field of epilepsy surgery. The main point relates to the concept of epileptogenic zone (EZ), definable as the "the site of the beginning and of primary organization of the epileptic seizures" (Munari and Bancaud, 1985). A number of milestone papers have faced the issue of assessing the EZ at a single-subject level, proposing that correct localization and resection of the EZ relates to significant chances of seizure freedom (Lüders *et al.*, 1993; Chauvel 2001; Kahane *et al.*, 2006). Whatever the approach or mental scheme - French or the anglophone - there is general agreement that structural epileptogenic lesions and the ultimate EZ does not always spatially coincide in the brain. Therefore, even when a FCD is visible, the choice between simple lesionectomy or larger resection must be driven by a coherent hypothesis on the correlations between clinical signs, EEG findings and anatomy. Do ictal symptoms suggest a specific ictal onset zone? Which propagation pathways are likely involved? Are interictal and ictal recordings topographically congruent with clinical semiology? Where is the lesion? Is lesion location compatible with clinical and EEG semiology? If we consider illustrative case 1, the decision of performing a simple lesionectomy was supported by coherent anatomo/electrical/clinical correlations. Moreover, the radiological aspect strongly suggested a FCD II, an intrinsically epileptogenic lesion. That usually is itself the site of seizure onset. Finally, due to the proximity of eloquent cortex, it would be unreasonable to plan a larger resection because it would likely impair motor and sensory functions. In contrast, illustrative case 4 has taught us that a well-visible lesion can be totally "innocent". The clinical symptoms and the EEG pointed to the right temporal lobe (where, in fact, there was a hippocampal sclerosis), while the location of the MRI-visible suspected FCD was not coherent with patient's history and ictal semiology. The simple resection of the suspected malformation would simply have failed.

Therefore, the method originally proposed and developed by Bancaud and Talairach at Sainte-Anne Hospital, Paris, remains the main rule to be followed. The multimodal definition of the EZ, as rigorous as possible, is crucial. All techniques are just part of the method and must be secondary in our mental hierarchy, even if many are crucial to surgical planning.

This chapter is aimed at briefly summarizing the method implemented at "Claudio Munari" Center for Epilepsy Surgery, Milan, for the surgical treatment of FCD, including the basics of planning. Moreover, we present the results of a retrospective analysis of our surgical series of histologically-proven FCD cases.

Patients, methods, results and discussion

Which results are currently obtained? Is there any difference between FCD types? Is the timing of surgery relevant? Are there other significant predictors of the outcome related to seizure control? Which improvements can be expected?

• Analysis of results on seizures and predictors of outcome

In order to answer these questions, we have retrospectively analyzed our surgical series.

In the period between May 1996 and December 2017 we have operated on 2226 patients suffering from drug-resistant partial epilepsy. Seven-hundred eighty-nine (789) had a histological diagnosis of FCD from at least one of the resected specimens. After 2011, the diagnosis was made according to the classification proposed by the International League Against Epilepsy (ILAE) (Blümcke *et al.*, 2011). Between 2004 and 2011, it was made according to the classification proposed by Palmini and co-workers (Palmini *et al.*, 2004). Between 1996 and 2004, Taylor-type FCD were diagnosed according to the original description published in 1971

(Taylor *et al.*, 1971), while all other FCD were labelled according to then current terminology (e.g., microdysgenesis). For the present analysis, types IIA and IIB from the three periods were considered equivalent. All other types of FCD were classified as ILAE type I (without any subtypes), or as ILAE type III when FCD was associated with another main lesion (with subtypes).

From these 789 patients, we further selected the 641 followed for longer than 5 years. This cohort led to two datasets:
• SURG641: a set of 641 patients with histologically-proven FCD (associated or not with other pathologies) followed for more than 5 years.
• SURG361: a subset of 361 patients, nested in SURG641, including only patients who had a histological diagnosis of FCD and no associated pathologies. Six patients who underwent hemispherotomy were excluded because the tissue samples were minimal and it is not reasonable to exclude the co-existence of associated pathologies. This dataset has been used only for multivariate analysis.

Cumulative result on seizures (i.e. assessed at the last available clinical outcome) is the dependent variable of our statistical inferential analyses. It is a binomial variable, categorized according to the absence or presence of disabling seizures after operation. Thus, statistical analyses were carried out to study the risk of postoperative seizures, categorized as a binary variable: absence (Engel's class I) or recurrence (Engel's classes II-IV) of disabling seizures (Engel *et al.*, 1993).

Uni/bivariate analysis was initially performed, and the subsequent multivariate regression analysis was carried out to identify predictors of seizure recurrence. Kruskal–Wallis rank sum test was used to analyze numerical variables, and Fisher's two-tailed exact test was computed for categorical variables. A multivariate logistic regression model was then fitted to assess the association of the explanatory variables with the outcome. Explanatory variables were manually selected with a multistep process. Relative risk (RR) was also calculated (Grant, 2014). $P < 0.05$ was considered significant. P-values between 0.05 and 0.1 were considered as trend towards significance. Statistical analysis was carried out using R 4.1.2.

Frequencies, proportions and univariate statistics for different FCD types are reported in **Table 1**. In line with other studies (Tassi *et al.*, 2002), we found a strong association between the type of FCD and outcome. Patients with FCD II B had a better outcome, with recurrence in only 12.5% patients. FCD II A was characterized by an intermediate rate of successful outcome, while 'pure' FCD I (i.e. not associated with any other pathologies) had the worst outcome, with 58.3% patients suffering from seizure recurrence. Interestingly, FCD III had a better outcome than FCD I, comparable to the outcome of the main associated pathologies. This finding is also coherent with papers previously published by our group (Cossu *et al.*, 2013, 2021; Tassi *et al.*, 2010).

Table 1

FCD type and outcome on seizures for SURG641: results of univariate statistical analysis (two tails Fischer's exact test).

FCD type	Frequencies (n. of cases)	SR (%)		P-value
		Yes	No	
I without associated pathologies	103	58.3	41.7	
I with associated pathologies (type IIIa+b+c+d)	234	21.8	78.2	
IIa without associated pathologies	88	29.5	70.5	
IIa with associated pathologies	30	33.3	66.7	<0.001*
IIb without associated pathologies	176	12.5	87.5	
IIb with associated pathologies	4	0	100	
I + II with associated pathologies	6	33.3	66.7	

SR: Seizure Recurrence; FCD: Focal Cortical Dysplasia.
* Statistically significant.

The lobar distribution of FCD found with unilobar surgeries is reported in **Table 2** and illustrated in **Figure 3**. These data are from the 453 patients who underwent a unilobar resection, excluding all the multilobar surgeries, whatever the size of the resection. Therefore, the lobar location of the FCD is certain for these patients. Of note, most associate FCD are located in the temporal lobe, while the vast majority of pure FCD is seated in all the other lobes with a strong prevalence of the frontal one. These findings are perfectly in line with a recent study reporting on a retrospective cohort of 580 patients with epilepsy attributed to FCD from 20 epilepsy centers worldwide (Wagstyl *et al.*, 2022).

Table 2

The distribution of resection topography in unilobar surgeries from our series. The majority of FCD were found in the temporal lobe, but most of them were associated with other pathologies. Differently, the vast majority of FCD located in all the other lobes were not associated with any other pathologies.

Lobe	FCD I	FCD III	FCD IIA	Associate FCD IIA	FCD IIB	Associate FCD IIB	Total
Temporal	22 (9.3%)	178 (75.4%)	7 (3%)	17 (7.2%)	10 (4.2%)	2 (0.8)	236 (100%)
Insular	0 (0%)	0 (0%)	0 (0%)	0 (0%)	1 (100%)	0 (0%)	1 (100%)
Frontal	31 (17.7%)	14 (8%)	33 (18.9%)	2 (1.1%)	94 (53.7%)	1 (0.6%)	175 (100%)
Central	1 (6.3%)	0 (0%)	2 (12.5%)	0 (0%)	13 (81.3%)	0 (0%)	16 (100%)
Parietal	3 (16.7%)	2 (11.1%)	0 (0%)	2 (11.1%)	11 (61.1%)	0 (0%)	18 (100%)
Occipital	1 (14.3%)	2 (28.6%)	2 (28.6%)	0 (0%)	2 (28.6%)	0 (0%)	7 (100%)
Total	58 (12.8%)	196 (43.3%)	44 (9.7%)	21 (4.6%)	131 (28.9%)	3 (0.7%)	453 (100%)

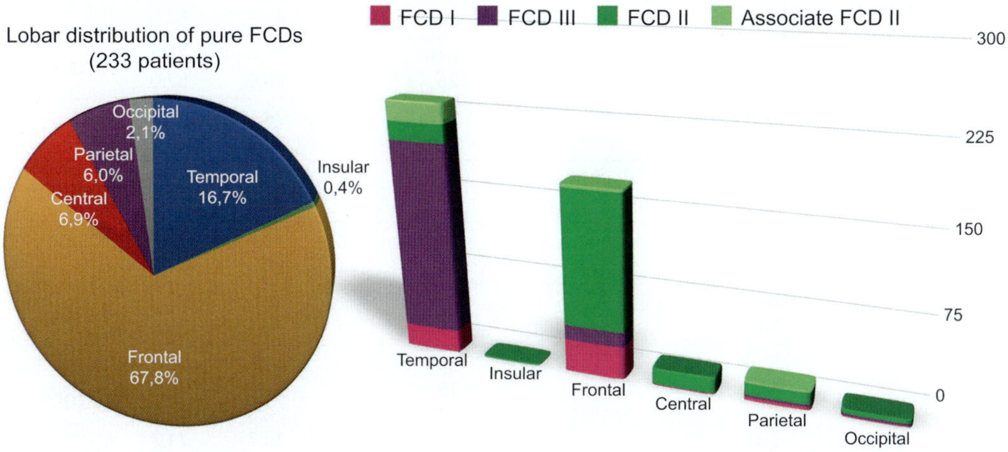

Figure 3

Distribution of FCD in unilobar resections

Graphs illustrating the lobar distribution of FCD from the 453 patients who underwent unilobar resection. The cake diagram illustrates the lobar proportions of all the pure FCD, including both types I and II. The histogram chart depicts the proportion of all the FCD, including also the ones associated to other pathologies, grouped by lobe.
Since the analyzed series includes only patients with follow-up longer than 5 years, surgeries performed in the last years are not reported. Actually, the proportion of FCD resected from the central region is certainly higher. Moreover, the percentage of FCD in rolandic region is under-estimated in this analysis also because the histological diagnosis of FCD is impossible when tissue specimens are very small, as typically happens when bottom-of-the-sulcus malformations are resected from eloquent cortex. Similar comments can be done for insular surgeries.

Frequencies, proportions and univariate statistics for categorical and numerical explanatory variables are reported in **Table 3** and **Table 4**, respectively (data are reported separately for the SURG641 and SURG361 datasets). Only variables with at least 10 occurrences are reported, and therefore a number of patients are missing (e.g., those associated with pleomorphic xanthoastrocytoma or polymicrogyria).

HS and ganglioglioma were the most frequent associated pathologies. A number of variables were significantly associated with outcome. Nonetheless, since univariate statistics do not control for confounders, multivariate analysis is shown in **Table 5**, where coefficients, OR and RR provide useful estimates of effect size.

It is interesting to note that out of the 274 patients with FCD associated to other pathologies, only 88 (32%) had a neuroradiological report suggesting the co-presence of the malformative abnormality. Therefore, the association of FCD to other pathologies was under-estimated at conventional MRI inspection.

Considering only patients with FCD not associated to other pathologies who did not undergo hemispherotomy (SURG361), 75/361 (21%) were MRI-negative. This proportion partially explains why half of these patients underwent SEEG, a percentage higher than in the general population of patients admitted to our center.

Table 3

Categorical variables and outcome on seizures: results of univariate analysis (two tails Fischer's exact test), from both datasets, SURG641 and SURG361. Only variables with at least 10 occurrences are reported.

Variable	Type	Categories	Frequencies (n. of cases)	SR (%)		P-value
				Yes	No	
SURG641						
FCD type	Multinomial	IIb	180	12.2	87.7	<0.001*
		IIa	118	30.5	69.5	
		I	337	32.9	67.1	
		I + II	6	33.3	66.6	
HS	Binomial	No	507	29.0	71.0	0.011*
		Yes	134	17.9	82.1	
PNH	Binomial	No	618	26.4	73.6	0.348
		Yes	23	34.8	65.2	
Ganglioglioma	Binomial	No	596	27.5	72.50	0.083°
		Yes	45	15.6	84.4	
DNT	Binomial	No	618	27.0	73.0	0.47
		Yes	23	17.4	82.6	
Glioneuronal Hamartoma	Binomial	No	618	26.9	73.1	0.81
		Yes	23	21.7	78.3	
Scars	Binomial	No	619	26.0	74.0	0.051°
		Yes	22	45.5	54.5	
Inflammatory pathologies	Binomial	No	616	25.8	74.2	0.02*
		Yes	25	48.0	52.0	
Resection side	Binomial	Left	270	28.1	71.9	0.47
		Right	371	25.6	74.4	
Topography of resection	Binomial	Unilobar (or small multilobar)	453	20.5	79.5	<0.001*
		Large multilobar	188	41.5	58.5	
Sex	Binomial	Female	283	23.7	76.3	0.15
		Male	358	29.0	71.0	
Predominantly sleep-related seizures	Binomial	No	469	27.5	72.5	0.48
		Yes	172	24.4	75.6	
Seizure frequency	Multinomial	Rare	51	11.8	88.2	0.06°
		Monthly	78	29.5	70.5	
		Weekly	230	26.5	73.5	
		Daily	282	28.7	71.3	
Neurological/Cognitive examination	Binomial	Normal	517	22.1	77.9	<0.001*
		Not normal	124	45.9	54.1	
MRI	Binomial	Positive	558	23.1	76.9	<0.001*
		Negative	83	50.6	49.4	
SEEG	Binomial	No	396	21.0	79.0	<0.001*
		Yes	245	35.9	64.1	
SURG361						
FCD type	Multinomial	IIb	173	11.6	88.4	<0.001*
		IIa	85	30.6	69.4	
		I	103	58.3	41.7	
Resection side	Binomial	Left	143	30.8	69.2	0.639
		Right	218	28.4	71.6	
Topography of resection	Binomial	Unilobar (or small multilobar)	232	22.8	77.2	<0.001*
		Large multilobar	129	41.1	58.9	

Variable	Type	Categories	Frequencies (n. of cases)	SR (%) Yes	SR (%) No	P-value
Gender	Binomial	Female Male	158 203	27.8 30.5	72.2 69.5	0.642
Predominantly sleep-related seizures	Binomial	No Yes	218 143	32.1 25.2	67.9 74.8	0.194
Seizure frequency	Multinomial	Rare Monthly Weekly Daily	28 31 92 210	14.3 41.9 35.9 26.7	85.8 58.1 64.1 73.3	0.044*
Neurological/Cognitive examination	Binomial	Normal Not normal	289 72	24.6 48.6	75.4 51.4	<0.001*
MRI	Binomial	Positive Negative	286 75	24.1 49.3	75.9 50.7	<0.001*
SEEG	Binomial	No Yes	179 182	21.8 36.8	78.2 63.2	0.002*

SR: seizure recurrence; FCD: focal cortical dysplasia; HS: Hippocampal Sclerosis; PNH: periventricular nodular heterotopy; DNT: dysembryoplastic neuroepithelial tumor; MRI: Magnetic Resonance Imaging; SEEG: Stereo-electroencephalography.
* Statistically significant.
° Trend toward significance.

Table 4

Comparison of numerical variables, grouped by results, with univariate statistical analysis (Kruskal-Wallis rank sum test), from both datasets, SURG641 and SURG361.

Variable	All patients median (IQ range)	Seizure Recurrence: Yes median (IQ range)	Seizure Recurrence: No median (IQ range)	P-value
SURG641				
Age at seizure onset (years)	5 (2 - 11)	4 (1 - 11)	6 (2 – 11.75)	0.059°
Epilepsy duration at surgery (years)	15 (7 - 24)	16 (9 - 25)	14 (7 - 24)	0.028*
Age at surgery (years)	24 (13 - 34)	24 (16 - 34)	24 (13 - 34)	0.387
SURG361				
Age at seizure onset (years)	5 (2 - 9)	4 (1 - 9)	5 (2 – 9.5)	0.144
Epilepsy duration at surgery (years)	14 (7 - 22)	16 (9 – 22.75)	13 (6 - 21)	0.084°
Age at surgery (years)	21 (13 - 34)	22.5 (14 - 32)	20 (10.5 - 32)	0.33

IQ = InterQuartile. *= Statistically significant. °= Trend toward significance.

The output of the fitted logistic regression models, SURG641 and SURG361, is reported in **Table 5**. SURG641 is the most important dataset because it was fitted from all available data, including patients who had histologically-proven FCD and associated lesions.

The first finding is that the predicting value of FCD type is confirmed. FCD IIB has been chosen as reference category because it had the best outcome. Surgery of all other types of FCD had an increased risk of seizure recurrence. The RR of FCD IIA is 2.31, meaning that, all other variables being equal, the risk of seizure recurrence is more than double that of type IIB. Similarly, the risk is more than quadruple when FCD is type I (RR = 4.24). These histopathological associations with outcome are independent from all other variables included in the model.

In contrast, the association of FCD with histologically-confirmed HS or ganglioglioma predicted outcome regarding seizure control in the opposite direction, with RRs of 0.40 and 0.49, respectively, indicating that the risk of seizure recurrence was reduced by about half when FCD was associated with these lesions.

The size of surgical resection was also statistically relevant: the need for large, multilobar resections doubled the risk of seizure recurrence, likely because of larger and more complex EZs. This finding confirms previous evidence that smaller lesions positively predicted postoperative seizure freedom (Fauser *et al.*, 2008; Chang *et al.*, 2011).

Furthermore, also in agreement with previous reports (Fauser *et al.*, 2008; Rácz *et al.*, 2021) and even more significantly, epilepsy duration proved a very important variable in outcome prediction (P = 0.003). The RR of 1.03 indicates that, all other variables being equal, the risk of seizure recurrence increased by 3% with every year[1] of disease, making it clear that the earlier the surgery, the higher the probability of post-operative seizure freedom.

Age at seizure onset should not have been included in the model because it was not significant[2]. However, we kept it to contrast its lack of significance with the crucial relevance of disease duration. In other words, a longer duration of epilepsy before surgery decreased the chance of postoperative seizure freedom not because seizures started at younger age but for some other "biological reason" such as the possibility of progressive enlargement of the EZ[3].

Moreover, neurological deficits or cognitive impairment before operation more than doubled the risk of recurrence. Some common clinical scenarios help explain this finding: motor deficits caused by epileptogenic lesions in the central lobe anticipate a high likelihood of incomplete resection of the FCD, whereas cognitive impairment may either be caused by an associated encephalopathy that affects the brain more widely than the FCD (Blackmon *et al.*, 2015) or the FCD is very extensive, making complete resection difficult.

Finally, the lack of MRI-visible abnormalities is another predictor of postoperative recurrence, also doubling the risk. A visible dysplastic lesion is extremely helpful to guide the delineation of the EZ, a finding that is also in line with other reports (Téllez-Zenteno *et al.*, 2005; Spencer and Hu, 2008; Rowland *et al.*, 2012).

A graphic illustration of these outcome associations is depicted in **Figure 4**.

We have also fitted a multivariate model from the smaller dataset SURG361, excluding patients with FCD associated to other main histological diagnoses. All variables that were significant in SURG641 (but HS and ganglioglioma, of course) were confirmed with similar effect sizes. Therefore, the positive predictive value of type IIB, unilobar resection, shorter duration of epilepsy, absence of neurological/cognitive deficits and positive MRI were confirmed.

Multivariate models are generally fitted with two goals. The first is to look for significant outcome predictors. The other is to exploit the output of the model to anticipate the probabilities of given outcomes. When a logistic multivariate model is fitted, it is therefore possible to estimate the probability of obtaining one or the other category of the binary output from the explanatory variables. In our SURG641 model, we can estimate the risk of postoperative seizure recurrence with different combinations of predictor values[4]. For instance, in case of a small FCD IIB visible at MRI visual inspection (and then histologically confirmed), with no associated pathologies, without any neurological deficits or cognitive impairment, with seizure onset at 4 years of age and surgery performed one year later, the probability of post-operative seizure recurrence was 5%. Under the same conditions, the risk of treatment failure increased to 10% if the patient was operated 25 years later (which is not infrequent).

1. This means that one year after epilepsy onset, the risk of disabling seizure recurrence is 3% higher than at baseline; at the end of the second year it is 3% higher than the first year, and so on.

2. In accordance to the Occam's razor principle, only significant variables should be maintained in the model.

3. It can also be underlined that age at seizure onset is significant at univariate analysis (see **Table 4**) and not at multivariate one due to a confounding effect. Since many (too many!) patients are still sent to presurgical evaluation after many years, the earlier the age at seizure onset, the longer the epilepsy duration. When both variables are included in the same multivariate model the confounding is controlled and only the true predictor remains significant.

4. The reader can play himself with the model output to estimate outcome probabilities with different combinations of predictor values. For instance, based on SURG641 model, it is necessary to edit a simple spreadsheet with the following columns: first column with all the tested variables (intercept, FCD IIA, type I FCD I, ...); second column with the coefficients; third column with the value for the single subject to be estimated (1 for the intercept, not changeable; 1 for FCD IIA when present, and similarly for all other categorical variables; the number of years for age at onset and epilepsy duration); fourth column with the products of columns 2 and 3. The Logit is the sum of all the values in column 4, and the OR for Seizure Recurrence (OR_{SR}) is the exponential of Logit. Finally, the probability of Seizure Recurrence is $OR_{SR}/(1+OR_{SR})$. Of note, the 0 value for each category means that the characteristic is absent, and thus the reference category is present. Therefore, if the patient has only type FCD IIB, all the three FCD categories in the spreadsheet must be set as 0.

Furthermore, if the FCD is type I instead of IIB, the risk of seizure recurrence increases to 35%. Finally, the worst situation occurred when MRI is negative, there was cognitive impairment and the resection zone is large and multilobar: in this situation, the probability of post-operative seizure freedom was only 10%.

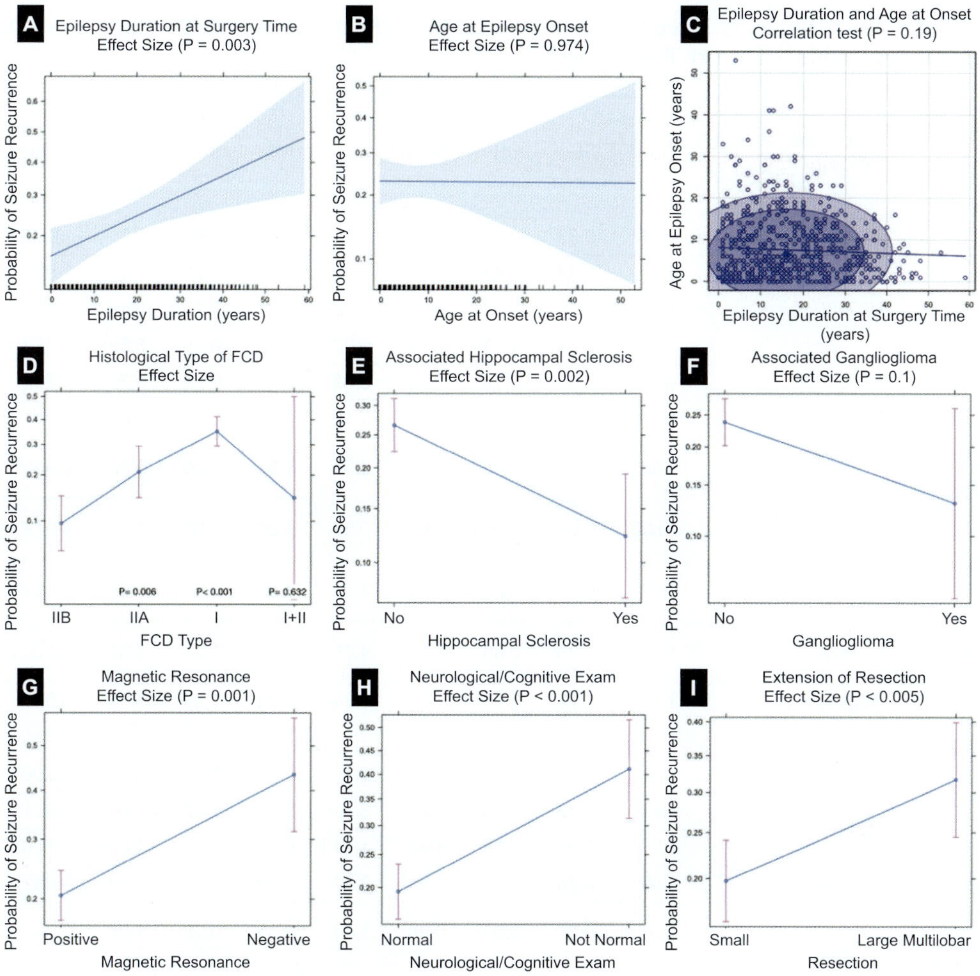

Figure 4

Graphs of effect sizes for independent variables included in model SURG641. A shows how a longer duration of epilepsy increased the probability of treatment failure, while age at onset was not significant (B). C shows that epilepsy duration and age at onset are independent, with wide dispersion of data. D, E and F show the association of histology with outcome. G, H and I illustrate the associations of MRI lesion identification, neurological deficits, cognitive impairment and extent of resection with prognosis.

The statistical analysis provides us also with the answer to the last question that opened this section: what can we do to improve the results on seizure control? We cannot change the patient-related predictors; hence we have to work on operator-dependent, modifiable variables. Every effort must be done to increase neuroradiological performance, adopting optimal protocols for imaging acquisition and using proper post-processing protocols whenever needed. Moreover, surgical treatment must be carried out as early as possible to improve probabilities of seizure freedom and also limit deleterious neurological, cultural, social and economic effects of a life with recurrent seizures and constant use of medication. The importance of early surgery has been highlighted mostly in pre-scholar aged children: seizure freedom, directly or indirectly, prevents younger patients from impaired adaptive and cognitive development (Loddenkemper *et al.*, 2007; Shurtleff *et al.*, 2015; Kadish *et al.*, 2019).

Unfortunately, the duration of epilepsy is a modifiable variable only when the patient is evaluated early. Sadly, it is still too common for patients to come for presurgical evaluation as much as 25-30 years after seizure onset. We cannot modify this variable for the specific patient we are seeing, nor the other nonmodifiable variables that should be carefully considered for indication for treatment and during presurgical counseling. For example, the patient (or his or her guardians) with drug-resistant epilepsy likely associated with an FCD should be aware that the likelihood of a successful diagnostic/therapeutic course is reduced if the MRI is not informative, or if cognitive performance is impaired, or if the EZ is presumed to be very large, or if the duration of the illness is very long.

Table 5

Output of the fitted logistic regression models for both the datasets, SURG641 and SURG361 (outcome variable = Seizure Recurrence).

Variable	Category	Reference category	Coeff	SE	OR	95% CIor		RR	95% CIrr		P-value
SURG641											
Intercept	–	–	-2.97	0.33	0.05	0.03	0.10	0.05	NA	NA	<0.001*
FCD type	FCD IIA	FCD IIB	0.91	0.33	2.47	1.30	4.76	2.31	1.28	4.02	0.006*
	FCD I		1.62	0.28	5.09	2.96	9.05	4.24	2.70	6.49	<0.001*
	FCD I + II		0.45	0.94	1.57	0.19	9.27	1.53	0.20	6.59	0.632
HS	YES	NO	-0.95	0.30	0.39	0.21	0.69	0.40	0.22	0.70	0.002*
Ganglioglioma	YES	NO	-0.74	0.45	0.48	0.18	1.10	0.49	0.19	1.09	0.1°
Topography of resection	Large Multilobar	Unilobar (or small multilobar)	0.63	0.23	1.88	1.21	2.93	1.81	1.20	2.68	0.005*
Age at seizure onset (years)	–	–	-0.001	0.01	1.004	0.99	0.97	1.00	0.97	1.03	0.974
Epilepsy duration at surgery (years)	–	–	0.03	0.01	1.03	1.01	1.05	1.03	1.01	1.04	0.003*
Neurological/Cognitive examination	Not normal	Normal	1.06	0.25	2.89	1.77	4.75	2.65	1.70	4.01	<0.001*
MRI	Negative	Positive	1.1	0.29	2.99	1.71	5.26	2.73	1.66	4.35	0.001*
SURG361											
Intercept	–	–	-3.01	0.40	0.05	0.02	0.11	0.05	NA	NA	<0.001*
FCD type	FCD IIA	FCD IIB	0.93	0.37	2.55	1.24	5.30	2.37	1.22	4.40	0.011*
	FCD I		2.22	0.34	9.18	4.80	18.23	6.62	4.07	10.05	<0.001*
Topography of resection	Large Multilobar	Unilobar	0.49	0.28	1.62	0.94	2.81	1.58	0.94	2.59	0.082°
Age at seizure onset (years)			-0.006	0.02	0.99	0.96	1.03	0.99	0.96	1.03	0.758
Epilepsy duration at surgery (years)			0.03	0.01	1.03	1.01	1.06	1.03	1.00	1.05	0.019*
Neurological/Cognitive examination	Not normal	Normal	1.19	0.34	3.28	1.69	6.44	2.96	1.64	5.12	<0.001*
MRI	Negative	Positive	0.83	0.33	2.29	1.20	4.38	2.16	1.19	3.78	0.012*

Coeff: coefficient; SE: standard error; OR: odds ratio; CI: confidence interval; RR: relative risk; FCD: focal cortical dysplasia; HS: hippocampal sclerosis; MRI: magnetic resonance imaging; NA: not available.

* Statistically significant.

° Trend towards significance.

The results of this retrospective analysis must be further commented. As far as we know, this is the largest series of FCD ever published by a single center, therefore data must be considered robust. Nonetheless, our analysis lacked a very important predictor, namely, the completeness of resection. Moreover, we have not included patients with clear FCD but without histopathological confirmation due to the use of techniques such as thermal ablation only. Finally, we have not studied the importance of FDG-PET scan findings and higher resolution, 3T MRI machines in lesion identification, which could have improved our results.

• Clinical methods actually used at "Claudio Munari" center

Non-invasive pre-surgical work-up

Our pre-surgical work-up includes family and personal history, with particular attention to ictal phenomena, neurological examination, neuropsychological testing, interictal (and ictal if available) scalp EEG and MRI.

Video-EEG long-term monitoring is performed in most patients to record at least one habitual electrical-clinical seizure.

All patients are scanned using an Achieva 1.5-T magnet (Philips Healthcare, Best, The Netherlands). For patients not undergoing SEEG investigation, major brain veins are imaged with an axial venous phase contrast angiography (PCA) sequence. Our MRI acquisition protocol was detailed elsewhere (Colombo *et al.*, 2012).

When needed, F-MRI and diffusion weighted images (DWI) are also obtained. Cortical activations and white-matter bundles are estimated with FEAT and FDT diffusion, dedicated tools included in the FSL software package (Behrens *et al.*, 2003; Jenkinson *et al.*, 2012).

Special techniques for image processing are often used to improve lesion detection, such as Voxel Based Morphometry (VBM) with MAP18 (Wagner *et al.*, 2011b). SUrface PRojected – FLAIR (SUPR-FLAIR), a surface-based analysis aimed at comparing cortical intensity values of the patient's FLAIR scan against comparable images from normal controls, is also used. This occasionally helped lesion detection when no obvious FLAIR hyper-intensities were seen with visual MRI inspection (Cardinale *et al.*, 2017a). Nowadays, such image processing techniques are routinely run on all patients' datasets.

FDG-PET scan is obtained only in collaborative patients with an integrated PET/computed tomography (CT) camera, Biograph TruePoint (Siemens Healthcare, Erlangen, Germany), starting from 2009. More recently, such metabolic images were acquired with a last generation Siemens Biograph scanner.

Invasive pre-surgical work-up

About one-third of our patients undergo SEEG investigation before resection or disconnection when non-invasive work-up does not allow clear definition of EZ. Minotti and coworkers have recently proposed the use of SEEG in some clinical scenarios involving temporal and extratemporal epilepsies. When temporal lobe (TL) epilepsy is suspected, SEEG would be indicated "when clinical and EEG data do not allow the existence of a mesial or neocortical TL generator to be ruled out, (...) when the combination of clinical data and presurgical investigations suggest the possibility of seizures arising independently from both TL, (...) in suspected pseudo-temporal lobe epilepsy when extra-temporal areas are involved early in the seizure according to non-invasive data". In suspected extra-temporal lobe cases, SEEG would be indicated when MRI is negative and "in the case of discordance between the topography of the lesion and the ictal clinical data, to define the respective roles of the lesion, the EZ and the eloquent cortex" (Minotti *et al.*, 2018).

The interpretation of SEEG recordings is a crucial step, of course. The main principles have been comprehensively resumed in a literature review (Bartolomei *et al.*, 2018). SEEG investigation is the highest-level implementation of the conceptual frame based on anatomo/electro/clinical correlation. Structural and functional anatomy must be carefully studied with multimodal imaging, and the exact location of every recording/stimulating contact must be carefully assessed by means of post-implantation imaging.

Qualitative analysis of SEEG traces must be carried out carefully, trying to define both the irritative and the EZ. The extension of the cortical areas generating spikes or spike/waves is of great interest but, as highlighted by Bartolomei and coworkers, the analysis of seizure onset is the most important step. Low voltage fast discharge is the most common seizure onset pattern but also patterns involving lower frequencies can be seen. However, the latter patterns can be recorded also from cortical structures involved by seizure spreading. Therefore, the definition of the EZ must be very cautious when low voltage fast discharges are not recorded before the onset of ictal symptoms. The possibility of inadequate sampling of the EZ should be considered in such cases.

The dynamic analysis of SEEG traces is also crucial: the propagation of the discharge across anatomo-functional systems should be carefully analyzed throughout the different phases of seizure onset, early and late propagation. Hopefully, the seizure dynamics should be found coherent with the sequence of clinical symptoms.

The possibility of electrical stimulation of brain tissue at both cortical and subcortical level allows accurate functional mapping in the sampled regions. Moreover, such stimulations are a powerful tool to contribute to the definition of the EZ, especially when a habitual seizure is elicited by means of low-frequency stimulations (Munari *et al.*, 1993; Trébuchon *et al.*, 2016, 2021). See the chapters by Chassoux and Bartolomei included in this textbook for a full discussion on the SEEG interpretation.

Since our epilepsy surgery program started in 1995, the use of SEEG progressively decreased in patients with MRI-visible lesions. The evidence that FCD are intrinsically epileptogenic (Palmini *et al.*, 1995; Chassoux *et al.*, 2000; Tassi *et al.*, 2012) has often led to resection without invasive investigations, particularly when the lesion can be clearly outlined on MRI images and is concordant with electrical-clinical signs. Even in rolandic FCD we prefer using intraoperative brain mapping or monitoring and 3D multimodal imaging (**Figure 5**). In fact, 3D reconstructions are very helpful in delineating gyral and sulcal patterns, and therefore allow better understanding of the convoluted brain anatomy for surgical planning (Cardinale *et al.*, 2015; Nowell *et al.*, 2015).

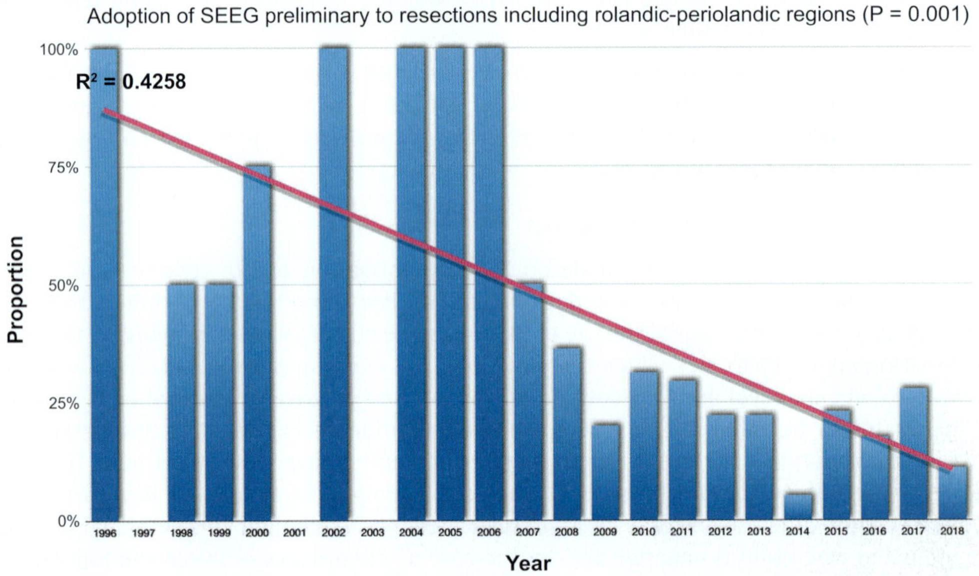

Figure 5

SEEG before resection over 20 years. Note diminished use in favor of intraoperative mapping and monitoring.

The use of SEEG includes a number of sequential steps: a hypothesis on the EZ topography based on non-invasive data is mandatory, followed by a coherent topographic strategy of implantation with the stereotaxic planning of the electrode trajectories. After implantation, video-SEEG long-term monitoring should allow definition of the EZ, which is followed by SEEG-guided surgical treatment, if any.

Our updated workflow for the implantation of SEEG electrodes, implemented since Fall 2008, was previously detailed (Cardinale *et al.*, 2013, 2015, 2017b). In summary, trajectories are planned on multimodal images merged with other images aimed at visualizing and reconstructing the brain vasculature. Between 2008 and 2020, 3D cone-beam-CT digital subtraction angiography (3D CBCT DSA) was obtained with O-arm (Medtronic; Minneapolis, Minnesota, USA), a mobile CBCT scanner. More recently, we are using Philips Azurion (Philips Healthcare, Best, The Netherlands). Two image datasets are obtained. The first (bone-mask) is registered to and subtracted from the subsequent one, obtained with iodinated contrast medium injected in the internal carotid artery. 2D stereoscopic images are also obtained, providing a high-quality (but non-stereotaxic) and pseudo-3D representation of the brain vasculature. All 3D datasets are processed (rigid registrations, thresholding, masking) with the tools provided by FSL (Jenkinson *et al.*, 2012), Freesurfer (Fischl *et al.*, 2012) and 3D Slicer (Fedorov *et al.*, 2012). Separated hemispheres, segmented vasculature and all other useful data are imported into the stereotaxic software package able to drive the robotic assistant. Entry points (EP) and target points (TP) are manually selected for every trajectory on both multiplanar reconstructions and 3D surface renderings of brain and vessels.

The electrodes (Microdeep Intracerebral Electrodes-D08; Dixi Medical, Besançon, France) are implanted under general anesthesia, with the help of the robot (Neuromate, Renishaw, Wotton-under-Edge, UK), which aligns the tool holder along each planned trajectory to assist the fixation of the guiding screw to the bone. Subsequently, the head-holder is removed and the electrodes are advanced into the brain under radioscopic control. A final intra-operative 3D CBCT is obtained to check the position of the implanted electrodes.

The complication rate of SEEG implantation is very low, especially with the new workflow implemented since 2008 (Cardinale *et al.*, 2019). We did not report any symptomatic bleedings with the implantation of 5181 electrodes in 232 SEEG procedures.

Spontaneous and electrically-induced seizures are recorded during long-term video-SEEG monitoring. Radio-Frequency THermal Coagulations (RF-THC) can be performed when intracerebral recordings demonstrate a very focal origin of the seizure, leading to seizure freedom in selected cases (Catenoix *et al.*, 2015; Cossu *et al.*, 2015, 2017; Bourdillon *et al.*, 2017; Cardinale *et al.*, 2019). In most cases, the temporary results of this ablation technique do not give long-term satisfactory results but can still be helpful for further definition of the EZ and better definition of the final open-surgery prognosis.

It is crucial to create interactive multimodal scenes with all available data, including 2D multiplanar views of all informative datasets, 3D reconstructions and results of post-processing (**Figure 6**). Once the electrodes are implanted, epileptologists must interpret SEEG findings looking carefully to the position of every recording lead relative to anatomical information. When SEEG monitoring is concluded, such multimodal scenes are again helpful for the final multidisciplinary staff meeting and planning the resection.

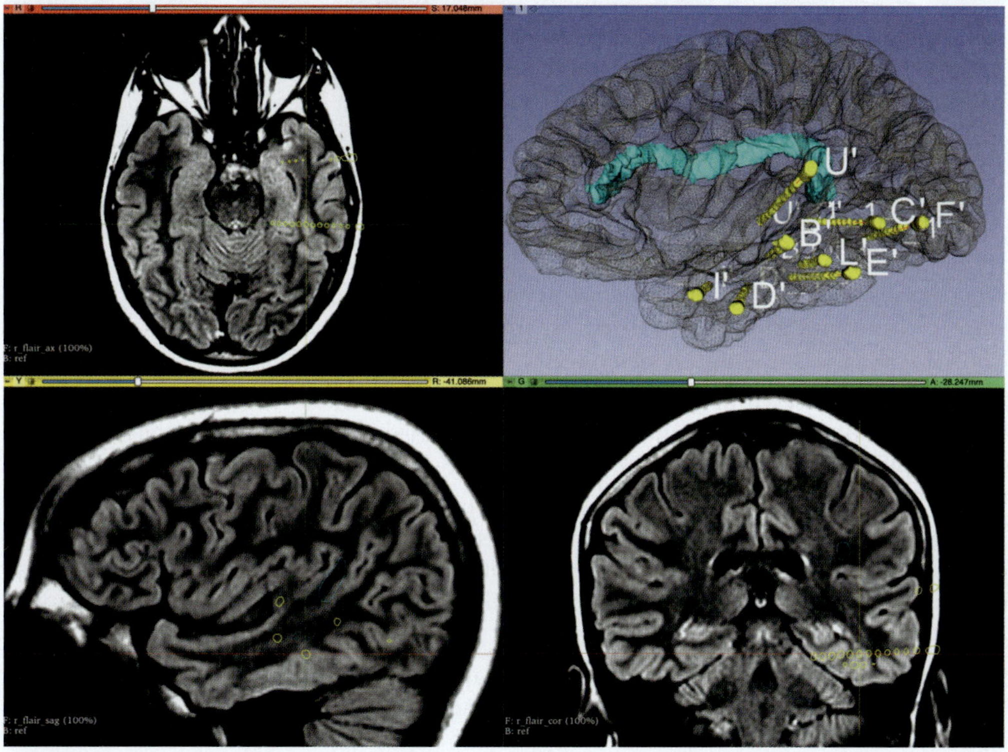

Figure 6

Illustrative patient 2.

Multimodal scene integrating data for SEEG interpretation. The model of the electrodes (yellow) is obtained computing an isosurface from the grey-scale thresholding of post-implantation CT, registered to MR. The position of every recording contact can be seen on both the 3D rendering and the multiplanar 2D views (yellow contours).

Open-surgery planning

3D multimodal scenes are obtained not only for patients who undergo SEEG, but also for those operated without invasive investigation (**Figure 7**). Most important veins are rendered with information from phase-contrast MRI angiography. Similar to SEEG-studied patients, catheter 2D stereoscopic angiography is obtained to visualize the arteries. This preliminary angiographic study is crucial to preserve the regional vascular pattern, especially in eloquent regions.

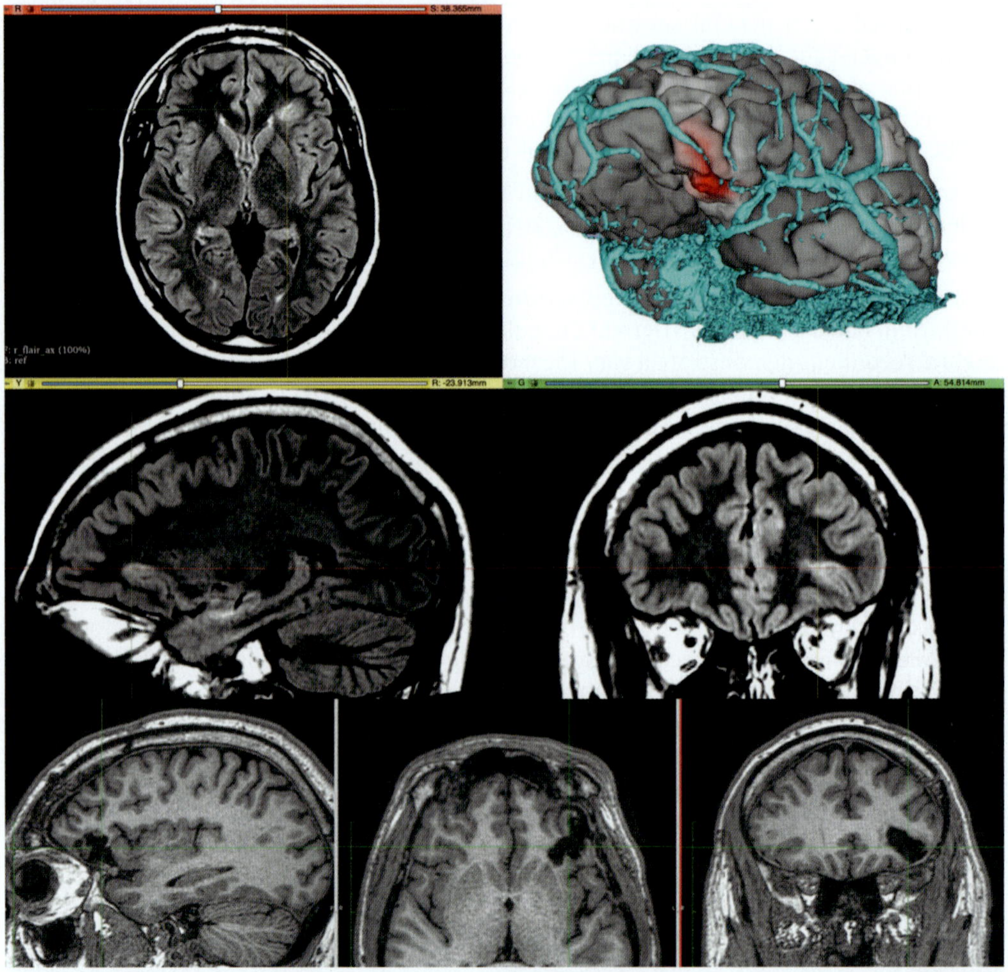

Figure 7

Multiplanar views of FLAIR scans show FCD at the bottom of the sulcus between the orbital part of the left inferior frontal gyrus, the lateral orbital cortex and the anterior part of the circular sulcus of the insula. 3D rendering depicts the reconstruction of brain surface, the red area of subtle peri-lesional FLAIR hyper-intensity (computed with SUPR-FLAIR statistical analysis) and the major veins segmented from phase-contrast MRI angiography. In the inferior row, multiplanar reconstructions of post-operative 3D T1-weighted scan show the successful resection of the FCD IIB. The patient is seizure free nine years after the surgery, without any drug-treatment.

Once the surgical plan has been completed, the patient is operated under general anesthesia with the assistance of the S7 neuronavigation system (Medtronic; Minneapolis, Minnesota, USA). One dose of antibiotics is administered just before the skin incision.

Intraoperative electrocorticography can help the 3D definition of the FCD borders, especially when supra-total resection is not possible due to proximity to eloquent regions. We find particularly helpful the use of SEEG electrodes, free-hand advanced into the brain tissue for a short distance (**Figure 8**).

Differently from grids or strips, SEEG electrodes allow recording not only from the surface of the brain. This is relevant especially when FCD is small and typically deep-seated in the bottom of the sulci. Resections are performed through subpial curettage and ultrasound aspiration.

Completeness of the resection is one of the main predictors of favorable seizure outcome (Alim-Marvasti *et al.*, 2022), thus accurate planning is crucial. However, it must be specified that radical lesionectomy is important only at the cortical level (Wagner *et al.*, 2011a).

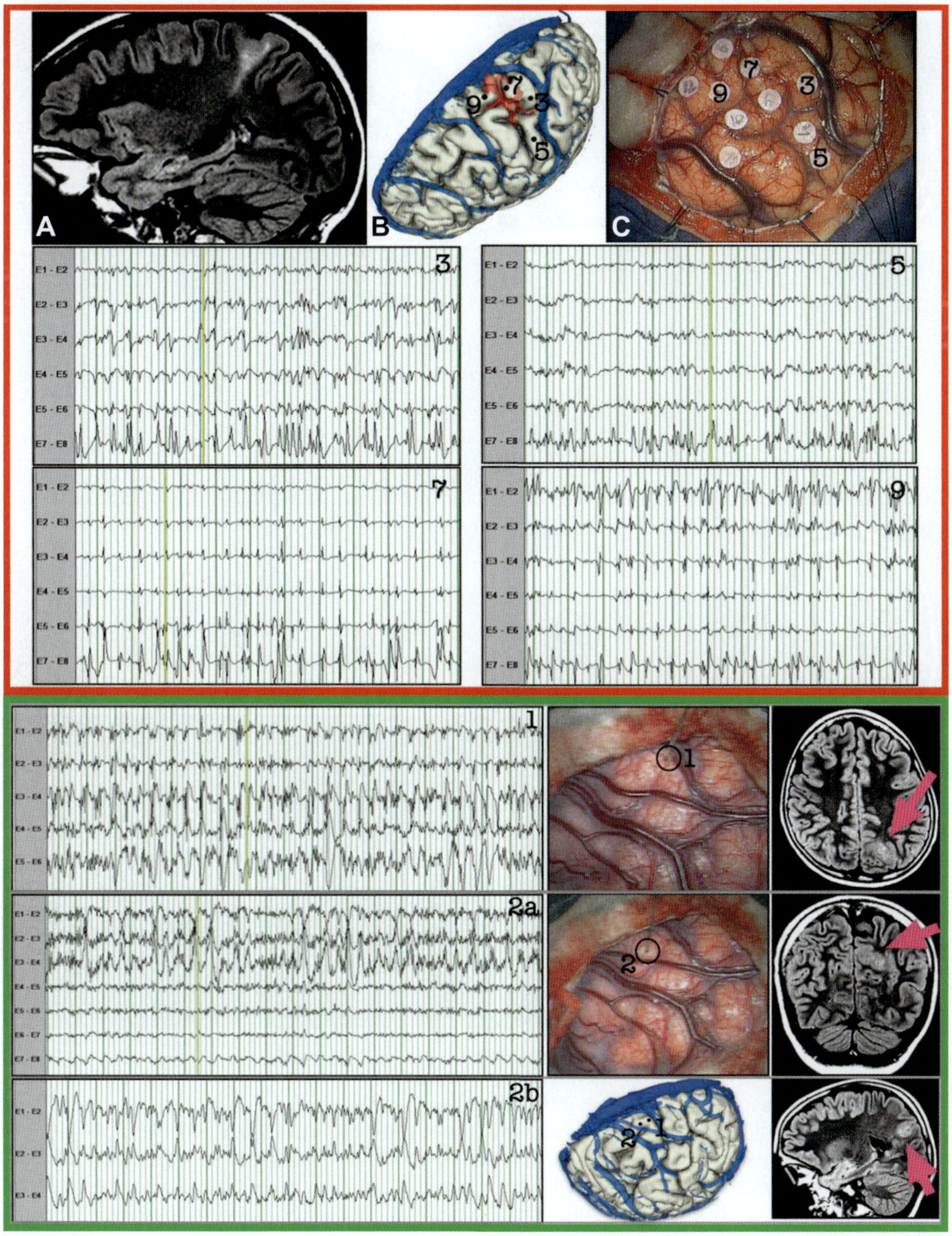

Figure 8

Electrocorticography of patient 6 (red frame). Intraoperative electrocorticographic mapping of a left post-central FCD IIB, carried out advancing an 8-contacts SEEG electrode into the brain tissue, in different positions. A. Sagittal FLAIR slice showing the FCD with its typical transmantle sign. B. 3D rendering showing the lesion (red) and the entry points of the SEEG electrode. C. Intraoperative picture of the surgical field with notifications labels on the cortex. Bipolar recordings obtained with the electrode introduced at sites 3, 7 and 9 show spikes-polyspikes and slow waves, without background activity, at 2-2.5 Hz. Recordings with the electrode at site 5 show physiological background activity and some single spikes coming from adjacent pathological cortex.

Illustrative patient 7 (green frame). First row: recordings obtained at site 1 show the core activity of a FCD IIB (indicated by the arrow on MRI): typical continuous polyspikes and slow waves at 2.5 Hz, without background activity, are visible. Second row: recordings obtained at site 2 before resection of the MRI visible lesion 2a. Continuous slow waves interrupted by fast activity (polyspikes?) are recorded from deeper contacts, at the FCD borders. Third row: recordings obtained at site 2 after the resection 2b. Fast activity is reduced but slow waves persist. Therefore, also the tissue at this site is resected, despite being external to the edges of the MRI-visible part of the lesion. In other words, electrocorticography has been used to delineate intraoperatively the borders of the FCD and thus allow delineation of the extent of the resection. It is important to perform recordings adjacent to the obvious lesion before and after the resection to ensure complete removal of epileptogenic tissue.

When MRI shows the typical trans-mantle sign, it is advisable not to follow it in the white matter, because it is not necessary and can be dangerous in the proximity of the most important tracts connecting eloquent corticol regions.

Intraoperative sleep mapping and monitoring with monopolar/bipolar stimulations of the cortical surface and underlying white matter is performed mainly for rolandic/peri-rolandic or opercular/insular resections. Of note, the cortical mapping of peri-dysplastic tissue can be difficult due to the spreading of pathological activity from the neighboring FCD (**Figure 9**).

The complication rate of our method is low, likely because of accurate topographic planning and angiographic studies. In 2019, we have detailed the complications occurred in a series of 1282 patients (thus including also non-FCD cases). Overall, 100 patients (7.8%) presented a severely complicated course. Older age at operation, multilobar surgery, resection in the rolandic/peri-rolandic and insular-opercular regions were found significant risk factors at multivariate analysis (d'Orio *et al.*, 2019). The risk of new neurological deficits for FCD surgery

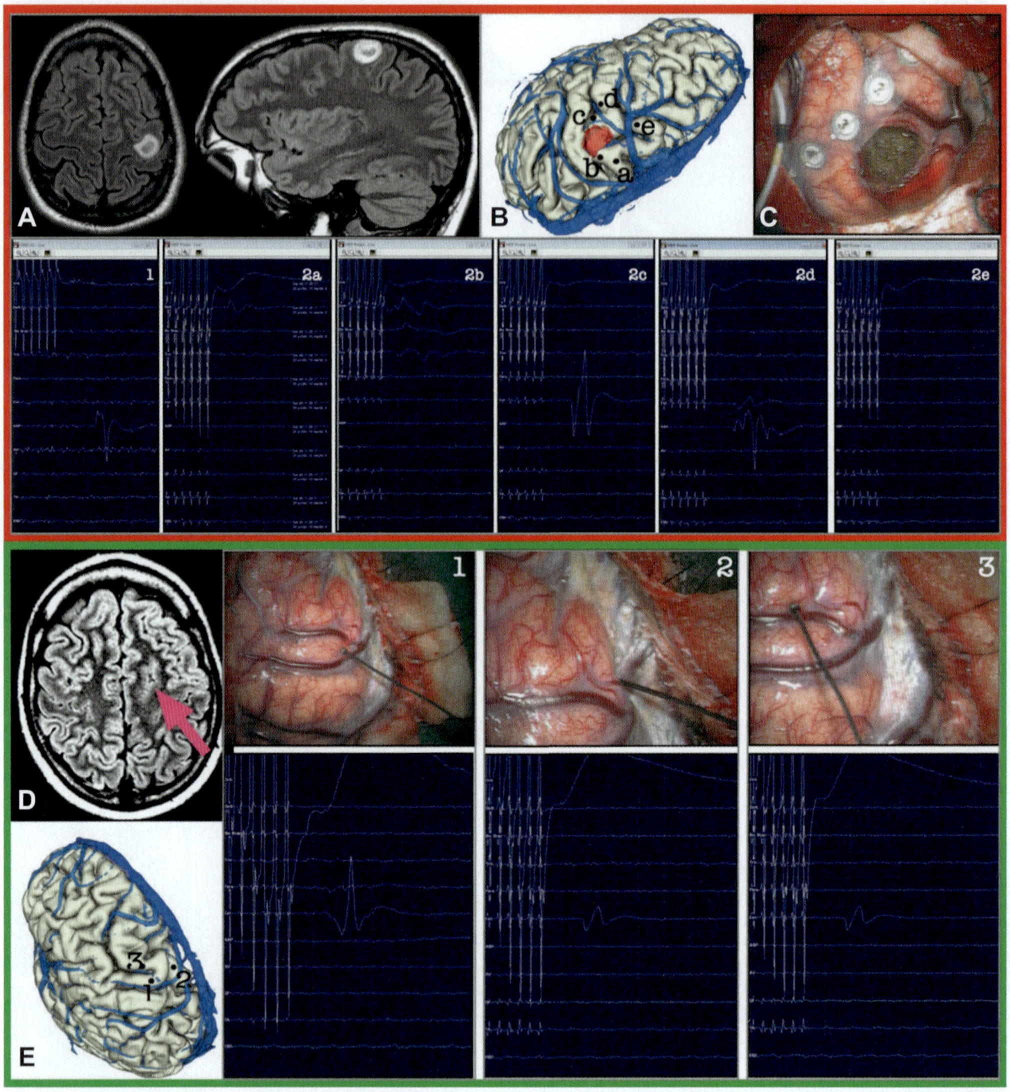

Figure 9.

Cortical mapping of peri-dysplastic tissue is different than in tumor cases.

Illustrative demonstration of mapping of patient 8 (red frame). MRI shows a hyper-intense lesion in the pre-central gyrus (diffuse astrocytoma grade II WHO). 3D rendering depicts the reconstruction of the tumor with surrounding veins and position of mono-polar stimulation aimed at recording motor-evoked potentials (MEP) for functional mapping. Picture shows the surgical field at the end of the resection and the position of the strip used for monitoring. 1. Cortical stimulation of contacts 2-3 of the grid: recorded MEPs from abductor brevis of thumb. 2. Cortical stimulation with monopolar probe along motor strip: MEPs from deltoid (2a), brachial biceps and triceps (2b), carpus extensor (2c) and abductor brevis of thumb (2d). No MEPs in pre-motor cortex (2e).

Illustrative demonstration of mapping of patient 9 (green frame). MRI shows the lesion in the posterior third of the superior frontal gyrus (FCD IIA). 3D rendering depicts the reconstruction of the lesion with surrounding veins and the position of mono-polar stimulation aimed at recording motor-evoked potentials (MEP) for functional mapping. Columns 1, 2 and 3 show intraoperative pictures with the stimulating probe at the three different positions and the correspondent evoked-potentials on carpus extenso muscle. Position 1 (6.2 mA), motor cortex: MEP shows a physiological potential with diffusion of the activation on the adjacent muscles, with low current intensity. Positions 2 (13.2 mA) and 3 (14 mA) on supplementary motor area and pre-motor cortex, respectively evoked a monomorphic potential, atypical, undifferentiated, with a double current intensity. This is a "paradoxical" potential which is frequent in FCD of the rolandic/perirolandic region.

While the peri-neoplastic tissue can be mapped looking for physiological responses external to the lesion, in cases with FCD (especially in the perirolandic area) peri-lesional cortical mapping is contaminated by the electrical activity due to the spreading of pathological activity from the dysplastic lesion. Therefore, data must be carefully considered under the light of 3D anatomical reconstructions is certainly related more to the brain region than to the nature of the abnormality, therefore it is comparable to the risk assessed from our more global retrospective analyses. Certainly, the insular/opercular (including language areas) and the central regions are the zones at higher risk of deficits with hard impact on quality of life. Particular attention must also be paid to the posterior regions to preserve the integrity of the visual pathways. The basal temporo-occipital passage and the intraparietal sulcus region must also be given special attention in the dominant hemisphere for language.

One more time, we want to underline the value of careful planning to avoid unexpected complications. Multiplanar 2D views, 3D reconstructions of the brain surface with its vasculature, cortical thickness mapping, probabilistic estimation of the most important white matter bundles (cortico-spinal and thalamo-cortical tracts, arcuate fasciculus, optic radiations) and f-MRI are the key points of multimodal planning aimed at preserving most important functional networks. Intraoperatively, the careful adoption of the subpial technique remains the safest way to resect the cortical ribbon preserving the vessels running in the sulcal subarachnoid space, as it was taught us a long time ago, when epilepsy surgery was born (Horsley 1886). Moreover, the continuous comparison of the surgical field with multimodal scenes helps the neurosurgeon not to get lost when, due to brain shift, navigation is no longer accurate. As already mentioned, careful intraoperative mapping and monitoring are also crucial. Finally, the rigorous respect of all the basic neurosurgical standards is mandatory to reduce the risk of major bleedings or infections. Indeed, the only death in our series, occurred in a 16-year-old girl suffering from an orbito-frontal FCD, was caused by a very small area of meningitis followed by a Waterhouse-Friderichsen syndrome.

Conclusion

The retrospective analysis carried out in our series of histologically-proven FCD cases (the largest ever published by a single center) has indicated that the histological type, lesion visualization on MRI, size of resection, presence of neurological deficits or cognitive impairment, association with hippocampal sclerosis or ganglioglioma and the duration of epilepsy before surgery significantly predicted outcome on seizures. Duration of epilepsy is operator-dependent, and thus modifiable. The larger the disease duration, the higher the risk of postoperative seizure recurrence. Therefore, earlier surgery is advisable. Also, the analysis of MRI should go beyond simple visual inspection. Post-processing techniques can increase the sensitivity of neuroradiological examination, favoring reinterpretation of image datasets and thus reducing the proportion of MRI-negative patients.

In conclusion, the rigorous respect of the method developed by Talairach and Bancaud to define the epileptogenic zone, advanced imaging analysis, shortening of epilepsy duration and a careful surgical planning are key to improve results in the surgery of focal cortical dysplasias.

References

Alim-Marvasti A, Vakharia VN, Duncan JS. Multimodal prognostic features of seizure freedom in epilepsy surgery. *J Neurol Neurosurg Psychiatry* 2022; 93: 499-508.

Bartolomei F, Nica A, Valenti-Hirsch MP, Adam C, Denuelle M. Interpretation of SEEG recordings. *Clin Neurophysiol* 2018; 48: 53–7.

Behrens TE, Johansen-Berg, Woolrich MW *et al.* Non-invasive mapping of connections between human thalamus and cortex using diffusion imaging. *Nat Neurosci* 2003; 6: 750–7.

Blackmon KE, Kuzniecky RI, Barr WB *et al.* Cortical Gray-White Matter Blurring and Cognitive Morbidity in Focal Cortical Dysplasia. *Cerebral Cortex* 2015; 25: 2854–62.

Bourdillon P, Isnard J, Catenoix H *et al.* Stereo electroencephalography-guided radiofrequency focal epilepsy: Results from a 10-year experience. *Epilepsia* 2017; 58: 85–93.

Blümcke I, Thom M, Aronica E *et al.* The clinicopathologic spectrum of focal cortical dysplasias: a consensus classification proposed by an ad hoc Task Force of the ILAE Diagnostic Methods Commission. *Epilepsia* 2011; 52: 158–74.

Cardinale F, Cossu M, Castana L *et al.* Stereoelectroencephalography: surgical methodology, safety, and stereotactic application accuracy in 500 procedures. *Neurosurgery* 2013; 72: 353–66.

Cardinale F, Pero G, Quilici L *et al.* Cerebral angiography for multimodal surgical planning in epilepsy surgery: description of a new three-dimensional technique and literature review. *World Neurosurg* 2015; 84: 358–67.

Cardinale F, Francione S, Gennari L *et al.* SUrface-PRojected FLAIR analysis: a novel tool for advanced imaging of epilepsy. *World Neurosurg* 2017a; 98: 715–26.

Cardinale F, Rizzi M, d'Orio M *et al.* A new tool for touch-free patient registration for robot-assisted intracranial surgery: application accuracy from a phantom study and a retrospective surgical series. *Neurosurg Focus* 2017b; 42: E8.

Cardinale F, Rizzi M, Vignati E *et al.* Stereoelectroencephalography: retrospective analysis of 742 procedures in a single centre. *Brain* 2019; 142: 2688–704.

Catenoix H, Mauguière F, Montavont A, Ryvlin P, Guénot M, Isnard J. Seizures Outcome After Stereoelectroencephalography-Guided Thermocoagulations in Malformations of Cortical Development Poorly Accessible to Surgical Resection. *Neurosurgery* 2015; 77: 9–15.

Chabardès S, Abel T, Cardinale F, Kahane P. Commentary: Understanding Stereo-electroencephalography: What's Next? *Neurosurgery* 2018; 82: E15–6.

Chang EF, Wang DD, Barkovich AJ *et al.* Predictors of seizure freedom after surgery for malformations of cortical development. *Ann Neurol* 2011; 70: 151–62.

Chassoux F, Devaux B, Landré E *et al.* Stereoelectroencephalography in focal cortical dysplasia: a 3D approach to delineating the dysplastic cortex. *Brain* 2000; 123: 1733–51.

Chauvel P Contributions of Jean Talairach and Jean Bancaud to epilepsy surgery. In Lüders HO and Comair YG (editors) *Epilepsy Surgery*, Second Edition, pp 35–41. Philadelphia: Lippincott Williams & Wilkins, 2001.

Colombo N, Tassi L, Deleo F *et al.* Focal cortical dysplasia type IIa and IIb: MRI aspects in 118 cases proven by histopathology. *Neuroradiology* 2012; 54: 1065–77.

Cossu M, Fuschillo D, Bramerio M *et al.* Epilepsy surgery of focal cortical dysplasia-associated tumors. *Epilepsia* 2013; 54(Suppl 9): S115–22.

Cossu M, Fuschillo D, Casaceli G *et al.* Stereoelectroencephalography-guided radiofrequency thermocoagulation in the epileptogenic zone: a retrospective study on 89 cases, *J Neurosurg* 2015; 123: 1358–67.

Cossu M, Cardinale F, Casaceli G *et al.* Stereo-EEG-guided radiofrequency thermocoagulations. *Epilepsia* 2017; 58(Suppl 1): S66–S72.

Cossu M, d'Orio, Barba C *et al.* Focal Cortical Dysplasia IIIa in Hippocampal Sclerosis-Associated Epilepsy: Anatomo-Electro-Clinical Profile and Surgical Results From a Multicentric Retrospective Study. *Neurosurgery* 2021; 88: 384–93.

d'Orio P, Rizzi M, Mariani V *et al.* Surgery in patients with childhood-onset epilepsy: analysis of complications and predictive risk factors for a severely complicated course. *J Neurol Neurosurg Psychiatry* 2019; 90: 84–9.

Engel Jr J, Van Ness PC, Rasmussen T, Ojemann LM. Outcome with respect to epileptic seizures. In Engel Jr J (ed) *Surgical Treatment of the Epilepsies*, Second Edition, pp. 609–21. New York: Raven Press, 1993.

Fauser S, Bast T, Altenmüller DM *et al.* Factors influencing surgical outcome in patients with focal cortical dysplasia. *J Neurol Neurosurg Psychiatry* 2008; 79: 103–5.

Fedorov A, Beichel R, Kalpathy-Cramer J *et al.* 3D Slicer as an image computing platform for the Quantitative Imaging Network. *Magn Reson Imaging* 2012; 30: 1323–41.

Fischl BR (). FreeSurfer. *NeuroImage* 2012; 62: 774–781.

Grant RL (). Converting an odds ratio to a range of plausible relative risks for better communication of research findings. *BMJ* 2014; 348: f7450.

Horsley V. Brain-Surgery. *BMJ* 1886; 2: 670–5.

Jenkinson M, Beckmann CF, Behrens TEJ, Woolrich MW, Smith SM. Fsl. *NeuroImage* 2012 ; 62: 782–90.

Kadish NE, Bast T, Wagner K *et al.* Epilepsy Surgery in the First 3 Years of Life: Predictors of Seizure Freedom and Cognitive Development. *Neurosurgery* 2019; 84: E368–77.

Kahane P, Landré E, Minotti L, Francione S, Ryvlin P. The Bancaud and Talairach view on the epileptogenic zone: a working hypothesis. *Epileptic Disord* 2006; 8(Suppl 2): S16–S26.

Loddenkemper T, Holland K, Stanford LD, Kotagal P, Bingaman WE, Wyllie E. Developmental outcome after epilepsy surgery in infancy. *Pediatrics* 119: 930–5.

Lüders HO, Engel J Jr and Munari C. (1993): General Principles. In Engel J Jr (editor) *Surgical Treatment of the Epilepsies*, Second Edition, pp 137–153. New York: Raven Press, Ltd, 2007.

Minotti L, Montavont A, Scholly J, Tyvaert L, Taussig D *et al.* Indications and limits of stereoelectroencephalography (SEEG). *Neurophysiol Clin* 2018; 48: 15–24.

Munari C and Bancaud J. The role of stereo-electroencephalography (SEEG) in the evaluation of partial epileptic seizures. In Porter RJ and Morselli PL (eds) *The Epilepsies*, pp 267–306. Bodmin: Butterworth & Co. (Publishers) Ltd, 1985.

Munari C, Kahane P, Tassi L *et al.* Intracerebral low frequency electrical stimulation: a new tool for the definition of the "epileptogenic area"?. *Acta Neurochir Suppl* 1993; 58: 181–5.

Nobili L, Cardinale F, Magliola U *et al.* Taylor's focal cortical dysplasia increases the risk of sleep-related epilepsy. *Epilepsia* 2009; 50: 2599–604.

Nowell M, Rodionov R, Zombori G *et al.* Utility of 3D multimodality imaging in the implantation of intracranial electrodes in epilepsy. *Epilepsia* 2015; 56: 403–13.

Palmini A, Gambardella A, Andermann F *et al.* Intrinsic epileptogenicity of human dysplastic cortex as suggested by corticography and surgical results. *Annals of Neurology* 1995; 37: 476–87.

Palmini A, Najm IM, Avanzini G *et al.* Terminology and classification of the cortical dysplasias, *Neurology* 2004; 62(Suppl 3): S2–S8.

Rácz A, Becker AJ, Quesada CM *et al.* Post-Surgical Outcome and Its Determining Factors in Patients Operated on With Focal Cortical Dysplasia Type II—A Retrospective Monocenter Study. *Front Neurol* 2021; 12: 666056.

Rowland NC, Englot DJ, Cage TA, Sughrue ME, Barbaro NM, Chang EF. A meta-analysis of predictors of seizure freedom in the surgical management of focal cortical dysplasia. *J Neurosurg* 2012; 116: 1035–41.

Shurtleff HA, Barry D, Firman T *et al.* Impact of epilepsy surgery on development of preschool children: Identification of a cohort likely to benefit from early intervention. *J Neurosurg Pediatr* 2015; 16: 383–92.

Spencer SS and Huh L Outcomes of epilepsy surgery in adults and children. *Lancet Neurol* 2008; 7: 525–37.

Tassi L, Colombo N, Garbelli R *et al.* Focal cortical dysplasia: neuropathological subtypes, EEG, neuroimaging and surgical outcome. *Brain* 2002; 125: 1719–32.

Tassi L *et al.* Type I focal cortical dysplasia: surgical outcome is related to histopathology. *Epileptic Disord* 2010; 12: 181–91.

Tassi L, Garbelli R, Colombo N *et al.* Electroclinical, MRI and surgical outcomes in 100 epileptic patients with type II FCD. *Epileptic Disord* 2012; 14: 257–66.

Taylor D and Falconer MA Focal dysplasia of the cerebral cortex in epilepsy'. *J Neurol Neurosurg Psychiatry* 1971; 34: 369–87.

Téllez-Zenteno JF, Dhar R and Wiebe S Long-term seizure outcomes following epilepsy surgery: a systematic review and meta-analysis. *Brain* 2005; 128: 1188–98.

Trébuchon A and Chauvel P. Electrical Stimulation for Seizure Induction and Functional Mapping in Stereoelectroencephalography. *J Clin Neurophysiol* 2016; 33: 511–521.

Trébuchon A, Racila R, Cardinale F *et al.* Electrical stimulation for seizure induction during SEEG exploration: a useful predictor of post-surgical seizure recurrence? *J Neurol Neurosurg Psychiatry* 2021; 92: 22–26.

Wagner J, Urbach H, Niehusmann P, von Lehe M, Elger CE, Wellmer J. Focal cortical dysplasia type IIb: completeness of cortical, not subcortical, resection is necessary for seizure freedom. *Epilepsia* 2011a; 52: 1418–24.

Wagner J, Weber B, Urbach H, Elger CE, Huppertz HJ. Morphometric MRI analysis improves detection of focal cortical dysplasia type II. *Brain* 2011b; 134: 2844–54.

Wagstyl K, Whitaker K, Raznahan A *et al.* Atlas of lesion locations and postsurgical seizure freedom in focal cortical dysplasia: A MELD study. *Epilepsia* 2022; 63: 61–74.

CHAPTER

20. Surgery for FCD without invasive monitoring: the role of ECoG

Eliseu Paglioli, Andre Palmini, Francine Hehn

Key points

- Higher rates of FCD identification by imaging and accumulated experience with resective strategies may revive the interest on acute intraoperative ECoG recordings to fine tune resection of the EZ.
- Although presurgical evaluation and resective strategies are often rooted in paradigmatic perspectives of how to delineate and remove the EZ, it is becoming clear that many patients with FCD may not need ictal recordings with chronically implanted intracranial electrodes.
- Acute ECoG using flexible, ball-pointed electrodes, allows sequential recordings leading to stepwise resections of relevant epileptogenic tissue in FCD surgery.
- Identification of frequent spiking and other highly epileptogenic patterns by acute intraoperative ECoG in tissue at variable distances from a visible FCD lesion may help to effectively tailor resections.

Introduction

The whole issue of the surgical treatment of focal cortical dysplasias revolves around delineating the tissue that should be resected to control seizures in the long term – and then, being able to remove it. The unending debates on how best to achieve such delineation are fuelled by several facts. One is that FCD is perhaps the most common neocortical pathology associated with drug resistant seizures and, therefore, in need of a surgical solution. The picture is compounded by the fact that there is a large variety of FCD scenarios, involving histopathological type, anatomical location, degree of spatial restriction and visibility by structural imaging (Palmini and Holthausen, 2013; Guerrini *et al*, 2015). Moreover, the tissue prone to seizure generation in many subtypes of FCD can extend beyond the margins of the visible lesion, and how to fully determine this tissue is both a key step in the surgical treatment and a major focus of debate. Finally, FCD can colocalize with functionally indispensable cortical regions, posing a final challenge: even when everything is 'perfect' in terms of delineating the EZ, it may not be entirely resected for functional reasons. These intermixed ingredients pertaining to the realm of FCD have occupied epileptologists and epilepsy neurosurgeons for the last 30 years and experience has accumulated accordingly. However, because experience also means perfectioning along given paths of procedures and reasoning (ie, getting better and better with a given approach), specialists often delineate the tissue that should be removed with the methods they are best acquainted.

A crucial step in the pursuit of the tissue that should be resected to control seizures in FCD is the valuation of electrographic findings, both ictal and interictal, either registered from the scalp, the surface or the deeper portions of the cortex. In this chapter we will propose that, indeed, there is a variable degree of relevance of electrographic patterns or findings in pointing to the relevant epileptogenic tissue ie, cortical tissue whose resection should control seizures not only in the short or middle, but in the long term (Palmini and Paglioli, 2019). We will discuss the possibility that despite being essentially an 'interictal method', a judicious cortical exploration with acute ECoG may help to delineate tissue that may cause seizures in FCD, even as delayed relapse after surgery. In other words, we believe the ECoG-based concept of tertiary localization put forth by Rasmussen should be revisited in this era of advanced imaging, to help delineate not only the current EZ, but also the potentially EZ, ie, the epileptogenic area that must be excised to produce a satisfactory long-term reduction of the patients' seizure tendency (Rasmussen, 1983). In a sense, this adds to the concept that the EZ (specially as indexed by the

lesion (**Figure 2**). As such, the acute ECoG may unveil relevant portions of the irritative zone that could be missed even by invasive methods (Tandon *et al*, 2019; Nascimento *et al*, 2021) and prompt a more extensive resection, crucial for successful epilepsy surgery *in the long term.*

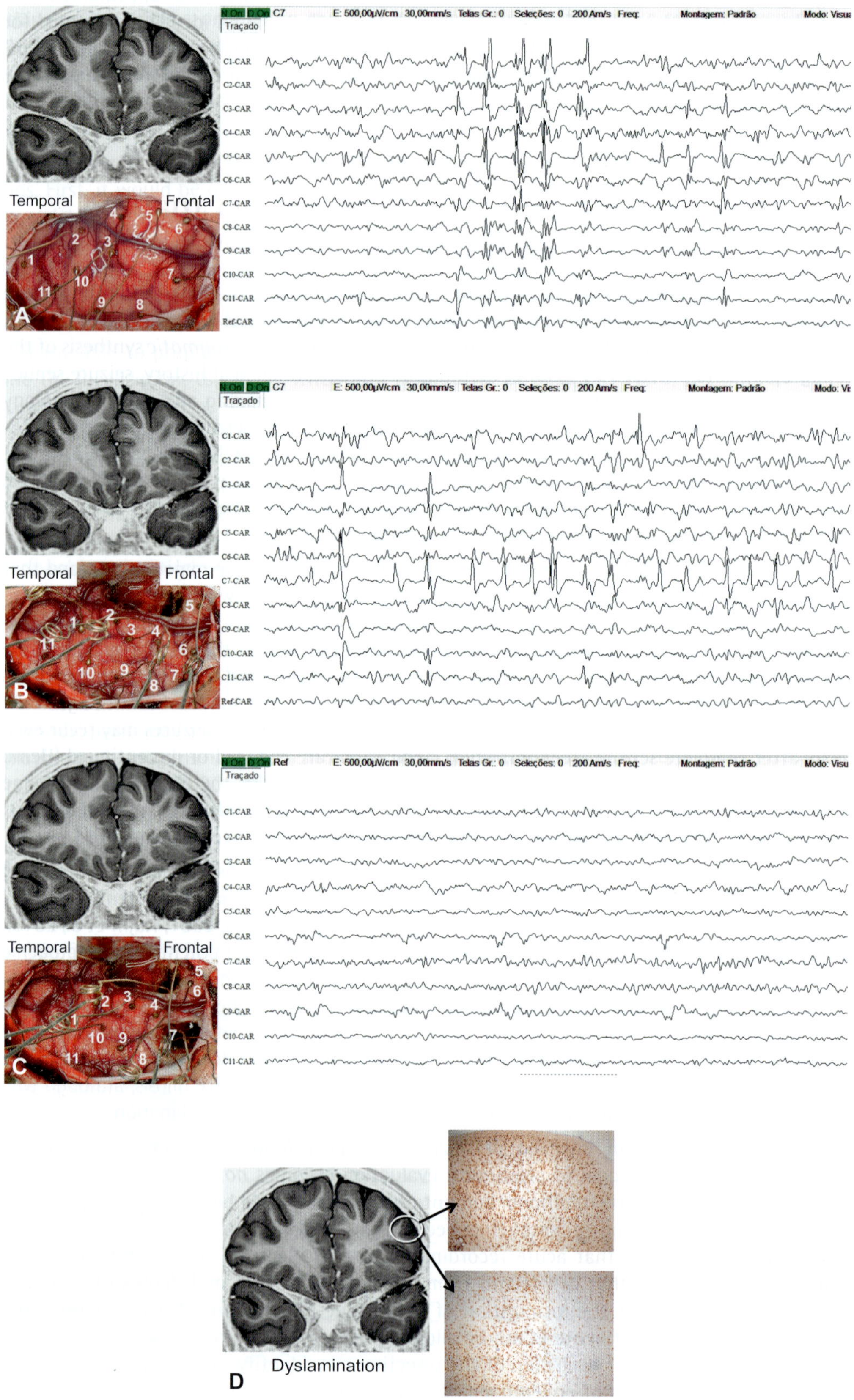

Figure 2

Example of relevant epileptogenic tissue non-adjacent to a visible dysplastic lesion identified by sequential recordings through acute intraoperative ECoG in a 15 year-old girl with FCD I. 2A shows recurrent spikes with a lead at electrode #5, over the left frontal dysplastic lesion; 2B is an ECoG sample following resection of the lesion and the region with lead spikes. Note 'resurgence' of frequent spiking at a distance from the lesion, centered at electrode position #7 (this area was mostly silent before initial resection); 2C is ECoG after final stepwise resection. Note infrequent, low voltage sharp waves in electrode positions #6 and #9, that are much less impressive than the ones before the second resection; 2D shows dyslamination in the non-adjacent cortical region with frequent spiking, identified by post-resection ECoG.

Such tissue that potentially has a lower epileptogenic threshold as identified by acute ECoG, takes into account that interictal spikes differ in *amplitude, rhythmicity, frequency and association with background rhythms*. Hence, different ECoG spikes have distinct significance as markers of cortical regions with tendency to generate seizures in the short and the long term and as we reviewed previously (Palmini, 2006; Palmini and Paglioli, 2019) this realization led Theodore Rasmussen to propose the concept of 'green' and 'red' spikes, referring to those less and more likely to index epileptogenically relevant tissue (Rasmussen, 1983).

Experience since accumulated has confirmed that frequent, at times continuous, rhythmic, or bursting spikes, and also spikes of high amplitude or associated with background abnormalities tend to indicate cortical regions that are part of the *actual or latent* EZ (Palmini *et al.*, 1995), extending beyond the visible lesion (**Figure 3**). Moreover, the association of spikes with background abnormalities points to a *convergence of the irritative zone with one measure of the zone of cortical dysfunction*. Hence, in the interpretation of the acute ECoG close attention should be

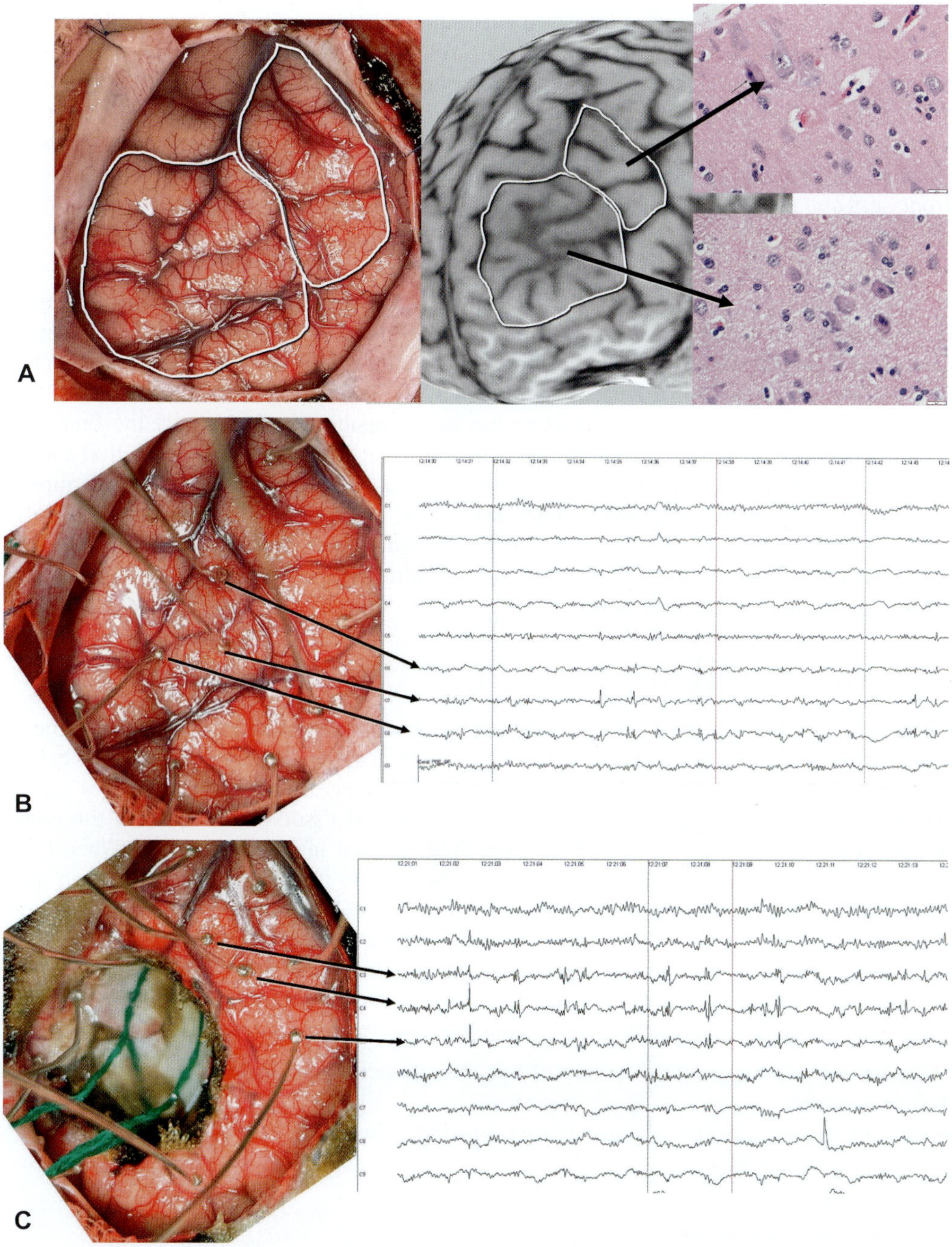

Figure 3

Another example of acute ECoG exploration of cortical regions in the same lobe of a visible dysplastic abnormality. 3A shows the lesion in a 3-dimension reformatting with a dimple in the middle of a 'rosette-like appearance' (center). On the **left** is the corresponding surgical picture and on the **right** the FCDII histopathology both over the lesion and over what appeared to be a non-lesional portion of an interconnected gyrus; 3B is the spiking and polyspiking over the visible lesion; 3C is the first post-resection ECoG showing appearance of intense spiking in an interconnected gyrus, not immediately adjacent to the lesion. These spikes did not appear in the pre-resection recording. Extention of resection to include this second area led to seizure freedom.

paid not only to spikes, but also to background rhythms, particularly absence of physiological fast rhythms and focal slow wave activity. Hence, the interpretation and planning of resection based upon acute ECoG departs from the 'chasing of spikes', and demands an hierarchization of spike patterns and background rhythms with variable probability of indexing the tissue relevant to current and 'future' seizure generation.

The ECoG strategy

• The relevance of the ECoG method of recording

Semantically, ECoG refers to the *direct* recording of electrical cortical activity by whatever method, ie, through individual (ball-pointed), subdural or intracerebral electrodes. A*cute ECoG* refers to the use of any of these types of electrodes only during the operation; hence, for such recordings, patients do not need to be chronically implanted. A clear distinction, however, should be made between acute ECoG recordings performed with individual (ball-pointed) electrodes from those performed with subdural electrodes. The former allows acute probing of electrical activity from the surface, lateral banks and depths of gyri in sequential fashion during resection, and electrode positioning can be customized at each stage under direct visualization of the gyri being explored. This is not the case with subdural electrodes, which allow only exploration of the superficial cortex, with a predetermined inter-electrode distance. *All recordings in Porto Alegre are performed with individual (ball-pointed) electrode sets and the discussion that follows refers to this specific type of electrodes.*

• ECoG patterns related to relevant epileptogenic tissue.

A comprehensive discussion on these patterns is found in the chapter by Palmini and Paglioli in this volume. Here, just a few points will be highlighted. It is known that spikes may be generated from pathologic cortical tissue or from regions connected with these and such differentiation is crucial. Both from acute ECoG and SEEG (Rasmussen, 1983; Palmini *et al*, 2005, Chassoux *et al*, 2000) such differentiation has been possible, particularly by the finding in FCD of virtually continuous, pacemaker-like discharges. It is also our experience that shorter trains of rhythmic spikes, even without a prolonged pacemaker-like appearance (**Figure 2**) and spikes over slow waves (FEDOIS; Holthausen *et al*, 1995) also indicate relevant epileptogenic tendency – even if nonadjacent to the lesion. Finding such nonadjacent highly epileptogenic patterns (**Figures 2 and 3**) through exploration of exposed gyri is the quintessential advantage of the ball-pointed, acute ECoG.

ECoG-based surgery for FCD

Needless to say, the first step is to plan the operation with a localization hypothesis garnered from seizure semiology, scalp EEG and the best imaging possible. At times, blurring may extend further than the obvious area of increased signal, for instance, or either EEG spikes or seizure semiology may suggest epileptogenic relevance of cortical tissue nonadjacent to the visible lesion, either in a different gyrus of the same lobe or even in a different lobe. When ECoG shows highly epileptogenic patterns, pathology often shows that FCD is present in such non-adjacent areas, that may or may not have been interconnected within an epileptogenic network (**Figures 2 and 3**). Crucially, the notion that 'MRI-invisible' dysplastic tissue may be present at some distance from a clear lesion seen on the MRI (particularly in FCD I and FCD IIA) must be kept in mind to plan a correct ECoG evaluation. These aspects are important to plan the craniotomy which, in ECoG-based FCD surgery, should encompass these potentially relevant areas.

Then, the main strategy is further identifying, then resecting cortical regions displaying:

- continuous or
- bursting spiking patterns and also cortex showing either:
  - trains of spikes (even short);
  - polyspikes;
  - spikes over slow waves.

Such resection, however, need not be in a single stage. The initial resection targets the lesion and the highly epileptogenic cortex in the same or adjacent gyri. Then, ECoG is again performed to look for two things:

- the disappearance of epileptogenic abnormalities found in the first recording, which likely represented propagation and not pathological tissue;
- the appearance of previously unidentified epileptogenic cortex, ie, cortex that did not show spikes or one of the highly epileptogenic patterns mentioned above in the first recording but was possibly disinhibited following initial resection of a part of the epileptogenic network.

As illustrated in **Figure 2B**, the possibility that such acute epileptogenic disinhibition may in fact 'mark' relevant epileptogenic tissue would be a major asset of acute ECoG – and particularly that performed with ball-pointed electrodes allowing free exploration of the vicinities of the 'main focus'.

Finally, the question often arises on whether cortical regions displaying *discontinuous, less frequent* interictal spikes, unaccompanied by abnormal background should be included in the resection. The relevance of these spikes is still unclear. Although cortical regions displaying any type of spike should be ideally resected, results have been conflicting and confounded by incomplete resections not only of the spiking cortex, but also of the visible dysplastic lesions themselves. The series from King's College, for instance, suggests that persistence of these spikes in post-resection ECoG - following complete lesion resection - does not correlate with surgical outcome (Ferrier *et al.*, 2001). Our experience is that frequent spikes in a given cortical region that are persistently recorded, even after resection of the lesion and regions with I/CEDs, are likely relevant and these cortical regions should be included in the resection, if at all possible. Less relevant spikes ('the green spikes' of Rasmussen; Rasmussen *et al*, 1983) often disappear or become very infrequent after resection of the more epileptogenic areas (**Figure 2C**).

Conclusion

Semantics may at times lead to confusion. Because the term 'ECoG' refers broadly to direct cortical recording – and that is almost always performed with subdural electrodes with limited ability to sequentially explore superficial and deep-seated cortical regions - its used has been relegated. We believe it is high time to revive the Montreal Neurological Institute-championed ECoG apparatus with ball pointed electrodes allowing free and sequential exploration of superficial and deep cortical regions under direct visualization of the surgeon – thus leading to sequential resections of epileptogenic tissue. Using this ECoG methodology, we propose that the tissue to be resected can be adequately delineated in many patients with visible FCD lesions combining semiology, scalp EEG, imaging and acute ECoG. When MRI is negative, of course, the question of how to proceed with presurgical evaluation is more complex. When semiology, scalp EEG and FDG-PET (and/or MEG) are clearly convergent to a specific cortical region, some Centers such as ours would still consider 'direct' surgery, with further refinement of the resection according to acute ECoG. Other Centers would not consider this possibility and use intracranial recordings, mostly SEEG. A number of highly epileptogenic patterns have been described and may index relevant epileptogenic tissue with the potential to generate seizures either at the time of presurgical evaluation and epilepsy surgery or even years later, due to reduced threshold. Expanded use and research with the adequate ECoG apparatus may be an important asset to identify such tissue and lead to long term seizure control, particularly in FCD II cases without sharply delineated imaging abnormalities.

References

Bancaud J, Dell MB. Technics and method of stereotaxic functional exploration of the brain structures in man (cortex, subcortex, central gray nuclei). *Rev Neurol* 1959;101: 213-27

Bartolomei F, Trébuchon A, Bonini F, *et al.* What is the concordance between the seizure onset zone and the irritative zone? A SEEG quantified study. *Clin Neurophysiol.* 2016; 127: 1157-62.

Chassoux F, Devaux B, Landré E, *et al.* Stereoelectroencephalography in focal cortical dysplasia. A 3D approach to delineating the dysplastic cortex. *Brain* 2000; 123: 1733-55.

Fauser S, Essang C, Altenmüller DM, *et al.* Long-term seizure outcome in 211 patients with focal cortical dysplasia. *Epilepsia.* 2015; 56: 66-76.

Ferrier CH, Alarcon G, Engelsman J, *et al.* Relevance of residual histologic and electrocorticographic abnormalities for surgical outcome in frontal lobe epilepsies. *Epilepsia* 2001; 42: 363-71.

Guerrini R, Duchowny M, Jayakar P, *et al.* Diagnostic methods and treatment options for focal cortical dysplasia. *Epilepsia.* 2015;56: 1669-86.

Guerrini R, Cavallin M, Pippucci T, *et al.* Is focal cortical dysplasia/epilepsy caused by somatic MTOR mutations always a unilateral d isorder? *Neurol Genet.* 2020; 7: e540.

Hemb M, Palmini A, Paglioli E, *et al.* An 18-year follow-up of seizure outcome after surgery for temporal lobe epilepsyand hippocampal sclerosis. *J Neurol Neurosurg Psychiatry* 2013; 84: 800-805.

Holthausen HH, Teixeira V, Tuxhorn I, *et al.* Epilepsy surgery in children and adolescents with focal cortical dysplasias. In: Tuxhorn I, Holthausen H, Boenigk H, eds. *Paediatric Epilepsy Syndromes and Their Surgical Treatment*, John Libbey and Company, Ltd.: London, 199-215, 1997.

Holthausen H, Coras R, Tang Y, Bai L, Wang I, Pieper T, *et al.* Multilobar unilateral hypoplasia with emphasis in the posterior quadrant and severe epilepsy in children with FCD ILAE Type 1A. Epilepsia. 2022; 63: 42-60.

Jasper HH. Electrocorticography. In: Penfield W, Erickson TC, eds. *Epilepsy and Cerebral Localization,* Charles C. Thomas Publisher: Springfield, Il, 380-454, 1941.

Jasper HH, Arfel-Capdeveille G, Rasmussen T. Evaluation of EEG and cortical electrographic studies for prognosis of seizures following surgical excision of epileptogenic lesions. *Epilepsia* 1961; 2: 130-7.

Jehi L. The Epileptogenic Zone: Concept and Definition. *Epilepsy Currents.* 2018; 18: 12-16.

Luders HO, Engel J, Munari C. General principles. In: Engel J Jr (ed*), Surgical Treatment of the Epilepsies* (2nd ed.). New York: Raven Press, 1993: 137–153.

Lüders HO, Najm I, Nair D, Widdess-Walsh P, Bingman W. The epileptogenic zone: general principles. *Epileptic Disord.* 2006;8 Suppl 2: S1-9.

Najm I, Jehi L, Palmini A, Paglioli E. Temporal patterns and mechanisms of epilepsy surgery failure. *Epilepsia*, 2013; 54: 772-82.

Nascimento FA, Srinivasan VM, Sheth SA, Gavvala JR. In the pursuit of the epileptogenic zone - listen carefully and look deeply. *Epileptic Disord.* 2021; 23: 667-73.

Palmini A, Gambardella A, Andermann F, *et al.* Intrinsic epileptogenicity of human dysplastic cortex as suggested by corticography and surgical results. *Ann Neurol* 1995; 37: 476-87.

Palmini A. The concept of the epileptogenic zone: a modern look at Penfield and Jasper's views on the role of interictal spikes. *Epileptic Disorders* 2006; 8 (Suppl. 2): S1- S6.

Palmini A, Holthausen H. Focal malformations of cortical development: a most relevant etiology of epilepsy in children. *Handb Clin Neurol.* 2013;111: 549-65.

Palmini A, Paglioli E. The irritative zone and seizure onset zone in acute ECoG: the quest for the relevant epileptogenic tissue. In: Lhatoo SD, Kahane P, Luders H (eds). *Invasive Studies of the Human Epileptic Brain: Principles and Practice.* New York: Oxford University Press, 2019.

Rasmussen T. Characteristics of a pure culture of frontal lobe epilepsy. *Epilepsia* 1983; 24: 482-93.

Rosenow F, Lüders H. Presurgical evaluation of epilepsy. *Brain.* 2001; 124: 1683-700.

Talairach J, Bancaud J, Bonis A, Szikla G, Tournoux P. Functional stereotaxic exploration of epilepsy. *Confin Neurol.* 1962;22: 328-31.

Tandon N, Tong BA, Friedman ER, *et al.* Analysis of morbidity and outcomes associated with use of subdural grids vs stereoelectroencephalography in patients with intractable epilepsy. *JAMA Neurol.* 2019;76: 672-81.

Tassi L, Colombo N, Garbelli R, *et al.* Focal cortical dysplasia: neuropathological subtypes, EEG, neuroimaging and surgical outcome. *Brain.* 2002; 125: 1719-32.

CHAPTER 21. Surgery for FCD with invasive monitoring

Jorge Álvaro González Martínez

Key points

- Extra-operative invasive EEG may be required in FCD surgery to localize the epileptogenic zone, demarcate the anatomical boundaries for the surgical treatment and/ or identify eloquent cortex in proximity with the cerebral areas responsible for the primary organization of the epileptiform activity.
- Subdural grids can be used when the FCD is superficial or extends into the cortical surface. Each anatomical region has specific technical nuances related to the implantation of SDG electrodes in the "FCD scenario".
- SEEG-guided resections have gained increased popularity and utilization in recent years, mainly due to the possibility of defining the three-dimensional aspects of seizure organization.
- The SEEG method is particularly suitable for the diagnosis and treatment of FCD since the highest epileptogenicity is in general located in the deeper parts the cortex. Thus, it is likely the method of choice to study patients with lesional epilepsies associated with FCD.

Introduction

In 1971, Taylor, Falconer and Corsellis published the paper entitled Focal Dysplasia of the Cerebral Cortex in Epilepsy (Taylor *et al.*, 1971). They discussed 10 cases of patients with epilepsy operated on by Murray Falconer (8 cases) in the Guy's – Maudsley – King's Neurosurgical Unit and 2 other cases treated at other Institutions. Every case was exceptionally detailed both from the clinical and surgical point of view. Schematic drawings clearly depicted the typical aspect of the cortex thickening and blurring whose image could only be seen pre-operatively decades later after the introduction of magnetic resonance imaging into clinical practice. They also described at microscopic examination the characteristic "...disruption of the normal cortical lamination and an excess of large aberrant neurons scattered randomly through all but the first layer... the most characteristic feature, therefore, was the disorganization both of the cortical architecture and of many of its individual neurons. In seven of 10 cases the anarchy was aggravated by the addition of malformed cells of uncertain origin with large, sometimes multiple, nuclei surrounded by an excess of opalescent pseudopodic cytoplasm".

Although some authors had already published isolated cases of the same pathology, Taylor's work is an original contribution in the sense that he correctly stressed the main features of the disease and described typical clinical features and image correlates. The impact of that publication in the field of epilepsy surgery has been paramount.

FCD represents the most common etiological entity concerning epilepsy surgical cases in children, amounting roughly to a third of all cases and a significant number of cases in the adult population. Its variegated mode of presentation and protean character from patient to patient justifies this publication aimed at pointing the major advances in the presentation at diagnosis, indications and results of surgery. Epilepsy surgery remains most successful for "lesional" epilepsy, and removal of the lesion, with or without adjacent tissue resection is sufficient to permanently control the epileptic activity in some patients. Nevertheless, in a significant number of patients, the removal of a dysplastic lesion is not sufficient to arrest the occurrence of debilitating recurrent seizures. MRI anatomic and signal abnormalities have been described in FCD, but despite significant MRI abnormalities in most cases of FCD, up to 25% of patients with "normal" MRI had histopathologic changes in focal lesions. Consequently, a sizable number of patients with FCD do not achieve a good outcome even after the apparently complete resection of the hypothetical epileptogenic zone lesion (defined by electroencephalographic and metabolic images). These results suggest that current imaging (and evaluation) techniques may not accurately map the extent of dysplastic and epileptogenic regions in FCD and stress the fact that image-based surgery in MRI visible FCD will result in suboptimal seizure outcome. The exception for this statement is the Taylor type FCD (FCD II), where the complete removal of the MRI visible dysplastic lesion is associated with permanent seizure control (Chassoux *et al.*, 2022).

GENERAL concepts in epilepsy surgery in the "FCD scenario"

The main goal and basic principle of curative epilepsy surgery is the arrest of the epileptic activity by the complete resection (or complete disconnection) of the cortical areas responsible for the primary organization of the EZ. As the EZ can eventually coincide with functional cortical areas (eloquent cortex), preservation of these fundamental brain functions is another goal of any curative surgical resection in patients with medically refractory epilepsy (MRE) (Adelson, O'Rourke, & Albright, 1995; Cossu *et al.*, 2008; Jayakar, 1999; Jayakar, Duchowny & Resnick, 1994; Rosenow & Luders, 2001; Winkler *et al.*, 1999; Wyllie *et al.*, 1988). The principle can be generally applied and disregard the epilepsy syndrome etiology. Medically intractable epilepsies caused by suspected or confirmed FCD are not exceptions.

As successful FCD related epilepsy surgery relies on accurate preoperative localization of the EZ, the appropriate pre-surgical evaluation is fundamental to obtain the widest and most accurate spectrum of information from clinical, anatomical, neurophysiological and neuropsychological aspects, with the primordial goal of performing an individualized, tailored and safe resection. The non-invasive methods of seizure localization and lateralization (scalp EEG, magnetoencephalography-MEG, positron emission tomography-PET, ictal single photon emission computed tomography-SPECT, functional MRI, diffusion tensor imaging) are complementary and results are interpreted in conjunction and never in isolation, in the attempt to compose a hypothesis of the anatomical location of the EZ. If the anatomical hypothesis is precisely delineated, there is no need for further studies and surgery may be carried on accordingly. This is pertinent to "lesional epilepsies", where FCD II lesions are located in cortical areas that correspond to the localization hypothesis (Chassoux *et al.*, 2022). In this scenario, the complete treatment of the EZ, which overlaps the lesion, is associated with a high degree of success. In general, extra-operative invasive monitoring is not required and intraoperative monitoring, as ECoG, may be applied as an adjuvant method to guide the resection. Nevertheless, when the non-invasive data is insufficient to define the EZ, extra-operative invasive monitoring may be indicated (**Figure 1**).

Regarding the different methods of extra-operative invasive monitoring, indications of subdural grid (SDG) recording and SEEG most often do not overlap. The two- versus tri-dimensional brain sampling dictates a quite different strategy for phase I goals as well as for data analysis. The "pre-surgical" attribute bears distinct meaning for SDG, which in most cases immediately leads to surgical resection to take advantage of the craniotomy, whereas SEEG evaluation leaves a period between removal of the electrodes and operation, so that an eventual contra-indication for surgery can still be decided.

The subdural grid method

A general principle is that the SDG method must be performed when an epileptogenic structural lesion has not been adequately identified with noninvasive testing. This situation may occur if:

- the data is discordant, raising the possibility that seizures emanate from more than one area
- or the data are insufficiently localizing to confidently define the location of the EZ.

A theorical example of discordant data would be the circumstance in which seizure semiology suggested a left frontal seizure onset, but the interictal spikes emanated from the left frontal and anterior temporal regions, and MRI was negative. Another indication of

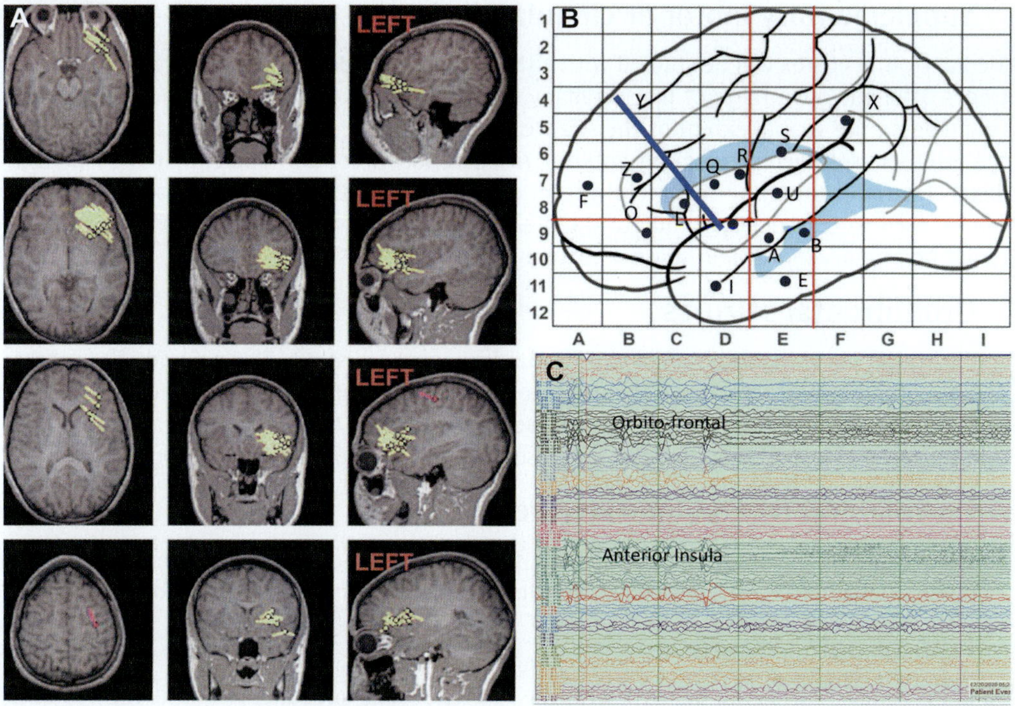

Figure 1

Pre-surgical evaluation in "FCD scenario"

A. MEG scan in patient with non-lesional medically refractory focal epilepsy showing the presence of MEG dipoles in cluster, located in the left anterior perisylvian/insula areas. B SEEG exploration from the same patient, demonstrating an anterior perysilvian SEEG exploration with orthogonal (dots) and oblique electrodes (line) targeting the pre-implantation hypothesis, which includes the frontal/temporal/insula and parietal areas. C. Interictal and ictal SEEG recordings demonstrating the presence of epileptiform interictal activity in the orbito-frontal and anterior insula areas, transitioning to ictal patterns, with low amplitude and high frequencies recordings located in similar cortical areas. The transition between the interictal and ictal recordings was characterized by the emerging of the ictal semiology (autonomic symptoms of tachycardia and nausea).

SDG is when the epileptogenic region has been localized, but surgery poses risk of causing a neurological deficit because the FCD lesion overlaps with functional cortex. As an example, let us consider a patient whose seizures begin with tonic posturing of the right hand with scalp EEG showing left frontal interictal spikes, left frontal seizure onset, and left rolandic hyperperfusion on SPECT or SISCOM). The EZ is undoubtedly located in the left frontal lobe, but proximity with the primary motor cortex poses a risk of motor deficit. One could proceed directly to surgery, map the primary motor cortex and excise cortex immediately anterior to motor cortex, using ECoG to additionally localize interictal discharges that might help to define the resection boundaries. Alternatively, one could proceed with extra-operative mapping of the irritative and ictal onset zones and mapping of functional cortex using SDG.

Proper planning needs a careful and detailed history and neurological examination, followed by scalp interictal and ictal EEG, MRI scan, PET, neuropsychological testing, and various other tests such as fMRI or DTI, SPECT, and MEG. If a lesion consistent with possible FCD is visible on pre-implantation MRI, the placement of the SDG must take into account the anatomical localization of the lesion and the surrounding cortex that may harbor microscopic FCD, not apparent on imaging. Each anatomical region has specific technical nuances related to the implantation of SDG electrodes in the "FCD scenario".

Frontal lobe epilepsies

The frontal lobes contain several discrete cortical areas which produce a variety of distinct types of seizures with different semiology. When the hypothesis of implantation is directed to particular areas, a suitable strategy for placing intracranial electrodes can be suggested. One should always avoid focusing electrode placements in a too restricted area, since the clinical hypothesis might be incorrect. Sampling from adjacent areas or lobes often improves confidence in localization and helps prevents surprises.

Supplementary motor or cingulate seizures

Medial frontal cortex can be studied with either subdural or depth electrodes. Subdural electrodes offer the advantage of placing many contacts in one or both hemispheres and allow for mapping the spatial extent of the seizure onset. Electrode strips or grids can be placed in the interhemispheric cortex in an anterior to posterior direction, supplemented by parasagittal electrodes to define the lateral extent of resection. In this region, the same electrodes can be used to electrically stimulate the brain and record somatosensory evoked potentials to define primary motor and sensory cortex.

Orbitofrontal seizures

Orbitofrontal cortex can be sampled with subdural grids or strips. Placing grids has greater potential for morbidity because of the need to mobilize the frontal lobe. Defining the anterior-posterior extent of an orbitofrontal epileptogenic zone can be challenging. The anterior perforated space is a natural boundary for any resection and investigation in this region.

Dorsolateral frontal lobe seizures

Subdural grids are ideally suited for sampling from large areas of dorsolateral frontal lobe, and mapping of eloquent cortex with electrical stimulation and somatosensory evoked potentials.

Frontal pole seizures

Subdural strips or grids can be used, with the former usually adequate to define the posterior margins of any resection.

• Parietal lobe epilepsies

Smaller than the frontal lobes, both medial and dorsolateral parietal cortex can be studied with subdural electrodes. Parietal lobe regions are often included in the sampled cortex when the frontal lobes are studied with intracranial EEG. In mesial and dorsolateral parietal seizures, the technique to place subdural electrodes is identical to that employed for medial and dorsolateral frontal seizures.

• Occipital lobe epilepsies

The occipital lobes have anatomic connections with both parietal and temporal lobes due to ontogeny, with superior occipital regions projecting preferentially to the parietal lobe, while the inferior portions (below the calcarine sulcus) project to the temporal lobe. Hence, areas in these lobes should usually be evaluated when occipital seizures are studied.

Lateral occipital lobe seizures

The technique is the same as for lateral cortical foci in frontal and parietal lobes. Subdural grids or strips may be used.

Medial and basal occipital lobe seizures

Interhemispheric and basal strips or grids can be used. Seizure onsets can be more easily mapped with grids, but surgeons infrequently excise striate cortex for epilepsy, so the intracranial EEG technique should not be overly aggressive if resection will not be done in that area.

• Temporal lobe epilepsies

Mesial temporal lobe seizures

Subdural electrodes can be used to record from the parahippocampal gyrus, but amygdala and hippocampus are internal structures, less accessible to the subdural grid method. Hence, depth electrodes are better suited for intracranial EEG recording from mesial temporal structures in most circumstances and a combination of SDG and semi-stereotactic placement of depth electrodes is applied.

Basal temporal lobe and temporal pole neocortical seizures

Subdural electrode strips are ideally suited to record from these regions. While one could use a subdural grid, this is usually not necessary.

Posterior temporal lobe neocortical seizures

Subdural grid electrodes are well suited to map the seizure onset zone and define areas critical for language (Wernicke's area). Arrays of subdural strips can also be used, but intra-operative language mapping more often requires larger grids due to gaps in sampling from cortex with strip electrodes. Specifically for focal cortical dysplasia, the main advantage of the subdural grid method is in the clinical scenario associated with Taylor type dysplasia in close proximity with highly eloquent cortex.

SBG-guided resection strategy

The subdural grid resection strategy is intimately related to the interpretation of the interictal and ictal recordings and the close proximity with functional cortical and subcortical areas. Specifically in the subdural grid method, the analysis of the interictal patterns is highly considered (Wyllie *et al.*, 1988). As a working hypothesis, it is assumed that brain tissue will only produce interictal epileptiform spikes (primary or secondary) where its excitability is significantly increased. Nevertheless, it is important to understand that the extend of interictal activity commonly larger than the epileptogenic zone and it should not be the only criteria to define the extend of resection. Spike frequency and certain interictal and ictal spiking patterns have been correlated with pathological findings related to specific subtypes of cortical dysplasia. Palmini *et al.* (1995) reported striking differences in EcoG patterns recording from FCD. The authors founded that "repetitive electrographic seizures" and continuous or quasi-continuous rhythmic spiking occurred in frequent association with the EZ and in consequence, the resection of these patterns is associated with optimal seizure control outcome. Resection of repetitive spiking, commonly associated with FCD II is the exception for interictal-based resection strategy.

Regarding the ictal activity, identification of the area(s) of earliest change in background activity and correlation with clinical manifestations are major aspects in defining the plan of resection. The plan of resection will combine information regarding the ictal, interictal, and functional data to better define the safe borders of resection. The plan of resection should also consider the distribution of cytoarchitectonic areas and the vascular structures in close association with the targeted cortical areas. The presence of high frequency oscillations at seizure onset is considered a measure of proximity of the recording electrodes to the EZ and should be considered for resection if there is a positive correlation with the patient's semiology.

The SEEG method

The SEEG is a modality of extra-operative invasive method that can be utilized in patients with focal MRE associated with FCD pathology, to anatomically define the EZ and its relation to adjacent eloquent cortex. The SEEG method and SEEG-guided resections and associated techniques have gained increased popularity and utilization in recent years, mainly due to the possibility of defining the three-dimensional aspects of seizure organization with a less invasive procedure. The author has the opinion that SEEG is the method of choice to study patients with non-lesional focal epilepsies and lesional epilepsies associated with FCD. The rationale for favoring SEEG method in detriment to other methods of extra-operative invasive investigation are explained in the following paragraphs.

The method was originally developed by Jean Talairach and Jean Bancaud during the 1950's (Bancaud & Dell, 1959) and has been mostly applied in Europe, initially France then in Italy, as the method of choice for invasive monitoring in MRE (Avanzini, 1994; Bancaud *et al.*, 1970; Bancaud, Favel, *et al.*, 1970; Bancaud & Talairach, 1973; Bancaud *et al.*, 1976; Bancaud, *et al.*, 1968, 1969; F. Bartolomei *et al.*, 2001; Battaglia *et al.*, 2006; Baucaud *et al.*, 1991; Biraben *et al.*, 2001; Cabrini, *et al.*, 1975; Cossu *et al.*, 2006; Cossu *et al.*, 2008; Engel *et al.*, 1990; Geier, Bancaud, Talairach, & Enjelvin, 1973; Guenot & Isnard, 2008a, 2008b; Musolino *et al.*,1990; Sindou *et al.*, 2006; Talairach *et al.*, 1992; Tassi *et al.*, 2005; Wendling & Chauvel, 2001a, 2001b).

In France, after the development of the stereotactic techniques, including frames and associated devices, initially applied for surgery of abnormal movement disorders, Jean Talairach devoted most of his activity to the field of epilepsy surgery, along with the neurologist Jean Bancaud, who joined him in 1952 at Sainte-Anne Hospital in Paris. This new methodology led them to depart from the surgical approaches limited to the superficial cortex and guided by interictal recordings. With SEEG it was possible to record the intracortical epileptiform activity and the seizure patterns, with their 3D characteristics of primary organization: regions of ictal onset, early and late propagation patterns. Their innovative thinking was to implement a working methodology for a comprehensive analysis of the morphological and functional cerebral space. The stereotactic atlas, authored by Tailarach and first published in 1967, perfectly illustrates the new anatomical concepts for stereotaxis (Talairach & Tournoux *et al.*, 1988).

The debut of SEEG was in 1957, when the first implantation of intracerebral electrodes for epilepsy was performed on May 3rd in Sainte-Anne Hospital. By departing from the current methods of invasive monitoring at the time, such implantations have allowed us to explore the activity of different brain structures and to record patients' spontaneous seizures.

Currently, the principle of SEEG methodology remains similar to those originally described by Bancaud and Talairach, which is based on anatomo-electroclinical correlations (AEC) with the main aim to conceptualize the 3-dimensional spatial-temporal organization of the epileptic discharges within the brain (Bancaud, Angelergues, *et al.*, 1970; Bancaud, Favel, *et al.*, 1970; Bancaud & Talairach, 1973; Bartolomei *et al.*, 2001; Battaglia *et al.*, 2006; Biraben *et al.*, 2001; Cossu *et al.*, 2006; Cossu *et al.*, 2008; Devaux *et al.*, 2008; Gonzalez-Martinez *et al.*, 2013; Guenot & Isnard, 2008a, 2008b; Isnard *et al.*, 2018; Sindou *et al.*, 2006; Tassi *et al.*, 2005; Wendling *et al.*, 2001a, 2001b). In the FCD scenario the implantation strategy is individualized, with electrode placement based on pre-implantation hypotheses that takes into consideration patient's seizures electroclinical correlations and their relationship with a suspected lesion. For these reasons, the pre-implantation AEC hypotheses formulation is the single most important element in the process of planning the placement of SEEG electrodes. If the pre-implantation hypotheses are incorrect, the placement of the depth electrodes will be inadequate and the interpretation of the SEEG recordings will not provide an accurate anatomical definition of the EZ.

The SEEG method is particularly suitable for the diagnosis and treatment of FCD since 1) the highest epileptogenicity is in general located in the deep part the cortex, as in depth of sulcus dysplasia, and 2) electroclinical correlations always point to a specific brain location. For these reasons, Talairach and Bancaud were available to identify FCD before the era of imaging, as described in the first SEEG paper for FCD and to cure 2/3 of the patients (Chassoux *et al.*, 2000).

The planning of the SEEG implantation is the beginning of the resection strategy as it requires a clear formulation of precise AEC hypotheses to be tested and the possible surgical treatment strategies that the investigation will provide. These hypotheses are typically generated during a multidisciplinary patient management conference based on the results of various non-invasive tests. A final tailored implantation strategy is generated during a separate pre-surgical implantation meeting. Intracerebral depth electrodes sample the dysplastic lesion (if identified), the more likely structure(s) of ictal onset, the early and late spread regions and the interactions with the functional (cognitive, sensori-motor, behavioral etc.) networks, based on a clear and well-articulated hypothesis of implantation. A three dimensional "conceptualization" of the network nodes upstream and downstream from the hypothesized epileptogenic network is an essential component of the pre-surgical implantation strategy. Initially, by analyzing the available non-invasive data and the temporal evolution of the ictal clinical manifestations, a hypothesis of the anatomical location of the EZ is formulated (Chauvel & McGonigal, 2014). The location of the hypothetical EZ may be congruent, partially congruent, or incongruent with the location of the potential dysplastic lesion. Adequate knowledge of the possible functional networks involved in the primary organization of the epileptic activity is mandatory in order to formulate sound hypotheses. It is also important to take into account the three-dimensional aspects of depth electrode recordings, which despite a limited coverage (largely compensated by the interpolation process made possible by the electrophysiological methodology: frequencies, spatial relations and latencies analyses), enable an accurate sampling of the structures along its trajectory, from the entry site to the final impact point. Therefore, the trajectory is as important as the target or entry point areas. Consequently, the investigation may include lateral and mesial surfaces of different lobes, as well as deep-seated cortices such as the depths of sulci, the insula, posterior orbitofrontal cortex, and areas in the inter-hemispheric cortical surface. The implantation should also consider the different cortical cytoarchitectonic areas involved in seizure organization patterns and their likely connectivity to other cortical and subcortical areas. It is important to emphasize that the implantation strategy aims to explore epileptogenic networks, which, in general, involve multiple lobes. Furthermore, exploration strategies should also take into consideration possible alternative hypotheses of localization (Cardinale *et al.*, 2013; Cardinale & Lo Russo, 2013; Gonzalez-Martinez *et al.*, 2014).

Lastly, the aim to obtain all the possible information from the SEEG exploration should not be pursued with an excessive number of electrodes that could increase the morbidity of the implantation. In general, implantations that exceed 15 depth electrodes are rare and likely not necessary. In addition, the possible involvement of eloquent regions in the ictal discharge requires their judicious coverage, with the two-fold goal to assess their role in the seizure organization and to define the boundaries for a safe surgical resection.

In addition to the meticulous analysis of seizure semiology and non-invasive data, the basic principles of adequate SEEG implantations and guided resection are based on:

- generic anatomo-functional cortical and subcortical organization,
- the 3D recognition of fine sulco-gyral anatomy using sub-segmentation in sulcal roots,
- the critical role played by the limbic structures.

Specifically, the basic knowledge about anatomical circuitry should be taken into account in the SEEG planning. Some practical examples are highlighted below:

When a dysplastic lesion located in the **temporal pole** is suspected, our group tends to systematically place electrodes in the posterior paralimbic part of the orbital frontal cortex (Brodman Area [BA] 13) and orthogonal lateral electrodes in the anterior insular, limen insulae and sub-callosal cingulate areas, which are all paralimbic cortices highly connected to the pole of the temporal lobe. In addition, to better define the involvement (or not) of the adjacent amygdaloid complex and hippocampus formation, depth electrodes are also placed in these respective regions, in an orthogonal fashion. Variations of these implantation plans depend primarily on seizure semiology and secondarily on the results of other pre-implantation methods of localization.

When the hypothesis of implantation (in addition to the dysplastic neocortex) involves the **mesial temporal lobe structures,** in addition to an electrode in the amygdaloid complex, the head, the body and the tail of the hippocampus, electrodes are systematically implanted in the peri-rhinal and entorhinal cortex through the collateral fissure because of the known role of these structures in subtypes of mesial temporal lobe epilepsy (MTLE) (Bartolomei *et al.*, 2005; Bartolomei *et al.*, 1999) with projections to the frontal cortex. It is important to take into consideration that the amygdaloid complex has dense connectivity to the anterior perisylvian areas, as well as the rostral portions of the superior temporal gyrus (Planum Polare) and frontal opercular areas. Consequently, these cortical areas should be explored in patient whose semiology indicates amygdala and peri-amygdala onset.

When involvement of the supplementary motor area and Frontal Eye Field (BA 6-8) is suspected, our group systematically implants electrodes in the posterior parietal operculum (BA 40) and the anterior border of the superior parietal lobule and rostral positions of the intraparietal sulcus (BA 7A). These three structures are known to be densely connected and, on several occasions, rapid propagation of the ictal discharge between these three distant structures has been observed.

SEEG-guided resection strategy

In the FCD scenario, the SEEG method is in general reserved for the non-lesional setting. Here, the resection strategy in the SEEG method significantly differs from the strategy defined by the SBG method. In addition to the location of the EZ, the surgical strategy requires planning the anatomic limits of the resection. As the EZ in a given patient is defined by the involved electrode lead space, if two leads in the same gyrus are involved, the entire gyrus will be, by extension, considered epileptogenic. The space between involved electrodes, as well as the distance between involved and non-involved electrodes, constitute the basis for defining the resection boundaries. In addition, the functional consequences of the corticectomy represent the ultimate safeguard and must take into consideration. The strategy is to extend the resection up to the vicinity of the functional area or the limits of a specific cytoarchitectonic area. If adjacent function and vascular anatomy allows, the resection should be extended until the topographic location of the least involved electrode, assuring the complete resection of the EZ. The identification of a MRI lesion suggestive of FCD II influences the final resection strategy and, in fact, it is statistically associated with a higher probability of seizure freedom. In this scenario, invasive monitoring can be avoided, and direct resection, guided or not by intra-operative EcoG can be contemplated, mainly when a clear anatomo-electroclinical correlation is identified in the pre-operative non-invasive data set (Chassoux *et al.*, 2022).

The anatomical electroclinical correlation hypothesis may not be congruent with the anatomical location of the identified lesion and a more careful discussion to define the surgical strategy is essential. If the imaging characteristics are typical for FCD II and congruent PET abnormalities are observed, direct surgical resection of the anatomically defined lesion is advocated. In this scenario, the utilization of the SEEG methodology may provide a distorted demarcation of the EZ, if electrodes are inadequately placed or the hypothesis of localization is wrongly formulated. Nevertheless, if image characteristics are not convincing of FCD II and not associated with PET abnormalities, SEEG is indicated. In this scenario, the careful evaluation of the imaging characteristics, and the identification of clear FCD features, are essential to define the surgical strategy: Direct resection versus SEEG evaluation.

In the non-lesional scenario or in lesional cases where MRI characteristics are unclear for FCD II, the SEEG methodology and associated resections are strongly related to the concept of epileptogenic network, as opposed to the concept of focus (SBG method) and an MRI lesion is not enough to define the EZ. First, the EZ may be not strictly organized around the location of the lesion. Second, even if the EZ were organized around the lesion, this information is not enough to determine the limits of the EZ. Third, the demonstration of the organization of seizures around the lesion is not incompatible with the involvement of remote cortical structures in the EZ. Nevertheless, the EZ is more likely to be related to the topology of the lesion in the case of a FCD II, and SEEG is in general not indicated.

Early postictal findings should be taken into account when defining the surgical strategy for FCD investigated through the SEEG method. Particular attention is paid to those cortical areas demonstrating, at the termination of seizures, major electrical attenuation and/or suppression of the background activity. Recovery time is another important feature that needs to be considered when defining the extend of the EZ. Post ictal spikes have less localizing significance, but early reappearance rhythmic spikes is highly correlated with high epileptogenicity. The results of electrical stimulation during SEEG evaluation in FCD scenario are fundamental to define the plan of resection. By definition, any component of the EZ is able to synchronize the whole epileptogenic network. It works as a validation of a method that, by nature must tolerate the fact that brain sampling is highly incomplete and bias. Moreover, when seizure onset is made of quasi-simultaneous "fast" activities in a large cortical area, likely more extensively than the EZ, electrical stimulation will discriminate which areas are associated with the EZ and which are not. To distinguish what is the (primary)

EZ from those areas "activated" only from a spread pattern, direct electrical stimulation will demonstrate how these different components are linked and how each of them contributes to early and late clinical semiology and, consequently, what areas showed be surgically treated (former) or not disturbed (later).

SEEG guided resections in the FCD scenario

The author reported 200 patients undergoing 2,663 SEEG electrode implantations for the purposes of invasive intracranial EEG monitoring, in accordance with a tailored pre-implantation hypothesis to investigate, localize and anatomically characterize the extent of the EZ (Serletis *et al.*, 2014). The most common pathological diagnosis in this group was FCD I (61.1%). The studied group was challenging due to the paucity of non-invasive data and/or the possibility of a more diffuse pathology suggested by a previous failed invasive monitoring exploration: nearly one-third of the studied patients (29.0%) had undergone prior surgical intervention for medically refractory epilepsy, resulting in post-op recurrent seizures. Despite this challenging and discouraging clinical scenario, the SEEG method was able to confirm the EZ in 154 patients (77.0%). Of these, 134 patients (87.0%) underwent subsequent craniotomy for SEEG guided resection. Within this cohort, 90 patients had a minimum post-operative follow-up of at least 12 months; therein, 61 patients (67.8%) remained seizure-free (i.e. Engel I outcome). Complications were minimal, with the total morbidity rate of 2.5% (**Figure 2**).

Results in terms of seizure outcome and complications are compatible with results from other groups. Munari and collaborators (Munari *et al.*, 1994) reported on their experience with SEEG in 70 patients undergoing a collective total of 712 electrode implantations. A tailored surgical resection was performed in 60 patients (85.7%). Moreover, the authors reported an asymptomatic intracerebral hematoma following the removal of one SEEG electrode (accounting for a morbidity rate of 1.4%, or 0.1% per electrode). More recently, Guenot and collaborators (Guenot *et al.*, 2001) presented a series of 100 patients collectively undergoing 1,118 SEEG electrode implantations for invasive EEG monitoring. SEEG was deemed helpful in 84 patients (84%) by either disproving or confirming (and additionally, in the latter case, guiding) the feasibility of surgical resection of the EZ. Moreover, SEEG indicated the possibility of resection in 14 cases (14%) that could not be resolved based on non-invasive work-up. These authors reported 5 complications (5% of cases), including 2 infections at the electrode site (0.2% per electrode), 2 fractures of the electrode (0.2% per electrode) and 1 intracerebral hematoma resulting in death (accounting for a mortality rate of 1% in the study). In a large series, Cossu and collaborators al. reported a morbidity rate of 5.6%, with severe permanent deficits from intracerebral hemorrhage in 1% (Cossu *et al.*, 2005). In another study, Tanriverdi and collaborators/ (2009) summarized their experience with a subgroup of 491 patients with refractory epilepsy collectively undergoing 2,943 depth electrode implantations (Tanriverdi *et al.*, 2009). They identified 4 patients (0.8%) with an intracranial hematoma at the electrode site (0.07% per electrode) and 9 patients (1.8%) with an infection arising from electrode placement (0.2% per electrode), but no mortality. Finally, Cardinale and Lo Russo presented their experience with 6,496 electrodes stereotactically implanted in 482 epilepsy patients with refractory epilepsy (Cardinale & Lo Russo, 2013). They identified 2 patients (0.4%, or 0.03% per electrode) with permanent neurological deficits; 14 patients (2.9%, or 0.2% per electrode) with hemorrhagic complications; 2 patients (0.4%, or 0.03% per electrode) with infection; and one mortality (0.2%) resulting from massive brain edema and concomitant hyponatremia. More recently, Cardinale *et al.* reported a retrospective series of 742 SEEG procedures. Resective surgery was indicated for 570 patients (79.9%). Two-hundred and seventy-nine of 470 patients operated on (59.4%) were free of disabling seizures at least 2 years after resective surgery. Negative magnetic resonance and post-surgical lesion remnant were significant risk factors for seizure recurrence, while FCD II, balloon cells, were significantly associated with seizure freedom (Cardinale *et al.*, 2019).

In a recent metanalysis review, Willard at al. (2022) identified 3,745 references reporting results associated FCD surgery. Many of these references were related to the utilization of extra-operative invasive monitoring for the localization and anatomical demarcation of the

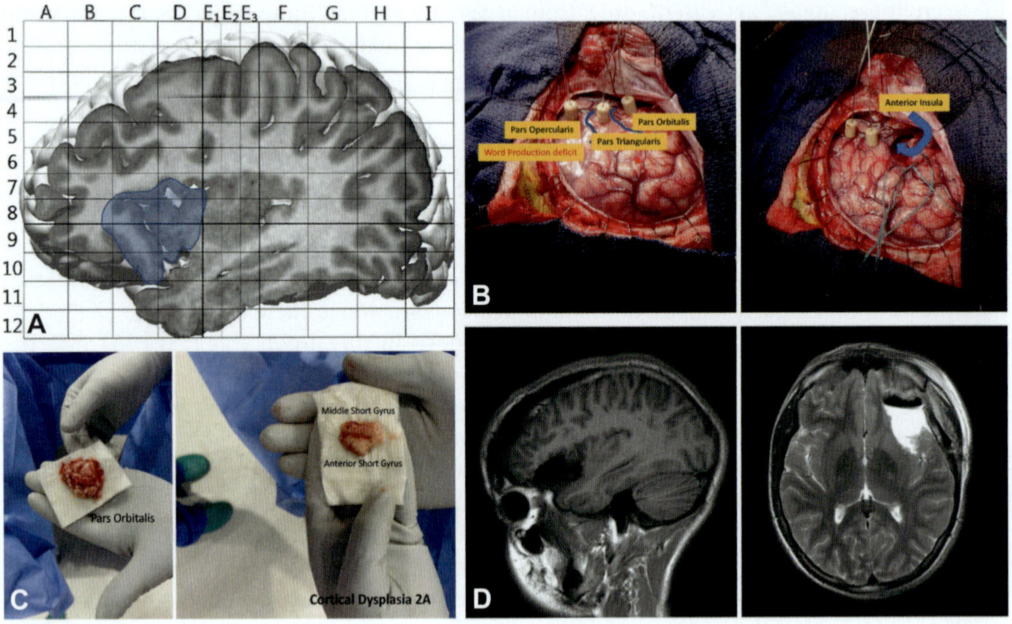

Figure 2

Surgical strategy in non-lesional medically intractable focal epilepsy in FCD scenario (patient illustrated in **figure 1**).

A. Demarcation of the resection areas in stereotaxic space. The blue shallow illustrates the anterior insula and posterior orbito-frontal areas as defined by the SEEG exploration. B. Intraoperative pictures demonstrating the anatomical exposure of the frontal opercular area during adjuvant ECoG recordings with depth electrodes. The functional mapping performed during the SEEG evaluation demonstrated the presence of word production deficits in par-opercularis. Initially, the par-orbitalis was resected, exposing the anterior face of the insula, which was resected through the open surgical corridor created by the frontal resection. C demonstrates the resected portions of the pars-orbitalis (left) and anterior insula (right). Surgical pathology from the respective specimens reviewed FCD IIA in the anterior insula specimen and no pathological findings in orbito-frontal segment. D demonstrate the post-operative MRI (sagittal T1 and axial T2), showing the resection cavities in the anterior insula and posterior orbito-frontal areas. Patient had an optimal outcome (Engel Ia) with no neurological deficit.

epileptogenic zone. Of these, 35 studies (total of 1,353 patients) were included. Most studies (89%) followed up patients for ≥24 months after surgery. The overall postsurgical favorable outcome rate was 70% (95% confidence interval [CI] 64-75). There was high interstudy heterogeneity. Favorable outcome was associated with complete resection of the FCD lesion (risk ratio [RR] 2.42 [95% confidence interval (CI) 1.55-3.76], $p < 0.001$) and location of the FCD lesion in the temporal lobe (RR 1.38 [95% CI 1.07-1.79], $p = 0.013$) but not lesion extent, intracranial EEG use, or FCD histologic type (Willard *et al.*, 2022).

Conclusion

The topographic and functional relationships between MRI-revealed FCD and the EZ are far from clear and unequivocal: neither all FCD nor all components of a FCD are necessarily epileptogenic. The exception is the Taylor type FCD (FCD II), where the EZ is located within the limits of the identified MRI lesion and an invasive monitoring phase may not be required. For other types of FCD, mainly in the non-lesional clinical scenario, where mild forms of FCD are suspected, extra-operative invasive monitoring is suggested to define the locations and the anatomical limits of the EZ. Among the different methods of invasive monitoring in non-lesional cases, the SEEG method provides an adequate understanding of the epileptic networks by providing a 3D view of the epileptic cortical areas based on anatomo-clinical correlations. This concept is at the center of the decision-making process regarding surgical strategies for FCD. The main clinical and surgical challenge for the near future remains in the further refinement of specific selection criteria for the need of invasive monitoring and different methods of invasive monitoring, with the ultimate goal of comparing and validating the results (long-term seizure free outcome) obtained from different surgical methods applied in the FCD scenario.

References

Adelson, P. D, O'Rourke, D. K, Albright, A. L. Chronic invasive monitoring for identifying seizure foci in children. *Neurosurg Clin N Am* 1995; 6: 491-504.

Avanzini, G. Discussion of stereoelectroencephalography. *Acta Neurol Scand Suppl* 1994; 152: 70-3.

Bancaud, J, Angelergues, R, Bernouilli, C, *et al.* Functional stereotaxic exploration (SEEG) of epilepsy. *Electroencephalogr Clin Neurophysiol* 1970; 28: 85-6.

Bancaud, J, Dell, M. B. Technics and method of stereotaxic functional exploration of the brain structures in man (cortex, subcortex, central gray nuclei). *Rev Neurol* 1959; 101, 213-27.

Bancaud, J, Favel, P, Bonis, A, *et al.* Paroxysmal sexual manifestations and temporal lobe epilepsy. clinical, EEG and SEEG study of a case of epilepsy of tumoral origin. *Rev Neurol (Paris)* 1970; 123: 217-30.

Bancaud, J, Talairach, J. Methodology of stereo eeg exploration and surgical intervention in epilepsy. *Rev Otoneuroophtalmol* 1973; 45: 315-28.

Bancaud, J, Talairach, J, Geier, S, *et al.* Behavioral manifestations induced by electric stimulation of the anterior cingulate gyrus in man. *Rev Neurol (Paris)* 1976; 132(10), 705-24.

Bancaud, J, Talairach, J, Waltregny, P, Bresson, M, Morel, P. Stimulation of focal cortical epilepsies by megimide in topographic diagnosis (clinical EEG and SEEG study). *Rev Neurol (Paris)* 1968; 119: 320-5.

Bancaud, J, Talairach, J, Waltregny, P, Bresson, M, Morel, P. Activation by megimide in the topographic diagnosis of focal cortical epilepsies (clinical EEG and SEEG study). *Electroencephalogr Clin Neurophysiol* 1969; 26: 640.

Bartolomei, F, Khalil, M, Wendling, F, *et al.* Entorhinal cortex involvement in human mesial temporal lobe epilepsy: an electrophysiologic and volumetric study. *Epilepsia* 2005; 46: 677-87.

Bartolomei, F, Wendling, F, Bellanger, J. J, Regis, J, Chauvel, P. Neural networks involving the medial temporal structures in temporal lobe epilepsy. *Clin Neurophysiol* 2001; 112: 1746-60.

Bartolomei, F, Wendling, F, Vignal, J, *et al.* Temporal lobe epilepsies: identification of subtypes using coherence analysis in stereoelectroencephalography. *Clin Neurophysiol* 1999; 110, 1741-54.

Battaglia, G, Chiapparini, L, Franceschetti, S, *et al.* Periventricular nodular heterotopia: classification, epileptic history, and genesis of epileptic discharges. *Epilepsia* 2006; 47: 86-97.

Baucaud, J, Talairach, J, Munari, C, Giallonardo, T, Brunet, P. Introduction to the clinical study of postrolandic epileptic seizures. *Can J Neurol Sci* 1991; 18(4 Suppl), 566-9.

Biraben, A, Taussig, D, Thomas, P, *et al.* Fear as the main feature of epileptic seizures. *J Neurol Neurosurg Psychiatry* 2001; 70: 186-191.

Cabrini, G. P, Ettorre, G, Marossero, F, *et al.* Surgery of epilepsy: some indications for SEEG. *J Neurosurg Sci* 1975; 19(1-2), 95-104.

Cardinale, F, Cossu, M, Castana, L, *et al.* Stereoelectroencephalography: Surgical methodology, safety, and stereotactic application accuracy in 500 procedures. *Neurosurgery* 2013; 72: 353-366; Discussion 366.

Cardinale, F, Lo Russo, G. Stereo-electroencephalography safety and effectiveness: some more reasons in favor of epilepsy surgery. *Epilepsia* 2013; 54: 1505-6.

Cardinale, F, Rizzi, M, Vignati, E, *et al.* Stereoelectroencephalography: retrospective analysis of 742 procedures in a single centre. *Brain* 2019; 142: 2688-704.

Chassoux, F, Devaux, B, Landre, E, *et al.* Stereoelectroencephalography in focal cortical dysplasia: a 3d approach to delineating the dysplastic cortex. *Brain* 2000; 123 *(Pt 8)*, 1733-51.

Chassoux, F, Mellerio, C, Laurent, A, *et al.* Benefits and risks of epilepsy surgery in patients with focal cortical dysplasia type 2 in the central region. *Neurology* 2022.

Chauvel, P, Mcgonigal, A. Emergence of semiology in epileptic seizures. *Epilepsy Behav* 2014; 38, 94-103.

Cossu, M, Cardinale, F, Castana, L, *et al.* Stereo-EEG In Children. *Childs Nerv Syst* 2006; 22: 766-78.

Cossu, M, Cardinale, F, Colombo, N, *et al.* Stereoelectroencephalography in the presurgical evaluation of children with drug-resistant focal epilepsy. *J Neurosurg* 2005; 103(4 Suppl), 333-43.

Cossu, M, Chabardes, S, Hoffmann, D, Lo Russo, G. Presurgical evaluation of intractable epilepsy using stereo-electro-encephalography methodology: principles, technique and morbidity. *Neurochirurgie* 2008; 54: 367-73.

Devaux, B, Chassoux, F, Guenot, M, *et al.* Epilepsy Surgery In France. *Neurochirurgie* 2008; 54: 453-65.

Engel, J, Jr, Henry, T. R, Risinger, M. W, *et al.* Presurgical evaluation for partial epilepsy: relative contributions of chronic depth-electrode recordings versus FDG-PET and scalp-sphenoidal ictal EEG. *Neurology* 1990; 40(11), 1670-7.

Geier, S, Bancaud, J, Talairach, J, Enjelvin, M. Radio-Telemetry In EEG And SEEG. Technology And Material. *Rev Electroencephalogr Neurophysiol Clin* 1973; 3: 353-4.

Gonzalez-Martinez, J, Bulacio, J, Alexopoulos, A, Jehi, L, Bingaman, W, Najm, I. Stereoelectroencephalography in the "difficult to localize" refractory focal epilepsy: early experience from a North American Epilepsy Center. *Epilepsia* 2013; 54: 323-30.

Gonzalez-Martinez, J, Mullin, J, Vadera, S, *et al.* Stereotactic placement of depth electrodes in medically intractable epilepsy. *J Neurosurg* 2014; 120: 639-44.

Guenot, M, Isnard, J. Epilepsy and insula. *Neurochirurgie* 2008a; 54: 374-381.

Guenot, M, Isnard, J. Multiple SEEG-Guided Rf-Thermolesions Of Epileptogenic Foci. *Neurochirurgie* 2008b; 54: 441-7.

Guenot, M, Isnard, J, Ryvlin, P, *et al.* Neurophysiological monitoring for epilepsy surgery: the talairach seeg method. stereoelectroencephalography. indications, results, complications and therapeutic applications in a series of 100 consecutive cases. *Stereotact Funct Neurosurg* 2001; 77(1-4), 29-32.

Isnard, J, Taussig, D, Bartolomei, F, *et al.* French Guidelines On Stereoelectroencephalography (SEEG). *Neurophysiol Clin* 2018; 48: 5-13.

Jayakar, P. Invasive EEG monitoring in children: when, where, and what? *J Clin Neurophysiol* 1999; 16: 408-18.

Jayakar, P, Duchowny, M, Resnick, T. J. Subdural monitoring in the evaluation of children for epilepsy surgery. *J Child Neurol* 1994; 9 *Suppl* 2, 61-6.

Munari, C, Hoffmann, D, Francione, S, *et al.* Stereo-Electroencephalography methodology: advantages and limits. *Acta Neurol Scand Suppl* 1994; 152, 56-67, Discussion 68-59.

Musolino, A, Tournoux, P, Missir, O, Talairach, J. Methodology of "in vivo" anatomical study and stereo-electroencephalographic exploration in brain surgery for epilepsy. *J Neuroradiol* 1990; 17: 67-102.

Rosenow, F, Luders, H. Presurgical evaluation of epilepsy. *Brain* 2001; 124 (Pt 9), 1683-700.

Serletis, D, Bulacio, J, Bingaman, W, Najm, I, Gonzalez-Martinez, J. The stereotactic approach for mapping epileptic networks: a prospective study of 200 patients. *J Neurosurg* 2014; 121: 1239-46.

Sindou, M, Guenot, M, Isnard, J, Ryvlin, P, Fischer, C, Mauguiere, F. Temporomesial epilepsy surgery: outcome and complications in 100 consecutive adult patients. *Acta Neurochir (Wien)* 2006; 148: 39-45.

Talairach, J, Bancaud, J, Bonis, A, *et al.* Surgical therapy for frontal epilepsies. *Adv Neurol* 1992; 57, 707-32.

Talairach, J, Tournoux P. Co-planar stereotaxic atlas of the human brain: 3-dimensional proportional system: an approach to cerebral imaging. Stuttgard New York: Georg Thieme Verlag, 1988.

Tanriverdi, T, Ajlan, A, Poulin, N, Olivier, A. Morbidity in epilepsy surgery: an experience based on 2449 epilepsy surgery procedures from a single institution. *J Neurosurg* 2009; 110: 1111-23.

Tassi, L, Colombo, N, Cossu, M, *et al.* Electroclinical, MRI and neuropathological study of 10 patients with nodular heterotopia, with surgical outcomes. *Brain* 2005; 128 (Pt 2), 321-37.

Wendling, F, Bartolomei, F, Bellanger, J. J, Chauvel, P. Identification of epileptogenic networks from modeling and nonlinear analysis of SEEG signals. *Neurophysiol Clin* 2001a; 31: 139-51.

Wendling, F, Bartolomei, F, Bellanger, J. J, Chauvel, P. Interpretation of interdependencies in epileptic signals using a macroscopic physiological model of the EEG. *Clin Neurophysiol* 2001b; 112: 1201-18.

Willard, A, Antonic-Baker, A, Chen, Z, *et al.* Seizure outcome after surgery for mri-diagnosed focal cortical dysplasia: a systematic review and meta-analysis. *Neurology* 2022; 98: E236-48.

Winkler, P. A, Herzog, C, Henkel, A, *et al.* Noninvasive protocol for surgical treatment of focal epilepsies. *Nervenarzt* 1999; 70(12), 1088-93.

Wyllie, E, Luders, H, Morris, H. H, 3rd, *et al.* Subdural electrodes in the evaluation for epilepsy surgery in children and adults. *Neuropediatrics* 1988; 19: 80-86.

CHAPTER 22. Surgery for FCD in eloquent cortex

Bertrand C. Devaux

Key points

- Surgery of FCD II in eloquent areas remains a challenge, but should no longer be a restriction for epilepsy surgery.
- Precise knowledge of the functional anatomy of each patient is crucial.
- Resective surgery remains the gold standard, but alternative techniques may also be offered with satisfactory results.
- Surgery of FCD II is a sulcal or a gyral procedure in most cases.
- Careful microdissection of the dysplastic cortex, using neuronavigational guidance and cortical/subcortical electrical stimulations is the procedure of choice.
- Complete FCD II resection without any surgical damage is associated with the best seizure-free outcome.
- Patients should accept a transient neurological deficit.
- There is a risk of permanent postoperative deficits, although most are mild and acceptable considering the expected benefits.
- Seizure recurrence is mainly due to incomplete resection for which reoperation should be considered.

Introduction

Cumulative information about FCD has demonstrated preferential location according to their subtype. Frontal predominance has been reported for FCD II from previous single center studies (Palmini *et al.*, 1995, Kuzniecky *et al.*, 1995, Chassoux *et al.*, 2000) and confirmed in large multicentric cohorts based on nearly 10,000 patients, while other FCD subtypes are mainly located in the temporal lobe (Blumcke *et al.*, 2017). This dichotomous location was also found in a recent multicentric series including 580 patients with FCD, reporting a propensity for FCD II to localize in the superior frontal sulcus, frontal pole, temporal pole, and superior temporal gyrus (Wagstyl *et al.*, 2022). In this study, involvement of eloquent cortex, ie, visual, motor, premotor and language areas led to a low percentage of seizure-free patients (30–40%), however the incidence of lesions in these specific locations was not indicated. In our experience, based on 150 patients operated on for epilepsy due to FCD II, we found that they were located in – or immediately adjacent to – an eloquent cortical area of the brain in more than half of the cases, especially in the sensorimotor area (Chassoux *et al.*, 2022).

Surgical resection in eloquent cortex is particularly challenging, carrying two opposite risks that must always be balanced:

- failing to control the seizures to preserve function, because of an inadequate resection that spares the functional cortex and pathways but leaves unresected a part of the dysplastic cortex,
- damaging the surrounding functional cortex to control the seizures, causing major permanent deficit, if a large resection is performed to provide the best chances of a seizure-free outcome.

For these reasons, surgical resection in highly functional regions have been reported as less favourable than in other brain areas (Kloss 2002, Pondal-Sordo *et al.*, 2006, Benifla *et al.*, 2009, Wagstyl *et al.*, 2022), although other studies, including ours, report higher rates of seizure freedom (Marnet *et al.*, 2008, Chassoux *et al.*, 2012, Gopinath *et al.*, 2016, Ostergard *et al.*, 2019).

The concept of inoperability has then evolved over the past decades as a result of:

- advances in brain imaging,
- improved knowledge and identification of epileptogenic lesions,
- refined microsurgical techniques and availability of new surgical tools,
- accumulated experience of epileptogenic brain lesions successfully operated in functional areas.

Functional structures, both cortical areas and subcortical pathways are better identified and spared during the resection, while functional compensation mechanisms and cerebral plasticity allow for improved functional recovery (Vitali *et al* 2008, Duchowny 2009, Barba *et al.* 2012, Duffau, 2014).

In this chapter, we will review current concepts of functional network and the relationships between FCD and functional cortex and pathways. As our experience is mainly based on FCD II, we will focus on the principles of resection in eloquent areas, with emphasis on the measures to prevent postoperative deficits, and the current less invasive alternatives to resection.

Eloquent cortex, functional networks and plasticity

Eloquent cortex usually refers to cortical areas of the brain necessary for language, motor and sensory function, or to areas of cortex that—if removed—will result in loss of sensory processing, linguistic ability\ or paralysis (Marusic *et al.*, 2002; Lachhwani *et al.*, 2004). The most common areas of eloquent cortex are in the dominant temporal and frontal lobes for speech and language, bilateral occipital lobes for vision, bilateral parietal lobes for sensation, and bilateral motor cortex and supplementary motor area (SMA) for movement. Beyond those primary functional cortical areas, many other territories are devoted to higher integrative functions, such memory encoding and storage, multiple cognitive, affective and behavioural functions, and performance. Although not usually considered as eloquent areas, surgical injury of these secondary functional areas may also cause disabling consequences for the patient's life. Eloquent cortex may also be defined as a cortical area whose electrical stimulation produces a reproducibly change in a particular neurological function (Lachhwani, 2004). Similarly, resection or ablation of the insular cortex does not produce neurological disability in itself, although its adjacent eloquent cortices and dense vascular network makes open surgery at risk for motor, sensory or language deficits.

Functional networks are based, both anatomically and functionally, on the connection between discrete areas of cortex through interconnecting subcortical white matter pathways. The basic concept of the localization-related functionality of brain areas remains valid, however eloquent areas of the brain should no longer be considered as static and purely related to their anatomical location, but as parts of functional dynamic networks (Engel *et al.*, 2013, Pessoa, 2014). An always pressing question is whether untouched parts of these anatomical networks would sustain function or facilitate recovery of function following resection of a key node.

White matter pathways and association fibres provide the connections between cortical nodes and are therefore necessary to sustain a given function. Their surgical injury - mechanical or ischemic - may cause complete and permanent disruption of a particular network leading to irremediable functional deficits (Duffau, 2014). Crucially, the functionality of cortical areas is not uniform among individuals, and there is an important inter-individual anatomo-functional variability. As an example, the functional map of the anterior bank of the central sulcus (motor cortex) shows a highly variable representation in different subjects (Burneo *et al.*, 2004, Farrell *et al.*, 2007). Functional imaging studies, as well as cortical and subcortical mapping in humans during surgery, have demonstrated an overlap of territories and spread of motor units over a much wider area than the anterior bank of the central sulcus (Farrell *et al.*, 2007).

Brain plasticity is a highly dynamic process acting at different spatial and time scales. Dynamic interaction between regions, changes in functional connectivity and dynamic reorganization of brain circuits provide adaptive mechanisms capable of maintaining a given function after a cerebral damage (Duffau, 2014). Ipsilateral non-primary motor areas – SMA, premotor, cingulate, parietal areas – as well as contralateral recruitment of motor and non-motor cortex via dynamic network changes (Chamoun *et al.*, 2007) allow for delayed recovery. Post-operative plasticity has been observed after resection in eloquent cortex, by remapping of functional areas (Barba *et al.*, 2012, Duffau, 2014, Jeong *et al.*, 2016), as we have observed in several of our patients – supported by functional imaging of the recovery processes.

Therefore, eloquent areas should be seen as a part of permanently modulated networks, involving connectivity between dedicated cortical areas - rather than fixed structure/function units supported by unique cytoarchitectonic localization. These observations strongly suggest that surgical resection or ablation of a discrete cortical lesion which spares the underlying pathways should not be associated with permanent functional deficits, because dynamic neuronal network connections and the recruitment of secondary cortical areas act towards functional recovery.

FCD II and functional areas

Based on our experience in surgery of FCD II, the involvement of eloquent cortex was found in 85 patients among 150 (57%) operated on between 2000 and 2021 for FCD II (**Figure 1**). Notably, the central region, defined as both banks of the central sulcus, was mostly involved while visual and associative language areas were rarely implicated. This singular tropism for the sensorimotor cortex has been previously reported but may represent a bias of recruitment, as our group developed a special interest for surgery in this functional area (Talairach *et al.*, 1992; Chassoux *et al.*, 1999; Devaux *et al.*, 2005; Marnet *et al.*, 2008).

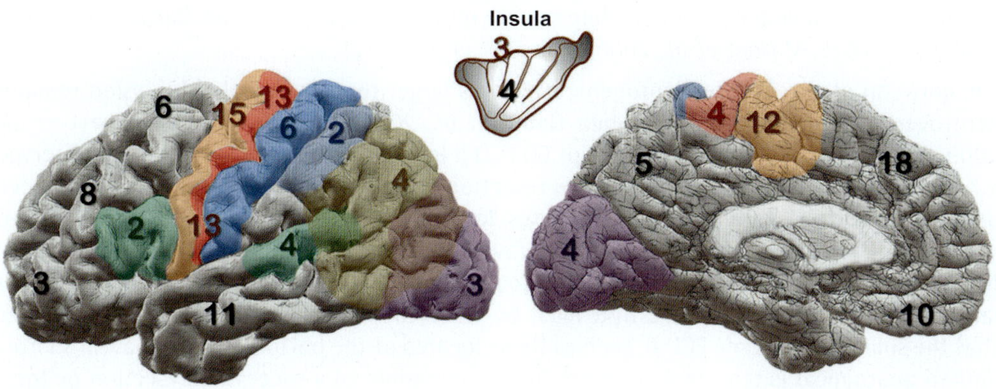

Figure 1

Frequency locations of FCD II in eloquent areas. Data from our personal series over a 21-years period. The number of patients in each location of FCD II is represented on the image. FCD II were found in eloquent areas in 85 patients (57%), over a total of 150 patients operated for FCD II during this period. The number of cases in each eloquent area are in color: sensorimotor operculum (13), central sulcus (13), mesial motor cortex (4), precentral gyrus (15), SMA (12), post-central gyrus (6), lateral parietal cortex (2), dominant inferior frontal gyrus (pars opercularis/ Broca's area)(2), dominant superior temporal gyrus (posterior part)(4), lateral occipital cortex (3), mesial occipital cortex (4), insulo-opercular cortex (3) and multilobar (temporo-occipito-parietal cortex) (4). The numbers of cases in non-eloquent areas are in black.

FCD II occurs during early stages of brain development and these lesions have both structural and functional abnormalities (Duchowny, 2009, Guerrini *et al.*, 2010, Besseling *et al.*, 2016). As other malformations of cortical development, FCD II is currently considered a neural network disorder, integrating multiple abnormalities including anatomical, histological, biochemical, functional, electrophysiological and clinical peculiarities (Duchowny, 2009, Guerrini *et al.*, 2010, Engel *et al.*, 2013, Pessoa, 2014). Intralesional aberrant connectivity profiles, mixing hyper- and hypo-connectivity, abnormal neuronal connections and synaptic transmission, and disturbed anatomical and functional networks have been observed (Jeong *et al.*, 2014, Besseling *et al.*, 2016, Hong *et al.*, 2017). However, the high rate of seizure freedom obtained after a focal resection limited to the dysplastic tissue suggest that FCD II is a highly focal epileptogenic lesion and differ from other malformations of cortical development. Reorganization of functional networks adjacent to the FCD II and atypical representation of functional areas, especially for sensorimotor and language functions, have been previously reported (Burneo *et al.*, 2004, Duchowny, 2009, Guerrini *et al.*, 2010). It has been stated that the higher the disruption of cortical lamination, the lower the ability of the cortex to subserve function (Guerrini *et al.*, 2010). However, the question of the retained functionality of the dysplastic tissue in areas normally devoted to specific brain functions still persists. Extensive studies from functional MRI (fMRI), and other imaging or neurophysiological tools have provided controversial data regarding persistence or absence of function in the dysplastic cortex. While some studies suggest an overlap of dysplastic and functional tissue (Marusic *et al.*, 2002; Janszky *et al.*, 2003, Bingaman, 2004, Cohen-Gadol *et al.*, 2004, Duchowny, 2009), others demonstrate the absence of functionality in FCD II (Burneo *et al.*, 2004, Barba *et al.*, 2012, Eldin *et al.*, 2015; Guerrini *et al.*, 2010).

Our observations, based on fMRI, intraoperative stimulation mapping and surgical results support the hypothesis that FCD II lacks intrinsic functionality. First, we never observe activations within imaging-defined FCD II on sensory-motor fMRI (60 patients), while activations close to the FCD II were found in 59% of the cases, and minor reorganisation was observed in 41% of patients (**Figures 2 – 4**); second, we did not elicit motor responses on stimulation of the dysplastic cortex during surgery of central region FCD II, while responses could be obtained on stimulation of adjacent cortex and subcortical white matter; third, recovery following initial severe postoperative deficits observed after resection of FCD II in the central region illustrates the phenomenon of brain plasticity but also support the notion of an absence of intrinsic function within the dysplastic lesion (Chassoux *et al.*, 2022). Moreover, intra and interhemispheric reorganisation was mostly seen in the few cases involving visual and language areas (personal observations). These data allow to consider surgery more favorably in eloquent areas despite the risks inherent to these locations.

FCD II resection: a gyral and a sulcal procedure

Since FCD II has intrinsic epileptogenicity (Palmini *et al.*, 1995, Chassoux *et al.*, 2000, Bingaman, 2004, Guerrini *et al.*, 2015), their resection must be complete. If one assumes that this abnormal cortex has no intrinsic function, complete removal may then be feasible, providing the best chances for complete seizure relief (Burneo *et al.*, 2004, Barba *et al.*, 2012; Eldin *et al.*, 2015, Marnet *et al.*, 2008, Chassoux *et al.*, 2022).

The question of extensive epileptogenic networks larger than the visible MRI lesion remains controversial (Bingaman, 2004, Cohen-Gadol *et al.*, 2004, Duchowny, 2009, Aubert *et al.*, 2009, Englot *et al.*, 2016). In our series of 60 FCD II located in the central region, we observed a high seizure-free outcome (88%) after resections limited to the dysplastic cortex defined on imaging and SEEG in MRI- negative cases. In contrast, failure was related to insufficient resection of the dysplastic cortex, with a favorable outcome after complete FCD removal (Chassoux *et al.*, 2022). These results do not support the view of epileptogenic networks larger than the dysplastic tissue that must be resected for seizure-freedom. We emphasize that the small size of some FCD II, such as those located at the bottom of sulci, have a sharply limited anatomical extent, making them highly accessible to a successful resection or focal ablation (Wellmer *et al.*, 2018, Chassoux *et al.*, 2022). Overall, the high seizure-free outcome after resection limited to the dysplastic tissue argue on the fact that complete resection is not only necessary but also sufficient for a favorable outcome.

Importantly, whereas in less eloquent areas the resection may encompass the limits of the identified dysplasia and extend to adjacent sulcal margins, this strategy cannot be performed in eloquent areas and resection must be restricted to the dysplastic tissue to prevent permanent injury of functional structures. Therefore, the main issue is the intraoperative identification of the limits of the dysplastic cortex and those of surrounding functional cortex and underlying pathways. Preoperative investigations including high resolution MRI sequences, PET-MRI, and SEEG in cases with insufficient concordant data, must lead to a clear surgical resection planning that will guide the extent of resection, along with intraoperative surgical tools and microscopic feedback. In most cases, intraoperative guidance only needs a neuronavigation equipment (we use both Medtronic Stealth Station, Medtronic, Minneapolis, MN, USA, and BrainLab Curve platform, BrainLab, Munich, Germany) and a cortical/subcortical stimulation device (we use Inomed Osiris, Inomed Medizintechnik GmbH, Emmendingen,

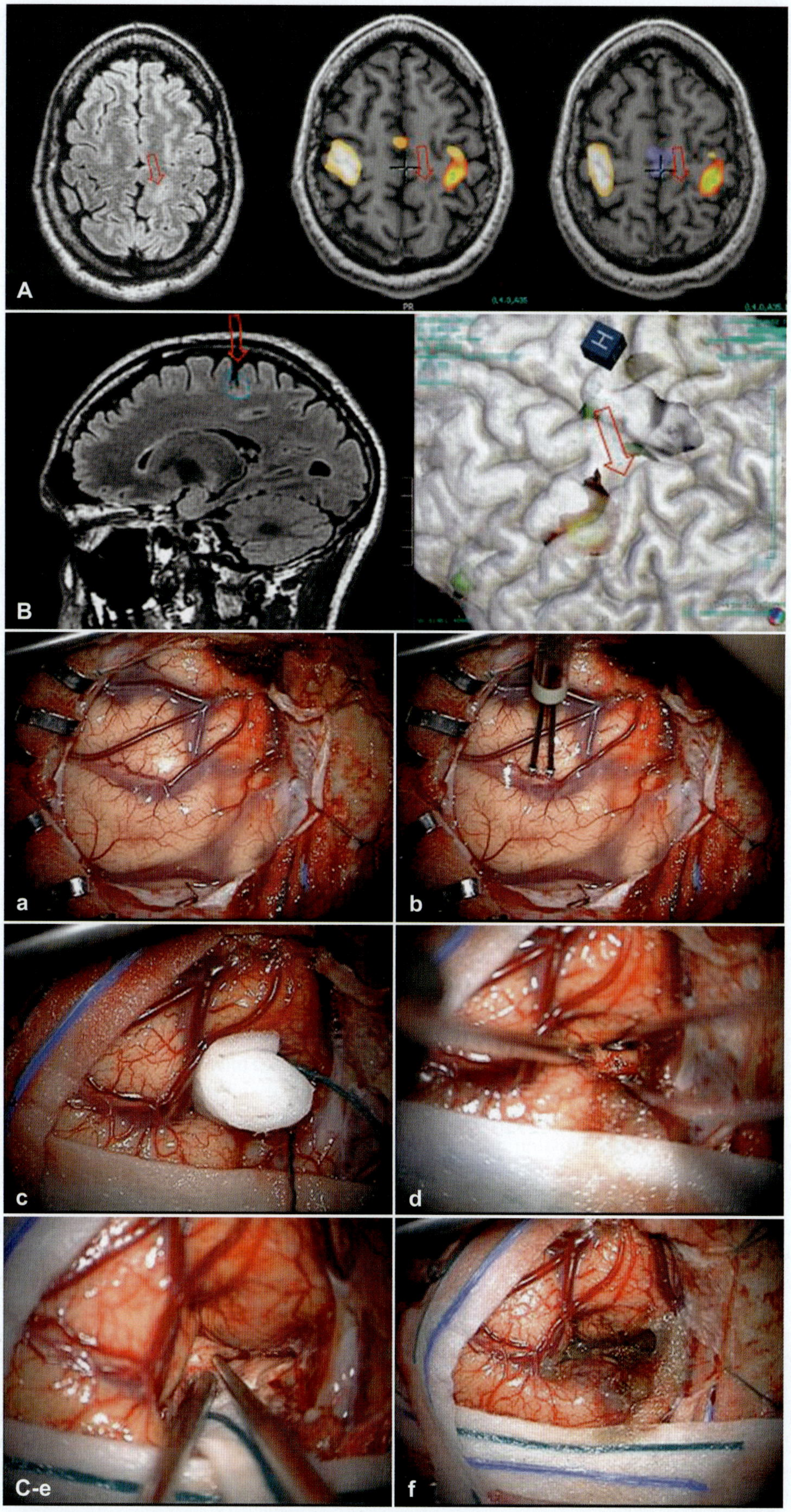

Figure 2

General strategy for a safe resection of a FCD II in eloquent areas. Example of a FCD II located in the deep upper aspect of the left central sulcus, in a 34-yrs old male patient.
A. Axial FLAIR MR sequence and motor fMRI (orange areas: bilateral hand activation; blue areas: bilateral foot activation) showing no activation in the dysplasia (red arrows);
B. Planning of the surgical access (red arrows) and planned extent of resection (yellow outline) from sagittal FLAIR and 3D reconstruction from fMRI;
C. Operative images: circular craniotomy and exposure of the upper part of the central sulcus and adjacent pre- and post-central gyri (a); bipolar cortex stimulations before sulcus opening and neuronavigation accuracy visual control (b); microdissection opening of the sulcus and gentle enlargement with a cotton pattie (c); piecemeal resection using a micro-forceps, and neuronavigation control (d); end of resection (hemostasis with Surgicel®) (e).

Germany). Mode B ultrasound generator, displaying a hyperechogenic area corresponding to the dysplastic tissue, is rarely useful because of an important image distortion and limited resolution.

Intraoperative electrocorticography (ECoG) with grids or strips is of limited use in our experience, first because the large size of ECoG contacts prevent placement in a surgically opened sulcus and surface recordings cannot precisely localize a deep-seated FCD, and also because absence of residual spikes after resection is not always predictive of a seizure-free outcome. However, an optimal use of ECoG is discussed in the chapter by Palmini and Paglioli. Moreover, ECoG may be helpful to reveal spread of after-discharges associated with intraoperative deficits in patients operated in awake conditions. Nevertheless, most surgeries may be performed under general anesthesia, since the resection does not extend beyond the dysplastic cortex. Motor cortex and pathways are mapped using cortical/subcortical electrical stimulations, avoiding the use of prolonged curare injection. Lesions located in or close to the sensory and visual cortex and pathways may be resected using repeat somesthesic and visual evoked potentials to preserve their functionality.

The role of SEEG in the surgical management of FCD II in eloquent areas has become, in our experience, limited to patients without MRI visible lesion. Among 85 FCD located in eloquent areas, 47 (55%) were operated without the need for a SEEG. As long as FCD II can be identified on high-resolution MRI, the extent of surgical resection is based on preoperative identification of dysplastic margins (including PET/MRI coregistration) and intraoperative surgical findings. In patients with MRI negative FCD II, the SEEG will provide, when electrodes are appropriately implanted within the lesion, the area delineating the dysplastic cortex and more often correlating with the epileptogenic zone. As previously described, typical FCD II pattern combines interictal continuous rhythmic spikes, ictal low-voltage rapid discharge with a transitional phase between interictal and ictal activity and followed by a localized depression of activity, and usual seizures elicited by low frequency electrical stimulations (Chassoux *et al.*, 2000). All these neurophysiological criteria combined with PET data and surgical findings will guide the resection extent.

The general strategy of surgical resection in eloquent areas preserving surrounding functional structures is illustrated in Figures 2, 3, and 4. The case presented in **Figure 2** describes the different steps during the resection of a FCD II located in the depth of the central sulcus. Minimal surgical access, to limit any brain shift, associating linear incision and a 1.5 to 2-inch circular craniotomy centred by the neuronavigation device, and X-shape dural opening, allows for an optimal cortex exposure. Accuracy of the neuronavigation system is visually controlled through easily identified superficial structures, and initial cortical stimulations (using a bipolar electrode, biphasic current set at 60 Hz, and increasing intensity from 1 to 4 mA, with 0.5 mA steps, to search for the response threshold) are performed to elicit functional responses – contralateral motor contractions for FCD II located in the sensorimotor area. Then, under microscope magnification, microsurgical opening of the sulcus at the bottom of which the FCD II is located – or of sulci adjacent to the dysplastic gyrus – is performed, using micro-forceps and blunt dissector. Care is taken to avoid vessel coagulations, especially crossing arteries and draining veins running towards the sagittal sinus; only micro branches that ends in the cortex that will be resected can be coagulated; opening the sulcus usually induces some degree of venous bleeding; this micro-bleeding is easily stopped by temporarily placing a small cotton at the sulcal edge. The sulcus is opened down to its depth, unveiling its three-dimensional anatomy, an essential step to understand how the resection will be made in the confined space. The use of cottons may help to hold the sulcus opened during the FCD II resection (**figure 2 c**). Repeat cortical stimulations are performed before any resection, during and after the resection, using similar parameters, on both banks and at the bottom of the sulcus. Once absence of responses from the suspected dysplastic cortex is confirmed, an incision is made on the pial surface of the sulcus bank until the underlying white matter is reached. Resection is subpial, using a micro-dissector and a micro-curette following each bank of the sulcus at the FCD-brain interface, progressing from the surface down to the bottom, until reaching the abnormal rubbery white matter, which confirms the presence of the dysplasia. This surgical consistency feedback has

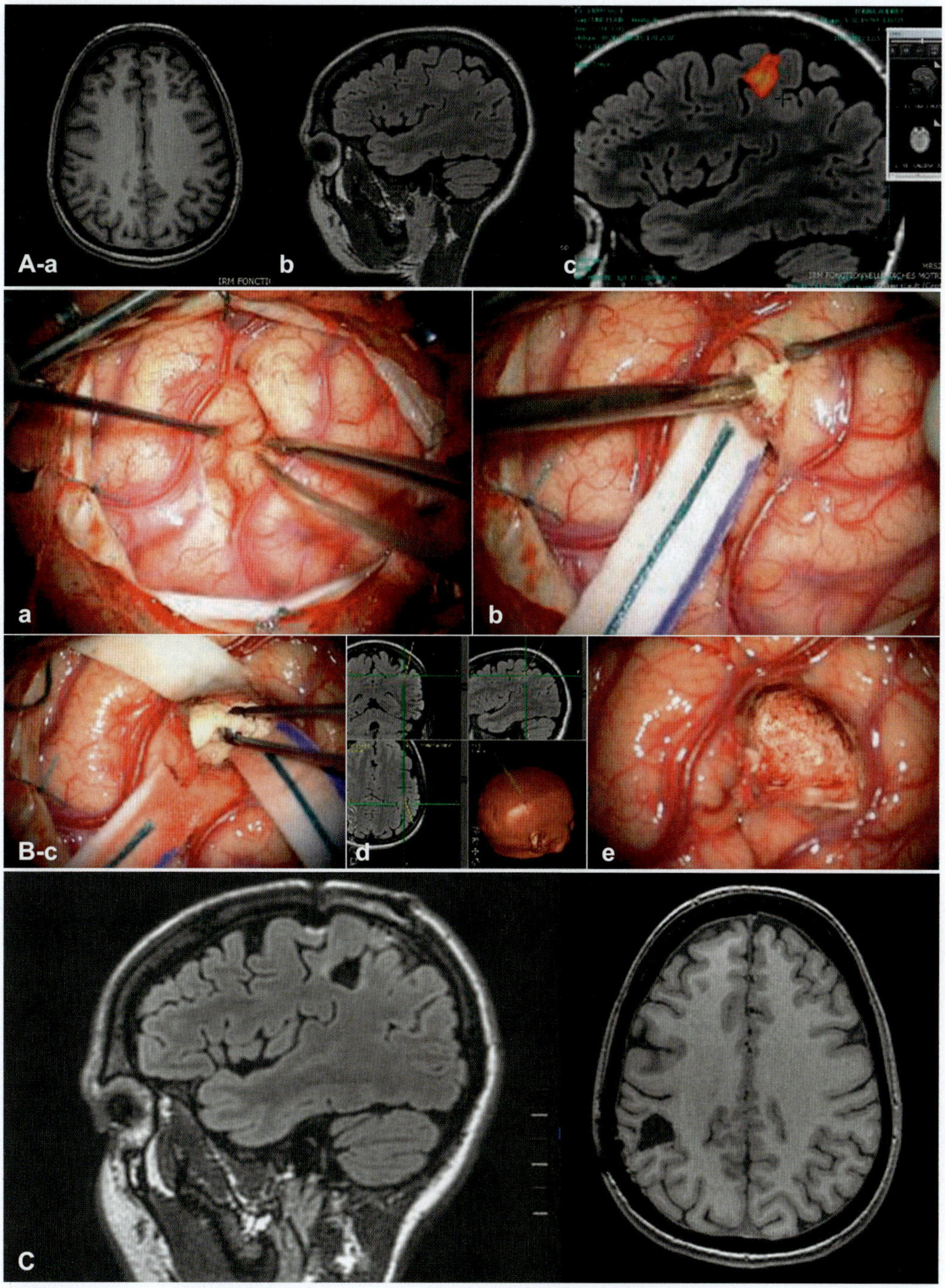

Figure 3

FCD II located in the right post-central sulcus.

A. Preoperative T1 (a) and Flair (b) MRI showing the typical appearance of a FCD II at the bottom of the right post-central sulcus; c) motor fMRI demonstrates a strong activation in the central sulcus anteriorly to the FCD.

B. Operative views: a) microdissection of the postcentral sulcus; b) blunt dissection of the dysplasia using a micro-dissector and c) a micro-forceps, under d) neuronavigation control; e) surgical cavity at the end of dissection.

C. 7 month postoperative control MRI, demonstrating no residual dysplasia, in a seizure-free and neurologically intact patient with a 8-year follow-up.

always been observed when the FCD II lesion was visible on MRI. Microsurgical resection of the dysplastic gyrus – or bottom of sulcus – is stopped once the dysplastic rubbery white matter lying underneath the sulcus is reached, using the tactile feedback. At this point, a deeper resection in the white matter is not necessary for a seizure-free outcome and carries a high risk of injury to functional pathways. Regularly, the neuronavigation pointer is used to control the limits of the resection, until considered complete. A last session of cortical and subcortical stimulations is performed to ensure that responses similar to the pre-resection are still observed, thus confirming preservation of motor pathways. When a stimulation-induced seizure is observed, cold saline solution is irrigated onto the brain surface until seizure cessation.

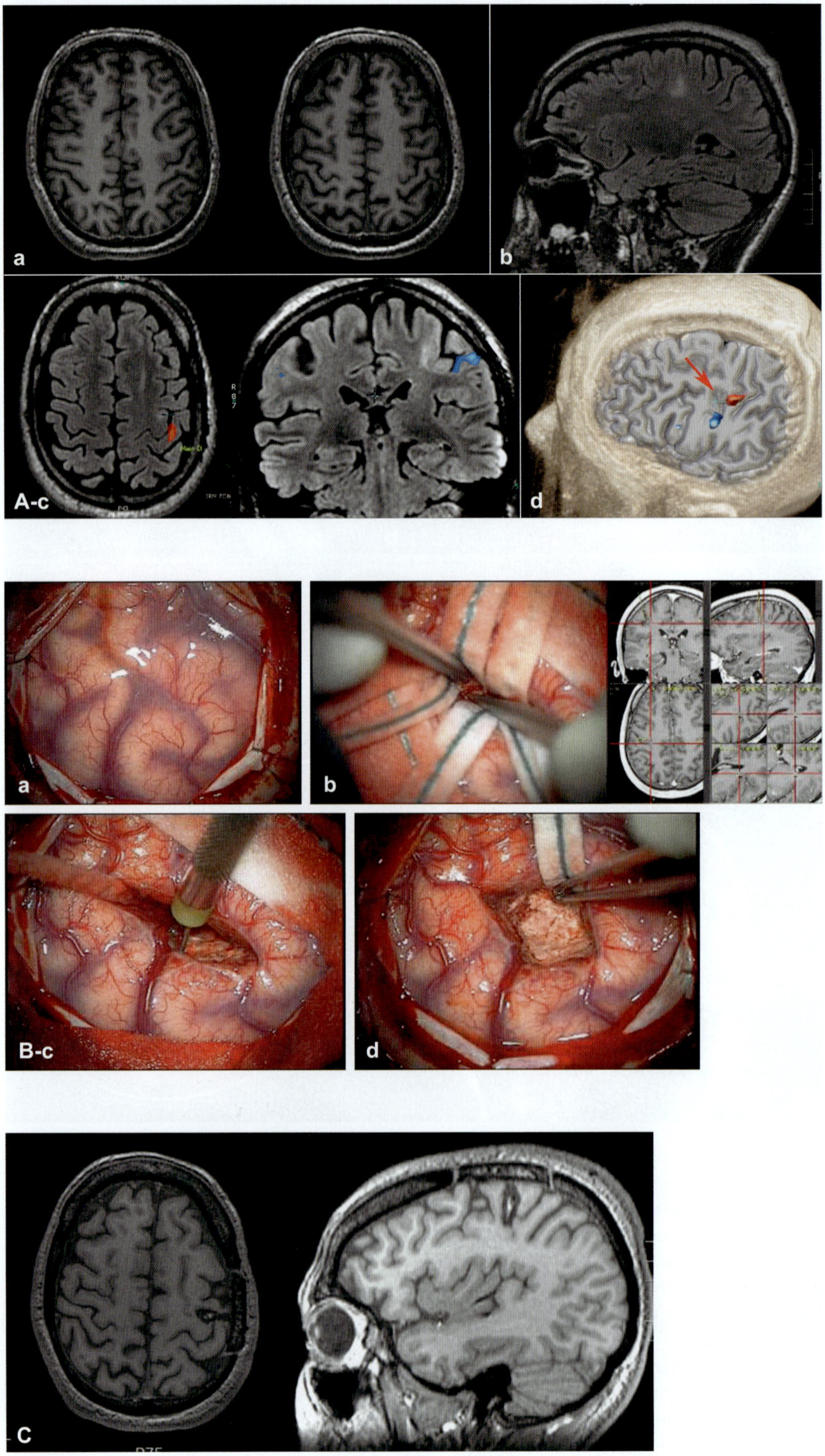

Figure 4

FCD II located in the left central sulcus.

A. Preoperative MRI: a) T1-weighted axial images showing the localized thickened cortex on the anterior bank of the central sulcus; b) Flair sagittal image showing the hyperintensity in the subcortical central area; c) motor functional MRI, showing activation area of the right hand (red) and face (blue) adjacent to the FCD; d) 3D reconstruction of the fMRI, the arrow indicates the abnormal sulcus corresponding to the FCD;
B. Operative views: a) a circular craniotomy unveils the cortical surface, with the central sulcus (thick arrows) and the dysplastic sulcus (thin arrow); b) microdissection of the abnormal sulcus, under neuronavigational control; c) subcortical bipolar stimulations dis not elicit any response in the dysplastic tissue; d) complete macroscopic removal of the dysplasia.
C. Six-month postoperative MRI, demonstrating a complete resection, in a patient seizure-free for 9 years and without permanent postoperative deficit.

Importantly, all surgical specimen should be sent for pathological examination to confirm the diagnosis of FCD II in negative MRI cases. Therefore, the use of Cavitron® ultrasonic aspirator is not recommended.

Beyond the use of described surgical tools – i.e. surgical microscope, neuronavigation equipment, cortical and subcortical stimulation device – many surgical teams use intraoperative ECoG recordings to assess the limits of the dysplastic cortex. In these patients, the resection includes the image-defined and the epileptogenic cortex defined by abnormalities found on ECoG (Bingaman, 2004, Pondal-Sordo *et al.*, 2006, Fauser *et al.*, 2015, Duchowny, 2009, Ostergard *et al.*,2019). The advantage of this technique is extensively discussed in the chapters by Palmini and Paglioli in this volume.

In patients who present an early or late seizures recurrence, a reoperation should be discussed. A repeat presurgical workup is necessary to analyse the cause of failure. In most cases, dysplastic tissue which was unidentified during the first resection remained in place. If suggested by non-invasive investigations, a second surgery may be offered to the patient and often achieve seizure freedom (Sacino *et al.*, 2017, Guerrini *et al.*, 2015, Chassoux *et al.*, 2022). If necessary, invasive monitoring of recurrent seizures (SEEG) may confirm a persisting abnormal discharge pattern typical for FCD II and guide a second surgery. Alternative techniques (see following paragraph) may also be offered as a complement to the initial surgery. In our experience, a second surgery was needed in 25% of patients operated in eloquent areas, and led to seizure-free outcome (Chassoux *et al.*, 2022).

The rules to avoid major permanent postoperative deficits

Major and permanent postoperative deficits are caused by an inadequate resection of functional cortex, mechanical surgical injury of functional cortex and/or subcortical functional pathways, or by an unwanted ischemic or haemorrhagic complication. Careful attention to some specific measures, however, may reduce these risks.

The position of the head during surgery is important, to avoid increased venous pressure and brain tension, that would render the micro-dissection difficult and increase the risk of collateral injury. Small circular craniotomy and minimal cortex exposure increases the reliability of the neuronavigation control and is sufficient for most focal resections under general anesthesia. Awake surgery is rarely indicated in our experience since few FCD are located in areas involving language functions. In addition, perioperative stimulations often elicit after-discharges or seizures making the functional responses difficult to interpret (**Figure 5**) and can falsely limit the extent of the resection.

In FCD II located at the bottom of sulci, the surgeon could be tempted to dissect and remove the abnormal sulcus as a single specimen, encompassing both banks and the bottom, without opening the sulcus; however, without identification of the passing vessels in the sulcus, they would be indistinctively coagulated and sectioned, carrying a risk of adjacent ischemia involving both cortex and white matter tracts (Ostergard *et al.*, 2019). I personally recommend opening the sulcus and control the sulcal vessels before dissecting the sulcal edges. Using a smooth micro-dissector under microscopic magnification and optimal illumination, the dissection is performed at the grey-white matter junction. Neuronavigation helps to understand the local anatomy, especially when the dissection reaches the deeper part of the sulcus and its 3D shape is complex. Extending the resection beyond the limits of the dysplastic cortex is unnecessary, in particular the resection of the transmantle extension that may contain abnormal neurons. It carries the risk of injury to functional pathways and white matter ischemia. The white matter underlying a FCD II is particularly hard, easily recognized and must be spared by the resection. It also provides a 'tactile limit of the resection', complementing the subtle change in tissue colour seen at high magnification of the microscope. As previously described, in case of small vessels bleeding during the dissection, haemostasis using mild compression by cottons is preferable to bipolar coagulation.

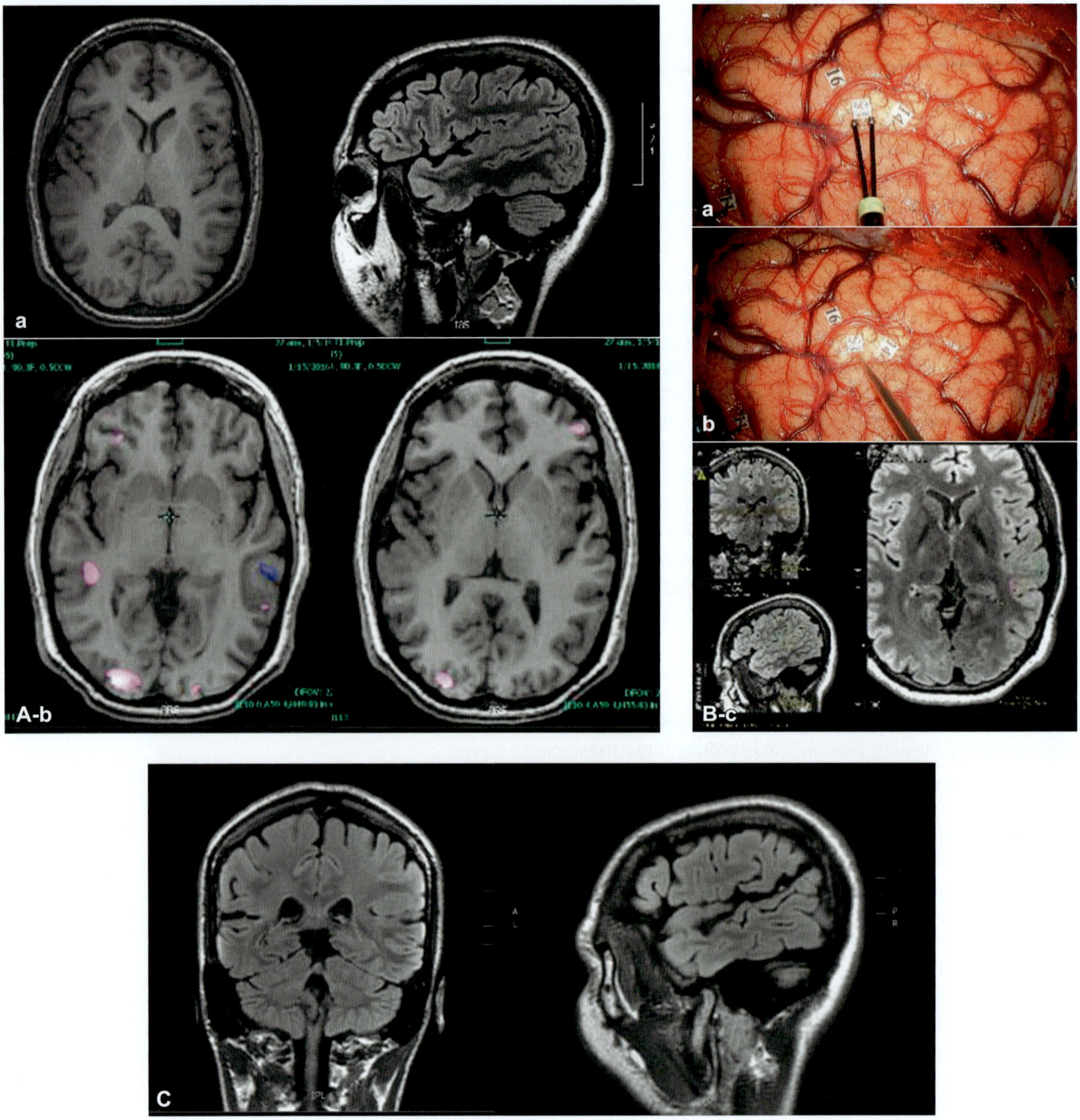

Figure 5

FCD II located in the posterior part of the right superior temporal gyrus in an ambidextrous patient with atypical (bilateral) dominance for language.

A. Preoperative MRI: a) T1-weighted and Flair MR images showing abnormal grey-white matter blurring in the posterior part of the superior temporal sulcus typical for FCD II; b) language fMRI showing no activation within the dysplasia and underlying activation of the middle temporal gyrus;

B. Operative views: a) bipolar stimulation of the abnormal superior temporal gyrus cortex elicited a speech arrest, b) while neuronavigation confirmed the presence of the dysplasia at the responsive spots; although electrocortical recordings demonstrated a discharge spread beyond the limits of the dysplasia, extending to the area of language activation on functional MRI; c) a safe resection of the FCD II was performed, ensued by a mild and transient language disturbance;

C. postoperative imaging at 6 months, showing the extent of resection.

Finally, the identification of functional motor cortex and subcortical pathways using repeat high-frequency stimulations, before, during and after the resection remains the best surgical tool to avoid unwanted injury of the functional structures. Obtaining similar responses at the same intensities before and at the end of resection ensures that these structures are spared. Although a postoperative deficit is frequently observed, a complete recovery or persistence of a non-disabling minor deficit will occur in most patients.

Outcome after resection of FCD II in eloquent cortex: excellent on seizures, without major functional compromise

Although the chances of a seizure-free outcome are still reported as poorer when FCD II is located in an eloquent brain area (Pondal-Sordo *et al.*, 2006, Wagstyl *et al.*, 2022), a more favorable outcome has been also reported, with 59 % to 92 % of patients being seizure-free (Benifla *et al.*, 2009, Sarkis *et al.*, 2010, Delev *et al.*, 2014, Gopinath *et al.*, 2016, Ostergard *et al.*, 2019). Our experience of surgical resections of FCD II in eloquent areas confirmed that excellent results (88% of seizure-free- outcome) may be obtained (Devaux *et al.*, 2005, Devaux *et al.*, 2008; Marnet *et al.*, 2008; Chassoux *et al.*, 2012, Chassoux *et al.*, 2022).

Regarding functional outcome, severe postoperative deficits are commonly described. In a recent meta-analysis including 280 patients, an immediate postoperative deficit was described in 58% and a permanent deficit in 23% (Ostergard *et al.*, 2019). Similar results were reported in series focusing on FCD II located in rolandic or perirolandic cortex, in which permanent deficits occurred in 28% to 59% of patients (Sarkis *et al.*, 2010, Delev *et al.*, 2014). In our series, immediate postoperative functional deficits occurred in 87 % of the patients, mainly after resection in the primary motor cortex and the SMA. All but three patients improved during the two first postoperative months. At follow-up, 47% of patients had a normal neurological examination, while a mild, non-disabling motor or sensory disturbance was observed in 32%, a moderate in 15% and a severe in 5%. These data may help to assess the benefit/risk ratio and to inform patients and their relatives during presurgical counselling.

Reports on specific functional outcomes following surgical resection of FCD II in eloquent regions other than the perirolandic cortex are less clear. Location of FCD II in language, visual or insular areas are infrequent. Occipital location accounts for 2.4 % to 3.6% and insular for 0.5% to 1.5% of all FCD II in large series (Wagstyl *et al.*, 2022), similarly to our data. As previously mentioned, local or remote functional reorganization demonstrated by fMRI is helpful for performing adequate resections without permanent neurological deficits. Of note, most FCD II located in the insular cortex were treated with an alternative surgical technique, such as multiple stereotaxic HF thermocoagulations (Mullatti *et al.*, 2019).

Finally, seizure outcome following resection of FCD II in eloquent regions compares favorably with other series of FCD II in any locations, suggesting that eloquent areas of the brain should no longer be seen as limiting successful resections, provided 1) no intraoperative injury is made to subcortical pathways nor to adjacent vessels, 2) no postoperative complications occur, and 3) a transient postoperative deficit and the risk of a mild or moderate permanent deficit are accepted by the patient and family (see below).

Factors related to functional recovery

Transient immediate postoperative deficits following resection in an eloquent area are likely due to a disruption of connections of adjacent cortex via short and mid-distance fibers and local intracortical millimiter -scale networks, even if intraoperative cortical and sub-cortical stimulations elicited functional responses throughout the whole procedure. Severity and duration of such deficits depend on the importance of the resection area. If functional white matter pathways have been severed by a mechanical or ischemic injury, a corresponding neurological deficit is likely to persist.

Progressive recovery is usually observed within the first postoperative weeks and continues over a few months (Chassoux *et al.*, 1999; Ostergard *et al.*, 2019). Resections of the perirolandic neocortex inferior to the thumb area, corresponding to the opercular part of the precentral gyrus and adjacent central sulcus, do not usually result in long-lasting postoperative deficits, since bilateral fibers coming from both facial motor areas project onto the pyramidal tract (Lehman *et al.*, 1994). However, persisting facial paresis and dysarthria have been reported, likely due to extensive resection and fiber tract injury (Ostergard *et al.*, 2019)

Abnormal functional networks associated with FCD II – as described in previous paragraphs – and dynamic functional reorganization of networks, including new synaptic connections and extra-synaptic transmission occurring at early and late stages at local and large-scale networks, underpin early and late recovery of immediate postoperative deficits. Such recovery is more or less complete, depending upon:

- the level of preoperative reorganization of primary and associative functions,
- the extent of cortical resection,
- the degree of injury of subcortical white matter tracts, the occurrence of a surgical complication (Chassoux *et al.*, 2022).

Importantly, functional outcome was significantly better in children than in adults, with fewer severe early deficits and total recovery (Benifla *et al.*, 2009, Sacino *et al.*, 2016, Chassoux *et al.*, 2022). Following resection in the central or precentral area, the proximal part of the superior limbs usually recovers before the distal part and persisting upper limb deficits are limited to a dysfunction of the fine motor control (Ostergard *et al.*, 2019). Fewer data are available about lower limb recovery, which is more challenging regarding functional outcome. Recovery of lower extremity deficit often allow independent walking, however some degree of disabling limp is observed after a more severe initial deficit. Major deficits occurring after SMA resection dramatically improve in a few weeks with no or only minor permanent deficits (Chassoux *et al.*, 1999).

Immediate unmasking of adjacent secondary motor cortex during surgery for low-grade tumors has been described, suggesting the existence of latent motor redundant circuits and the capacity of the brain to make short-term changes in local motor maps (Duffau, 2001). Hence, recruitment of adjacent ipsilateral premotor and primary sensory areas, as well as contralateral remote cortical areas such as premotor, motor or cingular areas, illustrates the diffuse nature of neuronal circuits capable of motor function restoration and the huge potential of brain plasticity.

• Alternatives to cortical resections: a risk to be suboptimal

Small FCD II located in the bottom of a single sulcus can be ablated without the necessity of an open surgical procedure. Minimally invasive techniques have thus been developed and performed in patients considered at risk for open surgery, either as a first surgical procedure or as complement in case of failure to control the seizures.

SEEG-guided thermocoagulations were initially developed as a palliative procedure at the end of the SEEG exploration in patients considered at risk or not candidates for a resective procedure (Guenot *et al.*, 2011). Several thermolesions performed from SEEG electrode contacts recording low-amplitude fast activity or spike wave discharges at the onset of seizures led to significant reduction of seizure frequency in half the patients (Guenot *et al.* , 2011).

Multiple stereotactic radiofrequency thermocoagulations (RFTC) consist in a volumetric thermal ablation of a discrete lesion or cortical area defined as epileptogenic from presurgical investigations, using a stereotactically guided monopolar electrode and an RF lesion generator (Cosman RFG-3B, Radionics Corp, Burlington, MA). Among the 19 patients treated with RFTC, 10 patients had a FCD II and 7 of them (70%) were rendered seizure-free (mean follow-up: 5.4 yrs); 3 had a transient minor postoperative deficit (Mullatti *et al.*, 2019). Similar results after RFTC performed with a curative perspective for small-size FCD II have been reported (Wellmer *et al.*, 2018).

Laser-assisted thermo-ablation of epileptic foci has been a rapidly expanding technology as an alternative surgical treatment for intractable temporal as well as extra-temporal epilepsy (Lewis *et al.*, 2015; Bandt *et al.*, 2016). Reported series include mainly MTLE patients. Very few cases of FCD treated by laser ablation have been reported, mostly in children, with favourable results in some cases (Lewis *et al.*, 2015). This well tolerated procedure is based on a similar principle as RFTC, ie, volumetric ablation by thermal necrosis precisely outlined, with the additional benefit of real-time temperature monitoring and lesional volume estimation using short sequences MRI and dedicated software. It could eventually replace RFTC, however at a significantly higher cost.

Multiple subpial transections (MSTs) is a disconnective procedure for patients presenting with seizures originating from an eloquent area, carrying a lower risk a permanent neurological deficit than resection, but with inconstant results (Spencer *et al.*, 2002). In FCD II surgery, they are usually performed in addition to a limited resection of the dysplasia and guided by intraoperative ECoG recordings, mostly in the sensorimotor area (Pondal-Sordo *et al.*, 2006, Delev *et al.*, 2014, Gopinath *et al.*, 2016, Ostergard *et al.*, 2019). Seizure outcome is better when MSTs are performed in association with a resection than as a stand-alone procedure but remains poorer than in other locations (Spencer *et al.*, 2002, Rolston *et al.*, 2018,).

Radiosurgery has been reported in a very limited number of patients with a FCD II, with unfavourable results (Aubert *et al.*, 2009; Boström *et al.*, 2016). However, new modalities of low-dose radiosurgery or hypofractionated stereotactic radiotherapy, with likely less long-term complications, could be an alternative option in selected patients (Boström *et al.*, 2016).

Neuromodulation techniques include deep brain stimulation (DBS) of selected subcortical targets - anterior nucleus, centromedian-parafascicular nucleus, of the thalamus, subthalamic nucleus - (Klinger *et al.*, 2016) and direct responsive neurostimulation (RNS) of one or two seizure foci (Bergey *et al.*, 2015; Jobst *et al.*, 2017). Although palliative by nature, both modalities have some efficacy in patients not candidates for resective surgery. Seizure outcome in patients with FCD II treated with subcortical DBS targets are not precisely described, but the average seizure reduction varies according to the selected target from 30 to 80%, with an average of 50-60% in most studies (Bergey, *et al.*, 2015). Similarly, RNS, a close-loop direct stimulation of epileptogenic foci through permanently implanted intracranial electrode(s) when abnormal ECoG activity is detected by the subdural recording electrode, has been evaluated in large clinical trials, enrolling patients with temporal lobe and neocortical epilepsy, including seizures onset from eloquent cortex. The mean percent of seizure reduction is 44 to 66% at 1 to 3 years after implantation (Bergey *et al.*, 2015, Jobst *et al.*, 2017).

Therefore, if seizure freedom is expected, neuromodulation techniques should not to be recommended as primary procedures in patients with FCD II in eloquent areas. However, in case of surgical failure, selected patients not considered candidates for reoperation could benefit from those techniques. Focused ultrasounds (fUS), a less invasive, incision-free, technique is currently offered to patients presenting with movement disorders as an alternative to deep brain stimulation (*see review in* Quadri *et al.*, 2018). This technique is also under evaluation in other functional diseases and could be applied as a neuromodulation technique in focal epilepsy.

How to improve seizure and functional outcome?

First of all, the preoperative investigation step is essential. Experienced neurologists, neurosurgeons, neurophysiologists and neuroradiologists, should work closely together to carefully review all data obtained from clinical, neurophysiological and imaging examinations and establish in every patient a clear and precise surgical resection planning (Guerrini *et al.*, 2015). Intra- surgical procedures to identify the dysplastic cortex to be removed and the functional structures to be spared, do not replace or compensate an imprecise presurgical planning. Optimized preoperative imaging, using high-field MRI and PET co-registration (for example, improved detection of FCD II on current MRI units at 3T and 7T), will reduce the rate of image-negative FCD II and provide better surgical guidance to achieve seizure freedom.

However, the favorable results obtained after FCD II resections can be further improved and thus reduce the need for reoperation in patients with relapses due to excessively prudent and insufficient resection. The completeness of resection is the main predictive factor of seizure-free outcome (Kloss *et al.*, 2002, Krsek *et al.*, 2009, Rowland *et al.*, 2012, Fauser *et al.*, 2015), therefore the first goal of the neurosurgeon is to precisely identify the entire volume of dysplastic tissue in the complex gyral or sulcal anatomy. The second is to do the same with the close or surrounding functional cortex. Once again, a careful and detailed preoperative workup must be undertaken to understand the position and three-dimensional organization of the FCD II lesion and functional cortical and subcortical structures.

A major aspect of the surgery is to avoid any operative and postoperative complication. Severe permanent deficits may occur in patients who experience intraoperative (oedema, coagulation ischemia) or postoperative (hematoma of the surgical site, ischemia of surrounding cortex due to excessive coagulation or to vasospasm) complications. These can be limited by performing blunt dissections, avoiding repeated micro-coagulations and white matter tractions.

As previously discussed, the balance between the risks of surgery of FCD II in eloquent areas should guide the surgical resection in a prudent rather than a risky manner. According to the experience of the neurosurgeon and his analysis during the procedure, he or she may prefer stopping the resection rather than damaging perilesional normal cortex and white matter. Planning a two-step procedure may be a reasonable choice, giving more chances of preserving functional structures while optimizing the resection. In case of seizure recurrence, a repeat investigation procedure may lead to a reoperation or an alternative procedure. The recovery mechanisms and the recruitment of adjacent cortex may render the second procedure more respectful to the functional structure while improving seizure control. Once again, this decision strategy must be explained to the patient and family before surgery.

What do we expect from emerging technologies to guide surgery and improve the outcome?

Current and coming intraoperative technologies are expected to better guide the surgical procedures. As already discussed, the key point for the neurosurgeon is the spatial identification of the dysplastic cortex, its anatomical limits, and that of functional cortical and subcortical structures. The question of the interface between the dysplastic and functional cortex is poorly understood and still debated; a clear margin between both is less likely than some overlap, however allowing a complete resection that, although encompassing a small area of functional cortex, will not lead to permanent deficit.

Therefore, there is a need for high-resolution imaging of the gyral and sulcal cortex, at a millimetric and sub-millimetric resolution. The spatial resolution of intraoperative high-field MRI appears too low to answer this latter issue. In addition, artifacts due to brain and air interface at the resection site and image distortion may hide dysplasia remnants after apparent complete resection. However, increased detection of FCD remnants after apparent complete resection using intraoperative MRI images has been reported (Sacino *et al.*, 2016) - with impact on the operative decision making.

Intraoperative identification of increased echogenicity using shear-wave ultrasound may help disclose and localize a FCD II underlying an apparently normal brain surface, and proves to be superior for detection of FCD II compared to standard B-mode ultrasound (Mathon *et al.*, 2021). However, once resected, the capability of sonic imaging to identify potential residual dysplastic cortex has not been demonstrated.

Micro-neurophysiological investigations using multi-electrode arrays (MEAs), that provide the possibility to stimulate and simultaneously record the field potentials and action potentials from multiple neurons from different layers of a cortical area, have been experimentally used to study the interictal, ictal and evoked seizure-like events from human epileptic cortical slices, and mechanisms underlying seizure onset and propagation (Dossi *et al.*, 2014). Similar technique could be applied during surgery to identify the limits of the dysplastic tissue at a small-scale cortical level.

Optical imaging techniques are capable to produce high resolution images at a cellular level, allowing detailed tissue identification. Two different and complementary techniques - full-field optical coherence tomography (ff-OCT) and biphotonic autofluorescence of nervous tissue - are under evaluation and could find a future place in the operating room to discriminate normal and abnormal tissue, and to collect architecture and metabolic images of the target tissue at a cellular level.

Alternative therapeutic techniques, as previously described, are expected to enlarge the surgical armamentarium. Once reaching sufficient safety and efficacy, they could be used to treat FCD II lesions, either as a sole or an additional procedure, or even in combination with several techniques. After precise tridimensional identification of dysplastic and functional tissue, the use of laser-induced hyperthermia (Lewis *et al.*, 2015) or focused ultrasonic tissue hyperthermic modulation (Quadri *et al.*, 2018) may increase our capability to safely ablate or control an epileptogenic lesion such as FCD II.

Conclusion

Surgery of FCD II in eloquent areas should not remain an overcoming challenge. Surgical technique does not differ from surgery of FCD II in other brain regions, however a more careful attention is necessary to identify and preserve functional cortical and subcortical structures, as well as surrounding vessels. Functional imaging and neurophysiologic data suggest redistribution of commonly accepted localization-related functions and reorganization of functional networks in view of the lack of function of the dysplastic tissue and the huge potential of cerebral plasticity subserving the recovery processes. This knowledge serves as a base for successful surgical resection with a low and acceptable permanent functional morbidity, after appropriately resected or ablated FCD, as long as no complication from surgery occurs. New tools will help to improve the functional outcome and minimize the risks.

References

Aubert S, Wendling F, Regis J, *et al.* Local and remote epileptogenicity in focal cortical dysplasias and neurodevelopmental tumours. *Brain* 2009; 132: 3072-86.

Bandt S.K, Leuthard E. Minimally invasive neurosurgery for epilepsy using stereotactic MRI guidance. , *Neurosurg Clin N Am.* 2016; 27(1): 51-8.

Barba C, Montanaro D, Frijia F, *et al.* Focal cortical dysplasia type IIb in the rolandic cortex: Functional reorganization after early surgery documented by passive task functional MRI. *Epilepsia* 2012; 53: e141-5.

Benifla M, Sala F, Jane J, *et al.* Neurosurgical management of intractable rolandic epilepsy in children: role of resection in eloquent cortex. *J Neurosurg Ped* 2009; 4: 199-216.

Bergey G.K, Morrell M.J, Mizrahi E.M, *et al.* Long-term treatment with responsive brain stimulation in adults with refractory partial seizures. *Neurology*, 2015, 84: 810-7.

Besseling R.M, Jansen J.F, de Louw A.J, *et al.* Abnormal profiles of local functional connectivity proximal to focal cortical dysplasias. *Plos One* 2016,; 11(11): e0166022,1-15.

Blumcke I, Spreafico R, Haaker G, *et al.* Histopathological Findings in Brain Tissue Obtained during Epilepsy Surgery. *N Engl J Med* 2017; 377: 1648–56.

Bingaman W.E. Surgery for focal cortical dysplasia. *Neurology* 2004; 62(Suppl.3): s30-4.

Boström J.P, Delev D, Quesada C, *et al.* Low-dose radiosurgery or hypofractionated stereotactic radiotherapy as treatment option in refractory epilepsy due to epileptogenic lesions in eloquent areas – Preliminary report of feasibility and safety. *Seizure* 2016; 36: 57-62.

Burneo JG, Kuzniecky RI, Bebin M, Knowlton RC. Cortical reorganization in malformations of cortical development – A magnetoencephalographic study. *Neurology* 2004; 63: 1818-24.

Chamoun RB, Mikati MA, Comair YG. Functional recovery following resection of an epileptogenic focus in the motor hand area. *Epilepsy Behav* 2007; 11: 384–8.

Chassoux F, Devaux B, Landre E, *et al.* Stereoelectroencephalography in focal cortical dysplasia. A 3D approach to delineating the dysplastic cortex. *Brain* 2000; 123: 1733-51.

Chassoux F, Devaux B, Landré E, *et al.* Postoperative motor deficits and recovery after cortical resections. *Adv. Neurol* 1999; 81: 189-99.

Chassoux F, Landré E, Mellerio C, *et al.* Type II focal cortical dysplasia: Electro-clinical phenotype and surgical outcome related to imaging. *Epilepsia* 2012; 53: 349-58.

Chassoux F, Mellerio C, Laurent A, Landré E, Turak B, Devaux B. Benefits and risks in epilepsy surgery for focal cortical dysplasia type 2 in the central region. *Neurology in press.*

Cohen-Gadol A.A, Ozduman K, Bronen RA, Kim JH, Spencer DD. Long-term outcome after epilepsy surgery for focal cortical dysplasia. *J Neurosurg* 2004; 101: 55-65.

Delev D, Send K, Wagner J, *et al.* Epilepsy surgery of the rolandic and immediate perirolandic cortex: surgical outcome and prognostic factors. *Epilepsia* 2014; 55: 1585-93.

Devaux B, Chassoux F, Landré E, *et al.* Surgical resections in functional areas: Report of 89 cases. *Neurochirurgie* 2008, 54: 409-17.

Devaux B, Chassoux F, Landré E, Turak B, Beuvon F, Rodrigo S. Central region resections for intractable epilepsy associated with Taylor type focal cortical dysplasia. Is a seizure-free outcome possible after resection without functional compromise? *Epilepsia* 2005, 46 (Suppl. 6): 55.

Dossi H, Blauwblomme T, Nabbout R, Huberfeld G, Rouach N. Multi-electrode array recordings of human epileptic postoperative cortical tissue. *J Vis Exp* 2014, 92: e51870.

Duchowny M. Clinical, functional, and neurophysiologic assessment of dysplastic cortical networks: implications for cortical functioning and surgical management. *Epilepsia* 2009, 50(Suppl. 9): 19-27.

Duffau H. Acute functional reorganisation of the human motor cortex during resection of central lesions: a study using intraoperative brain mapping. *J Neurol Neurosurg Psychiatry* 2001; 70: 506-13.

Duffau H. The huge plastic potential of adult brain and the role of connectomics: new insights provided by serial mappings in glioma surgery. *Cortex* 2014; 58: 325-37.

Eldin SS, Iwasaki M, Nishio Y, Jin K, Nakasato N, Tominaga T. Resection of focal cortical dysplasia located in the upper pre-central gyrus. *Epileptic Disord* 2015; 17: 479-84.

Engel J, Thompson P.M, Stern J.M, Staba R.J, Bragin A, Modi I. Connectomics and epilepsy. *Curr. Opin. Neurol* 2013; 26(2): 186-94.

Englot D.J, Konrad P.E, Morgan V.L. Regional and global connectivity disturbances in focal epilepsy, related neurocognitive sequelae, and potential mechanistic underpinnings. *Epilepsia* 2016; 57(10): 1546-57.

Farrell D, Burbank N, Lettich E, Ojeman G. Individual variation in human motor-sensory (Rolandic) cortex. *J Clin Neurophysiol* 2007; 4(3): 286-93.

Fauser S, Essang C, Altenmüller D.M, *et al.* Long-term seizure outcome in 211 patients with focal cortical dysplasia. *Epilepsia* 2015; 56(1): 66-76.

Gopinath S, Roy A.G, Vinayan K.P, *et al.* Seizure outcome following primary motor cortex-sparing resective surgery for perirolandic focal cortical dysplasia. *Int J Surgery* 2016; 36(Pt B): 466-76.

Guenot M, Isnard J, Catenoix H, Mauguière F, Sindou M. SEEG-guided RF-thermocoagulation of epileptic foci: A therapeutic alternative for drug-resistant non-operable partial epilepsies. *Adv Tech Stand. Neurosurg* 2011; 36: 62-78.

Guerrini R, Barba C. Malformations of cortical development and aberrant cortical networks: epileptogenesis and functional organization. *J Clin Neurophysiol* 2010; 27(6): 372-9.

Guerrini R, Duchowny M, Jayakar P, *et al.* Diagnostic methods and treatment options for focal cortical dysplasia. *Epilepsia* 2015; 56: 1669-86.

Hong S.J, Bernhardt B.C, Gill R.S, Bernasconi N, Bernasconi A. The spectrum of structural and functional network alterations in malformations of cortical development. *Brain* 2017; 140: 2133-43.

Janszky J, Ebner A, Kruse B, *et al.* Functional organization of the brain with malformations of cortical development. *Ann Neurol* 2003; 53: 759-767.

Jeong W, Jin S.H, Kim M, Kim J.S, Chung C.K. Abnormal functional brain network in epilepsy patients with focal cortical dysplasia. *Epil. Res* 2014: 108: 1618-26.

Jeong J.W, Asano E, Juhasz C, Behe M.E, Chugani H.T. Postoperative axonal changes in the contralateral hemisphere in children with medically refractory epilepsy: a longitudinal diffusion tensor imaging connectome analysis. *Hum Brain Map* 2016; 37: 3946-56.

Jobst B.C, Kapur R, Barkley G.L, *et al.* Brain-responsive neurostimulation in patients with intractable seizures arising from eloquent and other neocortical areas. *Epilepsia* 2017; 58(6): 1005-14.

Klinger N.V, Mittal S. Clinical efficacy of deep brain stimulation for the treatment of medically refractory epilepsy. *Clin Neurol Neurosurg* 2016; 140: 11-25.

Kloss S, Pieper T, Pannek H, Holthausen H, Tuxhorn I. Epilepsy surgery in children with focal cortical dysplasia (FCD): results of long-term seizure outcome. *Neuropediatrics* 2002; 33: 21-26.

Krsek P, Maton B, Jayakar P, *et al.* Incomplete resection of focal cortical dysplasia is the main predictor of poor postsurgical outcome. *Neurology* 2009; 72: 217-23.

Kuzniecky R, Morawetz R, Faught E, Black L. Frontal and central lobe focal dysplasia: clinical, EEG and imaging features. *Dev Med Child Neurol* 1995; 37: 159-66.

Lachhwani D.K, Dinner D.S. Cortical stimulation in the definition of eloquent cortical areas. *In* Presurgical assessment of the epilepsies with clinical neurophysiology and functional imaging. *Handbook of Clinical Neurophysiology*, Vol.3. Rosenow F. & Lüders H.O, Eds. Elsevier, 2004; pp 273-86.

Lehman R, Andermann F, Olivier A, Tandon PN, Quesney LF, Rasmussen TB. Seizures with onset in the sensorimotor face area: clinical patterns and results of surgical treatment in 20 patients. *Epilepsia* 1994; 35: 1117-24.

Lewis E.C, Weil A.G, Duchowny M, Bhatia S, Ragheb J, Miller I. MR-guided laser interstitial therapy for pediatric drug-resistant lesional epilepsy. *Epilepsia* 2015, 56(10): 1590-8.

Marnet D, Devaux B, Chassoux F, *et al.* Surgical resection of focal cortical dysplasias in the central region. *Neurochirurgie* 2008, 54: 399-408.

Marusic P, Najm IM, Ying Z, *et al.* Focal cortical dysplasias in eloquent cortex: functional characteristics and correlation with MRI and histopathologic changes. *Epilepsia* 2002; 43: 27-32.

Mathon B, Clemenceau S, Carpentier A. Intraoperative ultrasound shear-wave *elastography J Clin Med*, 2021; 10(5): 1049.

Mullatti N, Landré E, Mellerio C, *et al.* Stereotactic thermocoagulation for insular epilepsy: lessons from successes and failures. *Epilepsia* 2019, 60: 1565-79.

Ostergard TA, Miller JP. Surgery for epilepsy in the primary motor cortex: A critical review. *Epilepsy Behav* 2019; 91: 13-9.

Palmini A, Gambardella A, Andermann F, *et al.* Intrinsic epileptogenicity of human dysplastic cortex as suggested by corticography and surgical results. *Ann Neurol* 1995; 37: 476-87.

Pessoa L. Understanding brain networks and brain organization. *Phys Life Rev* 2014; 11(3): 400-35.

Pondal-Sordo M, Diosy D, Téllez-Zenteno JF, Girvin JP, Wiebe S. Epilepsy surgery involving the sensory-motor cortex. *Brain* 2006; 129: 3307-14.

Quadri S.A, Waqas M, Khan I, *et al.* High-intensity focused ultrasound: past, present and future in neurosurgery. *Neurosurg Focus* 2018, 44(2): E16,1-9.

Rowland N.C, Englot D.J, Cage T.A, Sughrue M.E, Barbaro N.M, Chang E.F. A meta-analysis of predictors of seizure freedom in the surgical management of focal cortical dysplasia. *J Neurosurg* 2012; 116: 1035-41.

Sacino M.F. Ho C.Y, Murnick J, Tsushida T, *et al.* Intraoperative MRI-guided resection of focal cortical dysplasia in pediatric patients: technique and outcomes. *J Neurosurg Ped* 2016; 17(6): 672-8.

Sacino M.F, Ho C.Y, Whitehead M.T, *et al.* Repeat surgery for focal cortical dysplasias in children: indications and outcomes. *J Neurosurg Ped* 2017; 19(2): 174-81.

Sarkis RA, Jehi LE, Bingaman WE, Najm IM. Surgical outcome following resection of rolandic focal cortical dysplasia. *Epilepsy Res* 2010; 90: 240-7.

Spencer S.S, Schramm J, Wyler A, *et al.* Multiple subpial transection for intractable partial epilepsy: an international meta-analysis. *Epilepsia* 2002; 43(2): 141-5.

Talairach J, Tournoux P, Musolino A, Missir O. Stereotaxic exploration in frontal epilepsy [Review]. *Adv Neurol* 1992; 57: 651-88.

Vitali P, Minati, L, D'Incerti L, *et al.* Functional MRI in malformations of cortical development: activation of dysplastic tissue and functional reorganization. *J. Neuroimaging* 2008; 18: 296-305.

Wagstyl K, Whitaker K, Raznahan A, *et al.* Atlas of lesion locations and postsurgical seizure freedom in focal cortical dysplasia: a MELD study. *Epilepsia* 2022; 63: 61-74.

Wellmer J. Lesion focused radiofrequency thermocoagulation of bottom-of-sulcus focal cortical dysplasia type IIb: Conceptual considerations with regard to the epileptogenic zone. *Epil Res.* 2018; 142: 143-8.

CHAPTER

23. Surgery for FCD in children

Georg Dorfmüller

Key points

- In addition to seizure relief, epilepsy surgery in infants and children has an additional positive effect on recognitive development and behavior.
- In infants and young toddlers under the age of 2 years pathologies responsible for very early epilepsy onset are mostly visible on structural MRI
- In multilobar FCD, surgical disconnection may be the preferred technique to avoid removing a very large amount of brain tissue, thus reducing complications, particularly in very young children
- Resection boundaries or line of disconnection will be in many cases adjusted during surgery, taking into account the electrodes involved in seizure generation, the anatomical structures within and surrounding the epileptic lesion/tissue, the macroscopic aspect of the cortex, intraoperative ECoG epileptiform patterns and nearby eloquent areas
- Surgery of children with FCD I can be challenging, because preoperative MRI and macroscopic aspect of the presumed dysplastic brain tissue are less clear. Decision on the margins of the resection or disconnection will be based on non-invasive and invasive EEG data and, occasionally, on functional imaging studies.
- Repeat surgery in children previously operated for FCD should be systematically considered when seizures persist or reoccur.

Introduction

Among the causes of drug-resistant epilepsy in children, FCD is the prevailing pathologic substrate, presenting mostly from the first two years of life on (Harvey *et al.*, 2008). The negative consequences of uncontrolled epilepsy, particularly during the critical period of brain maturation in early childhood, have led to a growing interest and focus, which is reflected by a worldwide growing number of sites offering a comprehensive pediatric epilepsy surgery program. Its main intentions are to guide eligible candidates without delay to a presurgical evaluation process and to provide adapted surgical treatment options. Early successful surgery that significantly reduces or eliminates seizure burden will enable an improved neurodevelopment and reverse the psychosocial impact thus far. Furthermore, published data have consistently confirmed that achieving seizure freedom is more likely in children with a shorter duration of epilepsy.

Patients with cortical dysplasia constitute approximately 14% of all patients undergoing epilepsy surgery (Mathern *et al.*, 2009) but this proportion is considerably higher in children, being the most frequent etiology of epilepsy surgery cases. In previous larger pediatric multicenter series, resection of the epileptogenic zone revealed cortical dysplasia in about 40% of the operated children and even 60% in the age group under 4 years-of-age, reflecting the very early manifestation of uncontrolled seizures in this pathology (Harvey *et al.*, 2008, Blümcke *et al.*, 2017).

Differences between surgery for FCD in children vs. adults

The foremost difference distinguishing surgery for FCD and other etiologies of focal drug-resistant epilepsy in infants and children when compared to adults is the additional positive effect of successful surgery with seizure relief on their cognitive development and behavior. As a general rule, the shorter the delay from seizure onset to the time of surgery during childhood, the better will be the cognitive and behavioral outcome when surgery is successful and drugs can be withdrawn.

According to the ILAE multicenter survey on pediatric epilepsy surgery cases in 2004, 46% of the children had seizure onset within the first year of life, and 68% within the first 3 years (Harvey *et al.*, 2008). Whereas a small FCD can become symptomatic with focal seizures at any time during childhood, adolescence or even adulthood, large FCD on a lobar, multilobar or hemispheric scale will clinically manifest with daily seizures in infancy or early childhood (**see Table 1**). Moreover, it has been confirmed that cortical dysplasia occupying a larger part of the brain that presents with early and frequent seizures has a deleterious effect on the cognitive and behavioral development that could be considerably improved if early surgery is able to achieve seizure freedom (Klein *et al.*, 2000, Freitag & Tuxhorn *et al.*, 2005, Berg 2012, Kimura *et al.*, 2014, 2019).

Table 1

Age characteristics of pediatric epilepsy surgery patients for the 2004 ILAE survey

Children 4 years or less were more likely to: undergo large resective operations (hemispherectomy and multilobar procedures); have cortical dysplasia, hemimegalencephaly, and TSC as their etiology; have daily seizures. By comparison, children 8–18 years were more likely to undergo lobar and focal resections for tumors, cortical dysplasia, and hippocampal sclerosis. Modified from: Harvey AS *et al.* Defining the spectrum of international practice in pediatric epilepsy surgery patients. Epilepsia 49: 146-155, 2008

	Birth to 4 years	Over 4 – 8 years	Over 8 – 12 years	Over 12 – 18 years
Cortical dysplasia ($p < 0.0001$)				
Hemimegalencephaly	23%	0%	0%	0%
Hemispheric CD	17%	13%	11%	2%
Multilobar CD	26%	18%	15%	13%
Lobar/focal CD	34%	68%	74%	85%

Presurgical evaluation of pediatric surgical candidates with FCD and drug-resistant epilepsy

Once drug-resistance in epilepsy of presumed focal onset is confirmed, the process of presurgical evaluation will bring together all clinical, electrophysiological and structural imaging data, and if necessary and available, certain functional imaging examinations, in order to decide if this phase one evaluation will be sufficient to directly propose (or reject) curative resective epilepsy surgery. It may also conclude that invasive EEG is needed in the next step to confirm and refine the hypothesis of a suspected epileptogenic focus and its localization.

There are two main age-dependent limitations in the presurgical evaluation process in children:
- Functional MRI, for lateralization and localization of language, requires active participation of the awake child, and therefore usually cannot be applied in children below school age and those with an important developmental impairment.
- If invasive EEG is necessary, Stereo-EEG cannot be proposed for infants and young toddlers under the age of about two years, since a minimum bone thickness of 2mm is required to firmly hold the anchor bolts of the intracerebral electrodes.

Beside the option to perform structural MRI, FDG-PET or magnetoencephalography (MEG) under sedation or general anesthesia in the very young or non-cooperating children (Schwartz 2008, Juhasz 2020), alternative functional imaging evaluations have been recently evaluated, such as fMRI motor cortex activation during passive hand and foot movement (Choudri 2015), passive language mapping in MEG during sleep (Van Poppel 2012), or the use of resting state MRI, even under anesthesia, for different functional pathways and localization of functional units, such as the language network (Pur 2021).

In infants and young toddlers under the age of 2 years, unable to undergo Stereo-EEG recording, the necessity for an invasive EEG study is less likely since the pathologies responsible for a very early epilepsy-onset are mostly visible on structural MRI. This will allow to compare the lesion and its anatomical extent with the result of a long-term Video-EEG, that should include several seizures. We systematically add an FDG-PET scan to our routine presurgical evaluation protocol. Other non-invasive studies currently in use may be added if further confirmation of the hypothesis of the EZ and its localization is required.

If resective surgery has been decided after this non-invasive evaluation, intraoperative ECoG can be an additional option to explore the lesion, its boundaries and even the cortical areas beyond, in order to define the extent of the interictal epileptic activity and guide the necessary amount of cortical resection (**see Figure 1 and the text below**).

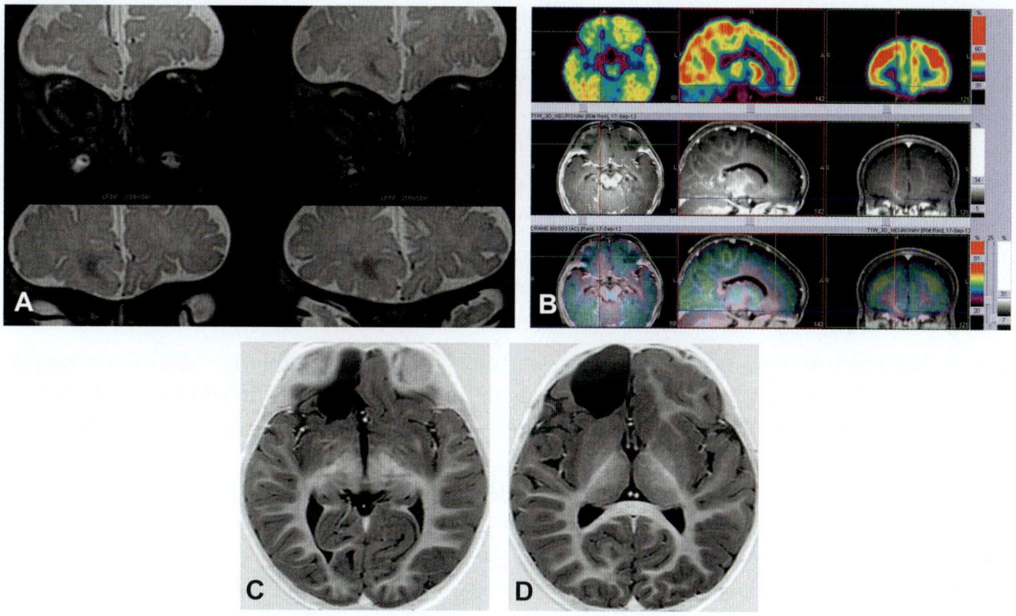

Figure 1

Frontobasal resection

Infant with seizure onset at 3 months, A. Right frontobasal dysplastic lesion well demarcated on the coronal T2 MRI, with overlapping focal hypometabolism on FDG-PET (B) and a corresponding seizure onset on prolonged Video-EEG. Focal surgery of the lesion with intraoperative electro-corticography (ECoG) was performed at the age of 10 months, histology of the epileptogenic tissue revealed an FCD IIA. C. MRI (axial T1-IR) control at 3 months postoperatively, demonstrating the resected volume. The young child has been seizure free and without medication for over 5 years, with a normal development.

Only if:

- there turns out to be a major conflict between all non-invasive evaluations as to the approximate localization of the epileptogenic zone,
- repeated MRI remains apparently normal,
- or primary functional cortex is within or in the vicinity of the EZ,
- invasive cortical EEG exploration with a subdural grid of electrodes that can be combined with additional depth electrodes should be considered as the next step.

Beside the direct intracranial recording over a large surface and with a dense distribution of the electrode contacts, this technique allows even in the youngest age group under two years-of-age a reliable localization of the primary motor cortex through cortical electrode stimulation mapping.

Otherwise, we use DTI tractography for motor and visual pathway localization, as well as fMRI under sedation or general anesthesia with passive hand and foot movements. In addition, the central sulcus and primary sensorimotor cortex can be identified intraoperatively using the phase reversal of somatosensory evoked potentials, and with cortical or subcortical stimulation-motor evoked potentials during the surgery, although the latter may be less reliable in very young children due to incomplete myelination and thus a higher threshold of stimulus intensity necessary to evoke motor responses.

When cortical and subcortical language areas are affected, awake surgery can be a valuable option for cooperative children from an age of about 10 years on. It requires a dedicated team of a neurosurgeon, anesthetist, neuropsychologist, and neurophysiologist with a particular expertise for this type of procedure. To achieve the best possible compliance of the child during the surgery, the preparation should include an age-adapted presurgical evaluation and training for this procedure (Balogun *et al.*, 2014, Delion *et al.*, 2015).

Intraoperative electrocorticography recording

This technique which was pioneered by Penfield and Jasper at the Montreal Neurological Institute in the early 1950s (Jasper 1954), allows to perform EEG recording over the exposed cortex during surgery, provided that a previous EEG has demonstrated a sufficient amount of IED. Today, there are principally two electrode types for intraoperative ECoG in use: either a rigid wire set of multiple metal electrodes fixed on a stable frame around the craniotomy, or in the form of a flexible multi-contact strip or grid, as used for extra-operative chronic recording. In addition to the presurgical multimodal evaluation that should have identified the approximate extent of the EZ, the aim of intraoperative ECoG is to obtain further information on the epileptogenicity of the targeted cortex and its vicinity in order to better define the limits of resection (Keene *et al.*, 2000, Yang *et al.*, 2014). This is particularly useful in children explored with non-invasive pre-operative diagnostic methods since they may have a more widespread area of dysplasia than the lesion recognized on MRI. But even for children following SEEG exploration, the refinement of the resection margins can in certain patients be obtained with additional ECoG during surgery.

The recording can be carried out, once the dura is opened and the cortical surface below exposed. A relatively large craniotomy centered over the epileptogenic lesion should be provided, allowing to expose as well cortical areas in the larger vicinity.

Beside the macroscopic identification of anatomical surface landmarks, MRI-based neuronavigation will help localize the preoperatively defined EZ and guide the additional placement of depth electrodes if indicated. The characteristic interictal EEG markers of epileptogenicity are spikes, slow waves and, notably in FCD II, continuous rhythmic or pseudo-rhythmic spike or polyspike patterns (Palmini *et al.*, 1995, Chassoux *et al.*, 2000). More recently, high frequency oscillations of 250-500 Hz during ECoG recording have been found to be an additional and perhaps more specific marker of epileptogenic brain tissue (van't Klooster *et al.*, 2017). Since the quality of the ECoG signal is strongly influenced by the given anesthetic drugs, a specific anesthesia protocol should be applied to avoid signal suppression of the cortical EEG activity.

Once the presurgically defined cortical resection has been realized, a second ECoG recording over the resection margins and beyond can be undertaken, which should confirm the absence of epileptic cortical activity or reveal its persistence. The latter may result in an additional limited cortical resection as long as eloquent cortex is spared.

We always perform the first ECoG following dural opening and before any intradural surgical procedure. This first recording will serve as a baseline for consecutive recordings during the same surgery after a partial or complete brain tissue removal or disconnection. However, the anatomic extension of interictal epileptic EEG activity during this first recording should be interpreted with caution. We frequently have found a normalization of the EEG signal over cortical areas beyond the actual EZ, as preoperatively delineated, once the EZ has been removed, which reflects the larger interictal network beyond the EZ margins. As a consequence, this emphasizes the utility of staged ECoG recordings during a single surgery, in order to avoid tissue removal beyond the minimum necessary and sufficient to obtain seizure-freedom.

Surgical resective and disconnective techniques

Once the anatomo-functional organization of the EZ has been understood, i.e., the area of seizure onset and the early ictal spread in spatiotemporal terms, and its extension delineated, the goal of curative surgery is to remove or, in the cases of large frontal or posterior multilobar FCD extensions, to isolate all epileptogenic tissue through a complete disconnection. Despite a thorough presurgical evaluation, the exact resection boundaries will be in many cases adjusted during surgery. This intraoperative decision process is based on the anatomical structures within and surrounding the the epileptic lesion/tissue, its macroscopic aspect during the resection, and potential nearby eloquent cortex and their corresponding subcortical fibers. Additionally, it can be supported and refined by ECoG mapping during surgery, although its utility is limited by the fact that recording frequent interictal epileptiform activity in general correlates with the area of epileptogenic cortex, but may expand well beyond the EZ proper, i.e., the minimum neuronal network necessary to generate and maintain the seizures.

Surgery for FCD in children can be very different in terms of localization and volume of brain tissue to be removed:

- very limited resections of a single gyrus or even parts of it;
- larger areas of resection within one lobe;

- resection of parts of two or three adjacent lobes, e.g., the paracentral lobule, the fronto-insular junction, the parieto-temporal, parieto-temporo-insular or temporo-occipital junction;
- cerebral lobectomies;
- resection and/or disconnection of two or three cerebral lobes (multilobar surgery proper);
- hemispherotomy.

Hemispherotomy will be indicated in unilateral extensive multilobar cortical dysplasias, when multilobar surgery that can spare eloquent cortex and thus preserve residual function within the affected hemisphere is unlikely to achieve seizure freedom.

The technique of subpial resection (sometimes referred to as endopial resection) is indicated for epileptogenic lesions within a single gyrus, resection in the vicinity of eloquent cortex, and near surface or in-depth sulcal vessels that must be spared to avoid vascular injury-induced functional deficits. This is the case in resections of FCD neighboring or including parts of the primary sensorimotor cortex, the opercular cortex, the insular cortex, where middle cerebral artery branches within the sulci have to be preserved (**Figure 2**). This technique consists in coagulating the vessel-free dome of the targeted gyrus, opening the pia parallel to the adjacent sulci over the surface and resecting subpially the cortex and white matter within this gyrus without surpassing the pial borders and the depth of the

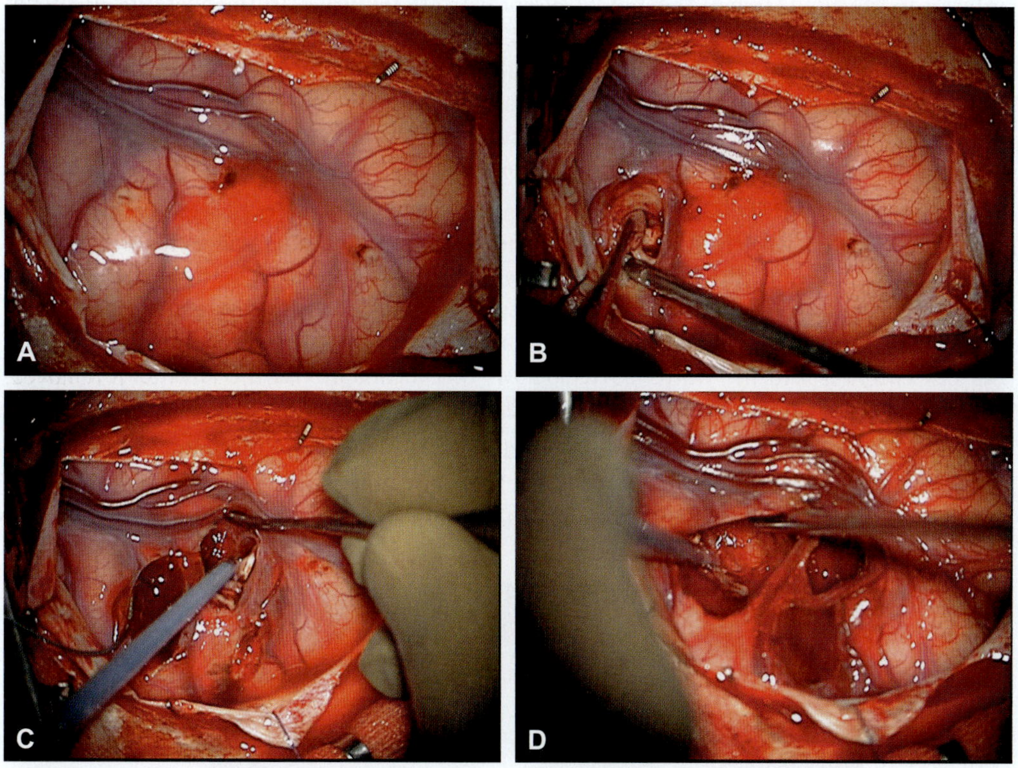

Figure 2

Technique of intervascular subpial resection

Intervascular subpial resection of an FCD confined to parts of the suprasylvian opercular cortex and underlying white matter. The extent of this resection was based on the result of an SEEG having explored the perisylvian and insular cortex of the right hemisphere.

A. Exposition after dural opening, with 3 visible entry points of the former SEEG electrodes. B. Intervascular subpial resection with the cavitron ultrasonic aspirator of the motor opercular cortex until exposition of the underlying insula. C and D. Subpial resection of the parietal operculum just behind, preserving all major superficial and interopercular vessels. The underlying insular cortex was left intact since the FCD was confined to the suprasylvian opercula. This technique significantly reduces the risk of vessel injury, in particular in this case in between the opercular gyri which contain the precentral and central branches of the middle cerebral artery that are ascending to supply the primary sensorimotor and the perirolandic cortex above. Histology confirmed a FCD IIB in the precentral opercular part of the gyrus. An incomplete postoperative hemifacial palsy regressed over the next few weeks.

sulcus. Whether for larger resections, we systematically use the cavitron ultrasonic surgical aspirator with a low setting of vibration amplitude and suction, the dysplastic cortical tissue can best be separated from the pial border with the aid of a blunt Penfield dissector. This allows better preservation and quality of the removed tissue samples for pathology analysis and research purposes.

When surgery of a larger epileptogenic lesion is required, the extent of resection will include several gyri and sulci. Each sulcal septum including smaller intrasulcal vessels is coagulated. Major arteries as well as larger cortical veins over the convexity that may drain cerebral territories beyond the area to resect have to be spared.

When the EZ comprises only parts of a cerebral lobe, the surgical technique remains in general a complete resection of the epileptogenic tissue, whereas disconnective techniques are not considered (**Figure 1**). Only for the large frontal lobe can a less-than-lobar surgical disconnection be reasonable, in particular, when the EZ comprises the anterior and basal frontal lobe, including the superior, middle and inferior frontal gyrus. In that case, an anterior frontal disconnection can be proposed that spares the posteriorly located premotor cortex and the supplementary motor area. The disconnection for a complete or anterior frontal lobe disconnection is in a coronal orientation, starting over the convexity downward to the pia over the dura that covers the posterior part of the anterior skull base, just anterior to the main stem of the middle cerebral artery (**Figure 3**). If the posterior premotor part of the frontal lobe is included in the EZ, the precentral gyrus containing the primary motor cortex has to be clearly identified with intraoperative MRI-based neuronavigation and the neurosurgeon's macroscopic identification of the related gyral, sulcal and vascular landmarks. But this should be additionally supported by electrophysiological techniques, such as direct motor cortex stimulation and/or somatosensory evoked potentials for central sulcus localization (Simon, 2013).

In several children with frontal lobe FCD, the epileptogenic lesion can extend into anterior parts of the insula. In these cases, following disconnection or resection of the frontal lobe, the anterior insula can be directly accessed below its pial covering and resected in an antero-posterior direction. Attention has to be paid in remaining within the cortical layer and not entering into the white matter below. This technique has the advantage of minimizing the risk of injury to the overlying middle cerebral artery branches.

If the FCD responsible for the seizures includes two or even three cerebral lobes, surgical disconnection may be the preferred technique, similar to the indication for hemispherotomy in children with a vast but unilateral multifocal epilepsy. This will avoid removing a very large

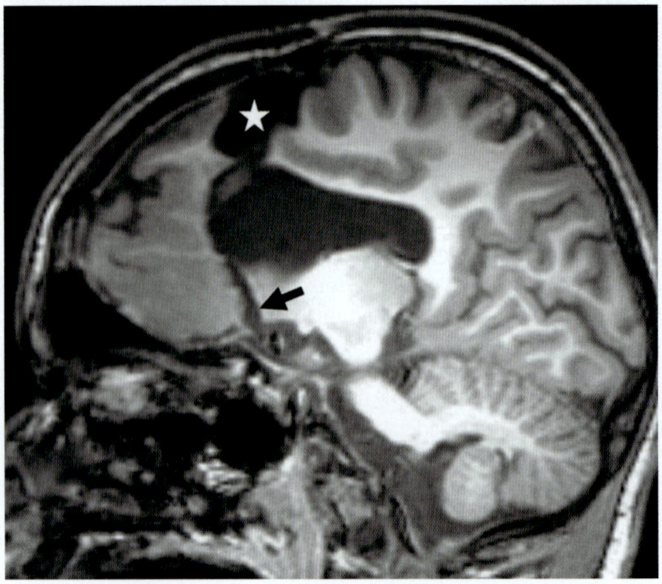

Figure 3

Frontal disconnection

Postoperative T1 MRI in the sagittal plane showing an anterior frontal lobe disconnection in a 7-year-old child with frontal FCD IIA (anterior disconnected part to the left) and drug-resistant epilepsy from infancy on. A certain amount of cortical and subcortical resection (white asterisk) in the beginning of the procedure is helpful to better visualize the deeper part of the disconnection downward to the posterior part of the anterior skull base (black arrow). For all disconnection procedures, either frontal or posterior, it is essential to additionally perform a partial callosotomy along the otherwise disconnected lobe(s).

amount of brain tissue, thus reducing the size of craniotomy, volume of blood loss, duration of surgery, and related complications. This is particularly important for very young children who are by far more often candidates for these extensive surgeries.

On the other end of the age spectrum, completed maturation of functional cortical and subcortical pathways in older children and adolescents may be a contraindication for multilobar disconnections, proposing rather surgical procedures of more limited cortical resections.

Going for resective or disconnective surgery, one must have a clear idea of the approximate volume and boundaries of the EZ, including cortex and subcortical white matter, which should have been elucidated by the non-invasive and, in part, invasive presurgical evaluation. This also includes a meticulous study of the structural MRI to evaluate all potential neurological and vascular risks.

If an SEEG has been part of the presurgical evaluation, a former CT scan after electrode implantation should be included and fused with the MRI that will serve for the intraoperative neuronavigation. This will help the surgeon localize all former electrodes and their contacts within and at the border of the EZ, so that he can better appreciate the three-dimensional extent of the volume to be removed.

Importantly, even when the results of a preceding invasive EEG study have supported the initial hypothesis and helped define the EZ, the exact borders of the epileptogenic cortex necessary to remove are not always as clear. This lies in the nature of the available techniques of invasive exploration, either with grid electrodes covering a large area of cortical surface or with multiple SEEG electrodes exploring more selectively larger cortical areas from surface to depth. The intraoperative decision where to define the margins of resection or line of disconnection is principally based on the identification of all electrode contacts within and bordering the EZ, as has been decided on preoperatively, taking as well into account potential eloquent cortex that should be preserved. But this decision may be furthermore modified by the surgeon's macroscopic appreciation of the pathological brain tissue which will be included or not in the volume of resection/disconnection, and delimitations related to anatomic landmarks. In addition, intraoperative ECoG can serve as a useful tool, in particular for FCD giving a characteristic interictal EEG pattern of continuous, rhythmic or pseudo-rhythmic spike or polyspike patterns that are a strong biomarker for underlying FCD, particularly of type II (see paragraph on ECoG above).

Intraoperative real-time imaging control

Besides the routine use of intraoperative neuronavigation, based on a recent MRI, real-time image-based supports used in recent years are intraoperative MRI and ultrasound. Following the intended resection, these additional diagnostic tools are helpful to exclude or to discover suspected dysplastic tissue at the border of the cavity, thus improving the completeness of resection and improving seizure outcome (Sacino *et al.*, 2016, Akeret *et al.*, 2018). Whereas an MRI within a dedicated operating room is only available in few centers, requires MRI-compatible anesthesia equipment, and the time-consuming procedure of moving the patient under general anesthesia into the scan and back, ultrasound systems are less expensive, mobile and easily applicable by the surgeon himself. As a more recent development, shear-wave elastography is an ultrasound technique that examines the elasticity values of the cerebral tissue and seems to be superior to standard ultrasound which examines the echogenicity in order to differentiate normal brain tissue from intracerebral lesions, such as FCD (Mathon *et al.*, 2021).

How to define the extent of resection in FCD1

Surgery for FCD I is more challenging for several reasons.

In children carrying this type of cortical dysplasia, the lesion is radiographically more likely to be normal or to demonstrate more subtle or diffuse and ill-defined abnormalities as compared to FCD II, even on high-resolution MRI and with a specific epilepsy imaging protocol. Therefore, children with FCD I more likely will be explored by invasive EEG during their presurgical evaluation. During surgery, these lesions are more difficult to identify based on their macroscopic aspect, and it has been shown that surgery has a lower likelihood to achieve seizure freedom (Krsek *et al.*, 2008, 2009a). There is consequently a higher tendency for children with this FCD type to undergo repeat exploration and/or repeat surgery.

The surgeon facing FCD I can therefore rely less on the preoperative MRI during intraoperative neuronavigation concerning the lesion and also less on the macroscopic aspect of the presumed dysplastic brain tissue. Instead, the decision on the actual margins of the resection or disconnection will be more based on all non-invasive and invasive EEG data, and perhaps the result of additional consistent functional imaging studies.

When the FCD is neighboring or within eloquent cortex

Beside the anatomical identification of the functional cortex and related subcortical fiber tracts on high-resolution MRI, the most reliable methods nowadays to obtain a functional cartography in children are electrical stimulation mapping during chronic invasive EEG recording, fMRI and MEG (Jayakar *et al.*, 2018). There are in general the following surgical options when the FCD is neighboring or even implying eloquent cortex, such as the primary motor cortex, language network, verbal memory-related mesial structures, or post-geniculate visual fiber tracts and cortex.

• Function-sparing resection

Based on the structural and functional imaging data, the extent of resection/disconnection will be partial or subtotal when compared to the total EZ volume, in order to preserve function and avoid neurological sequelae. In consequence, the probability of seizure freedom will be inferior to complete resection and secondary anti-seizure drug withdrawal unlikely.

• Awake surgery

In children from 10 years and above who are cooperating and without a considerable cognitive impairment, the technique of awake surgery can be considered (see above). The main indication is intraoperative language mapping, but motor function can also be closely monitored to allow a maximum resection of the dysplastic tissue while preserving function.

• Multiple subpial transections

Completeness of resection of the dysplastic cortex constituting the EZ is an important factor for long-term seizure freedom. In turn, incomplete resection has been confirmed to be a strong predictor of unfavorable seizure outcome, and one of the main reasons is the intentional avoidance of complete resection when eloquent cortex is located within or in the imminent vicinity of the EZ (Krsek *et al.*, 2009b). In this situation, multiple subpial transsections (MST) which is a palliative technique that was initially proposed by Morrell in 1989 can be proposed alone or in addition to cortical resection, to partially inactivate the eloquent area and to prevent at the same time undesirable and irreversible loss of function (**Figure 4**). It consists of performing multiple linear and parallel intracortical cuts perpendicular to the cortical surface, which will interrupt the horizontal interneuronal connections but will leave the vertical columnar arrangement of the central cortex intact, thus disrupting the seizure spread along the horizontal plane and preserving at the same time cortical function. Obviously, dysplastic cortex treated with this technique will lead to an incomplete inactivation of seizure onset and propagation, and all published results thus far have reported a seizure reduction but are inferior as compared to complete resection of the EZ. Nevertheless, MST may present a complementary and safe procedure to further improve seizure outcome when loss of function is not an option (Benifla *et al.*, 2006, Hufnagel *et al.*, 1997).

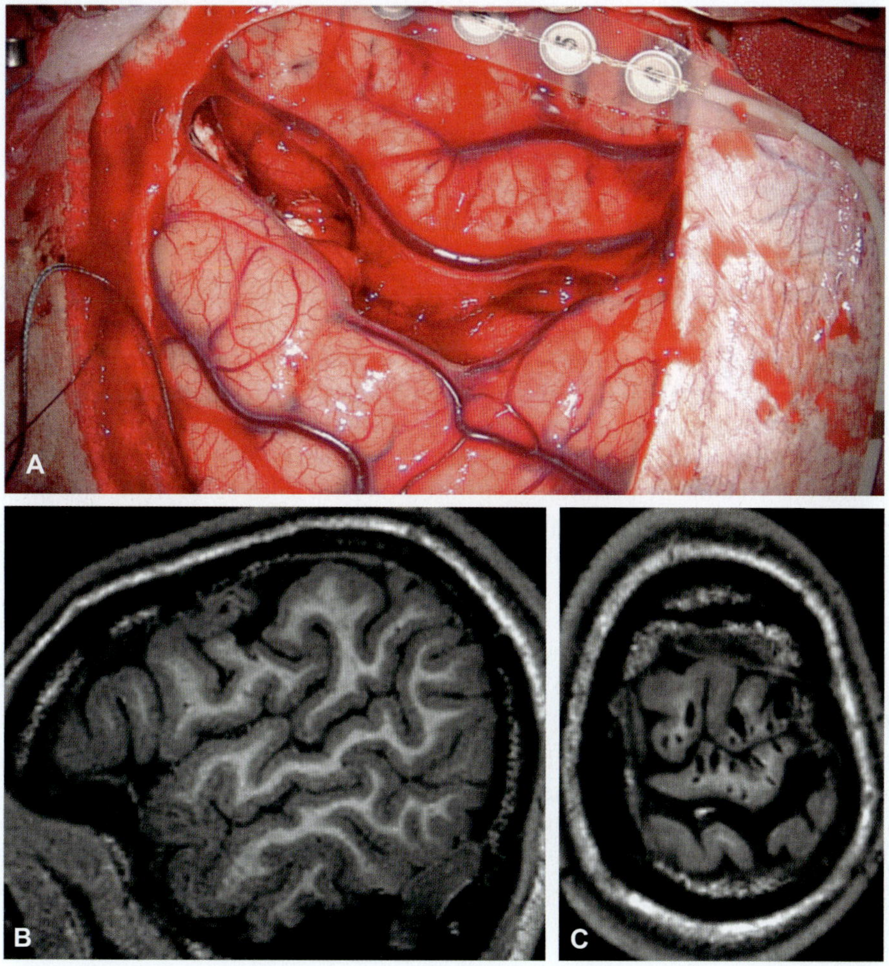

Figure 4

FCD of the primary sensorimotor cortex

Refractory focal epilepsy of the left primary sensorimotor cortex as confirmed with SEEG. A. Intraoperative photograph: following intraoperative electro-corticography, the postcentral gyrus is resected while exposing the central sulcus, followed by multiple subpial transections of the precentral gyrus and the posterior supplementary motor area. Histology revealed FCD IIA B. and C. T1 MRI of this patient at 3 months after surgery: the sagittal image (B) shows the focal resection of the postcentral gyrus and the axial plane, (C) the traces of the multiple subpial transections, perpendicular to the long axis of the gyri.

• Complete EZ resection including eloquent cortex

This will first imply a thorough discussion with the patient and his family, weighing the burden of persisting seizures and continued drug treatment against a new neurological deficit, the chances of improvement and its functional consequences. According to the result of this discussion, a joint decision may be taken to include eloquent but epileptogenic cortex in the planned resection. Evidently, a complete surgical removal of the EZ has a higher chance to achieve seizure freedom and subsequently drug arrest. However, the patient will most probably sustain the expected neurological deficit, with a variable degree of amelioration over time, depending also on the age at surgery.

Surgery-related complications in children operated for FCD

As for cortical and intracerebral resection procedures for other epilepsy-related pathologies and patient age groups, there are several types of complications one has to be aware of that are listed below (Behrens *et al.*, 1997, Bjellvi *et al.*, 2015):

- Infection
- Postoperative hematoma
- Postoperative edema
- Vascular accidents:
  - vessels within the resection volume
  - vessels outside the resection volume

- Functional neurological deficits
- Subdural hygroma
- Hydrocephalus

Risk of surgery-related infection, such as wound infection and meningitis and postoperative bleeding into the resection cavity are general complications that may occur in all types of neurosurgical interventions. They depend on factors such as duration of the procedure, the individual patient's immune defense, potential underlying coagulopathies, the quality of surgical hemostasis, among others.

More specific to the surgery of FCD are edema formation and vascular accidents, which may be caused by impairment of the venous drainage and from damaged arterial supply. These complications may be prevented by systematically studying the vascular anatomy within and adjacent to the area of the EZ before surgery on MR or CT angiography sequences. This will help to decide during surgery if a particular vessel within the cortex to be removed can be sacrificed or should be preserved? In the case of larger veins overlying the cortical surface, cortical resection should be performed separately on both sides of the vein, thus preserving it. Beside the focal surgical technique of subpial resection (**Figure 2**), disconnecting techniques for large EZ of lobar or multilobar extension offer a major advantage: most of the arterial supply and venous drainage within the EZ can be preserved without difficulty, since the process of resection will only concern the limited area of the disconnection cleft over the cerebral convexity and be then further pursued subpially toward the skull base or the midline, leaving all larger vessels at the deep line of the disconnection behind an intact pial envelope (**Figures 3, 5 and 6**).

Neurological deficits due to cortical or subcortical fiber damage have been discussed above in the case of proximity of eloquent zones and the dysplastic cortex. Beside the aforementioned vascular accidents, unintentional extension of the area to be removed towards eloquent cortex and/or corresponding subcortical fibers may be the cause. Here again, it is essential to study before surgery the functional anatomy neighboring the epileptogenic tissue to

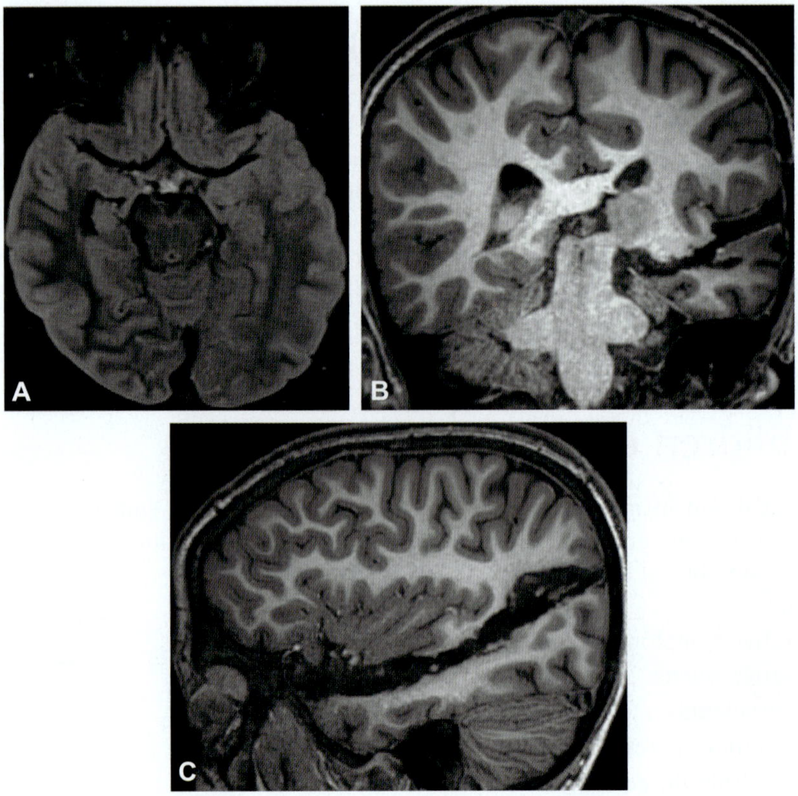

Figure 5

Temporo-Occipital Disconnection

Child with left-sided drug-resistant focal epilepsy from the age of 2 years on, with concomitant stagnation of the cognitive and psychosocial development. A. Preoperative Axial T2 FLAIR MRI demonstrating left temporo-occipital extension of a supposed cortical dysplasia, SEEG confirmed the extent of the EZ comprising both lobes but sparing the parietal and insular cortex. This child underwent disconnection of the left temporal and occipital lobe. T1 MRI 3 months after surgery, in the coronal (B) and the sagittal (C) plane demonstrating the line of disconnection. Histology revealed an FCD IIA, surgery resulted in seizure freedom and a spectacular improvement for cognitive and psychosocial functions.

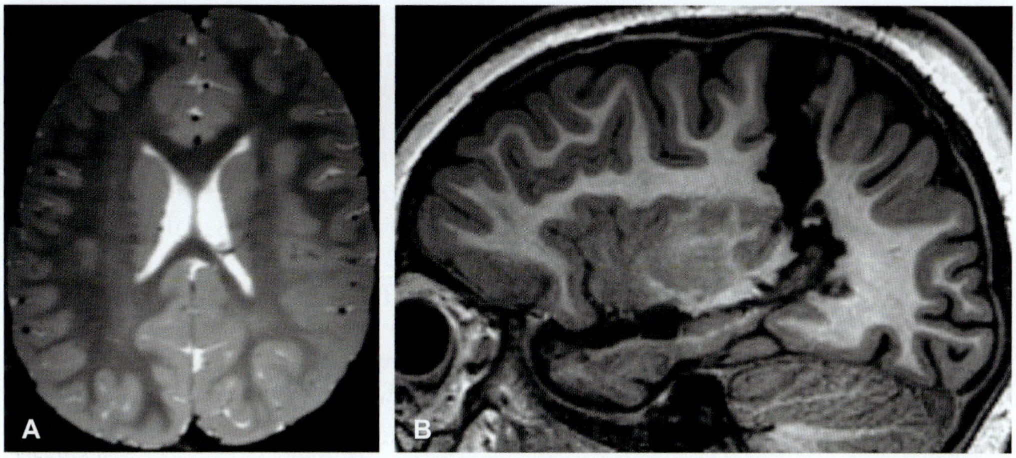

Figure 6

Temporo-parietal-occipital (TPO or posterior quadrant) disconnection

A. Axial T2 MRI in a 4-year-old child demonstrating left parietal and occipital cortical dysplasia. Seizure-onset was at 7 months, with concomitant developmental delay. An SEEG exploration found the left temporal lobe to be in addition part of the epileptogenic zone; B. Sagittal T1 MRI showing the trace of a posterior disconnection comprising the temporal, occipital and parietal lobe, Histology confirmed FCD IIA, postoperative seizure freedom paralleled with developmental improvement.

be removed. Furthermore, epilepsy surgery today takes routine use of image-based intra-operative neuronavigation, allowing to visualize at any moment the structural and functional images during the entire procedure.

Postoperative subdural hygroma formation may occur in larger cerebral volume resection and do not pose in itself a problem. They should be followed, however, by imaging controls since in a few cases there can be a tendency for growth over time, subsequently necessitating surgical evacuation, together with external or subduroperitoneal drainage. Postoperative hydrocephalus can occur when the ventricular system has been opened during surgery, allowing blood to enter the ventricles, with subsequent clot formation and potential impairment of CSF circulation. An external ventricular drainage may be indicated during the first postoperative days and in case of persisting shunt dependence a permanent ventriculoperitoneal shunt.

Repeat surgery for FCD in children

Repeat surgery in children previously operated for FCD should be systematically considered when seizures persist or reoccur. In children with proven incomplete resection of the epileptogenic lesion on postoperative MRI which does not imply eloquent cortex, and a postoperative scalp Video-EEG that is compatible with the remaining epileptogenic lesion, a second complementary surgery should be considered and will in many instances improve the outcome.

In other clinical settings, a more extended than the originally planned and performed surgery may be considered. In specific cases, an invasive EEG study should be either repeated or firstly performed if the first surgery was based on non-invasive data, with an electrode implantation hypothesis that should cover the areas adjacent to the first resection but as well specific anatomo-functional remote landmarks that may be involved in the actual seizure propagation. Other non-invasive studies that had not been realized during the first presurgical evaluation might be necessary to add information before a planned invasive EEG or repeat surgery (Muthaffar *et al.*, 2017, Sacino *et al.*, 2017).

If the reason for incomplete resection during the first surgery had been nearby located eloquent cortex, the secondary treatment strategy may be more complex. The remaining seizure burden and continuing medical treatment have to be balanced against a potential functional deficit following a second, more extensive resection. Other options, such as awake surgery or the additional palliative technique of multiple subpial transections may be considered as well to improve outcome (see above). Each option and its respective potential consequences have to be thoroughly evaluated with the patient and his family, in order to come to a common consent in favor of or against a second surgery.

Minimal invasive surgical techniques

• SEEG-guided RF thermocoagulation

This technique was first reported by the epilepsy surgery group in Lyon (Guenot *et al.*, 2004) and can be proposed during or at the end of a video-SEEG recording, where one or several spatially limited foci of seizure-onset have been identified, or rhythmic spike or polyspike activities, typically observed during the interictal EEG over the electrodes in the direct proximity of FCD II, have been frequently recorded.

The idea is to produce multiple bipolar radiofrequency thermocoagulations (RF-TC) of the electrode contacts identified to cover the indicated zone by delivering an adequate current that results in a coagulation of the targeted brain tissue. Each of the thus produced small ovoid necrotic lesions measures about 4 to 6 mm, clearly visible on a later MRI control.

Before and a couple of minutes after these SEEG-guided thermocoagulations, an EEG of the concerned electrodes can be recorded to confirm the decrease or disappearance of the spike activity.

The advantage of this technique is twice: No additional RF-TC probe insertion is necessary, since all SEEG electrodes are in place at the end of the recording period and before removing all electrodes, thus not adding any additional morbidity. Furthermore, eloquent cortex can be located through an electrical stimulation protocol before deciding which electrode contacts to use for thermocoagulation. In selected cases, the video-SEEG can be continued after the realization of the thermocoagulations, to study their effect on the entire epileptic network as reflected by the SEEG, and perhaps to propose a second series of coagulations in a next step, before definitive electrode ablation.

With respect to a permanent seizure relief, the results have been in general disappointing so far. But it has been demonstrated that several patients with anatomically very confined FCD or with nodular subcortical heterotopias may be better candidates for curative purpose. On the other side, it has been shown that a positive response following RF-TC, i.e., significant seizure reduction or arrest over a period of several months or longer, indicates that a subsequent resection of the indicated epileptogenic zone has a higher likelihood to achieve seizure-freedom (Bourdillon *et al.*, 2017, Cossu *et al.*, 2017). This technique thus may be indicated in two clinical settings: a curative purpose in patients with very focal FCD, in particular when difficult to approach or located close to eloquent cortex, subcortical targets such as nodular heterotopias, and as a presurgical test with a positive predictive value for a favorable outcome following subsequent surgical resection.

Most published series on SEEG-guided RFTC until now have been performed in adult patients. Our own recent series has confirmed the feasibility and safety aspects of this technique and found a positive predictive value for a favorable later surgical outcome in those who had a transient positive response following SEEG-guided thermocoagulations (Chipaux *et al.*, 2019) (**Figure 7**).

• Stereotactic RF Thermocoagulation

The more classical approach to focal RFTC of epileptogenic lesions such as FCD is by stereotactic means independent of SEEG-recording. The stereotactic approach for functional neurosurgery in the human had been first developed and propagated by Spiegel and Wycis in the late 1940s (Spiegel *et al.*, 1948). Stereotactic RFTC in drug-resistant epilepsy has been used for well circumscribed but difficult to access epileptogenic lesions, such as FCD II of different locations such as bottom-of-sulcus-lesions or within the insular cortex, periventricular nodular heterotopias, or hypothalamic hamartomas (Mullatti *et al.*, 2019, Kameyama *et al.*, 2016, Wellmer *et al.*, 2014).

In contrast to coagulation lesions produced by SEEG electrodes, the TC probe is rigid, has a larger diameter, and a longer probe tip. According to the probe type, monopolar or bipolar coagulations can be realized, being able to produce larger volumes of coagulation necrosis and thus cover larger targets.

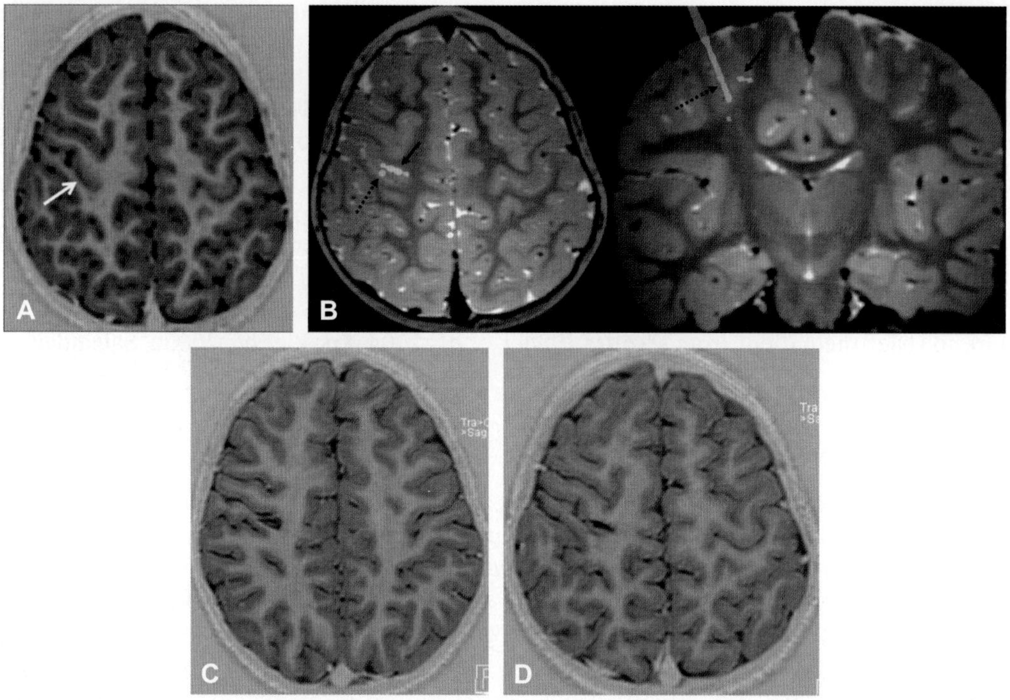

Figure 7

SEEG-guided radiofrequency thermocoagulation

6y-old child with a radiologically diagnosed right central FCD of the primary motor cortex primarily concerning the hand area. Drug-resistant epilepsy with onset at 3 years and recent progressive clumsiness of the left hand.

A. T1-IR MRI showing a subtle FCD in the right precentral gyrus bordering the central sulcus (white arrow). An SEEG was performed to confirm the seizure-onset and to perform a motor function mapping. Several contacts of three of the SEEG electrodes were covering this lesion and the surrounding epileptogenic cortex:

B. Fusion of a CT scan following SEEG electrode placement with the preoperative MRI, T2 sequence in the axial (left) and coronal (right) plane, showing two of the three electrodes implied in the seizure onset and immediate propagation, one in an oblique direction (black dotted arrow) and one in an orthogonal direction along the dysplastic segment of the precentral gyrus (black arrow). Bipolar RF-induced thermal lesions were performed through all involved contacts of the three electrodes within the epileptogenic zone, covering the MRI-visible cortical dysplasia and its vicinity.

C and D. The MRI at 3 months post lesioning shows the very focal destruction within this motor cortex FCD. The child has been seizure-free for more than 5 years and has a normal development, but remains under anti-seizure drug treatment. A thermocoagulation-induced temporary worsening of her preexisting left-hand paresis recovered within a few months and has since further improved.

• MR-guided stereotactic laser ablation

MRI-guided stereotactic laser ablation (SLA) is a recently developed minimally invasive technique in neurosurgery. It allows to precisely destruct a defined intracerebral tissue volume by photo-thermically induced irreversible cell injury, by means of a stereotactically inserted fiberoptic laser probe to the target. The process of photo-thermic tissue coagulation is performed under quantitative real-time thermometry in the MRI. The exact extent of ablation can thus be estimated and tissue damage adjacent to the target volume avoided. In children, SLA has been successfully applied in recent years to different types of solitary low-grade or high-grade brain tumors of supra- or infratentorial location, and to distinct epileptogenic lesions (Fayed *et al.*, 2018, Arocho-Quinones *et al.*, 2020, Zeller *et al.*, 2021). This technique seems to be of particular interest in difficult-to-approach-lesions, such as hypothalamic hamartomas associated with refractory epilepsy, which represents the most frequent indication for the SLA approach in pediatric epilepsy cases thus far (Curry *et al.*, 2018, Xu *et al.*, 2018, Hoppe *et al.*, 2020).

Application of SLA for focal cortical dysplasia in children has been reported as well (Hale *et al.*, 2019, Lewis *et al.*, 2015). In the series of Lewis *et al.* on SLA treatment in 17 children with a drug-resistant lesional epilepsy, 11 patients had focal cortical dysplasia as the underlying substrate. After a mean follow-up of 16 months, only 36% became seizure-free and 45% had a favorable outcome, which reflects a result inferior to previously published series on open resection for FCD.

For pediatric as for adult focal epilepsy, more data from larger prospective studies focusing on surgery-related morbidity and long-term outcome rates have to be awaited in order to definitely assess its role as compared to open surgery. For FCD as for other epileptogenic lesions, it has been well demonstrated that incomplete resection is a strong predictor of failure to relief the patient from seizures (Hader *et al.*, 2004, Krsek *et al.*, 2009b, Salemdawod *et al.*, 2021).

Conclusion

Focal cortical dysplasia is the most common cause of drug-resistant focal epilepsy in children, more frequently found in an extratemporal location and with a greater variability in size as compared to adults. The majority will present with seizure onset under the age of two years, and multilobar or hemispheric surgery for very large or multifocal cortical dysplasia is mostly performed in infants and young toddlers with very early onset of daily seizures.

High-resolution MRI and standardized epilepsy imaging protocols will identify the dysplastic cortical and subcortical lesions in most cases but the exact extent and boundaries may remain unclear, which is more frequently the case for FCD I. Invasive EEG will be indicated if the MRI and video-EEG recording of the seizures, as well as additional non-invasive studies will conclude with contradictory results as to the approximate anatomical localization of the seizure focus, or if eloquent cortex in the vicinity requires a functional mapping with intracranial electrode stimulation.

The greater variability in size of FCD in children is also reflected by a large spectrum of surgical techniques applied to this pathology, from subpial resections within a single dysplastic gyrus, to tailored disconnective approaches being the preferred technique in the youngest age group with FCD of multilobar extension, that will reduce surgery-related morbidity as compared to complete tissue removal, but maintaining the same results on seizure outcome.

The particularity of surgery for FCD with refractory epilepsy in children is the developmental aspect: Although frequent seizures from early childhood on will have a deleterious effect on the cognitive and behavioral development during the ongoing period of brain maturation, early successful surgery with a shorter delay from seizure-onset will have a positive influence on the further psychosocial development of the child. Repeat presurgical evaluation in case of persisting or recurring seizures, even when the child has improved form the time before surgery, should be systematically considered and a repeat surgery may lead to seizure freedom and additional cognitive improvements.

Recent minimal invasive surgical techniques applied for FCD, such as SEEG-guided radiofrequency thermocoagulations or MRI-guided stereotactic laser ablation, need to be further evaluated in prospective studies with larger patient cohorts and a longer follow-up to better assess their role in the surgical management of FCD in children.

References

Akeret K, Bellut D, Huppertz HJ, *et al.* Ultrasonographic features of focal cortical dysplasia and their relevance for epilepsy surgery. *Neurosurg Focus* 2018; 45(3): E5.

Arocho-Quinones EV, Lew SM, Handler MH, *et al.* Magnetic resonance-guided stereotactic laser ablation therapy for the treatment of pediatric brain tumors: a multiinstitutional retrospective study. *J Neurosurg Pediatr* 2020; 26: 13-21.

Balogun JA, Khan OH, Taylor M, *et al.* Pediatric awake craniotomy and intra-operative stimulation mapping. *J Clin Neurosci* 2014; 21: 1891-94.

Behrens E, Schramm J, Zentner J, *et al.* Surgical and neurological complications in a series of 708 epilepsy surgery procedures. *Neurosurgery* 1997; 41: 1-9.

Benifla M, Otsubo H, Ochi A, *et al.* Multiple subpial transections in pediatric epilepsy: indications and outcomes. *Child's Nervous System* 2006; 22: 992-8.

Berg AT, Zelko FA, Levy SR, *et al.* Age at onset of epilepsy, pharmacoresistance, and cognitive outcome: a prospective cohort study. *Neurology* 2012; 79: 1384-91.

Bjellvi J, Flink R, Rydenhag B, *et al.* Complications of epilepsy surgery in Sweden 1996-2010: a prospective, population-based study. *J Neurosurg* 2015; 122: 519-25.

Blümcke I, Spreafico R, Haaker G, *et al.* Histopathological findings in brain tissue obtained during epilepsy surgery. *N Engl J Med* 2017; 377: 1648-56.

Bourdillon P, Isnard J, Catenoix H, *et al.* Stereo electroencephalography-guided radiofrequency thermocoagulation (SEEG-guided RF-TC) in drug-resistant focal epilepsy: Results from a 10-year experience. *Epilepsia* 2017; 58: 85-93.

Chassoux F, Devaux B, Landré E, *et al.* Stereoelectroencephalography in focal cortical dysplasia: a 3D approach to delineating the dysplastic cortex. *Brain* 2000; 123: 1733-51.

Chipaux M, Taussig D, Dorfmuller G, *et al.* SEEG-guided radiofrequency thermocoagulation of epileptic foci in the paediatric population: Feasibility, safety and efficacy. *Seizure* 2019; 70: 63-70.

Choudhri AF, Patel RM, Siddiqui A, *et al.* Cortical activation through passive-motion functional MRI. *AJNR Am J Neuroradiol* 2015; 36: 1675–81.

Cossu M, Cardinale F, Casaceli G, *et al.* Radiofrequency-guided Stereo-EEG thermocoagulations. *Epilepsia* 2017; 58 Suppl 1: 66-72.

Curry DJ, Raskin J, Ali I, *et al.* MR-guided laser ablation for the treatment of hypothalamic hamartomas. *Epilepsy Res* 2018; 142: 131-4.

Delion M, Terminassian A, Lehousse T, *et al.* Specificities of Awake Craniotomy and Brain Mapping in Children for Resection of Supratentorial Tumors in the Language Area. *World Neurosurg* 2015; 84: 1645-52.

Fayed I, Sacino MF, Gaillard WD, *et al.* MR-Guided Laser Interstitial Thermal Therapy for Medically Refractory Lesional Epilepsy in Pediatric Patients: Experience and Outcomes. *Pediatr Neurosurg* 2018; 53: 322-9.

Freitag H, Tuxhorn I. Cognitive function in preschool children after epilepsy surgery: rationale for early intervention. *Epilepsia* 2005; 46: 561-7.

Guenot M, Isnard J, Ryvlin P, *et al.* SEEG-guided RF thermocoagulation of epileptic foci: feasibility, safety, and preliminary results. *Epilepsia* 2004; 45: 1368-74.

Hader WJ, Mackay M, Otsubo H, *et al.* Cortical dysplastic lesions in children with intractable epilepsy: role of complete resection. *J Neurosurg* 2004 (2 Suppl Pediatrics): 110-7.

Hale AT, Sen S, Haider AS, *et al.* Open Resection versus Laser Interstitial Thermal Therapy for the Treatment of Pediatric Insular Epilepsy. *Neurosurgery* 2019; 85: E730-6.

Harvey AS, Cross JH, Shinnar S, *et al.* Defining the spectrum of international practice in pediatric epilepsy surgery patients. *Epilepsia* 2008; 49: 146-55.

Hoppe C, Helmstaedter C. Laser interstitial thermotherapy (LiTT) in pediatric epilepsy surgery. *Seizure* 2020; 77: 69-75.

Hufnagel A, Zentner J, Fernandez G, *et al.* Multiple subpial transection for control of epileptic seizures: effectiveness and safety. *Epilepsia* 1997; 38: 678-88.

Jasper H. Electrocorticography. In: *Epilepsy and the Functional Anatomy of the Human Brain* (Eds: W. Penfield H. Jasper). Boston, Little Brown, 1954: pp. 692-738.

Jayakar P, Jayakar A, Libenson M, *et al.* Epilepsy surgery near or in eloquent cortex in children – practice patterns and recommendations for minimizing and reporting deficits. *Epilepsia* 2018; 59: 1484-91.

Juhász C, John F: Utility of MRI, PET, and ictal SPECT in presurgical evaluation of non-lesional pediatric epilepsy. *Seizure* 2020. 77: 15-28.

Kameyama S, Shirozu H, Masuda H, *et al.* MRI-guided stereotactic radiofrequency thermocoagulation for 100 hypothalamic hamartomas. *J Neurosurg* 2016; 124: 1503-12.

Keene DL, Whiting S, Ventureyra EC. Electrocorticography. *Epileptic Disord* 2000; 2: 57–63.

Kimura N, Takahashi Y, Shigematsu H, *et al.* Developmental outcome after surgery in focal cortical dysplasia patients with early-onset epilepsy. *Epilepsy Res* 2014; 108: 1845-52.

Kimura N, Takahashi Y, Shigematsu H, *et al.* Risk factors of cognitive impairment in pediatric epilepsy patients with focal cortical dysplasia. *Brain Dev 2019*; 41: 77-84.

Klein B, Levin BE, Duchowny MA, *et al.* Cognitive outcome of children with epilepsy and malformations of cortical development. *Neurology* 2000; 55: 230-5.

Krsek P, Pieper T, Karlmeyer A, *et al.* Different presurgical characteristics and seizure outcomes in children with focal cortical dysplasia type I or II. *Epilepsia* 2009a; 50: 125-37.

Krsek P, Maton B, Jayakar P, *et al.* Incomplete resection of focal cortical dysplasia is the main predictor of poor postsurgical outcome. *Neurology* 2009b; 72: 217-23.

Krsek P, Maton B, Korman B, *et al.* Different features of histopathological subtypes of pediatric focal cortical dysplasia. *Ann Neurol* 2008; 63: 758-69.

Lewis EC, Weil AG, Duchowny M, *et al.* MR-guided laser interstitial thermal therapy for pediatric drug-resistant lesional epilepsy. *Epilepsia* 2015; 56: 1590-8.

Mathern GW. Challenges in the surgical treatment of epilepsy patients with cortical dysplasia. *Epilepsia* 2009; 50: 45-50.

Mathon B, Clemenceau S, Carpentier A. Intraoperative Ultrasound Shear-Wave Elastography in Focal Cortical Dysplasia Surgery. *J ClinMed* 2021; 10: 1049.

Morrell F, Whisler WW, Bleck TP. Multiple subpial transection: a new approach to the surgical treatment of focal epilepsy. *J Neurosurg* 1989; 70: 231-9.

Mullatti N, Landre E, Mellerio C, *et al.* Stereotactic thermocoagulation for insular epilepsy: Lessons from successes and failures. *Epilepsia* 2019; 60: 1565-79.

Muthaffar O, Puka K, Rubinger L, *et al.* Reoperation after failed resective epilepsy surgery in children. *J Neurosurg Pediatr* 2017; 20: 134-40.

Palmini A, Gambardella A, Andermann F, *et al.* Intrinsic epileptogenicity of human dysplastic cortex as suggested by corticography and surgical results. *Ann Neurol* 1995; 37: 476-87.

Pur DR, Eagleson R, Lo M, *et al.* Presurgical brain mapping of the language network in pediatric patients with epilepsy using resting-state fMRI. *J Neurosurg Pediatr* 2021; 27: 259-68.

Sacino MF, Ho CY, Murnick J, *et al.* Intraoperative MRI-guided resection of focal cortical dysplasia in pediatric patients: technique and outcomes. *J Neurosurg Pediatr* 2016; 17: 672-8.

Sacino MF, Ho CY, Whitehead MT, *et al.* Repeat surgery for focal cortical dysplasias in children: indications and outcomes. *J Neurosurg Pediatr* 2017; 19: 174-81.

Salemdawod A, Wach J, Banat B, *et al.* Predictors of postoperative long-term seizure outcome in pediatric patients with focal cortical dysplasia type II at a German tertiary epilepsy center. *J Neurosurg Pediatr* 2021; 29: 83-91.

Schwartz ES, Dlugos DJ, Storm PB, *et al.* Magnetoencephalography for pediatric epilepsy: how we do it. *AJNR Am J Neuroradiol* 2008; 29: 832-7.

Simon MV. Intraoperative neurophysiologic sensorimotor mapping and monitoring in supratentorial surgery. *Clin Neurophysiol* 2013; 30: 571-90.

Spiegel EA, Wycis HT, Freed H, Lee AJ. Stereoencephalotomy. *Trans Am Neurol Assoc* 1948; 73(73 Annual Meet.): 160–3.

Van Poppel M, Wheless JW, Clarke DF, *et al.* Passive language mapping with magnetoencephalography in pediatric patients with epilepsy. *J Neurosurg Pediatr* 2012; 10: 96-102.

van 't Klooster MA, van Klink NEC, Zweiphenning WJEM, *et al.* Tailoring epilepsy surgery with fast ripples in the intraoperative electrocorticogram. *Ann Neurol* 2017; 81: 664-76.

Wellmer J, Kopitzki K, Voges J. Lesion focused stereotactic thermo-coagulation of focal cortical dysplasia IIB: a new approach to epilepsy surgery? *Seizure* 2014, 23: 475-8.

Xu DS, Chen T, Hlubek RJ, *et al.* Magnetic Resonance Imaging-Guided Laser Interstitial Thermal Therapy for the Treatment of Hypothalamic Hamartomas: A Retrospective Review. *Neurosurgery* 2018; 83: 1183-92.

Yang T, Hakimian S, Schwartz TH. Intraoperative ElectroCorticoGraphy (ECog): indications, techniques, and utility in epilepsy surgery. *Epileptic Disord* 2014; 16: 271-9.

Zeller S, Kaye J, Jumah F, *et al.* Current applications and safety profile of laser interstitial thermal therapy in the pediatric population: a systematic review of the literature. *J Neurosurg Pediatr* 2021; 28: 360-7.

CHAPTER

24. Long-term outcome after surgery for FCD

Susanne Fauser

Key points

- Epilepsy surgery is the most successful treatment option for patients with FCD. Postoperative seizure freedom rates have improved over time. Nowadays, around 50-80% of patients become seizure-free.
- In case of seizure relapse, seizures mainly recur in the first postoperative year. However, late seizure relapse after a seizure-free period of more than one year is observed in few patients.
- Risk factors for (late) seizure recurrence are incomplete resection, preoperative FBTCS, FCD I, extratemporal location, non-lesional MRI and the need for invasive EEG recordings. Longer duration of epilepsy and older age at operation as well as preoperative multi-regional EEG patterns may also be negative predictors.
- Mechanisms for (late) seizure relapse are residual FCD tissue due to incomplete resection of the MRI-visible lesion, and possibly also lager networks beyond the borders of the FCD as well as somatic mutations in the mTOR pathway with widespread mutant cells below MRI resolution.
- AED reduction can be initiated in patients with complete resection of the MRI-visible FCD. Usually, AED tapering is started one year postoperatively. In patients with AED side effects, tapering may be safely started already six months after surgery.

Comparative cohort studies: a critical overview

There are a multitude of cohort studies investigating postoperative seizure outcome in patients with FCD. Post-surgical seizure outcome in FCD patients has improved over time. Epilepsy surgery in early FCD series operated before 2000 yielded poorer results with seizure freedom (Engel class I) in about 35-40% of cases (reviewed by Sisodiya, 2000). However, two studies already published between 2000 and 2004 (Chassoux *et al.*, 2000, Tassi *et al.*, 2002) showed better results (with around 65% seizure freedom one year postoperatively). The good results in these two latter studies are probably attributed to an invasive presurgical evaluation with SEEG in all or in the majority of investigated patients. More recent studies mainly reported good or excellent results with seizure-free outcome in 45-80% of patients. In this chapter cohort studies published between 2004 to 2021 were considered (**Tables 1a-c**). Interestingly, since 2004 post-surgical outcomes remained at a good/very good level, but have not substantially improved any more, reflected by numerous case series from different countries (**Table 1**) as well as by monocentric analyses (Rácz *et al.*, 2021). Initial overwhelming improvement is explained by an advancement of preoperative diagnostic methods and surgical techniques (reviewed by West *et al.*, 2016). In particular, more refined neurophysiological investigations with SEEG in conjunction with functional imaging have joined forces with MRI to achieve these significant better outcomes up to 90% seizure freedom rate (Guerrini *et al.*, 2015). The lack of further improvement as to seizure freedom rates despite further impressing advance in diagnostic methods and surgical techniques during the last 17 years may be explained by patient selection. Over time, the number of more complicated cases (e. g. MRI negative FCD, patients with need for invasive recordings) with per se reduced chances for postoperative seizure freedom have successively increased in surgical programs (Cloppenborg *et al.*, 2016).

Histologic classification of FCD was modified in the considered time period from 2004 to 2021. A practicable systematic classification of FCD was presented by Palmini *et al.*, 2004. A modification of this classification was published by Blümcke *et al.* in 2011. Whereas FCD II remained unchanged over the past 17 years, FCD I was differently defined, so that the FCD I subgroup is not exactly the same in older publication before 2011 and newer publications after 2011.

Table 1

A. Summary of larger retrospective cohort studies including adult and pediatric patients
B. Summary of larger retrospective cohort studies including only pediatric patients
C. Summary of retrospective cohort studies including only FCD II patients
Seizure-free postoperative outcome mainly corresponds to Engel class I. In studies analyzing Engel class Ia, this is indicated under particularities.
AED: antiepileptic drugs; APOS: acute postoperative seizures; ECoG: electrocorticography; EEG: electroencephalography; FCD: Focal Cortical Dysplasia; MRI: magnetic resonance imaging; po: postoperative (ly); SEEG: stereo-EEG; SGTCS: secondary generalized tonic-clonic seizure.

Table 1A

Outcome and predictors in cohorts comprising children and adults

Study	No of patients	Particularities	Engel outcome	Positive predictors	AED withdrawal
Alexandre, 2006	41		63%	• Temporal location • Regional ictal EEG onset	
Siegel, 2006	21	Patients >18y at operation	52%	• Absence of SGTCS (trend) • Short duration of epilepsy • Regional interictal discharges (trend)	
Widdess-Walsh, 2007	48	Only patients with subdural electrodes	45%	• Complete resection of the EZ • Unilateral EEG abnormalities • Only one seizure type	
Fauser, 2008	120	Outcome Engel Ia (12 months) po	53%	• Complete resection • Absence of SGTCS • No need for invasive EEG • Younger age at operation • Short duration of epilepsy • Unilobar extension	
Kim, 2009	166		57%	• Complete resection • Absence of SGTCS • Severe histologic features	
Fauser, 2015	211	Long-term outcome	1 year Engel I 65% Last follow up Engel I 60% (48% Engel Ia)	• Complete resection • Younger age at operation • Unilobar location	AED reduction in 40% Complete AED withdrawal in 21%
Jin, 2016	120	Long-term follow-up	1 year 73% 2 years 70% 5 years 65%	• Complete resection • No post-operative interictal discharges • No APOS	
Chaturvedi, 2018	52	Long-term outcome Engel Ia	2 years 70% 6 years 85%	• FCD II • Age <20y at operation • EEG (focal discharges without propagation) • No APOS	
Jayalakshmi, 2019	188	Long-term outcome (follow-up at least 2 years po)	Last follow-up 62%	Multivariate: • Complete resection • FCD II • Single seizure type • No APOS Univariate: • Younger age at surgery • Short duration of epilepsy • No daily seizures • No developmental delay • No eloquent cortex location	

Table 1B

Outcome and predictors in pediatric cohorts

Study	No of patients	Particularities	Engel outcome	Positive predictors	AED withdrawal
Hader, 2004	39		54%	• Complete resection	
Krsek, 2009	149	145 children/4 adults	55%	• Complete resection	
Phi, 2010	41	Outcome Engel Ia	1 year 49% 2 years 44%	• Complete resection • Visible MRI lesion	AED withdrawal in 91% after 5 years
Choi, 2018	58	Long-term outcome	2 years 62% 5 years 58% Last follow-up 53%	• Complete resection • FCD II • Visible MRI lesion	
Martinez-Lizana, 2018	113	Long-term outcome Engel Ia	2 years 56% 5 years 52% Last follow-up 50%	• Age older 9 years at operation	
Chen, 2019	92	Engel Ia	53%	• Complete resection • FCD II • No need for invasive EEG	
Choi, 2019	70		49%	• Complete resection • No postoperative interictal EEG discharges	AED withdrawal in 57% Seizure recurrence in 35% of them (57% while tapering, 43% after discontinuation)

Table 1C

Outcome and predictors in cohorts comprising only patients with FCD II

Study	No of patients	Particularities	Engel outcome	Positive predictors	AED withdrawal
Cohen-Gadol, 2004	22	Adults and children	73%	• Complete resection (trend) • Temporal location of FCD • Preoperative regional EEG discharges	59% monotherapy or no medication, 2 with seizures during drug modification
Tassi, 2012	100	Adults and children	83%	• Unilobar resection	46% stopped medication, in 30% medication was reduced
Noli, 2013	31	Only children Long-term follow-up (mean 4 years)	68%	• Epilepsy onset older than 2 years	
Harvey, 2015	32	Bottom of sulcus dysplasia	88%		62% discontinued medical treatment (4.1 year)
Sun, 2017	110	Only FCD IIA	1 year 65% 3 years 40%	• Complete resection • Temporal location • Preoperative ECoG • Lower seizure frequency	
Ramirez-Molina, 2017	106	Focused on early (< 6 years) and late (> 20 years)	73% (all) Age <6 years: 75% Age >20 years: 71%		AED withdrawal not influenced by age at operation
Wang, 2019	112	Only children Very early epilepsy onset (median 0.9 years)	Last follow-up 88%		
Racz, 2021	102	Adults and children Long-term outcome	1 year po: 84% (Engel Ia 71%) Last follow up (63 +/- 5 months) 69% (Engel Ia 54%)	• Long-term: • Complete resection • Absence of SGTCS • No positive family history (marginal)	
Jain, 2021	41	Bottom of sulcus dysplasia, only children Long-term outcome	Long-term-outcome (mean follow-up 4,3 years) 78%		
Salemdawod, 2021	50	Only children	Last follow-up: 76%	• Complete resection • Younger age at surgery • Shorter duration of epilepsy • Lower number of AED	Reduction of AED in 60% 24% with late seizure recurrence, half of them after reduction

Whereas earlier series mainly investigated the whole spectrum of FCD patients (Alexandre *et al.*, 2006; Siegel *et al.*, 2006; Fauser *et al.*, 2008; Kim *et al.*, 2009) studies published later than 2010 increasingly focused on subgroups or special aspects: pediatric cohorts (Phi *et al.*, 2010; Choi *et al.*, 2018, Martincz-Lizana *et al.*, 2018; Chen *et al.*, 2019; Choi *et al.*, 2019) (**Table 1b**), histologic subgroups - mainly FCD II - (Noli *et al.*, 2013, Sun *et al.*, 2017; Ramirez-Molina *et al.* 2017; Wang *et al.*, 2020, Racz *et al.*, 2021; Salemdawod *et al.*, 2021), and bottom of sulcus dysplasia (Harvey *et al.* 2015; Jain *et al.*, 2021) (**Table 1c**). Moreover, special surgical methods were published: e.g. primary motor sparing resections in peri-rolandic FCD (Gopinath *et al.*, 2016) or outcome depending on lesion volume and resection volume (Oluigbo *et al.*, 2015).

Over the years, outcome analyses in FCD patients increased in numbers. Such analyses are clinically relevant as it is crucial to select good surgical candidates based on prognostic factors for favorable surgical outcome.

Prognostic factors in surgically treated FCD: predicting the outcome accurately

Seizure outcome after surgery is dependent on several factors. In the literature since 2004 many potentially predictive factors were analyzed. Earlier studies mainly reported seizure outcome one year postoperatively. More recently, long-term outcome results became available (**Tables 1-3**).

The following influencing factors were analyzed in the literature:

FCD-related factors

- Histology (FCD I, FCD II, FCD III, mMCD)
- Location (temporal, extratemporal)
- Extension (unilobar, multilobar, hemispheric)

Age- and time-related factors

- Age at seizure onset
- Age at operation
- Duration of epilepsy

Diagnostic-related factors (preoperatively)

- Visibility on MRI (lesional, non-lesional)
- EEG characteristics (regional discharges, multi-regional, contralateral propagation)
- Need for intracranial EEG

Semiology/epilepsy-related factor (preoperatively)

- Occurrence of secondary generalized tonic-clonic seizures (SGTCS)/(FBTCS)
- Single versus multiple seizure types
- Seizure frequency
- Number of preoperative AED
- Positive family history for seizures/epilepsy

Epilepsy surgery related factors

- Completeness of resection

Postoperative factors

- Postoperative EEG (occurrence of epileptic discharges)
- Occurrence of acute postoperative seizures (APOS)

The heterogeneity of FCD patient series with respect to these factors may account for some inconsistencies in proposed predictive factors across various studies. Several of these factors revealed nevertheless to be consistently or at least in many studies predictive.

Complete resection (usually defined by MRI; rarely by intracranial EEG or histology) was the most consistent, very often analyzed and always positive prognostic factor (Chassoux *et al.*, 2000; Cohen-Gadol *et al.*, 2004; Hader *et al.*, 2004; Widdess-Walsh *et al.*, 2007; Fauser *et al.*, 2008; Kim *et al.*, 2009; Krsek *et al.*, 2009; Phi *et al.*, 2010; Fauser *et al.* 2015, Jin *et al.*, 2016; Sun *et al.*, 2016; Choi *et al.*, 2018; Jayalakshmi *et al.*, 2019; Chen *et al.*, 2019; Choi *et al.*, 2019; Rácz *et al.*, 2021; Salemdawod *et al.*, 2021).

Also, the absence of SGTCS/FBTCS was always a positive predictor (Siegel *et al.*, 2006; Fauser *et al.*, 2008; Kim *et al.*, 2009; Rácz *et al.*, 2021). Similarly, the presence of only one seizure type was a positive factor, however, not frequently analyzed (Widdess-Walsh *et al.*, 2007; Jayalakshmi *et al.*, 2019).

Temporal location of FCD was mainly a positive prognostic factor (Cohen-Gadol *et al.*, 2004; Alexandre *et al.*, 2006; Sun *et al.*, 2016). The influence of unilobar extension (versus multilobar extension) of the FCD was rarely investigated, but smaller extension limited to one lobe seems to be a favorable predictor (Fauser *et al.*, 2008; Fauser *et al.*, 2015).

FCD II was often described as a positive predictor for seizure-free outcome (Tassi *et al.*, 2012; Chaturvedi *et al.*, 2018, Choi *et al.*, 2018; Jayalakshmi *et al.*, 2019; Chen *et al.*, 2019). In earlier studies before 2012 the differences in outcome between FCD I and II, however, remained often not statistically significant (Hader *et al.*, 2004; Alexandre *et al.*, 2006; Siegel *et al.*, 2006; Fauser *et al.*, 2008). This difference may be explained by the fact, that earlier studies comprised a mix of FCD I cases, with a significant number of patients with temporal lobe seizures, reduced volume of the temporal pole and dyslamination under the microscope, and few cases with neocortical, multifocal or hemispheric type I. In this context, Tassi *et al.*, 2010, could show that patients with FCD I and associated hippocampal sclerosis had a very good outcome (88% class I), whereas patients with isolated FCD I did worse (46% class I). Recently, a large multicenter cohort also confirmed, that isolated FCD I was one of those entities with poor outcome (50% class I) (Lamberink *et al.*, 2020).

Lesional MRI was sometimes found a statistically significant positive prognostic factor (Phi *et al.*, 2010; Choi *et al.*, 2018). In contrast, other studies showed no statistically significant difference in outcome between lesional and non-lesional cases (Hader *et al.*, 2004; Siegel *et al.*, 2006; Widdess-Walsh *et al.*; 2007; Kim *et al.* 2009; Krsek *et al.*, 2009). One explanation of these different findings may be a selection bias in the criteria used to include patients in these studies. For instance, it might be that in some of these studies lesional cases often encompassed those in whom FCD involved eloquent cortex leading to incomplete resections and less favorable outcome. Additionally, within a grou p of non-lesional cases there might have been a significant number of patients with MRI-negative temporal lobe epilepsy, whose histopathology showed dyslamination and were reclassified as FCD I. If these two circumstances – only partially related to having or not having a lesional visible MRI – add up, then the final result in a multivariate analysis would be that having a visible lesion makes no difference. Another possibility is that studies not showing a difference had most MRI-negative patients studied with SEEG and only those in whom the EZ was reliably localized were operated.

No need for intracranial EEG recordings was usually found a positive predictor (Fauser *et al.*, 2008; Chen *et al.*, 2019). In one cohort comprising exclusively FCD IIA patients, preoperative electrocorticography was a positive predictor (Sun *et al.*, 2017). It is likely that more difficult cases, including those with negative MRI, are the ones usually selected for invasive monitoring.

Younger age at operation was sometimes mentioned as a positive prognostic factor. Most of these studies compared epilepsy surgery in adults to epilepsy surgery in children (Fauser *et al.*, 2008; Fauser *et al.*, 2015; Chaturvedi *et al.*, 2018; Jayalakshmi *et al.*, 2019), but few also within childhood (Salemdawod *et al.*, 2021). Another analysis in a pediatric cohort found better results at an age older than 9 years than in the very young children (Martinez-Lizana *et al.*, 2018). One study compared very early epilepsy surgery before the age of 6 years to late surgery (>20 years) in FCD II and found no difference in outcome (Ramírez-Molina *et al.*, 2017).

Similarly, shorter duration of epilepsy revealed to be a positive predictor in a few cohorts (Siegel *et al.*, 2006, Fauser *et al.*, 2008; Jayalakshmi *et al.*, 2019; Salemdawod *et al.*, 2021).

Presurgical focal/regional (interictal or ictal) epileptic discharges (compared to multiregional or bilateral epileptic discharges) were found to be a positive predictor in few studies (Cohen-Gadol *et al.*, 2004; Alexandre *et al.*, 2006; Siegel *et al.*, 2006; Widdess-Walsh *et al.*, 2007; Chaturvedi *et al.*, 2018).

Postoperative EEG without IED was associated with a positive long-term seizure outcome (Jin *et al.*, 2016; Choi *et al.*, 2019). Patients with no acute postoperative seizures (APOS) did better than those with APOS as to long-term outcome (Jin *et al.*, 2016; Chaturvedi *et al.*, 2018; Jayalakshmi *et al.*, 2019).

Rarely investigated factors which are possibly associated with better outcome are lower preoperative seizure frequency (Sun *et al.*, 2016; Jayalakshmi *et al.*, 2019), lower preoperative AED numbers (Salemdawod *et al.*, 2021), no overlap with eloquent cortex (Jayalakshmi *et al.*, 2019); no developmental delay (Jayalakshmi *et al.*, 2019), no positive family history (Rácz *et al.*, 2021).

A frequently investigated variable without significant prognostic value was age at epilepsy onset. There may be one exception: Epilepsy onset after 2 years of age compared to very early epilepsy onset was found a positive predictor in one study (Noli *et al.*, 2013).

Hierarchization of preoperative predictive factors

According to my personal view, the most important preoperative positive predictive factor is a circumscribed FCD visualized by MRI (or in "non-lesional" patients by FDG-PET) paired with a congruent semiology and a congruent focal EEG pathology (interictal and ictal). Semiology is more important than EEG because EEG may be normal in mesial frontal lobe FCD. Interictal discharges (in particular repetitive spiking patterns) are sometimes even more predictive than ictal onset patterns in surface EEG. In case this kind of FCD does not overlap with eloquent (language or motor) areas, an extended lesionectomy performed by an experienced neurosurgeon is the best guarantor for postoperative seizure freedom. Moreover, only one seizure type and the absence of FBTCS play a certain role, but are strictly speaking a mode of expression of a circumscribed focus and no independent factors. As FCD II more often meets the mentioned criteria than FCD I, FCD II is associated with a better prognosis. The need for invasive EEG is a negative predictor in FCD near to eloquent areas and in FCD with a diffuse MRI aspect. In contrast, if invasive EEG is performed to confirm an "non-lesional" FCD only visible in FDG-PET or with help of MRI postprocessing but not with "normal" MRI, invasive EEG is no negative predictor.

Temporal or extratemporal location plays a secondary role, as long as the lesion fulfills the above mentioned conditions. FCD II is mainly localized extratemporally, nevertheless the postoperative results are good or excellent.

An independent but possibly less crucial predictive positive factor is an age at surgery under 16 years.

Seizure frequency and number of preoperative AED are no strong negative predictors as long as the epileptogenic focus is circumscribed and well-resectable.

Outcome algorithms for epilepsy surgery as proposed by Jehi *et al.*, 2015, may be helpful and are applicable also in FCD patients (cause of seizures = malformation of cortical development). However, the importance of a circumscribed MRI lesion and focal preoperative EEG findings for FCD patients seem to be underestimated in this general outcome algorithm.

Relapse after seizure-free outcome: mechanisms and clinical implications

Most studies agree that seizure relapse mainly occurs within the first postoperative year. However, long-term outcome analyses showed a slight worsening tendency between 12 months and longest follow-up (Phi *et al.*, 2010; Fauser *et al.*, 2015; Jin *et al.*, 2016; Sun *et al.*, 2016; Choi *et al.*, 2018; Martinez-Lizana *et al.*, 2018; Rácz *et al.*, 2021).

Whereas many studies report postsurgical seizure outcome and possible prognostic factors in FCD patients, data on postoperative AED withdrawal strategies and the risk of seizure recurrence in FCD patients are rare. Detailed information is given in three larger studies: Choi *et al.* 2019 (pediatric series including FCD I, II, and III), Salemdawod *et al.*, 2021 (pediatric series including only FCD II); Fauser *et al.*, 2015 (pediatric and adult patients, including FCD I, II, and III). All three studies report a small number of late seizure recurrences. In some patients, seizure relapse seemed to be related to AED withdrawal (as seizures recurred while tapering AED), whereas in other patients, seizures recurred long time after AED discontinuation. The chance of regaining seizure freedom after AED reintroduction varied between the cohorts. However, all three studies report few cases in whom seizure freedom could not be achieved any more.

Which mechanisms could be responsible for late seizure recurrence (Figure 1)?

Late seizure recurrence (similar to early seizure recurrence) may be due to incomplete resection of the MRI visible lesion. Therefore, it is worthwhile to perform a postoperative MRI of high quality in order to verify whether the visible lesion was completely removed. In cases of incomplete resections, a second operation can be successful as to seizure freedom, especially if MRI lesion and preoperative EEG discharges were congruent (Sacino *et al.*, 2017).

Another mechanism may be the presence of a more widespread epileptogenic network reaching far beyond the histological boundaries of FCD in a subset of patients (e.g. Lee *et al.*, 2021). In temporal lobe epilepsy such extended networks proved to be predictive (Keller *et al.*, 2015). For FCD patients, a negative influence of widespread networks on postoperative outcome has not been shown so far. The negative predictive value of SGTCS/FBTCS and multi-regional (sometimes even bilateral) IED, however, hints in this direction. Patients with seizure relapse and with evidence for more widespread (unilateral) networks may benefit from more aggressive resections like multilobe lobectomy or hemispherectomy (Sacino *et al.*, 2017).

An interesting hypothesis for late seizure recurrence might also be the presence of mutations in the mTOR pathway. A single point mutation may occur in a neuronal progenitor cell. If this happens before hemispheric cleavage, mutant cells may even bilaterally (but asymmetrically) distributed in the two hemispheres. A visible area of FCD appears only in the region with highest concentration of mutant cells whereas only small foci of dysplastic tissue below MRI resolution are present where the percentage of mutant cells is low (Guerrini *et al.*, 2021). Moreover, the study by Rácz *et al.*, 2021 could show, that a positive family history for epilepsy was of marginal negative predictive value. In cases with positive family history or proven mutations and complete resection of the MRI-visible lesion a reoperation may be less successful than in "non-genetic" patients.

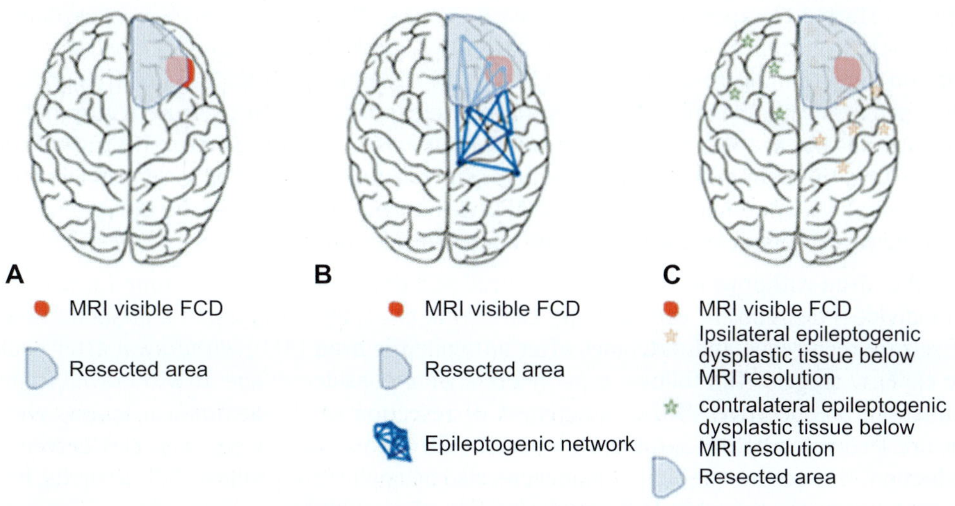

Figure 1.

Mechanisms for (late) seizure relapse

The figure schematically depicts theories of possible mechanisms:
A. Incomplete resection of an MRI-visible lesion.
B. Complete resection of an MRI-visible lesion but widespread epileptogenic network.
C. Complete resection of the MRI-visible FCD but somatic mTOR mutation with widespread distribution of mutant cells; mechanism c can be the reason for mechanism b.

Drug withdrawal after successful surgery: determing the best time

There are only few papers reporting drug withdrawal in patients with FCD. In the series reported by Fauser *et al.*, 2015, a relevant reduction of AED from polytherapy to monotherapy or complete withdrawal was performed in 83/211 patients (40%). Complete drug withdrawal was achieved in 43/211 (21%) patients. Seizure recurrences occurred mainly in the first postoperative year. Late seizure recurrences after initial seizure-free outcome for at least one year were observed in only 26/211 patients (12%).

Choi *et al.*, 2019 reported attempted drug withdrawal in 40/70 (57%) patients. 26/40 (65%) remained seizure free without AED and 8/40 (20%) with AED, 6/40 (15%) were not seizure-free despite AED treatment.

In the study by Fauser *et al.*, late loss of seizure control occurred during tapering of medication in nine patients (9/26, 35%). In another two patients, it was presumably caused by noncompliance in taking AED (8%). In 7 of these 11 patients (64%) with AED-tapering (or discontinuation) associated seizure recurrence, seizure control was regained by reestablishment of the initially successful anti-convulsive medication or by further modifications of the medication. However, four patients (4/11, 36%) did not become seizure-free again until the latest available postoperative outcome. In 13 patients (13/26, 50%) late seizure relapse occurred without a clear explanation under stable medication. In two additional patients, seizures reappeared several years after complete withdrawal of AED.

According to Choi *et al.*, 2019, seizures recurred in 14/40 (35%) of patients who started AED withdrawal. Seizure recurrence occurred significantly more often in patients with incomplete resection of the FCD and in patients with postoperative epileptic discharges in EEG. In contrast, the time of starting the AED taper did not play a significant role. Seizures recurred while reducing the AED dose in 8 patients and after discontinuation in 6 patients. Seizures recurred at a mean of 9.6 months after AED withdrawal (range, 20 days to 2.3 years) in patients who recurred while the AED dose was being reduced, and at a mean of 4.2 years after the start of AED withdrawal (range, 1.2–8.5 years) in those who experienced relapse after AED discontinuation. In 7/14 (50%) patients with postwithdrawal seizures, seizure freedom was regained after AED reinduction. The probability of regaining seizure freedom in patients with intractable FCD was lower than expected (compared to other entities).

Of interest is the relationship between recurrence rate and early AED withdrawal after surgery. Findings from adult studies have suggested that early drug withdrawal increases the likelihood of seizure recurrence (Park *et al.*, 2010). The risk of recurrence was also found to be increased in children who discontinued AED within 6 months after surgery (Lachwani *et al.*, 2008).

Choi *et al.*, 2019 found that the risk of recurrence in the long run was not increased when children started to taper AED from at least 6 months after surgery. This is in accordance to the TimeToStop study: Early withdrawal may only demasked recurrence earlier without influence on long-term outcome (Boshuisen *et al.*, 2012). Although in this seizure-free postoperative pediatric cohort earlier AED withdrawal increased the risk for seizure recurrence, this increase was not at the cost of seizure freedom or cure in the longer term. The authors concluded that the strongest negative predictor for seizure outcome and cure was incomplete resection of the anatomical lesion; early AED withdrawal seems safe in the group of patients with presumed complete resection of the anatomical lesion.

Whether drug withdrawal should be initialized and determining the best time for it remains an individual decision for each patient. Lamberink *et al.*, 2018 suggested a prediction model of seizure recurrence and outcomes after antiepileptic drug (AED) withdrawal after pediatric epilepsy surgery. The following parameters were considered: age at withdrawal, time to reduction, preoperative MRI, completeness of resection of the anatomical lesion, average seizure frequency before surgery, number of AED before surgery per day, EEG before AED reduction. This general prediction model can also be applied for pediatric FCD patients. It also might be useful in the adult FCD population (Lin *et al.*, 2020).

Next to the before mentioned relevant predictive factors, other circumstances should be considered such as the actual social situation (professional situation, driving license), side effects of the medication and the patient's wish. Although postoperative drug withdrawal remains a very individual decision, the following scheme may be helpful for clinicians (**Table 2**).

How AED should be reduced depends on the dosage and on the effects/side effects of the drug. It is reasonable to tapper first the medication with most side effects or with the lowest effect on seizure control. AED should be reduced slowly over months. If seizures recur, dosage should be increased to the last effective dosage.

Taken together, patients with low recurrence risk and social conditions in which seizure relapse does not have severe sequels for private and professional life are the best candidates for AED withdrawal. Usually, AED tapering begins one year after surgery. In prognostic good candidates with AED side effects, drug withdrawal can be initiated already within the first postoperative year.

Table 2.

Proposed scheme when and under what circumstances reduce antiepileptic drugs. Postoperatively four different conditions should be considered in respect with planning AED withdrawal.

Time after surgery	6 months postoperatively or earlier					12 months postoperatively or later			
Condition 1	seizure-free					seizure-free			
Condition 2	(severe) AED side effects				no AED side effects	+/– AED side effects			
	Eventually consider AED reduction				*Wait until 12 months*	*Eventually consider AED reduction*			
Condition 3	critical candidate		good candidate			critical candidate		good candidate	
	(e.g. incomplete resection, multifocal lesions in MRI, FCD I)		(e.g. complete resection, circumscribed MRI lesion, EEG congruent to lesion, FCD II)			(e.g. incomplete resection, multifocal lesions in MRI, FCD I)		(e.g. complete resection, circumscribed MRI lesion, EEG congruent to lesion, FCD II)	
	Be careful with AED reduction		*Still consider AED reduction*			*Be careful with AED reduction*		*Still consider AED reduction*	
Condition 4	no epileptic discharges in postoperative EEG and/ or favorable social circumstances	epileptic discharges in postoperative EEG and/or unfavorable social circumstances	no epileptic discharges in postoperative EEG and/ or favorable social circumstances	epileptic discharges in postoperative EEG and/or unfavorable social circumstances		no epileptic discharges in postoperative EEG and/ or favorable social circumstances	epileptic discharges in postoperative EEG and/or unfavorable social circumstances	no epileptic discharges in postoperative EEG and/ or favorable social circumstances	epileptic discharges in postoperative EEG and/or unfavorable social circumstances
	Balance risks and benefits of AED reduction	*AED reduction not recommended; think about AED modification*	*Initiate AED withdrawal*	*AED withdrawal is feasible, but thoroughly balance risks and benefits of AED reduction*		*Balance risks and benefits of AED reduction*	*AED reduction not recommended; in patients with AED side effects think about AED modification*	*Initiate AED withdrawal*	*AED withdrawal is feasible, but thoroughly balance risks and benefits of AED reduction*

AED: antiepileptic drugs.

Conclusion

Epilepsy surgery is an important treatment option in patients with FCD. Pre- and postoperative variables allow to predict postoperative seizure-freedom more precisely and prediction models can be used. This is important in counselling patients as to the benefit of planned epilepsy surgery and as to postoperative AED reduction. In candidates with complete resection of the MRI-visible lesion and with other mainly positive predictive factors, AED reduction and even complete withdrawal is feasible.

References

Alexandre V Jr, Walz R, Bianchin MM, *et al.* Seizure outcome after surgery for epilepsy due to focal cortical dysplastic lesions. *Seizure* 2006; 15: 420-7.

Blümcke I, Thom M, Aronica E, *et al.* The clinicopathologic spectrum of Focal Cortical Dysplasias: a consensus classification proposed by an ad hoc Task Force of the ILAE Diagnostic Methods Commission. *Epilepsia* 2011; 52: 158-74.

Boshuisen K, Arzimanoglou A, Cross JH *et al.* Timing of antiepileptic drug withdrawal and long-term seizure outcome after paediatric epilepsy surgery (TimeToStop): a retrospective observational study. *Lancet Neurol* 2012; 11: 784-791.

Chassoux F, Devaux B, Landré E, *et al.* Stereoelectroencephalography in Focal Cortical Dysplasia: a 3D approach to delineating the dysplastic cortex. *Brain.* 2000; 123: 1733-51.

Chaturvedi J, Rao MB, Arivazhagan A, *et al.* Epilepsy surgery for Focal Cortical Dysplasia: Seizure and quality of life (QOLIE-89) outcomes. *Neurol India* 2018; 66: 1655-1666.

Chen J, Huang Z, Li L et al Histological type of Focal Cortical Dysplasia is associated with the risk of postsurgical seizure in children and adolescents. *Ther Clin Risk Manag.* 2019; 15: 877-884.

Choi SA, Kim SY, Kim H, *et al.* Surgical outcome and predictive factors of epilepsy surgery in pediatric isolated Focal Cortical Dysplasia. *Epilepsy Res* 2018; 139: 54-59.

Choi SA, Kim SY, Kim WJ, *et al.* Antiepileptic drug withdrawal after surgery in children with Focal Cortical Dysplasia: Seizure recurrence and its predictors. *J Clin Neurol* 2019; 15: 84-89.

Cloppenborg T, May TW, Blümcke I *et al.* Trends in epilepsy surgery: stable surgical numbers despite increasing presurgical volumes. *J Neurol Neurosurg Psychiatry* 2016; 87: 1322-1329.

Cohen-Gadol AA, Ozduman K, Bronen RA *et al.* Long-term outcome after epilepsy surgery for Focal Cortical Dysplasia. *J Neurosurg* 2004; 101: 55-65.

Fauser S, Bast T, Altenmüller DM *et al.* Factors influencing surgical outcome in patients with Focal Cortical Dysplasia. *J Neurol Neurosurg Psychiatry* 2008; 79: 103-5.

Fauser S, Essang C, Altenmüller DM, et al Long-term seizure outcome in 211 patients with Focal Cortical Dysplasia. *Epilepsia* 2015; 56: 66-76.

Guerrini R, Duchowny M, Jayakar P *et al.* Diagnostic methods and treatment options for Focal Cortical Dysplasia. *Epilepsia.* 2015; 56: 1669-86.

Gopinath S, Roy AG, Vinayan KP *et al.* Seizure outcome following primary motor cortex-sparing resective surgery for perirolandic Focal Cortical Dysplasia. *Int J Surg* 2016; 36: 466-76.

Hader WJ, Mackay M, Otsubo H *et al.* Cortical dysplastic lesions in children with intractable epilepsy: role of complete resection. *J Neurosurg* 2004; 100: 110-7.

Harvey AS, Mandelstam SA, Maixner WJ *et al.* The surgically remediable syndrome of epilepsy associated with bottom-of-sulcus dysplasia. *Neurology* 2015; 84: 2021-8.

Jain P, Ochi A, McInnis C *et al.* Surgical outcomes in children with bottom-of-sulcus dysplasia and drug-resistant epilepsy: a retrospective cohort study. *J Neurosurg Pediatr* 2021; 2: 1-11.

Jayalakshmi S, Nanda SK, Vooturi S *et al.* Focal Cortical Dysplasia and refractory epilepsy: Role of multimodality imaging and outcome of surgery. *AJNR Am J Neuroradiol.* 2019; 40: 892-8.

Jehi L, Yardi R, Chagin K, *et al.*Development and validation of nomograms to provide individualized predictions of seizure outcomes after epilepsy surgery: a retrospective analysis. *Lancet Neurol* 2015; 14: 283–90.

Jin B, Wang J, Zhou J *et al.* A longitudinal study of surgical outcome of pharmacoresistant epilepsy caused by Focal Cortical Dysplasia. *J Neurol* 2016; 263: 2403-10.

Keller SS, Richardson MP, Schoene-Bake JC *et al.* Thalamotemporal alteration and postoperative seizures in temporal lobe epilepsy. *Ann Neurol* 2015; 77: 760-74.

Kim DW, Lee SK, Chu K *et al.* Predictors of surgical outcome and pathologic considerations in Focal Cortical Dysplasia. *Neurology* 2009; 72: 211-6.

Krsek P, Maton B, Jayakar P Incomplete resection of Focal Cortical Dysplasia is the main predictor of poor postsurgical outcome. *Neurology* 2009; 72: 217-23.

Lachhwani DK, Loddenkemper T, Holland KD *et al.* Discontinuation of medications after successful epilepsy surgery in children. *Pediatr Neurol* 2008; 38: 340-4.

Lamberink HJ, Boshuisen K, Otte WM *et al.* TimeToStop Study Group. Individualized prediction of seizure relapse and outcomes following antiepileptic drug withdrawal after pediatric epilepsy surgery. *Epilepsia* 2018; 59: e28-e33.

Lamberink HJ, Otte WM, Blümcke I *et al.* European Epilepsy Brain Bank writing group; study group; European Reference Network EpiCARE. Seizure outcome and use of antiepileptic drugs after epilepsy surgery according to histopathological diagnosis: a retrospective multicentre cohort study. *Lancet Neurol* 2020; 19: 748-57.

Lee DA, Lee H-J, Kim HC *et al.* Alterations of structural connectivity and structural covariance network in Focal Cortical Dysplasia. *BMC Neurol* 2021; 330.

Lin J, Ding S., Li X *et al.* External validation and comparison of two prediction models for seizure recurrence after the withdrawal of antiepileptic drugs in adult patients. *Epilepsia* 2020; 61: 115-24.

Martinez-Lizana E, Fauser S, Brandt A *et al.* Long-term seizure outcome in pediatric patients with Focal Cortical Dysplasia undergoing tailored and standard surgical resections. *Seizure* 2018; 62: 66-73.

Noli D, Bartuluchi M, González FS *et al.* Type II Focal Cortical Dysplasia: electroclinical study and surgical outcome in 31 pediatric patients. *Childs Nerv Syst* 2013; 29: 2079-87.

Oluigbo CO, Wang J, Whitehead MT *et al.* The influence of lesion volume, perilesion resection volume, and completeness of resection on seizure outcome after resective epilepsy surgery for cortical dysplasia in children. *J Neurosurg Pediatr* 2015; 15: 644-50.

Palmini A, Najm I, Avanzini G *et al.* Terminology and classification of the cortical dysplasias. *Neurology* 2004; 62: S2-8.

Park KI, Lee SK, Chu K *et al.* Withdrawal of antiepileptic drugs after neocortical epilepsy surgery. *Ann Neurol* 2010; 67: 230-8.

Phi JH, Cho BK, Wang KC *et al.* Longitudinal analyses of the surgical outcomes of pediatric epilepsy patients with Focal Cortical Dysplasia. *J Neurosurg Pediatr* 2010; 6: 49-56.

Rácz A, Becker AJ, Quesada CM, *et al.* Post-surgical outcome and its determining factors in patients operated on with Focal Cortical Dysplasia Type II-a retrospective monocenter study. *Front Neurol* 2021; 9; 12: 666056.

Ramírez-Molina JL, Di Giacomo R, Mariani V *et al.* Surgical outcomes in two different age groups with Focal Cortical Dysplasia type II: Any real difference? *Epilepsy Behav* 2017; 70: 45-9.

Sacino MF, Ho CJ, Whitehead MT *et al.* Repeat surgery for Focal Cortical Dysplasias in children: indications and outcome. *J Neurosurg Pediatr* 2017; 19: 174-81.

Salemdawod A, Wach J, Banat M *et al.* Predictors of postoperative long-term seizure outcome in pediatric patients with Focal Cortical Dysplasia type II at a German tertiary epilepsy center. *J Neurosurg Pediatr* 2021; 15: 1-9.

Siegel AM, Cascino GD, Meyer FB *et al.* Surgical outcome and predictive factors in adult patients with intractable epilepsy and Focal Cortical Dysplasia. *Acta Neurol Scand* 2006; 113: 65-71.

Sisodiya SM. Surgery for malformations of cortical development causing epilepsy. *Brain* 2000; 123: 1075-91.

Sun Y, Wang X, Che N *et al.* Clinical characteristics and epilepsy outcomes following surgery caused by Focal Cortical Dysplasia (type IIa) in 110 adult epileptic patients. *Exp Ther Med* 2017; 13: 2225-34.

Tassi L, Colombo N, Garbelli R *et al.* Focal Cortical Dysplasia: neuropathological subtypes, EEG, neuroimaging and surgical outcome. *Brain* 2002; 125: 1719-32.

Tassi L, Garbelli R, Colombo N *et al.* Type I Focal Cortical Dysplasia: surgical outcome is related to histopathology. *Epileptic Disord* 2010; 12: 181-91.

Tassi L, Garbelli R, Colombo N *et al.* Electroclinical, MRI and surgical outcomes in 100 epileptic patients with type II FCD. *Epileptic Disord* 2012; 14: 257-66.

Wang TS, Liu QZ, Liu M *et al.* Clinical features and surgical outcomes in young children with Focal Cortical Dysplasia type II. *CNS Neurosci Ther* 2020; 26: 270-7.

West S, Nolan SJ, Newton R. Surgery for epilepsy: a systematic review of current evidence. *Epileptic Disord* 2016; 18: 113-21.

Widdess-Walsh P, Jeha L, Nair D. Subdural electrode analysis in Focal Cortical Dysplasia: predictors of surgical outcome. *Neurology* 2007; 69: 660-7.

Conclusion

Francine Chassoux, Andre Palmini

A small series of 10 epileptic patients operated on for refractory seizures with "*histological abnormalities as a particular form of localized cortical dysplasia*", published before the era of brain imaging, was bound to pave the way for perhaps the most remarkable, pragmatic advance in epilepsy in the decades that followed. The description by Taylor and colleagues of FCD, the 50th anniversary of which inspired the organization of this book, already contained most of the electroclinical, anatomical and histological findings that characterize one of the most frequent epileptogenic lesions in pediatric and adult patients suffering from intractable focal epilepsy.

Careful clinical observation combined with original thinking and rigorous investigation lead research in the good direction. Where the long journey of FCD has led is the matter of this book, which reflects the collective efforts of the people who has advanced concepts, knowledge and strategies to improve the condition of these severely disabled patients. We believe the goal of curing many patients with severe epilepsies due to FCD is currently largely attainable, exactly because of the expertise of the authors of this book. Their generosity to share their experience, providing readers with the state of the art in the field, made this work possible.

Half a century after the first description, FCD II (Taylor-type) has stood the test of time with accumulating and robust evidence on its uniqueness, while more work on the spectrum of dyslamination is needed – hopefully aided by molecular genetic studies - before firm conclusions can be drawn upon subtyping FCD I/III on the basis of cortical architectural abnormalities. In contrast, FCD II is easy to identify by histology, as well as by characteristic clinical, electrical, and imaging features. More importantly, a favorable outcome is very often achieved when the lesion can be completely removed. The recognition of a unique neurophysiologic signature, characterized by a striking intralesional electrical activity, and the mechanisms of the high intrinsic epileptogenicity strongly support the view that the FCD model could open the way to major advances in all fields of epilepsy. Because a radiological signature was progressively identified, making visible the invisible has become the challenge of contemporary imaging, brilliantly resolved in large part and carefully detailed by the experts who author the neuroimaging chapters of this book. Finally, the clinical puzzle has been progressively resolved and we are now able to suspect a FCD II as one of the first diagnosis rather than an exceptional possibility. Typical electroclinical-imaging pictures must be readily identified by clinicians who take care of patients, as this may change their life.

Based on this clear phenotype, impressive and rapid advances have been achieved at the genetic and molecular level, firmly placing FCD II in the arborization of the mTor cascade, thus discovering many of its genetic causes. Keeping in mind that in most patients the brain is normal except for a small lesion, often limited to a single gyrus or even to a part of a gyrus, we are now ready for the next step, searching for more limited and less invasive approaches within the realm of individualized precision medicine.

Due to major progresses in imaging and surgical techniques, surgery remains today the most efficacious therapy, and many patients can be cured after resection safely performed, even in eloquent areas. A large part of this book has been reserved to experienced surgeons to share their practical experience in operating patients with FCD. We hope their detailed chapters will encourage neurosurgeons everywhere to master the techniques of epilepsy surgery for FCD, therefore leading to improved surgical outcome in a large pool of pediatric and adult patients. Notably, better outcome was largely demonstrated if the epilepsy duration was shorter, inviting clinicians to actively refer patients with FCD to surgery as soon as possible. Nevertheless, despite high technical standards, surgery remains an invasive procedure and we should expect more restricted approaches in a near future. New progress could be conceived such as correction of the molecular defect initiating epileptic activity either by local or systemic approaches. We do believe that the clinical and genetic chapters of this book demonstrate that such advances will be feasible more rapidly than previously thought. On the other hand, improvement on imaging, immunohistochemistry, genetics and clinical observations raise new challenges on the validity of subtypes FCD I and FCD III as truly representing dysplastic abnormalities, and hence considered epileptogenic lesions in themselves. This will be crucial to firmly establish these FCD subtypes as relevant entities – or abandon those that prove irrelevant form a clinical, imaging, genetic and decision-making standpoints.

Finally, we hope readers will appreciate a volume written by the people who has followed the steps of pioneers and produced the much-needed knowledge to cure patients with epilepsy due to FCD. We warmly thank all colleagues who accepted to contribute to this very special project. We also thank the patients who have trusted us and courageously built a part of their own healing.

Achevé d'imprimer en juin 2022 sur les presses de la Sepec 01960 Péronnas
Numéro d'impression : 25347220501 - Dépôt légal : juin 2022 - Imprimé en France

IMPRIM'VERT®